The New Midwifery

For Elsevier

Commissioning Editor: Mary Seager
Development Editor: Rebecca Nelemans
Project Manager: David Fleming
Designer: Andy Chapman
Illustrations: David Graham
Illustration Manager: Bruce Hogarth

The New Midwifery
Science and Sensitivity in Practice

SECOND EDITION

Edited by

Lesley Ann Page BA MSc PhD RM RN

*Joint Head of Midwifery and Nursing Women's Services,
Guy's and St Thomas' NHS Foundation Trust, London, UK*

*Visiting Professor of Midwifery, Nightingale School of
Nursing and Midwifery, King's College, London, UK*

*Adjunct Professor in the Faculty of Nursing, Midwifery
and Health, University of Technology, Sydney, Australia*

Rona McCandlish BA(Hons) MSc(Epid) RGN RMN RM

*Wellcome Trust Training Fellow in Clinical Epidemiology
National Perinatal Epidemiology Unit, University of Oxford, UK*

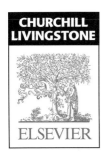

Contributors

Belinda Ackerman MA PGDip PGCEA ADM RN RM HV
Consultant Midwife, Guy's and St Thomas' NHS Foundation Trust, London, UK

Alok Ash MBBS(Cal) MD(Cal) FRCOG(UK)
Consultant Obstetrician, Guy's and St Thomas' NHS Foundation Trust, Honorary Senior Lecturer, King's College, London, UK

Pat Brodie BHSc DMid MN RM
Professor of Midwifery Practice, Development and Research, Sydney South West Area Health Service and University of Technology, Sydney, Australia

Jean Chapple MBChB MCommH FFPH FRCP DRCOG DCH
Consultant in Perinatal Epidemiology, Westminster Primary Care Trust, London, UK

Michael Corkett MSc
Senior Information Specialist, National Collaborating Centre for Women's and Children's Health, London, UK

Ruth Deery BSc(Hons) PhD RM RGN ADM
Research Leader in Midwifery, University of Huddersfield, Huddersfield, UK

Jacqueline Dunkley-Bent MSc PGCEA RGN RM ADM
Joint Head of Midwifery and Nursing, Women's Services, Guy's and St Thomas NHS Foundation Trust, London, UK

Nadine Edwards PhD
Researcher, Vice Chair, AIMS, Childbirth Educator, Edinburgh, UK

Carol Kingdon BA(Hons) MA
Research Fellow, University of Central Lancashire, Preston, UK

Mavis Kirkham BA MA PhD RM RGN
Professor of Midwifery, University of Sheffield, Sheffield, UK

Tina Lavender MSc PhD RM RGN
Professor of Midwifery and Women's Health, University of Central Lancashire, Preston, UK

Nicky Leap MSc DMid RM
Director of Midwifery Practice, South Eastern Sydney and Illawarra Area Health Service, Australia
Associate Professor of Midwifery, University of Technology, Sydney, Australia

Paul Lewis BSc(Hon) MSc DipN(Lond) ADM PGCEA RM RN RMN
Professor of Midwifery Practice and Development; Academic Head of Midwifery and Child Health, Bournemouth University, Bournemouth, UK

Rona McCandlish BA(Hons) MSc(Epid) RGN RMN RM
Wellcome Trust Training Fellow in Clinical Epidemiology, National Perinatal Epidemiology Unit, University of Oxford, UK

Christine McCourt BA PhD
Reader, Maternity Health and Social Science, Thames Valley University, London, UK

Mary Newburn BSc PGDip
Head of Policy Research, National Childbirth Trust, London, UK
Honorary Professor, Thames Valley University, Slough, UK

Lesley Page BA MSc PhD RM RN
Joint Head of Midwifery and Nursing Women's Services, Guy's and St Thomas' NHS Foundation Trust, London, UK
Visiting Professor of Midwifery, Nightingale School of Nursing and Midwifery, King's College, London, UK
Adjunct Professor in the Faculty of Nursing, Midwifery and Health, University of Technology, Sydney, Australia

Sally Pairman BA MA DMid RM RGON
Head of School of Midwifery and Group Manager Health, Otago Polytechnic, Dunedin, New Zealand; Chair of Midwifery Council of New Zealand

Maggie Redshaw BA PhD C Psychol
Social Scientist, National Perinatal Epidemiology Unit, University of Oxford, Oxford, UK

Jane Sandall BSC(Hons) MSc PhD RM RN HV
Professor of Midwifery and Women's Health, King's College, London, UK

Trudy Stevens MA(Cantab) MSc PhD PGCEA SRN SCM
Senior Lecturer in Midwifery, Anglia Ruskin University, Chelmsford, UK

Sally Tracy BNurs MA DMid RM RGON
Associate Professor of Midwifery Practice Development, Northern Sydney and Central Coast Area Health Service, Sydney, Australia
NH&MRC Post Doctoral Research Fellow, National Perinatal Statistics Unit, University of New South Wales, Sydney, Australia

Sara Wickham BA(Hons) MA PGCert RM
Independent Midwifery Lecturer and Consultant, Wickford, UK

Foreword

'Midwifery is a vocation in which a midwife's knowledge, clinical skills, and judgement are put in the service of bringing new life into the world, of protecting and restoring a mother's wellbeing. This purpose is realized through a partnership between mother and midwife, one based on mutual respect, individual responsibility, and appropriate accountability.

In their day-to-day practice, midwives are committed to:

- integrity
- compassion
- altruism
- continuous improvement
- excellence
- working in partnership with members of the wider healthcare team.

These values, which underpin the science and practice of midwifery, form the basis for a moral contract between the midwifery profession and society. Each party has a duty to work to strengthen the system of healthcare on which our collective human dignity depends.'

I have marginally changed these words to make them appropriate for the midwifery profession. The text is drawn from a report commissioned by the Royal College of Physicians whose working party I chaired.[1]

While working with my colleagues I was conscious how important it was to define the new professionalism. We live in a turbulent world. The NHS is in crisis, struggling to make ends meet. World-wide society's attitudes are fast changing. Scientific advances bring unrealistic expectations. Demography is working against us. In this maelstrom of change the anchor which secures, which enables us to continue and improve, is our professionalism. It is your 'set of values, behaviours, and relationships that underpins the trust the public will have in you'[1] which will ensure women have an experience which is life enhancing.

The New Midwifery, creatively edited by Lesley Page and Rona McCandlish, with their co-authors, inspires, illuminates, and illustrates how science and sensitivity can be put into practice. It is a remarkable book, based on solid evidence and experience by writers who are recognized as international leaders in the field. It is reaffirming and instructive for those who have already spent time in the profession but are open-minded, recognizing that updating is an essential part of being a professional. It is essential reading for those recently qualified and hungry to deepen their understanding of this remarkable and privileged position of being a professional midwife. For the rest of us it is a thoroughly good read and a mine of information.

I commend it highly.

Baroness Julia Cumberlege
Chairman of the Expert Maternity Group. Report: Changing Childbirth

---

(1) Doctors in society. Royal College of Physicians. Report of a Working Party, December 2005

Acknowledgements

The work presented in *The New Midwifery* brings together the experiences and knowledge of a huge array of people. These include women and their families who are at the centre of care and from whom all of us who work with them learn so much; midwives, doctors, politicians, researchers and leaders of maternity services who work to develop *The New Midwifery*; the wonderful authors who have contributed to both editions of this book; our editors and technical team at Elsevier, especially Rebecca Nelemans. We thank them all.

Many thanks to Jane Phillips, Gael Beddoes, Hester Lean and Laura Reed who have provided pictures and given us the privilege of a glimpse into their families, labour and the birth of their babies. These pictures really are worth a thousand words and we appreciate their contribution tremendously.

We wish to extend our appreciation of Patricia Percival who was assistant editor to the first edition. This second edition is developed on the very firm foundation that Patricia helped build. We would also like to thank Pauline Cooke, Barbara Mills, Patricia Percival, Lee Saxell and Trudy Stevens who were contributors to chapters in the first edition; their work was an important basis to the updated chapters in the second edition.

We thank our families, friends, and colleagues for their enduring support and care for us and for our work.

Introduction
The new midwifery: science and sensitivity in practice

Lesley Page and Rona McCandlish

INTRODUCTION

For us, to be a midwife means being able to work with a woman, in the sense of working alongside her, to ensure that the care we offer meets her individual needs and those of her family in the early weeks of family life. Being a midwife 'with the woman' implies a relationship of knowing each other, of mutual trust, of working in the best interests of the woman and her family and ensuring that their care is uppermost in midwifery work.

The essence of midwifery is to assist women around the time of childbirth, in ways that recognize that the physical, emotional and spiritual aspects of pregnancy and birth are equally important. Midwifery care is likely to have profound and long-term consequences not only physical outcomes, but also on personal and family integrity, and the relationship between mother and her partner and the baby. Of course a midwife must provide competent and safe physical care – but without sacrificing respect for the emotional and spiritual dimensions which give meaning to the whole individual and personal experience of pregnancy and birth.

In her everyday and intimate connection with birth, a midwife is the guardian of one of life's most important events, for each individual and for society as a whole. Being a midwife, being 'with woman', is a privileged role; one which a wealth of art and science, knowledge and expertise, humanity and spirit surround and which combine to bring a unique and irreplaceable approach to care.

However, simply believing that we do good is not sufficient and we must be prepared to ask questions of ourselves to find out whether midwifery care helps, harms, or makes no difference to women and families. Commitment to 'creative questioning' was one of the strong motivations for this second edition of *The New Midwifery: Science and Sensitivity in Practice*.

This edition of *The New Midwifery* has been written by contributors who all acknowledge that, in developed country settings, it has become more and more difficult to work 'with woman' to practice to the full potential of the midwifery role. All the chapters seek to address how practice can be developed by examining the following essential elements of midwifery:

- Working in a positive relationship with women.
- Being aware of the significance of pregnancy and birth and the early weeks of life as the start of human life and the new family.
- Avoiding harm by using the best information or evidence in practice.
- Having adequate skills to deliver effective care and support.
- Promoting health and wellbeing.

The new edition is divided into three sections:

- The transition to parenting and relationships in practice – working with women.

- Putting science into practice.
- Promoting healthy birth, midwifery skills and the organization of practice.

SECTION 1 TRANSITION TO PARENTING AND RELATIONSHIPS IN PRACTICE – WORKING WITH WOMEN

Woman-centred care requires some understanding of what individual women and communities of women require from midwives. The book starts appropriately with a chapter by Mary Newburn, Head of Policy Research, National Childbirth Trust (NCT), London and Honorary Professor, Thames Valley University, London, UK, called What Women Want from Care Around the Time of Birth. The chapter examines the difficulty of determining what women want from care because this is often influenced by existing care and expectations arising from that.

Making the important point, dealt with by many authors in the book, that the interests of the mother are intimately bound up with those of the baby, the chapter traces fifteen years of policy change culminating in the Standard for Maternity Care of the National Service Framework (NSF) for Children's, Young People and Maternity Services (Department of Health 2004). Twelve principles of the NCT's birth policy drawn from research provide detailed standards for the maternity services to work towards. Summarizing from some major surveys of women's needs and responses to their care the chapter indicates some of the changes evident in women's attitudes, particularly to labour, and the relationship of women's attitudes to interventions and the outcomes of their birth, over recent years. While there is some evidence of positive change in the quality of care in maternity services in the UK, the complexity of the cultural changes required to bring about care that is truly woman-centred makes such transformation difficult to achieve. A number of important issues are considered in this chapter, many of these are further explored in other chapters of the book. For example, the need for more information for women to be provided in a way that they can use, the importance of women being involved in making choices in their care and having a sense of control, and the need for equity when setting up continuity of care

schemes by providing these in the areas of greatest need.

The second chapter First Relationships and the Growth of Love and Commitment by Maggie Redshaw, Social Scientist, National Perinatal Epidemiology Unit, University of Oxford, Oxford, UK, draws on theories of, and research into, attachment. This chapter shows just how closely the interests of mother and baby are intertwined. The attachment relationship is key to survival of the individual and the first years of life are of critical importance to the long-term mental health of the individual. Midwives are facilitators not only of the physical birth but also have the potential to contribute to the birth of the parent–child relationship and of the birth of the family. Research is explored that sheds light on the connection between the sensitivity of early parenting and the subsequent developmental trajectory of the child. The midwife's role in facilitating early parent–child contact and in screening and interventions are examined. Contextual factors affecting the parent–child relationship are described. The potential impact on society of a child having an insecure relationship with parents and or caregivers is becoming clearer. For example, lack of a secure attachment may be associated with more negative relationship patterns over many years and also with victimization and aggression.

Moving from theories of and research in attachment, the next chapter focuses on the development of parenting. Becoming a Parent by Chris McCourt, Reader in Midwifery, in the Centre for research in Midwifery and Childbirth, Thames Valley University, considers the importance of family in support of the child, and the transitions that are required to make adjustments in awareness, roles and priorities in order to be able to be sensitive to the needs of the child/children and respond to them appropriately. A central theme of the chapter is the tendency for society and individuals to romanticize parenting and the importance of breaking the conspiracy of silence around this issue is discussed. Childbirth is examined as a social and cultural transition, by drawing on research from social, psychological and anthropological perspectives. The importance of informal and formal support for families themselves is considered. The negative effects of biomedicine and the fragmented production line approach of hospital-centred care and alternative approaches to the organization of maternity services that would provide better support for effective care and parenting are described. Overall there is strong evidence that the nature and quality of the support the midwife gives is very likely to have an effect on the development of effective sensitive families.

The next chapter goes to the heart of midwifery: The Relationship of a Midwife with a Woman. Sally Pairman, Head of the School of Midwifery and Group Manager Health, Otago Polytechnic, Dunedin New Zealand and Inaugural Chair of the Midwifery Council of New Zealand, starts her chapter, Midwifery Partnership: Working 'With' Women, with the statement 'Midwifery *is* the partnership between the woman and the midwife'. This relationship is the medium from which midwives practice. The development of partnership is a complex process and the chapter describes clearly the importance of the intentional nature of this process, through developing self-awareness and a stated philosophy of care. Important to the development of partnership, is the definition 'that [partnership] . . . is mutually defined and negotiated on an equal basis, with full participation of both partners and ensuring the protection of each, redressing imbalances through negotiation between partners'. These principles, including the idea of cultural safety, would be appropriately extended to other parts of the world where the recognition of the need to empower women around the time of birth is crucial to woman-centred care. Building and optimizing this partnership requires continuity of care, and independent autonomous practice.

The concept of partnership present throughout the midwifery world in New Zealand at policy and political level as well as in practice, is also explored in the next chapter by Nadine Edwards, Researcher, Vice Chair of Association for the Improvement of the Maternity Services (AIMS), Childbirth Educator, Edinburgh, UK, and Nicky Leap, Director of Midwifery Practice, South Eastern Sydney and Illawarra Area Health Service, Australia and Associate Professor of Midwifery, University of Technology, Sydney, Australia. As a consumer representative and a midwife, both have drawn from their experiences of birth as the inspiration for their work. The Politics of Involv-

ing Women in Decision-Making calls for a more nuanced examination of choice. The chapter refers to the context of oppression in the maternity services and women's lives, and criticizes the idea of informed choice that places the onus of control on the individual without recognizing that social inequalities are particularly powerful. Such malign influences mean that women are offered limited choices and are not truly involved in decision making. These limited choices give women the illusion of involvement and participation in decision making and serve to maintain the status quo. Focusing on the importance of continuity in the relationship between women and their midwives, and the difficulty of involving women in decision making they nevertheless provide very clear guidance for midwives in all types of service, whether fragmented or continuous care is provided, by drawing cameos to illustrate alternative approaches to communication and enabling choice. They describe the emotional engagement necessary and describe clearly the idea of 'real talk' that is part of more leisurely and less formal discussions, the value of story telling, and groups rather than classes for education and the building of community. This chapter together with Sally Pairman's provides a detailed picture of the politics underlying care, and the potential power of transformative change in the maternity services.

Woman-centred care then requires an understanding of women's general and individual needs, an awareness of the crucial importance of the support of the mother/parent carers for the baby through a secure attachment, the adjustment and support required by the parents to parent adequately. In turn women and their partners need a relationship of partnership with their midwives. But to work to their full potential midwives need support too. They need supportive managers, to support each other, and to work in a supportive environment if they are to give of their best.

However, the majority of midwives in the industrialized world work in large centralized maternity services, where this support is more difficult to provide and access. But a number of developments are now moving midwives into alternative and more effective structures. All the chapters so far have described the difficulty of providing woman-centred care in what is referred to as an industrialized model of care. Yet, as Ruth

Deery, Research Leader in Midwifery, University of Huddersfield, UK, and Mavis Kirkham, Professor of Midwifery, University of Sheffield, UK point out, the parallels between the devoted mother and the devoted midwife are obvious, as are the parallels in support they need. Their chapter Supporting Midwives to Support Women, draws on a range of research from different theoretical frameworks to explain how and why midwives in large organizations avoid the primary task of caring for childbearing women and rather concentrate on the task of getting through the work. Conflicting needs of the organization and of women and their families will often result in the evasion of relationship. Given the importance of relationship and support, described clearly in the previous chapters it is easy to see the frustration that may arise and that are described in this chapter, often leading to midwives leaving the work they love. Whereas in the UK midwives employed in the NHS seem to be crying out for help and support, they often seem to lack a coherent plan for resolution of their needs. By contrast independent midwives have consciously set up systems of support. There is a continuum of effective support, sustenance and development offered which can be charted from the large impersonal organizations to smaller ones. The experience of working in a smaller scale organization, can offer rewarding work such as home births, and is associated with a lower risk of burn out. The 'virtuous circle' that this creates spins off into positive relationships with childbearing women. Support and focus on the primary task are essential work for managers. This means that to achieve effective midwifery management the same emphasis on communication, interpersonal skill building and therapeutic proficiency is needed as required on mandatory skill building.

Working with Women: Developing Continuity of Care in Practice by Christine McCourt, Reader, Maternity Health and Social Science, Thames Valley University, London, Jane Sandall, Professor of Midwifery and Women's Health, King's College, London, Pat Brodie, Professor of Midwifery Practice, Development and Research, Sydney South West Area Health Service and University of Technology, Sydney, Australia and Trudy Stevens, Senior Lecturer in Midwifery, Anglia Ruskin University, Chelmsford, UK, brings together the earlier themes of responding to the needs of women, respecting the importance of the parents to the baby, developing relationships in which midwives are working with women, in a system that supports continuity of carer, rather than staffing wards and departments. The move to develop systems which provide continuity of carer, in an effort to move away from fragmentation, has happened in many parts of the world. The chapter looks at the role and definition of continuity, examining continuity as a hierarchical continuum, and gives a brief history of the development of continuity of care and carer. The changes in emphasis from provision of institutional care towards women and family-centred care are examined in the context of policy changes including the National Service Framework for Children, Young People and Maternity Services (Department of Health 2004). The results of research, including the methodological problems of evaluating complex interventions such as development of continuity of care are described. Why continuity is important to women and to midwives is discussed and practical issues concerned with setting up continuity of care are addressed. The chapter shows how the relationship between women and midwives has the potential to be more than transactional. When built on mutuality of understanding and trust this relationship transforms midwifery for women as well as midwives.

Meeting the challenge of the abundance of information and evidence about midwifery and maternity care is something faced every day by contemporary midwives. The skills to integrate a structured and systematic approach to evidence, with the knowledge, experience and 'gut instinct' gained from practice, and developing confident, open communication with other care professionals and with women and their families is at the core of sensitive effective midwifery. In the chapter Finding and Using Evidence, Lesley Page, Joint Head of Midwifery and Nursing Women's Services, Guy's and St Thomas's NHS Trust, London and Visiting Professor of Midwifery, Nightingale School of Nursing and Midwifery, King's College, London and one of the editors of this book, Michael Corkett, Senior Information Specialist, National Collaborating Centre for Women's and Children's Health, London, and Rona McCandlish, Research Fellow, at the National Perinatal Epidemiology Unit, Oxford University, Oxford, UK, also editor of this book, describe efficient accessible approaches to asking questions about practice, and ways to identify and appraise evidence and reflect on the importance and relevance of evidence to women accessing midwifery care. In the same way as midwives systematically carry out assessment of physical and psychological health and wellbeing they suggest using a structured framework to evaluate evidence.

Paul Lewis, Professor of Midwifery Practice and Development; Academic Head of Midwifery and Child Health, Bournemouth University, Bournemouth, UK, in his chapter The Birth of Twins: a Reflection on Practice, eloquently describes the personal and professional journey he made when he sought to support his sister-in-law, Ness, during her pregnancy and birth of her twin sons. He shares frankly the challenges thrown up by the fact that he was unable to practise as a midwife in the country where Ness was living. Using Lesley Page's five steps for effective midwifery practice (Page 2000) he describes how both the mother's wishes and needs as well as the available 'best evidence' are central to the process of care and constitutes a more rigorous way to ensure that the practice of midwives is both 'women-centred' and 'evidence-based'. His detailed presentation of important aspects of the care Ness received, the evidence base for it, and living the process of reflection on care and outcomes of care, is a powerful testament to his expert midwifery practice.

SECTION 2 PUTTING SCIENCE INTO PRACTICE

The first section of this book contains chapters which focus on transition to parenthood and midwives working with women by using relationship as a unifying concept, this second section highlights working with the woman in her best interests by basing information offered and clinical practice on the best evidence available.

Evidence-based Care and Twins by Belinda Ackerman, Consultant Midwife and Alok Ash Consultant Obstetrician, Guy's and St Thomas' NHS Foundation Trust, London, and Honorary Senior Lecturer, King's College, London, also uses Page's five steps of evidence-based midwifery (Page 2000) to tell the care story of a woman who wanted care that provided support for a physiological birth of twins in a large maternity service. As well as taking the reader through the current status of evidence on outcomes and interventions in multiple pregnancy the chapter shows how multi-disciplinary work and a team effort combined with good individual care provided the family with a positive experience in which their self-control was supported. The story gives an honest account of what it feels like for staff when the boundaries of usual or routine care are changed. This chapter also shows how the institutions in which most midwives practice, need to support individual practitioners to provide care appropriate to the needs of the individual, and challenge boundaries to care.

Jane Sandall, Professor of Women's Health and Midwifery, King's College, London and Rona McCandlish, Wellcome Trust Training Fellow in Clinical Epidemiology National Perinatal Epidemology Unit, University of Oxford, Oxford, UK, and editor of this book, are both 'research active' midwives. But their chapter, Why Do Research?, is not about 'how to do' research; it is about placing research in the context of real midwifery and highlighting how research for midwifery can only be really worth that title if all midwives get involved. They describe the huge change brought about by the opening up of access for women and families to information and knowledge about maternity care. This revolution changed the way that midwifery is learned, and practised, so that deference to 'expert' opinion is no longer acceptable to those who access, or those who offer, care. One way of ensuring that midwifery remains relevant and useful is for its research to be as strong as possible and for the evidence it generates to be used to make a positive difference. Jane and Rona want everyone to want to be involved in research and to know that this does not necessarily mean conducting research. Not every midwife will be a researcher, but every practicing midwife should, for example, feel confident to scrutinize whether or not a piece of research that she is being asked to give information to women about, is ethical. This chapter covers key questions to ask about the purpose, aim and objectives of any study. Resources that can keep midwives up to date with the fast changing world of research, ethical and governance are signposted – accessing and using these will help make sure that research for midwifery should never be the preserve of the 'experts'.

Sally Tracy, Associate Professor of Midwifery Practice Development, Northern Sydney and Central Coast Area Health Service, Sidney, Australia and NH&MRC Post Doctoral Research Fellow, National Perinatal Statistics Unit, University of New South Wales, Sydney, Australia, in her chapter, Risk: Theoretical or Actual?, deals with the complexity of risk and is aimed at helping midwives think about their practice in light of society's preoccupation with risk. While the actual risk of childbirth is lower than it has ever been in resource rich countries for women who aren't poor or from ethnic minority groups, the attempts to assess and quantify risk and control risk have become a subliminal form of social control. The interventions introduced with the intention of lowering it may actually constitute greater risk. Providing a wider view of changes in society including the development of biomedicine, genetic screening and the growth of digital data bases the pervasive influence of the surveillance and gaze of biomedicine is explored. Importantly, the evidence on scoring systems to quantifying risk indicates that they may not work as well as the judgement of an experienced clinician. The potential for social and judicial control of women's lifestyle are great, while the biggest influences on risk may be poverty, lack of education, unsafe housing and addiction to drugs, alcohol and smoking. The chapter concludes with comments on the cascade of intervention and the risk this creates, and ways of midwives working with women to help in making decisions, using an aid developed in New Zealand. The potential of midwives to promote women's self confidence, intuition and trust and the importance of these in reducing risk is highlighted.

Sara Wickham, a midwife in practice and independent midwifery lecturer and consultant, closes the section with: Jenna's Care Story: Post-term Pregnancy. In this chapter Sara takes the reader into the issues and challenges of working and connecting with each woman as an individual, while accessing and mobilizing professional knowledge. These issues resonate particularly with those covered in Chapter 5, the concept of 'real talk', and the knowledge that comes out of more 'informal' communications. Jenna's Care Story deals with a contentious issue, a 'prolonged' pregnancy, and takes the reader through the evidence in a constructive critical way. Jenna's values are clear throughout, and are an essential part of the information on which care is based and decisions made. The language used demonstrates respect not only for Jenna and her partner but also for their unborn baby. The clinical knowledge so important to evidence-based care is described, as are the many sources and types of knowledge that midwives need to draw on. Sara's personal philosophy is clearly stated and this chapter provides a vital example of a synergistic midwife–woman partnership in practice.

SECTION 3 PROMOTING HEALTHY BIRTH, USING MIDWIFERY SKILLS AND THE ORGANIZATION OF PRACTICE

The final section of the book illustrates how, as well as promoting health in individual women and families, midwives have a public health role in promoting health in populations of women, and in reducing the effects of inequalities on the outcomes of care and health.

A Public Health View of Maternity Services by Jean Chapple, Consultant in Perinatal Epidemiology, Westminster Primary Care Trust, London, UK, takes us from this individually oriented care to a view of women and families in populations. The chapter examines the common aims of personal and public health services. It describes how the community health needs of pregnant women are assessed, and how evidence-based policy of care provided by midwives acting as public health practitioners can help to improve the health of mothers, babies and families. Public health is defined and the process of setting priorities through health needs assessment is described. Epidemiology is an important tool for midwives in deciding where priorities lie. Risk is defined and the methods of identifying those at risk so that we may know which women may develop complications and when. Risks before conception, before, and during pregnancy and environmental factors from the external environment and in utero environment are explained. The decrease in the current perinatal mortality is shown to be affected by demographic factors. While public health is about populations the point is made that interventions need to be individual and tailored to specific needs. Some specific public health interventions such as smoking cessation, support for women with mental health problems through continuity of care, and support for increase in initiation and duration of breastfeeding, promotion of healthy diet and social support provide potential tools for midwives. Increasing access and uptake of services and more effective care for women from ethnic minorities and women who do not speak English may be enhanced by the use of interpreters/translators, link workers and bilingual advocates. There are a number of innovative ways for midwives to work with these services. The purpose, advantages and disadvantages of screening and the need for well thought through programmes are described with case studies provided. Finally, the difficulty of measuring relevant outcomes and the limitations of mortality rates as an indicator of the quality of a service are described.

Jacqueline Dunkley-Bent, Joint Head of Midwifery and Nursing, Woman's Services, Guy's and St Thomas, NHS Foundation Trust, London, brings the midwifery perspective to public health in the chapter Reducing Inequalities in Childbirth: the Midwife's Role in Public Health. Building on the perspectives of the previous chapter the important role and opportunity for midwives to be public health practitioners and to decrease inequalities in access and outcomes and break cycles of deprivation are explored in detail. Disadvantaged women often have disadvantaged babies and this chapter describes the possibility for midwives to work with other agencies, for example in Sure-Start schemes, aimed at bringing together early education, childcare, health and family support to deliver the best start in life for every child. As well as inequalities in health the needs of particularly vulnerable women are considered. These may be women experiencing domestic violence, asylum seeking women, women pregnant as a result of rape, female genital mutilation, post-traumatic stress disorder and acute stress reaction as well as teenage pregnancy and economic and social disadvantage. Although the examples are UK based the chapter provides examples of approaches that are likely to have universal application.

It is a part of the specialist role of the midwife to be able to support physiological processes while knowing when intervention is required. In Keeping Birth Normal by Tina Lavender, Professor of Midwifery and Women's Health, University of Central Lancashire, Preston, UK, and Carol Kingdon, Research Fellow, University of Central Lancashire, Preston, UK, the evidence, skills and personally sensitive approaches are intertwined to provide advice on the best ways of 'keeping birth normal'. The role of the midwife is to protect and support normal processes. In this chapter the concept of normal is analysed, the importance of positive memories of birth and the significance of the event is stressed. Topics include creating a positive atmosphere and arranging the furniture, the assessment of labour, assessment of the health of the fetus, mobilization and positions for labour, helping women to cope with the pain of labour, constant support and presence in labour. The importance of tuning in to women's needs is stressed.

The final chapter of the book, Being with Jane in Childbirth: Putting Science and Sensitivity into Practice by Lesley Page, Joint Head of Midwifery and Nursing Women's Services Guy's and St Thomas's NHS Foundation Trust and Visiting Professor of Midwifery to the Nightingale School of Nursing and Midwifery at King's College, London, and an editor of this book, provides an example from real life that will illustrate midwife support of normal processes. Using the five steps of evidence-based practice (Page 2000) the care story draws on a number of complex situations that faced Jane and Lesley, and gives results of a search for evidence that yielded surprising results. The chapter describes the politics as well as the clinical considerations in challenging usual approaches to care and reflections on developments in evidence since Lesley first wrote Jane's story.

We all know that the days are long gone when one book could answer all questions and tell a midwife everything she thought she needed to know! We hope that this edition of the New Midwifery will be a source book for a number of topics which are important to midwifery practice. We believe that effective midwifery requires a different approach to care. This approach needs midwives to be open to change, questioning, and challenge and involves continuing evolution, as a midwife, and as a human being. We want this book to be an aid to midwives in developing and sustaining themselves to take this approach to the new midwifery.

For us, personal sensitivity and an understanding of the science are at the basis of contemporary maternity care. An understanding of the meaning of pregnancy and birth in modern day society is worth striving for to achieve the new midwifery. Importantly, working this way as a midwife requires the enduring ability to think, to learn, to make decisions and to question. The integration of science and sensitivity in practice is the crux of the new midwifery, and the core for sustaining midwifery.

References

Department of Health 2004 National service framework for children, young people and maternity services. www.doh.gov.uk/nsf accessed October 2005

Page L (ed.) 2000 The new midwifery: science and sensitivity in practice. Churchill Livingstone, Edinburgh

SECTION 1

Transition to parenting and relationships in practice – working with women

'I take real delight in working for them, helping them to work together because it's their birth and I work quite a bit now at not being intrusive and supporting the husband to support the wife rather than just directly supporting the woman'

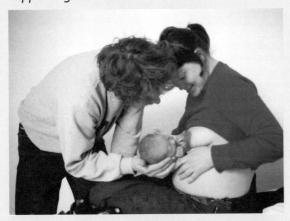

Chapter 1

What women want from care around the time of birth

Mary Newburn

> Women's reactions to care around the time of birth can affect the way they care for themselves and their baby and influence the contact they go on to have with care-givers . . .When things go well, women may feel more confident with the new baby and happier to ask for help and advice from caregivers. When things go badly, women may find themselves going over the events again and again in their minds and may be very anxious about another pregnancy.
>
> Garcia et al 1998, p. 4

It is important to question what women want from care around the time of birth, but not necessarily easy to come up with a satisfactory answer. There is some evidence to show what women *get* – or *don't get* – from the existing systems of maternity care, but it is quite a different matter to spell out convincingly what women *want* during the transition to motherhood and what they *want* from the maternity services.

In an unpublished review of parents' information and support needs around the time of birth, carried out by members of the National Childbirth Trust (NCT) in the 1990s, Taylor and Glossop noted that there was very little research that starts from first principles by asking pregnant women or new parents what they want at this time in their lives (Hames et al 1997). They argued that most of the available evidence relates to evaluations of services that are being used, and thus the agenda for 'what women want' is determined, and limited, by what is already provided. Similar arguments

have been made by Stadlen who discusses how our understandings about 'what mothers do' is limited and defined by people other than mothers themselves. She shows that the language used to describe mothering activities is often pejorative and disempowering, rather than reflecting the complexity and value of what is actually going on (Stadlen 2004).

However, the opposite problem is also a significant, and perhaps an equally limiting, one. That is, unless women have had the opportunity to experience a particular service, how can they know whether they would like it or how it might affect their labour and adjustment after birth? The chance to explore a choice or model of care not previously considered might alter their preferences for pregnancy and birth, or their feelings about motherhood.

A dramatic way to illustrate this is to highlight the apparent interest in and demand for home birth. In many areas of the UK the home birth rate is 2% (or less) of all births. In Peckham, in south London, however, the home birth rate is over 40% (Rosser 2003). Do women in Peckham have different aspirations and desires from other women? The answer is both yes and no. Their wishes are unlikely to be markedly different from other women of similar background in English cities but the maternity care they encounter is very different. The factors that seem to make such a big difference to the number giving birth at home include the expertise and confidence of their midwives in home birth, the opportunity not to have to decide where to give birth until labour is established, and the growing number of local women who have experience of home birth as safe and satisfying.

'What women want' might mean what a single 16-year-old mother, a mother of three with diabetes in Bradford, a 42-year-old who has had three miscarriages, an asylum seeker who does not speak English or know how the NHS works, a healthy woman of 31 worrying about work and childcare, or a mother with a premature baby might want. Ideally, we would want to be able to draw on a range of qualitative and quantitative studies that focus on a range of different geographical areas, and include women from different ethnic and cultural backgrounds and different kinds of families – young mothers, older mothers, lone parents, nuclear families, stepfamilies, extended families, lesbian mothers, etc.

The number of women in Peckham having a home birth demonstrates that the stereotypical idea about 'natural childbirth' being a middle class preoccupation is superficial. While women have a range of different needs and preferences, depending on their social circumstances at least as much as clinical considerations, these are not obvious and clear cut.

This chapter will particularly address what women want during labour or when planning for their birth, exploring research findings and drawing on the NCT's work to address women's experiences, needs and preferences. The first section will look at the policy agenda over the last 15 years, as this both reflects an understanding about what women want around the time of birth and is also a factor influencing the kind of services that have been developed. The qualities and standards identified in government policy documents have had a considerable impact on the questions addressed in recent evaluations of the maternity services in England. The second section will review some of the most relevant evidence on support and care and on women's views of interventions and coping with pain, drawing especially on the survey carried out for the Audit Commission in the 1990s (Audit Commission 1997, Garcia et al 1998) and the comparative study by Green and colleagues (Green et al 1998, 2003). In the concluding discussion, there is a summary of the key themes and issues.

THE POLICY AGENDA

Over a decade ago, the idea of 'woman-centred care' was established in the UK as the result of the UK parliament's Health Select Committee Inquiry into the Maternity Services (House of Commons Health Committee 1992a). The committee's conclusions, together with the volumes of written and verbal evidence, capture the emotions and personal testimonials of women, expert witness statements, reviews of evidence and accounts of key debates (House of Commons Health Committee 1991). The National Childbirth Trust, Maternity Alliance, AIMS and the Institute for Social Studies in Medical Care were among those who gave complementary accounts to the enquiry about women's experiences and needs around the time of birth.

Themes that emerged, included the need for each woman to be respected and treated as an individual. Most women, it was suggested, wanted to be better informed about what was happening during their personal journey into motherhood, to know about the options open to them, and be involved in decision-making. There was an emerging sense that women had been cajoled – some would say duped – into conforming with a system of care in which hospital doctors had decided what was best for them and their babies. The report still makes highly relevant reading.

Becoming a mother is not an illness. It is not an abnormality. It is a normal process that occurs during the lives of the majority of women and can indeed be seen as a manifestation of health. It is physically very demanding and is a time when women are vulnerable in many ways. They require help and support during the process of being pregnant, giving birth, and postnatally and some of this, though not all, needs professional help. In some circumstances the quality of the professional help is literally vital. But it is the mother who gives birth and it is she who will have the lifelong commitment that motherhood brings. She is the most active participant in the birth process. Her interests are intimately bound up with those of her baby.

House of Commons Health Committee 1992b

This philosophy and perspective – the belief that having a baby is usually a 'normal process' and that the woman is 'the most active participant' who 'gives birth', and whose interests are 'intimately bound up with those of her baby' – was a key underpinning principle for the idea of woman-centred care. If women were the ones having the babies, the maternity services should be paying attention to what they wanted and responding. The committee concluded that women wanted continuity of care and carer; choices about where they had their care, including where they gave birth; and 'the right to control over their own bodies at all stages of pregnancy and birth'.

The inquiry took place before health matters had been devolved from the UK Parliament in London to the Scottish Parliament and Welsh Assembly, so was relevant to health departments and ministers across the four countries of the UK. The initial government reply and the resulting policy for England and Wales, Changing Childbirth, confirmed that this perspective would be expected of the NHS in the years to follow (Department of Health 1993). Many of the key themes were also explored in Scotland (Scottish Executive 2001) and subsequently to some extent in Northern Ireland (Northern Ireland Department of Health 2002).

The new government policy represented a seismic shift, questioning the extent to which care had become routinely medicalized and impersonal. The evidence did not support the need for all women to be confined in hospital under the care of an obstetrician; women could give birth healthily and happily at home, in a community unit or with midwife-managed care. Changing Childbirth emphasized the need for consistent care and advice, with women receiving most of their care from a named individual, who would get to know them and become a familiar reassuring presence at times of stress or vulnerability. It was recognized that women with more complex pregnancies, and those who didn't have English as their first language often missed out on the continuing support of a midwife and their needs should be identified so that appropriate services could be developed in response.

When a woman is having a baby, nothing can replace the support of a known and trusted professional. Many women described to the Group the reassurance of seeing a familiar face at critical points, when they were anxious or when complications arose, but especially when they went into labour. Continuity of carer is seen as being one of the fundamental principles underpinning woman centred care.

Department of Health 1993 (2.3.1)

A little over a decade after Changing Childbirth was published a new National Service Framework (NSF) for NHS maternity services has been published both in England and in Wales and an agreed set of clinical standards for Scotland has been developed (Department of Health 2004, NHS Quality Improvement Scotland 2005, Welsh Assembly Government 2004). The emphasis on individualized care focusing on the needs of women, babies and the wider family has been reinforced with a particular emphasis on making services accessible and welcoming to those who are disadvantaged or socially excluded. There is also a specific commitment in England and in Wales to supporting normal childbirth:

We want to see women being supported and encouraged to have as normal a pregnancy and birth as possible, with medical interventions recommended to them only if they are of benefit to the woman or her baby.

Department of Health 2004

Birth is a normal physiological process in which medical intervention should only be offered if it can be demonstrated that there is proven benefit for the mother and/ or her child.

Welsh Assembly Government 2004

NCT birth policy and campaigns

The National Childbirth Trust (NCT) is the largest and best known childbirth and early parenthood charity in Europe. Consulted by key policy makers on all aspects of pregnancy, birth, baby feeding and early parenthood, the NCT works to improve maternity care, and ensure that high quality services and facilities are available for pregnant women and their families. The NCT raises awareness about the needs of new parents and works to ensure that their needs are met.

In 2002 the NCT published a policy paper covering 12 principles that should inform the care provided around the time of birth (Newburn 2002). The policy was developed following the commissioning of a discussion paper from Thames Valley University (Beake & McCourt 2001) and after consultation with NCT members and branches. A development group made up of NCT members and workers with divergent views came up with the key themes and approved the wording of the policy before it was tested on an outside audience and further revised. The principles of the policy together with the supporting beliefs and explanations are reproduced in full in Box 1.1. The policy addresses important elements of what women want from care around the time of birth. It compliments the NCT's baby feeding policy (National

---

Box 1.1   The National Childbirth Trust birth policy

1. *Birth and the transition to parenthood should be an experience that enriches parents' lives.* As babies are dependent on adults and cannot describe how they feel, we have a special responsibility to look after them. Birth should be as gentle, loving and protective as possible. As the foundation of family life, the significance for society of birth and early parenting is enormous.

2. *Maternity care should be a positive experience for women and make a significant contribution to public health, the wellbeing of families and the next generation.* Experiences of pregnancy, birth and the early weeks with a new baby can have a long-lasting impact on the family, affecting physical and mental health, social relationships and child development. It is important that women begin motherhood feeling good about themselves, and valued and supported by others. It is not sufficient simply to aim to reduce deaths and major illness. Positive experiences act as a buffer against later physical and emotional stress.

3. *Women need to feel as fit and well-prepared as possible if they are to look after their new baby, themselves and the rest of their family.* The birth is far from the end of the process of having a baby; it is an important beginning. Women need to be able to cope with personal and family changes at the same time as meeting the demands of a new baby. Women who have had a straightforward birth have a greater chance to start the next stage of their lives feeling fit and well.

4. *The maternity services should be developed and managed to increase the proportion of straightforward vaginal births.* With appropriate support and care, the vast majority of women can have a straightforward vaginal birth. Maternity services should provide one-to-one midwifery care for all women in labour. The NCT uses the term 'straightforward vaginal birth' to mean a birth that starts, progresses and concludes spontaneously, without major interventions, such as a caesarean or an instrumental delivery, or a series of other medical procedures. A large majority of women in the UK give birth in hospital and action should be taken to increase their opportunities to give birth without unnecessary interventions. For many of those women with a more complex pregnancy, requiring some medical care or ready access to emergency facilities, birth does not have to be a wholly medical event. It can be immensely rewarding for them to be actively involved in coping with contractions and pushing their baby into the world.

5. *The maternity services should be developed to provide women with easy access to a reliable home birth service and to midwife-led birth centres.* There can be important benefits for the whole family when a baby is born in a social rather than a medical environment. The birth is likely to be straightforward, without the need for drugs, and breastfeeding is usually established as a matter of course. The father can be fully involved and the baby is not separated from the family at any time. This

Continues

experience can be particularly beneficial for women who feel their autonomy may be threatened in hospital, for women with a disability, young mothers, those who are economically deprived, and women from ethnic minorities. Women without complications or high-risk factors who plan to have their baby outside of hospital are half as likely to have a caesarean section or an instrumental delivery compared with similar women who plan to have their baby in hospital. The baby is just as likely to be born safely. Women should have a right to a reliable home birth service. Currently, women cannot absolutely rely on a midwife being available for them in labour if those commissioning and providing services do not see this as a priority. This is unacceptable.

6. *The education of midwives, obstetricians, anaesthetists, GPs and other health professionals should involve observation of birth as a normal physiological process.* The place of birth, continuous midwifery support, freedom of movement, comforting massage, warm water, visualization and relaxation techniques, a peaceful, unhurried atmosphere, together with support from loving companions, are some of the factors that can help labour flow smoothly. Observation of births in different settings and cultures, either directly or by video, raises awareness of how much the physiological birth process can be supported or disturbed. Considering birth to be normal only in retrospect, which has been a traditional medical perspective, encourages clinicians to look for problems and find signs that are frequently interpreted as a cause for concern. Attention is then focused on managing potential problems rather than on the needs of the labouring woman. The primary focus in maternity care should be facilitating normality, with well organized contingency plans in place so that appropriate action can be taken if the pregnancy or labour ceases to be normal.

7. *Women's opportunities to experience a straightforward vaginal birth are dependent on midwives maintaining their knowledge of the physiological process of birth and practical midwifery skills.* Midwives must ensure that their knowledge and skills are maintained in clinical practice and developed through research. They have a key role in establishing new services and ways of working that help to meet the needs of families around the time of birth. They should work in partnership with medical colleagues, contributing equally to policy development, appraising evidence critically and confidently, and ensuring that midwifery skills are maintained.

8. *Parents should have ready access to evidence-based information to show how health outcomes vary with different kinds of care.* In deciding whether a treatment should be offered, advised or asked for, it is important to weigh up the possible benefits with the known costs, risks or side effects. There may be alternative treatments, or the choice between a treatment and 'watchful waiting'. If too little research has been done to show how different options compare, parents should be told. Pregnant women have the right to refuse unwanted treatment. The principle of informed consent has been strengthened by Article 8 of the Human Rights Act (1998); the right to respect for privacy and family life.

9. *All maternity services should be designed to enable women to get to know their main carer; and for healthy women with a straightforward pregnancy this should usually be a midwife.* Women value having care from midwives and doctors they can get to know. Their main carer should coordinate and provide the majority of their care, supported by a small number of colleagues. Women feel valued if they are known as an individual and their circumstances and wishes are understood. They are more confident to ask questions and confide their anxieties. All women need midwifery care and benefit from being able to form friendly, supportive relationships with a small number of midwives. Women

Continues

most in need, those living in socially disadvantaged areas, those with medical complications, or mental health problems should have priority when continuity of carer schemes are set up.

10. *Medical care can be invaluable for mothers and babies when there are complications or an increased chance of complications.* Those women and babies who need expert medical care should have access to well-resourced medical services with suitably trained staff. Women with a complex pregnancy are particularly likely to benefit from being able to get to know at least one of the team caring for them, so that their medical history is understood and there is no conflicting advice. The midwife is an important source of information and support, not only providing clinical care but also recognizing the woman's social and emotional needs.

11. *Individualized care is important; appropriate ways of providing support should be explored for each woman.* Many women have fears that can impinge on their pregnancy. They need opportunities to talk about their changing roles and relationships; help to address any problems with depression, domestic violence, social isolation or lack of support; and may need help in approaching agencies about debts, benefits, housing or childcare worries. Many women fear the birth process itself (coping with pain, pushing the baby out or getting back to normal afterwards) or have worries about the baby. Those who have experienced abuse may feel very threatened by the prospect of examinations or treatment which they cannot control. Women should have an opportunity to

talk through their anxieties with someone who is sympathetic and understanding, as well as confident in the birth process. Some fears can be overcome with acknowledgement and support, others amount to a clinical need and care should be tailored accordingly.

12. *The living conditions of pregnant women and families with babies must be improved.* Families with young children need adequate housing and warmth, sufficient income and nourishing food, protection from violence, access to healthcare, the opportunity to be together as a family and not suffer separation. Currently, in the UK, almost one child in three is born into a family living on means-tested benefits. Poverty leads to significantly higher risks of stillbirth, perinatal and infant death, and childhood illness. Disadvantaged babies have less chance of experiencing the benefits of breastfeeding and their mothers are more likely to experience postnatal depression. Targeted and responsive maternity and child health services can help to reduce these inequalities. However, reducing child poverty that causes these health inequalities requires other changes. The NCT, a member of the Maternity Alliance, lobbies for progressive social and economic policies to improve living conditions for families with young children.

NB Since the policy was published the number of children living in poverty in the UK has gone down, though a quarter of children are still affected. Child income poverty has been reduced from 4.2 million children (around one in three) In 1998/99 to 3.6 million in 2002/03 (close to one in four) (Department for Work and Pensions 2004).

Childbirth Trust 1999) and a policy on postnatal and parenthood issues (National Childbirth Trust 2005).

These policies have drawn on NCT workers' understandings of the opportunities and barriers that make a difference to parents, as well as drawing on published research. They have underpinned our subsequent lobbying and campaigning work, the results of which are evident in the current gov-

ernment commitment to 'promote the normality of childbirth', provide one-to-one care during labour, provide quiet, comfortable and relaxing birth environments, including access to home birth and the option of using a birth centre, and ensure that there are community-based support networks for breastfeeding mothers (Department of Health 2004, Welsh Assembly Government 2004a). On facilitating normal birth, the NSF for England says:

... the environment should be quiet, relaxed with comfortable 'home like' surroundings where [women] can progress through labour with the support of their birth partners ... [it should] enable women to do what feels right for them during labour and delivery with health professionals supporting their wishes wherever possible.

All staff [should] have up-to-date skills and knowledge to support women who choose to labour without pharmacological intervention; including the use of birthing pools, and in their position of choice.

Department of Health 2004

The NSF reflects growing recognition of the public health implications of the rising caesarean rate and the need for positive action to be taken if women's opportunities to have a normal birth are not to be further eroded. The NCT has made a major contribution to highlighting these issues through collaborative working with health professionals and their professional bodies, and with other voluntary organizations (National Childbirth Trust 2004a, National Childbirth Trust et al 2000, Royal College of Obstetricians and Gynaecologists et al 2001, 2002). The studies drawn on most by the NCT in developing its birth policy and lobbying for improved care during labour and birth include the Audit Commission's First Class Delivery (Audit Commission 1997) and work on women's expectations and experiences by Green and colleagues (Garcia et al 1998, Green et al 2003). The NCT's descriptive studies, carried out over a number of decades, have also enabled us to build up a picture of what may contribute towards or hinder 'woman-centred care'. Topics have included women's experiences of induced labour, (Kitzinger 1978) episiotomy, (Kitzinger & Walters 1981) rupture of the membranes (Borton et al 1989) and postnatal infection (Greenshields 1987).

Following publication of Changing Childbirth, the NCT Policy Research Department was funded to carry out three major studies, two for North Thames Regional Health Authority and one for the Department of Health. The first of these focused on childbirth options, information and choices available through the NHS maternity services in North Essex (Gready et al 1995). The follow up study, also carried out via the NHS in North Essex but also involving women using maternity services in West London, was a qualitative study of women's understanding and use of evidence-based information leaflets (Wiggins & Newburn 2004). This was followed by national surveys of women and men across the whole of the UK on their access to information and need for support during pregnancy and labour, and during the early months with a new baby (Singh & Newburn 2000a, 2000b). More recently, the NCT has been funded by primary care trusts to investigate the views of local communities regarding the provision of maternity services and possible solutions to reconfiguration issues (National Childbirth Trust 2004b; 2004c). Several of these will be referred to further later on.

RESEARCH ON WOMEN'S EXPERIENCES AND VIEWS

The Audit Commission study, First Class Delivery, was carried out in England and Wales a decade ago, in 1995. It is the most recent, comprehensive country-wide study of women's experiences during pregnancy, birth and the early postnatal period (Audit Commission 1997). The study followed four local surveys carried out in 1987 to test the Office for Population and Census Studies (OPCS) survey manual questionnaire from which many of the questions were taken. Altogether, 3570 women were invited to participate when their babies were around four months of age and 2375 (67%) responded describing their maternity care and expressing their views (Garcia et al 1998).

The study addressed how women evaluated their care in terms of kindness, support and respect, their confidence in the staff, information and communication, care options and choices, involvement in decision making and their views about continuity of carer, staff numbers and morale. These topics were selected as important for women as they had 'either emerged from previous research (or were) the focus of current policy' (Garcia et al 1998, p.34).

The majority of women rated their care as good. However, only a small majority were able to *agree strongly* with positive statements about their care.

This can be interpreted, therefore, either as most women getting the kind of care that they want, or that most women are being denied the kind of high quality, individualized care that would make all the difference to their start to mothering a new baby. Sometimes women who have had different models of care – or who have experienced particular interventions in previous pregnancies – are better able to identify what they value and explain why things matter to them (Garcia et al 1998). Some women who have nothing else with which to compare their care may find it more difficult to put their feelings into words. However, women who have used a service may have developed a sense of loyalty to the system they know, this too may affect what they say is important (Allen et al 1997).

The report concluded that:

Although women's needs and wishes vary a lot, there are some things that we can generalise about. Women want care that is technically good and well organised, where caregivers communicate well and respect each other. . . . They need, and want, good communication between their care-givers, enough information about what is happening, and the opportunity to find out more if they need to. They want to be treated with kindness and respect, and when they are in pain or frightened they want support and help.

Garcia et al 1998

A uniform approach is not the goal, since different places have different populations, and services will choose to give priority to different aspects of care. Equity, though, should be an important consideration when care is looked at nationally.

Garcia et al 1998, p.76

The authors noted that:

Those who work in the service also deserve fair treatment; poor staff morale is bad in itself and may lead to worse care for women.

Garcia et al 1998, p.76

Comparative studies enable differences in effect to be made evident. Work by Green and colleagues has added substantially to what is known about women's preferences for childbirth (Green et al 1990). In 2000, they set up a study to follow-up their earlier work to examine whether any changes had occurred in women's expectations and experiences of care during childbirth, focusing particularly on 'decision making', 'continuity', 'choice' and 'control' (Green et al 2003).

The first of these studies, Great Expectations was based on findings from research in four semi-rural areas in the south of England, carried out in 1987 and involving over 700 women (Green et al 1998). The authors concluded that having a sense of control was important for women, and was 'critical' to their 'subsequent psychological well-being'. The follow-up study involved women using the same four maternity units in 2000, plus women using four units serving similar semi-rural populations in the north of England. In all, six of the units were medium sized (around 2500 births per year), one was larger (3300 births) and one smaller (1600 births).

Some characteristics of the 1987 and 2000 samples reflected national trends over that period of time: the mean age of first-time mothers had increased form 25.7 years to 28.1 years. Fewer women left education at 16 years and more stayed on in education beyond 19 years. In the 2000 sample, 23% had a degree and 10% had no qualifications. Almost three quarters of the pregnant women (72%) were working in 2000, compared with around half (47%) in 1987, with the greatest rise among multiparous women (61% working, up from 26%). Unemployment rates were lower; in 1987 6% of women had an unemployed partner compared with 4% in 2000.

The findings showed a big change in pregnant women's attitudes to labour pain and anticipated ways of coping with pain during labour. More pregnant women felt 'very worried' about labour pain and there was a particularly marked increase among primiparous women, up from 9% in 1987 to 26% in 2000. Correspondingly fewer women said they were 'not at all worried'. In 2000, significantly more women expressed a preference for 'the most pain-free labour that drugs can give me' and fewer women said that they would ideally prefer 'to put up with quite a lot of pain in order to have a completely drug free labour' (see Table 1.1). However, it was still the case that four in five women wanted either no drugs or 'a minimum of drugs to keep the pain manageable'.

More pregnant women anticipated wanting to use an epidural for pain relief during labour, and – when the time came – more did have an epidural. Fewer women reported using breathing and relaxation techniques for coping with pain. In 1987, only 8% of primips and 11% of multiparous women said they did *not* use these techniques at all, but by 2000, over a quarter of women were *not* attempting these kinds of self-help techniques (29% primips, 26% multips). The authors suggest that this may be a result of fewer women attending antenatal preparation classes.

There was a positive correlation between what women wanted in terms of pain relief and what they got. However, many more women ended up using pain-relieving drugs than had wanted to. Over 60% of both multiparous and primiparous women had not actively favoured an epidural. In particular, many more women giving birth to their first baby resorted to an epidural, including over half of those who did not actively express a preference for one during pregnancy. This exposure to epidural anaesthesia for pain relief during labour is related to the way the women's babies were born. Only 41% of primiparous women who had an epidural had an unassisted vaginal birth, compared with 78% of those who did not have an epidural. For multiparous women, almost all of those who avoided an epidural had an unassisted vaginal birth (96%) compared to just two thirds (68%) of those who had one. The authors emphasize that while causality cannot be inferred from these data because many other factors may have played a part in influencing the mode of birth, the relationship is a highly significant one.

Women's expectations and preferences seemed to be an independent factor influencing what happened during their labour. Excluding those who expected to have an elective caesarean section, Green et al (2003) found that those pregnant women who favoured having an epidural were significantly less likely to have an unassisted vaginal birth (43% primips, 78% multips) than those who did not express this preference (59% primips, 93% multips). This is important because it highlights that we need to ask not only 'what do women want?' but 'do women know that some things tend to lead to another?'. Do women who want an epidural mind whether they reduce their chance of avoiding forceps or ventouse?

Green at al (2003) also reported that induction of labour was up from 16% in 1987, to 23% in 2000, and more women had their labour accelerated: 17% in 1987 and 28% in 2000. Acceleration of labour was particularly high among first-time mothers with an epidural, 60% of whom had oxytocic drugs for this purpose. Women were significantly more likely to have an epidural if their labour was induced. This evidence begs the same questions. Women's views about interventions might alter if they were given information about how different aspects of care influence each other. Perhaps healthcare professionals are not always clear themselves. Is it that stronger contractions, induced by oxytocin, mean that more women ask for or are given an epidural to cope with the pain,

Table 1.1   Preferences for coping with pain during labour – n (%)

	1987		2000	
	Primips n = 289	Multips n = 443	Primips n = 508	Multips n = 682
Most pain free possible	17 (6)	49 (11)	107 (21)	143 (21)
Minimum drugs	205 (71)	292 (66)	330 (65)	443 (65)
Drug free	66 (23)	102 (23)	66 (13)	95 (14)

Source: Green J M, Baston H, Easton S et al 2003 Greater Expectations? Inter relationships between women's expectations and experiences of decision making, continuity, choice and control in labour and psychological outcomes: summary report. Mother and Infant Research Unit University of Leeds, Leeds

or that more liberal use of epidural leads to a greater need for an oxytocic drug to achieve progress in labour? The processes may work differently in different maternity units according to varying policies and practices. For the purpose of this chapter, the point is, do women have this kind of information explained or discussed with them and, if they do not, can we truly know their views?

It became clear to the development group working on the NCT Birth Policy that this kind of information was not available to women. Those women – of whom there seem to be many – who want to have a straightforward labour and birth with a minimum of intervention are not routinely being given comprehensive information about what they can *do* (or seek to *avoid*) to make their chances of a straightforward labour more likely (Newburn 2002, Rosser 2002). Unless they have information about the kinds of birth environments, interventions and behaviour that may increase or reduce their chances of having the kind of birth they want, their chances of achieving what they want may be lower. More recently, the NICE caesarean section guideline has confirmed that healthy women with a straightforward pregnancy who plan for a home birth are less at risk of having a surgical delivery and yet they and their babies have equally good outcomes (National Collaborating Centre for Women's and Children's Health 2004).

The NCT has taken action to provide this kind of information for women, and encourage the MIDIRS and the Department of Health to do so too. We have also addressed some of the barriers that labouring women face. As part of the NCT birth environment survey we asked women who had recently had a baby how they rated a variety of facilities, equipment and opportunities for comfort and control during labour (Newburn 2003, Newburn & Singh 2003). Nine out of ten women felt that their physical surroundings could affect how easy or difficult it was to give birth. The three things that were considered highly important to the greatest number of women were having a clean room, being able to walk around and not being overlooked or within sight of other people. Then we specifically asked what if any physical aspects of the room they were in during labour they found 'helpful for encouraging the kind of

birth you wanted'. Starting with the factors mentioned by most women, the helpful aspects were:

- space for walking and moving around;
- a birth pool or large bath;
- en suite toilet/bathroom;
- a comfortable adjustable bed;
- low lights or adjustable lighting; and
- privacy and quiet.

Factors that the most women found unhelpful, starting with those mentioned most frequently, were:

- a clinical 'hospital room' atmosphere;
- a small room with little space to move around;
- a hard uncomfortable bed that was not adjustable or in an unhelpful position;
- lack of privacy;
- having to go into a public area to use the toilet;
- being too hot or too cold and unable to control the temperature.

Women who gave birth at home or in a midwife-led unit or birth centre had greater access to valued facilities and opportunities for comfort and privacy than those who gave birth in a traditional hospital unit. There was also an association between access to valued facilities and opportunities and a greater chance of vaginal birth. For example, we found that most of the women who had vaginal birth, had been able to walk around as much as they liked (75%) and around half had enough pillows, mats and beanbags (45%). In contrast only 45% of women whose labour had ended in an emergency caesarean section said they were able to walk around and only a quarter had enough pillows and mats (24%) to help them get comfortable. A high proportion of respondents were NCT members or had visited the NCT website, so they may not have been representative of all women.

One woman who gave birth in a midwifery led unit said

There was an exercise ball which I found invaluable for support, plenty of floor space and mats to move around easily as I laboured on the floor. There was an en suite toilet and shower which was great as I spent some time during the second stage on the loo.

Another commented

The only way I managed to have such a positive birth experience was by being totally focused on what I was doing (i.e. managing pain through breathing etc.). If anything distracts you, e.g. other external factors, this is less achievable. The room was large and spacious, so I was able to move around freely and change positions. There were various different seating / squatting / lying options available (e.g. beanbags, mats, chairs, tables, beds). There was calm music playing, calm colours and calm lighting. The midwives had a very personal flexible approach – I led the midwives followed.

Newburn & Singh 2003

A follow-up postal survey in 2005, based on questionnaires disseminated through NHS maternity units, was representative in terms of age, ethnic groups and place of birth. It replicates many of the earlier findings. Women valued having a clean, comfortable, homely-looking room that they could stay in throughout labour, and have the opportunity to stay in afterwards. They regarded having space to move around freely and use of a private toilet as high priorities. There continued to be a lack of facilities and equipment to help women to ease the pain of labour without using drugs or invasive procedures. The women wanted their midwife to praise and encourage them as this was highly motivating, and those midwives who encouraged women to try a variety of techniques for coping with pain during labour were especially highly regarded (Newburn & Singh 2005).

In 1987, Green and colleagues found that there was a clear correlation between women feeling they were able 'to get into the positions that were most comfortable' for them during labour and birth and positive psychosocial outcomes. Unfortunately, in 2000, significantly fewer women said that they could get into comfortable positions all the time (17% of primips compared with 39% in 1987). The authors attribute this change partly to increased use of epidurals and continuous electronic fetal monitoring (EFM). However, significant differences remained even when those variables were controlled for (Green et al 2003).

An 'attitude to intervention' score was constructed based on seven possible interventions (induction, acceleration, planned caesarean section, forceps, drugs for pain relief, episiotomy and continuous EFM). In 2000, women were found to have a greater willingness to accept interventions, especially those expecting their first baby. Those who were more willing to accept interventions were also more likely to have an unplanned caesarean or assisted delivery than those who were less willing. Analysis showed that an increase in the use of epidurals was a key factor and that the attitudes of women using different maternity units varied. This reinforces the argument that attitudes and beliefs in society, and also in local maternity services, make a difference to what women feel they need and say they want.

Clement et al (1999) have pointed out that studies of interventions during childbirth have tended to be based on investigators' perceptions of the significance of common procedures. To overcome this limitation, they asked women to rate a broad range of procedures that they had experienced, including use of a transcutaneous electrical nerve stimulation (TENS) machine for coping with pain, vaginal examinations, fetal scalp blood sampling and being sutured, in terms of the extent to which they rated each one as a 'medical procedure'. They wanted to know how women perceived the full range of things that might be done to them – or for them. While this approach may be limited, as the women were not asked separately about their sense of control, the invasiveness of each procedure, or about levels of stress or pain experienced, the study is useful. It suggested that certain procedures have been regarded as fairly insignificant by hospital staff but are not viewed this way by women on the receiving end. For example, women regarded artificial rupture of the membranes as a significant medical intervention, and they rated an epidural as equivalent to the use of forceps. While further descriptive work is needed to draw out women's perceptions in more detail, the point is well made that staff should not make assumptions about the physical or psychological impact of commonplace practices for women.

Shortly after Changing Childbirth (Department of Health 1993) was published, the NCT had an opportunity to explore what woman-centred care might encompass. The Birth Choices (Gready et al 1995) project looked at women's experiences and views about communication, information, involvement in decision-making, continuity of carer, and dignity and personal comfort. Like Clement et al (1999), we wanted to question assumptions about an activity that was commonplace on labour wards but might carry a very different meaning for women than for some members of staff. We asked women about vaginal examinations. While almost all women believed vaginal examinations were necessary, and nine out of ten felt they were reassuring, during labour, over half found them painful (Gready et al 1995). One said, 'I wish I'd had an epidural – not for the contractions, for the internals; . . . (the) midwife handled me like a piece of dead meat!'.

The interviews with women emphasized the value of having someone they could turn to who they knew wouldn't make them feel foolish for asking questions, preferably a midwife they knew well enough to be on friendly terms. Midwife-led units emerged as a setting in which there was more time for women and more support could be provided, yet women who could have used the units were often not given the option.

Green and colleagues (2003) also selected some of these aspects of care for evaluation. They found that more women in 2000 reported feeling able to 'be as assertive as they wanted' compared with 1987 (41% vs. 31%). More women described their carers as 'sensitive' (62% vs. 48%) and more felt that they had been given the right amount of information (76% vs. 68%).

Studies since the 1970s have shown consistently that women have wanted more information than was offered or easily available to them (Cartwright 1979, Fleissig 1993, Jacoby 1988). A recent large representative study reinforced that message (Singh & Newburn 2000a) and demonstrated that it was also the case for fathers (Singh & Newburn 2000b). Half of the women said they 'wanted to know as much as possible' about pregnancy, birth, and what to expect after they had had their baby. First-time and younger mothers were particularly keen to be able to find out more. The greatest unmet demand for more information came from women expecting their first baby and from women aged under twenty.

There were also high levels of anxiety with one in three 'very worried' about aspects of labour and birth or something being wrong with the baby.

There was a clear desire for more information to be provided at the first appointment with a health professional during pregnancy – especially what range of pregnancy care services were available, information about maternity benefits and employment rights, and the available choices about place of birth. At least 40% of women wanted more information about a number of key birth topics:

- what to expect from maternity services;
- reasons for, and what to expect with, assisted deliveries, caesareans, and inductions;
- self help and medical methods of pain relief;
- what to expect in labour; and
- moving around in labour.

Women from all kinds of backgrounds valued written information, that was:

- up to date,
- gave answers to common questions/problems,
- offered different options with the advantages and disadvantages of each,
- was based on research evidence, and
- included practical tips.

In an earlier longitudinal study, in which women were introduced to three MIDIRS (Midwives Information and Resource Service) Informed Choice, evidence-based leaflets on Support in Labour, Positions in Labour and Listening to Your Baby's Heartbeat During Labour as part of group discussions, they had a chance to consider where the evidence came from, what it might mean for them as an individual and whether they could use the information (Wiggins & Newburn 2004). Around a third of the women were 'resigned but regretful' feeling that they would like to move around and influence how their baby was monitored during labour, but believed that the opportunities to influence what happened to them during labour would be minimal. Interviewed for the second time before giving birth, one woman said, 'I thought the leaflets made you think you had choices that in reality weren't there. The health professionals controlled the show. I'm not saying the information isn't true, it just made you believe you had a choice when in my previous experience you don't'.

Another third of women felt they would like to use the information, of this group most were 'cautiously optimistic'; the others, whom we called 'crusaders', were determined that knowing the advantages and disadvantages described in the leaflets would enable them to be more assertive. A further third, were unmoved by the leaflets, anticipating neither regret not conflict as they were expecting to have an elective caesarean, happy to take health professionals' advice or were sceptical about the evidence.

The information did make a difference for some women, 10 of the 47 women who went into labour said the Positions leaflet – and discussions during pregnancy – had influenced their behaviour in labour. Others did not want to move around much but felt a sense of 'having more options'. Influencing aspects of clinical care proved more challenging; just four women said they had asked for and received intermittent fetal monitoring as a result of the reading and talking about the leaflet.

One of the reasons that women like to have a familiar midwife with them during labour is that they have fewer surprises. If they have developed a relationship during pregnancy, the midwife doesn't have to ask a lot of questions, but already understands a lot about what the woman wants. Almost half of the women in the Audit Commission survey (49%), carried out in 1995 (Audit Commission 1997), said that they were cared for at the time of the birth by someone they had met before. This was less than the Changing Childbirth target that 75% of women 'should know the person who cares for them', but considerably greater than the OPCS (Office for Population and Census Studies) pilot studies had found in 1987 (Garcia et al 1998). Half the women also said that one midwife had been able to stay with them throughout their labour. This was more likely for those women having a shorter labour and a normal vaginal birth. Half the women said it was *very important* to have the same staff throughout labour and a quarter said it was *very important* to have met the staff before.

Given the emphasis Changing Childbirth (Department of Health 1993) placed on the importance of having a known midwife providing care during labour, Green and colleagues expected there to be more evidence in 2000 that women valued having a midwife they knew. Although demand was significant, with half the women saying they wanted a known midwife with them in labour, compared with the 1987 findings, fewer

women wanted this (50% vs. 62%). The remaining women said they did not mind. Expectations were also lower, with only 16% anticipating that they were going to have care in labour from a midwife they knew, down from 24%. Only 4% were sure they would be cared for by a midwife they had met previously, compared with 7% in 1987 (Green et al 2003).

Indeed, in 1995 reports suggested that at some time during their labour two thirds of women had no midwife or other professional with them (Garcia et al 1998). This was not reported as a problem by everyone, but 17% of woman – one in six – were left by themselves, or with a friend or family member only, at a time when it worried them to be alone. The women interviewed by Hunt (2004) in her ethnography of poverty and pregnancy emphasized how important it was to have the support of a midwife during labour. Some of those who had had children before felt they were left to get on with it when they needed the comfort of a knowledgeable person with them.

This reduction in care from a known individual may reflect the move towards team midwifery that was introduced in many areas in the 1990s, replacing access for a small proportion of women to a 'domino' service. Domino care was usually provided by one or two named midwives who saw the woman in her home or local community during pregnancy, accompanied her to the maternity unit for the birth and then provided postnatal care at home. It was seen as a Rolls Royce service conferring disproportionate benefits on a small minority of usually socially advantaged women (those who were well informed, through reading and social networks who knew about the scheme and booked on it early). Team midwifery was introduced in many areas in an attempt to offer continuity of carer to all women using the service and overcome this example of the inverse care law – in which those who least need services are best at exploiting what is available. The result however, unless the teams were small and well integrated, was that women felt they never saw the same midwife more than once during pregnancy, so had less continuity in the antenatal period, and although they might have met the midwife who cared for them in labour, they might not know her well or have built up a rapport. Caseload midwifery in contrast, based on a self-managed, flexible, community-based way of working with regular on-call responsibilities, enables women to see the same midwife during pregnancy, at the birth and afterwards, but seems to have been implemented more slowly (see Chapter 7).

Lack of midwifery capacity, high turnover of midwives, high vacancy rates and reliance on 'bank' midwives may also be factors preventing implementation of new ways of working across whole NHS trusts.

Women's expectations of knowing their midwife may therefore have actually been reduced over the last 12 to 18 years rather than increased, despite the view expressed in Changing Childbirth (Department of Health 1993) that this was central to woman-centred care. Indeed, responses to Green and colleagues' (2003) postnatal questionnaire confirmed that only 19% had met any of the midwives caring for them in labour compared with 24% in 1987. Just over half of these women said that they knew the midwife well.

Fewer women in 2000 (Green et al 2003) said that they wanted – and also fewer women expected – to have one midwife responsible for their care throughout their labour. In 1987 (Green et al 1998), 87% of women had wanted this and 49% expected it; 13 years later a large majority still wanted this (78%) but a quarter rather than half expected it (24%). In practice, reports of having had one midwife throughout labour had not declined on average, though first-time mothers using the units in the south of England were less likely in 2000 to have care from the same midwife throughout their labour.

Discussing postnatal care, Garcia and colleagues said, 'More than two thirds of women said that it mattered to them to have met the community midwives before. Women who had met all the midwives before reported more consistent advice, more active support and more practical help with breastfeeding. They were also more likely to think it mattered a great deal to have met the midwives before the birth' (Garcia et al 1998, p. 61).

Making reference to the earlier NCT study which found a link between how midwives were organized and the care women received (Gready et al 1995), the authors recommended that 'knowing the caregivers involved in labour and birth is very important for some women'. And

they questioned whether it would therefore be a priority to provide continuity of carer selectively for 'those women who might benefit from it most, in places that do not aim to make it available for all women' (Gready et al 1995, p. 78). The NCT supports this approach; our birth policy states that 'Women most in need . . . should have priority when continuity of carer schemes are set up' (National Childbirth Trust 2002).

DISCUSSION

The idea that maternity care should be 'woman-centred' has been a central tenet for NHS maternity care now for almost 15 years. The authors of Changing Childbirth (Department of Health 1993) wanted women to have access to a service that, '. . . does not jeopardise safety, yet is kinder, more welcoming and more supportive to the women whose needs it is designed to meet' (Department of Health 1993, p. II).

This much is very widely accepted and there is evidence of positive change in favour of involving women. In some areas and for some women there also seems to be more respect for individual autonomy. However women living in poverty and others who are disadvantaged often feel criticized and told what to do (Hunt 2004) and even quite assertive women find it difficult to negotiate with some of the institutional assumptions they come up against. In 2000, Green and colleagues (Green et al 2003) found some evidence of positive change. Greater numbers of women wanted to be in control of decisions about their care, and the largest group of women said that 'staff had discussed things with me before making a decision', whereas in 1987 the largest group said that 'the staff made decisions but kept me informed'.

There has been debate about the central importance of each woman having an established, trusting relationship with a small number of carers, partly because this means changing the system in which midwives work and changing their working lives. Partly it is because the available evidence is limited and raises more questions than it can answer. The midwife's attitude towards the women she is looking after and the philosophy of care provided are two other central components of woman-centred care. Services that enhance continuity of carer also encourage positive attitudes and usually a particular philosophy of care, so it is difficult to separate out the different influences. More research is needed to show how different models of care work for women.

Undoubtedly, the use of drugs, drips and intensive monitoring has been increasing. Although more women have 'pain-free labour' these women are not the most content or confident. In fact, when describing the reality of their labour, more women in 2000 used the words 'frightened', 'powerless', and 'helpless' to describe how they felt, and fewer used the words 'confident' or 'involved', compared with responses in 1987 (Green et al 2003). If having a sense of control during labour is central to a woman's 'subsequent psychological well-being' as Green and colleagues (Green et al 2003) have suggested, it seems that providing what women need from care around the time of birth is proving somewhat illusive.

Despite the growing levels of fear, widespread use of anaesthesia, increasing caesarean rates over successive years and changing attitudes toward interventions, four in five women said that they would prefer either no drugs or 'a minimum of drugs to keep the pain manageable'.

Unless things have changed since 2000, or the units in the Greater Expectations (Green et al 2003) study were not typical, the system is not currently helping women to achieve what they want. More women ended up using pain-relieving drugs than had wanted to and only four out of ten first-time mothers who had an epidural went on to have a spontaneous vaginal birth. Women not only need to be told about how some decisions may have unanticipated or unwanted consequences, they also need to be offered alternative strategies that acknowledge and respond to their fears. This means providing more practical support from those with the appropriate skills and training; it undoubtedly means a coordinating midwife. It may also mean an NCT antenatal teacher or discussion leader, a massage instructor, doula or maternity assistant from the local community.

There was no explicit discussion in Changing Childbirth (Department of Health 1993) about the culture of maternity services – the beliefs, practices and 'ways of doing things around here' – that make up how an institution works. On reflection, some elements of the 'principles of good maternity care' may have over emphasized the potential of women's decision making. For example, it seems clearer now that providing women with reliable information about options is only one aspect of making 'informed choices'. One of the feisty, 'crusader' women in our study found, 'the whole thing was completely opposite to how I wanted it. I was strapped to the monitor for the whole time and then he had a head monitor which I said I was going to completely refuse . . . They wanted to monitor him, I don't know why, because they don't really explain a great deal to you'.

Access to reliable information is undoubtedly important, as is involvement in decision making, but neither is sufficient to ensure that women get the kind of care that they might want, nor to prevent unnecessary medical interventions. If the maternity service the woman is using has a high rate of interventions she will be more likely to get caught up in them despite having evidence-based information, even if she has a clear preference to avoid certain interventions. Information on its own is now known to be insufficient to change a maternity service culture without other measures being introduced to achieve different beliefs and attitudes (Kirkham & Stapleton 2001). During labour in particular, an over emphasis on information giving and making choices can detract from the need for a confident, quiet midwife providing empathic support and encouragement when necessary (Leap & Anderson 2004).

It is sad and surprising given the considerable demand for more information and the extent of anxiety about labour, that only a minority of women seem to attend antenatal classes or groups during pregnancy (Singh & Newburn 2000a). For those who did go to a class or group the main motivations were getting information, preparing for the birth, meeting other pregnant women, and preparing for being a parent. Some women said that they did not feel comfortable with the services available. They did not feel that they would fit in with the other women, or would prefer to speak to someone individually rather than in a group. First-time mothers, women under twenty, women from an ethnic minority, and those from lower socio-economic groups were more likely than others to feel that the available support services were not right for their needs (Singh & Newburn 2000a).

However, over many years NHS trusts seem to have been reducing the number of antenatal classes, sometimes cutting out all provision or charging parents a fee to attend. There have been good examples of social support and group work with pregnant women in Sure Start initiatives, particularly those that have prioritized services during the initial transition to parenthood. As Sure Start is phased out in England and Children's Centres are set up, it remains to be seen whether these examples of good practice will flourish or be swallowed up. As there is no ring-fenced funding for the health element of Children's Centres provision, local lobbying will be needed to ensure that resources are made available.

The Children's National Service Frameworks for England and Wales (Department of Health 2004, Welsh Assembly Government 2004), built on understandings spelt out in Changing Childbirth (Department of Health 1993), to move the policy agenda on further. They recognize the importance for women of giving birth in a place which is quiet, relaxed and home-like, having one-to-one support from a midwife and, overtly promoting the 'normality of childbirth'. Though there are many challenges ahead, the frameworks provide opportunities to introduce new systems of care which address lack of relationship, a task-oriented approach, intrusive monitoring, routine use of drugs and growing rates of surgical intervention.

Women seem to form quite clear ideas about what is likely or realistic, which influences their expectations; in turn their expectations seem to influence their expressed 'wants'. In order to understand what women want it is important to invest some time and explore beyond initial impressions. Anyone planning services for parents or wondering what kind of improvements are needed should spend time with new parents and get them to talk about their day-to-day lives, their experiences of labour and looking after their babies, and how they would like to see things change. Published research, particularly ethnographic work, can be a good source of information on what women and their partners may want, but the opportunity to talk directly, to question and reflect on what parents say, can provide another

dimension of understanding. Sometimes the emotional impact of parents' experiences is lost in academic studies.

Parent advocates have a key role to play too. They may be employed in health or social care or be recruited from the local community of parents. Parent representatives on maternity services liaison committees and labour ward forums have often had long experience of working with pregnant women and with mums and dads through NCT groups and Sure Start, or they may be part of the same community networks. Advocates with a knowledge of local people, services and politics, and those who know about national policies and research evidence have a key role to play in identifying key questions and helping to answer them.

PRACTICE POINTERS

- It is important to go back to first principles and explore with women and their partners what they want from services, not just to ask them what they think about what is currently available.
- Be aware that expectations are often low. Develop group work with pregnant women and new parents to give them permission to 'think outside of the box'.
- Unless you have experienced a service you won't really know how it feels. So, parents don't necessarily know what they would choose unless they had knowledge about all the options.
- It may be easier to imagine yourself having a main-stream option (e.g. a hospital birth) than a less usual option (e.g. a home birth) but if you have the chance to try the less usual option you might rate it highly.
- Options may include access to care from the same midwife during pregnancy, birth and the postnatal period (continuity of carer), use of a birth centre or a birth pool, skin-to-skin contact with your new baby; all aspects of care that are highly rated by most women and families who have had the chance to try them.
- Talking directly with other parents – or watching a DVD showing a range of parents who have had different experiences – can be really helpful.

References

Allen I, Dowling S K, Williams S 1997 A leading role for midwives? Evaluation of midwifery group practice development projects. Policy Study Institute, London

Audit Commission 1997 First class delivery. Improving maternity services in England and Wales. Audit Commission for Local Authorities in England and Wales, London

Beake S, McCourt C 2001 The social context of birth: a discussion paper to inform the development of the NCT birth policy. New Digest (12): 14[i]–14[iv]

Borton H, Newburn M, Moran Ellis J et al 1989 Rupture of the membranes in labour: a survey conducted by the National Childbirth Trust. National Childbirth Trust, London

Cartwright A 1979 The dignity of labour? A study of childbearing and induction. Tavistock, London

Clement S, Wilson J, Sikorski J 1999 The development of an intrapartum intervention score based on women's experiences. Journal of Reproductive and Infant Psychology 17(1): 53–62

Department for Work and Pensions 2004 Households below average incomes: an analysis of the income distribution from 1994/5 – 2002/3, 15th edn. Department for Work and Pensions, London

Department of Health 1993 Changing childbirth: Part 1. Report of the expert maternity group. HMSO, London

Department of Health 2004 National service framework for children, young people and maternity services. Department of Health and Department for Education and Skills, London

Fleissig A 1993 Are women given enough information by staff during labour and delivery? Midwifery 9(2): 70–75

Garcia J, Redshaw M, Fitzsimons B et al 1998 First class delivery. A national survey of women's views of maternity care. Audit Commission for Local Authorities in England and Wales, London

Gready M, Newburn M, Dodds R et al 1995 Birth choices: women's expectations and experiences. National Childbirth Trust, London

Green J M, Baston H, Easton S et al 2003 Greater expectations? Inter-relationships between women's expectations and experiences of decision making, continuity, choice and control in labour, and psychological outcomes: summary report. Mother & Infant Research Unit, Leeds

Green J M, Coupland V A, Kitzinger J V 1998 Great expectations: a prospective study of women's expectations and experiences of childbirth 2nd Edition. Books for Midwives, Hale, Cheshire

Green J M, Kitzinger J V, Coupland V A 1990 Stereotypes of childbearing women: a look at some evidence. Midwifery 6(3): 125–132

Greenshields W 1987 Postnatal infection: a survey conducted by the National Childbirth Trust. National Childbirth Trust, London

Hames P, Taylor J, Glossop C 1997 Parents' needs for information and support during pregnancy, labour and the first three years of parenthood (Internal report). National Childbirth Trust, London

House of Commons Health Committee 1991 Maternity services – preconception: Health Committee fourth report 1990–91. [Chairman Nicholas Winterton], Vol 1. Report together with the proceedings of the committee. HMSO, London

House of Commons Health Committee 1992a Maternity services. Health Committee second report 1991–92. [Chairman Nicholas Winterton], Vol 3. Appendices to the minutes of evidence. HMSO, London

House of Commons Health Committee 1992b Maternity services. Health Committee second report 1991–92. [Chairman Nicholas Winterton], Vol 1. Report together with appendices and the proceedings of evidence. HMSO, London

Hunt S 2004 Poverty, pregnancy and the healthcare professional. Books for Midwives, Edinburgh

Jacoby A 1988 Mothers' views about information and advice in pregnancy and childbirth: findings from a national study. Midwifery 4: 103–119

Kirkham M, Stapleton H (eds) 2001 Informed choice in maternity care: an evaluation of evidence based leaflets. CRD report 20. NHS Centre for Reviews and Dissemination, York

Kitzinger S 1978 Some mothers' experiences of induced labour. National Childbirth Trust, London

Kitzinger S, Walters R 1981 Some women's experiences of episiotomy. National Childbirth Trust, London

Leap N, Anderson T 2004 The role of pain in normal birth and the empowerment of women. In: Downe S (ed) Normal childbirth: evidence and debate. Churchill Livingstone, Edinburgh p 25–39

National Childbirth Trust 2004a Making normal birth a reality: sharing good practice and strategies that work. Transcriptions from the NCT Conference, Thursday 27 November 2003. MIDIRS, London

National Childbirth Trust 2004b Developing maternity services: what do local people think?. National Childbirth Trust, London

National Childbirth Trust 2004c Birth services in mid Sussex: what is most important to women? National Childbirth Trust, London

National Childbirth Trust 1999 NCT baby feeding policy report. National Childbirth Trust, London

National Childbirth Trust, Royal College of Midwives, Royal College of Obstetricians and Gynaecologists 2000 The rising caesarean rate – a public health issue. Report of a national conference organised by the NCT, the RCM and the RCOG; held in London 23 November 1999. Profile Productions, London

National Collaborating Centre for Women's and Children's Health 2004 Caesarean section: clinical guideline. NICE Clinical Guideline 13. RCOG Press, London

Newburn M 2002 A birth policy for the National Childbirth Trust. MIDIRS Midwifery Digest 12(1): 122–126

Newburn M 2003 Culture, control and birth environment. Practising Midwife 6(8): 20–25

Newburn M, Singh D 2003 Creating a better birth environment: women's views about the design and facilities in maternity units: a national survey. An audit toolkit. National Childbirth Trust, London

Newburn M, Singh D 2005 Are women getting the birth environment they need? Report of a national survey of women's experiences. National Childbirth Trust, London

NHS Quality Improvement Scotland 2005 Clinical standards – maternity services. NHS Quality Improvement Scotland, Edinburgh

Northern Ireland Department of Health, Social Services and Public Safety 2002 Developing better services: modernising hospitals and reforming structures. Northern Ireland Department of Health, Social Services and Public Safety, Belfast

Rosser J 2002 Help yourself to a straightforward birth. New Generation (February): 6–7

Rosser J 2003 How do Albany midwives do it? Evaluation of the Albany Midwifery Practice. MIDIRS Midwifery Digest 13(2): 251–257

Royal College of Obstetrics and Gynaecologists, Royal College of Midwives, National Childbirth Trust 2001 The rising caesarean rate – causes and effects for public health. Conference report of a one-day national conference organised by the RCOG, RCM, NCT held in London on 7 November 2000. National Childbirth Trust, London

Royal College of Obstetricians and Gynaecologists, Royal College of Midwives, National Childbirth Trust 2002 The rising caesarean rate – from audit to action. Report of a joint conference organised by the RCOG, RCM, NCT held in London on 31 January 2002. National Childbirth Trust, London

Scottish Executive 2001 A framework for maternity services in Scotland. Scottish Executive, Edinburgh

Singh D, Newburn M (eds) 2000a Access to maternity information and support: the experiences and needs of women before and after giving birth. National Childbirth Trust, London

Singh D, Newburn M 2000b Becoming a father: men's access to information and support about pregnancy, birth and life with a new baby. National Childbirth Trust, Fathers Direct, London

Stadlen N 2004 What mothers do, especially when it looks like nothing. Piatkus, London

Welsh Assembly Government 2004 National service framework for children, young people and maternity services in Wales: consultation document. Key points. Welsh Assembly Government, Cardiff

Wiggins M, Newburn M 2004 Information used by pregnant women and their understanding and use of evidence-based 'Informed Choice' leaflets. In: Kirkham M (ed) Informed choice in maternity care. Palgrave Macmillan, London

Chapter **2**

First relationships and the growth of love and commitment

Maggie Redshaw

FIRST RELATIONSHIPS: GROWING LOVE AND COMMITMENT

This chapter is based on the understanding that early experience matters and that the first years of life are of critical importance in the long-term mental health of the individual. As health professionals we have a role to play in the promotion of the long-term emotional and social health of women, children and their families. But what exactly is it about the parent–infant relationship we are aiming to encourage? Enjoyment, confidence, understanding, consistent care, appropriate stimulation for an infant's age and stage, an appreciation of individual differences, effective adaptation to the role of parent and a close and positive reciprocal relationship in which child and parent feel significant and valued.

A midwife is a facilitator not only of the physical birth of the individual, but also has the potential to contribute to the birth of the parent–child relationship and the family. She is in a unique and privileged position to play an active role in promoting maternal mental health and in the identification of parents and infants at risk of long-term social and emotional problems.

This chapter acknowledges the role of the midwife in helping to create the optimal circumstances for pregnancy, birth and the initiation of family relationships. The focus is on the influence of the early parent–child relationship on the long-term emotional and psychological health of the growing and developing infant. The human

infant's attachment to the mother or other primary caregiver has been seen as a prerequisite for survival and as a prototype for all the other close relationships that he or she will make in the future. Bowlby's attachment paradigm will be used to explore the concepts of the attachment system and of the development of early internal representational models of self, and of self in relation to others that form the template for the long-term mental health of the individual (Bowlby 1969, 1973, 1980). Research will be explored that may shed light on the connection between the sensitivity of early parenting and the subsequent developmental trajectory of the child. The midwife's role in facilitating early parent–child contact and attachment will be examined, as will her role in screening and interventions.

BIRTH AND THE FOUNDATION OF HUMAN RELATIONSHIPS

Birth can mark the beginning of the relationship between parents and their newborn infant (Klaus et al 1995, Stern 1977). However, for many women and their partners the relationship and feelings of emotional engagement often begin before birth (Condon 1993, Fonagy et al 1991, Winnicot 1987), though the relationship takes a different form at that stage. Early parent–infant interaction, embodied in a growing appreciation of infant signals and timing, and an intense period of learning and developing expectations, underpins in a fundamental way the form of this and other relationships. Evolution and biology have worked to ensure that the newborn human infant receives what it needs: the longest period of care and nurturing required by any species. Parents and infants are primed at birth to respond to each other: most new parents expect to love and care for their tiny newborn infant and most full-term healthy newborn babies are programmed with amazing capacities to capture the attention and commitment of their parents and caregivers. Despite an uncomfortable journey, healthy newborns are able to turn to the familiar voice of their mother; they gaze at faces and try to follow their movement, grip fingers placed in their tiny palms and, if given the opportunity, will attempt to crawl up their mother's abdomen to latch on to her nipple (Brazelton 1973, Brazelton & Nugent 1995). The cry of the newborn too is one that is difficult for an adult to ignore. The pitch, tone and intensity are such as to make us respond and attempt to soothe and quiet.

There are few parents who are not able to respond in some way to this small, dependent being that has emerged from the mother's body. The nine months of pregnancy and a mother's slowly altering body and changing identity have built within her a set of hopes and expectations for this child and their future relationship together (Klaus & Kennell 1982). By the time labour begins, a mother is usually anxious to deliver, to see, hold and get to know her new baby and the early postpartum period is commonly characterized by the power of this intense and intimate early relationship.

Clinicians and researchers have argued for the significance that the first hours and days of life can have for the developing parent–infant relationship (De Chateau & Wiberg 1984, Klaus & Kennell 1982). A range of reviews and research studies have demonstrated the significance of such factors as the support available and empowerment of parents during labour and delivery, and the provision of an atmosphere following birth that facilitates the natural process by which parents have direct contact with, get to know and become committed to their infants (Feldman et al 2002, Hodnett et al 2003, Tessier 1998, Whitelaw et al 1988).

However, we also know that the ability to maintain the commitment to an infant, to develop

appropriate skills and to sustain the patience, generosity and dedication that are necessary to raise a child to be a healthy, loving, sociable individual, takes more than the initial love and physiological changes associated with pregnancy, birth and the postnatal period. Like any human relationship, that between parent and infant is influenced by a multiplicity of factors (see Fig. 11.1). These include new parents' own experience of being parented, their lifelong history of relationships, their own ability to love and support each other, whether this baby is the first or later born, perinatal factors such as a difficult or 'at risk' pregnancy and environmental stress. The quality of the emotional and practical support received by parents, as well as infant factors such as health and temperament also contribute to the way the relationship develops. In fact, a variety of research and clinical studies have concluded that many of the factors occurring long before the birth of the infant have a profound effect upon the long-term quality of the parent–infant relationship (Fraiberg 1980, Fraiberg et al 1975, Lyons-Ruth et al 1990, Zeanah 1993). This same research also tends to demonstrate that the quality of the early parent–child relationship is a key influence on the long-term mental, emotional and social health of the individual (Fonagy et al 1996).

At this time, with increasing concern about child abuse and neglect, as well as recognition of the importance of social and emotional problems experienced by both children and adults, there is an obligation to examine the way in which, as health professionals involved in supporting early parent–child relationships, we can play a part in being aware and contributing to the prevention of mental health problems. This chapter is written on the premise that the quality of the early parent–child relationship is a key determinant of the long-term mental health of the individual. We will thus examine some of the factors that are thought to influence the ability of a parent to develop a bond with, nurture and be sensitive to his or her infant. This will be done in the context of relevant theoretical approaches and research evidence, primarily influenced by attachment theory (Bowlby 1988, Rutter 1995), which traces the impact of the early parent–child relationship on infant mental health, that of the older child and later the adult. We will explore the role that midwives might play in recognizing parents and infants who are at risk of developing problems in parenting and discuss possible interventions that are currently in use, in order to support positive parent–child relationships and interrupt the inter-generational transmission of destructive attachment patterns and parenting practices.

The principle underlying the focus of this chapter is the repeated finding that many of the factors strongly influencing the quality of the mother–child relationship are already in place long before pregnancy or labour begin. The focus on attachment theory and research is intended to reiterate the significance of the first years of life in determining the nature of the child's relational and developmental trajectory. Attachment research is also presented to demonstrate the link between the mother's history of relationships and her ability to provide the quality of parenting needed by her infant. The ultimate goal is to provide a theory base from which the midwife, together with other health professionals, can develop an approach in practice that can contribute to the primary prevention of problems in the early parent–child attachment.

ATTACHMENT THEORY AND RESEARCH

Attachment theory developed from the work of John Bowlby and Mary Ainsworth. Bowlby was a child psychotherapist who found current mental health theories of his day to be entirely inadequate for understanding and treating the problems he found in his own practice. Turning to the fields of ethology and psychoanalysis, as well as to his own practice and research, he formulated the basic outline and principles of attachment theory. His influential works, the three volumes of Attachment and Loss (Bowlby 1969, 1973, 1980), formed the basis for an approach to understanding the impact of an infant's early experience upon the development of self and relationship patterns. Over the same time period Ainsworth furthered the usefulness of attachment theory by testing some of its basic components with empirical study by developing instruments for infant observation (Ainsworth 1967, Ainsworth et al 1978).

Many others have contributed to the wider adoption of attachment concepts, to the development of attachment theory and to a broadening empirical base. Some have focused on assessing and updating the theory in the light of research evidence and social change (Rutter 1981), on children (Bretherton 1985, Dunn 1993, Stern 1977), on non-maternal child care (Belsky 2001), on adult relationships (Hazan & Shaver 1987, 1994), on intergenerational links (Rutter & Rutter 1993) and the application of theory and evidence to clinical practice (Fonagy et al 1994, Zeanah & Emde 1994).

This section will introduce the basic principles of attachment theory.

Attachment theory suggests that the quality of the early relationship between parent and child is an essential determinant of the long-term social and emotional health of the individual. Bowlby (1988) argued that the power of the attachment system arises from the absolute and long-term dependency of the human infant upon the caregiving figure. Because of this dependency, the attachment relationship is key to the survival of the infant. Since maintaining contact with a parent answers survival needs, an infant will over time adapt his or her behaviour and ways of being in the world to ensure that parental rejection or abandonment does not occur. For this reason, attachment relational patterns learned during this early preverbal stage of life are powerful and influential in determining future behaviour. Subsequently, the behavioural patterns that evolve from the early parent–child relationship reflect the infant's developing internal representational model of self and of self in relation to others. Bowlby proposed that these early internal models have a profound influence on the long-term interactional, exploratory and social behaviour of the individual over time.

Ainsworth's research (1967, 1973) extended our understanding of the interface between attachment and the quality of the mother–infant relationship. She followed mothers and infants in both the USA and Uganda, using detailed systematic observations over the first 18 months of life. Her findings provided a better understanding of the relationship between early maternal care and sensitivity and the ongoing relational pattern of her infant. From these early data, Ainsworth developed an observational assessment instrument (the Strange Situation procedure) that has allowed researchers to operationalize the concept of internal representational models and to track the stability of individual attachment patterns over time using other methods of assessment (Van Ijzendoorn 1992, Waters et al 2000).

The Strange Situation procedure consists of a standardized procedure, observation and assessment leading to categorization of attachment patterns of infants between 12 and 18 months of age. The procedure documents an infant's interactions with a caregiver during a series of observations in which the parent and infant are in a play situation, followed by a separation and then a reunion with the caregiver. The infant's response and interaction with the parent, particularly following reunion, are the basis for an infant's classification as secure or as having one of three different categories of insecure attachment. The assessment is usually carried out with the participation of a parent, but can involve a regular caregiver.

INTERNAL REPRESENTATIONS AND ATTACHMENT SECURITY

Attachment theory and research emphasize the role that children's experiences of interpersonal relationships have in their psychological development, that attachment and dependency are different and that the former can promote, in a substantial way, maturity in social functioning. Thus attachment is seen as contributing to the promotion of security, encouraging independence and takes place within the context of normal developmental processes. It is argued that the early mother–child relationship provides a prototype upon which all future intimate relationships are built. The way in which the mother or primary caregiver interacts with the child provides continuous feedback to the child of his or her lovability, worth and competence. Through interaction with the care-giving figure, an infant gradually forms an internal image or internal representational model of self, of others and of self in relation to others. This concept of an internal representational or working model is one of the most useful concepts within attachment theory, allowing researchers to operationalize attachment concepts (Shaver et al 1996). Ainsworth et al's (1978) research with the strange situation demonstrated

that infants form consistent internal representational models of attachment by the age of 18 months and that there are marked differences between individuals in this respect. An internal representational model is embodied in feelings, beliefs, expectations and behavioural strategies that are used by an individual in relation to himself and others. The value of internal working models, according to Shaver et al (1996) is that they explicitly recognize the role of active thought processes in mediating the effects of experiences and provide a mechanism for individual continuity and change. Thus working models serve a useful purpose for the developing child, making unnecessary the construction of a new set of expectations for each new situation. The child can use existing models to appraise and guide behaviour in new situations. For example, a child who has a working model of his mother as available when needed may spend less time monitoring her movements than a baby unsure of his mother's availability. Although Bowlby viewed working models as open to new input, he believed that because they tend to operate outside consciousness, they become increasingly resistant to change over time. Thus, even when working models are no longer appropriate or necessary in a relationship, they may remain influential, guiding an individual's behaviour in repetitive and even pathological ways.

For Bowlby, there is a direct relationship between the working model of self and the working model of relationship to the primary attachment figure, though relationships with a range of caregivers are also thought to be influential in this respect (Oppenheim et al 1988, Schaffer 1996). Individuals are seen as developing either secure or insecure attachments depending upon the sensitivity of their early care-giving experience. If a child experiences a positive early parenting relationship in which his or her needs are met with sensitivity and consistency, a secure attachment relationship is formed, and positive internal representational models are established. These representational models are of attachment figures as positive, available, safe, responsive and helpful. Similarly, the internal representational model of self is one of self as worthy, loveable and capable. In contrast, if early care is inconsistent, insensitive, hurtful or frustrating, an insecure attachment to the caregiver will develop. The resultant internal model will be of the self as unlovable, incapable and unworthy and the representational model of others in relationships will be of others as dangerous, hurtful, unpredictable or unreliable.

Thus, attachment theory suggests that the types of parent–infant relationship that are most likely to yield secure attachments and therefore emotionally healthy individuals are the ones in which the parent behaves in a consistent way, is sensitively receptive to the child's signals and contingently responsive to them. For secure attachment to be sustained, parental sensitivity alters as the child's needs for both security and for exploration change with development. Subsequent research by Ainsworth et al (1978) described parental sensitivity as parenting that is readily available to the child and freely giving of comfort and close bodily contact when requested, particularly when the child is frightened, ill or distressed.

In one of his later works, Bowlby (1991) wrote about the developmental trajectories that children's early attachment patterns set in motion. He described a variety of longitudinal research demonstrating that insecure attachments in infancy were found to predict disturbed developmental patterns, and thwarted potential in later life. Long-term studies have to some extent confirmed the link between the quality of early parenting and the child's ongoing mental health and relationship patterns (Colin 1996, George et al 1985, Troy & Sroufe 1987). However, the nature of the link between insecure attachment in infancy and later psychopathology has yet to be elucidated fully in the attempt to understand the role of attachment in relation to adverse outcomes. The next section will review selected studies concerning what is known about the relational and developmental impact of early attachment security over time.

SEQUELAE OF INFANT ATTACHMENT PATTERNS IN LATER CHILDHOOD

If, as Bowlby suggested, the early parent–infant attachment relationship serves as an internal, perhaps tacit, model for future relationships, one might expect the pattern to repeat itself in childhood relationships and in later parenting relation-

ships. This hypothesis has been tested in a number of studies, using the Strange Situation as the base and this section highlights some studies that have tracked relationship patterns from infancy into early and middle childhood, in 'normal' and maltreated populations.

Early studies sought to determine the stability and reliability of the Strange Situation classification at twelve months and then later in the second year (Ainsworth et al 1978). Greater stability was found in children categorized as securely attached and within middle-class families with minimal stress. Using the Strange Situation Instrument, Connell (1976) found that 81% of the infants in a sample received the same attachment security classification at 12 and 18 months of age. Similarly, Waters (1978) assessed 50 middle-class babies and found a 96% consistency in classification at 12 and 18 months old. Main and Weston (1981) also found a high level of consistency when following babies over this time period.

There have also been studies that have followed children over time in order to understand the developmental consequences following different kinds of parenting experiences, particularly insensitive early parenting and insecure attachment in infancy. One of the most well known of these is the Minnesota longitudinal study that followed 267 high-risk families from the prenatal period through childhood and beyond (Weinfield et al 2000). At the current time, the most recent data collection involves contacting the children who are now adults aged 28 years. The focus of the interviews at this age is on mental health issues, including anxiety and depression, use of mental health services, levels of stress, social support, and current work situation, education and romantic relationships.

As an earlier part of the Minnesota study, Troy and Sroufe (1987) examined the association between 38 preschool children's attachment histories and their interaction with their peers in a preschool setting. All the children (20 boys and 18 girls) had been previously assessed using the Strange Situation procedure at 12 months of age and were routinely in contact with each other in a preschool setting. After at least 6 weeks of preschool attendance, the children were observed playing in a specifically designated playroom for seven different sessions of 15 minutes each, spread over many weeks. The data were analysed comparing the play behaviour of different combinations of children with varying classifications of attachment security.

An analysis of the play using different observers showed a significant difference in the quality of play and quantity of aggression between dyads containing insecurely attached children and those containing securely attached youngsters. The analysis revealed that the presence of a child with an insecure attachment history was more likely to be associated with victimization related behaviours such as aggression, hurtful or coercive play. Five out of seven pairs in which at least one child had an insecure attachment history showed victimization, whereas none of the seven pairs without a history of insecure attachment showed victimization. In contrast, the presence in the dyad of a child with a secure attachment history was associated with a non-victimizing peer play relationship. None of eight such pairs showed victimization, whereas in five out of the six pairs containing exclusively insecurely attached children victimization was observed.

Studies like Troy and Sroufe's (1987) research shed light on some of the findings in the clinical abuse and attachment literature. It is accepted in abuse and neglect research that maltreated children are more likely than well-treated children to be the victims of further abuse or serious aggression (Egeland 1993, Kaufman & Ziegler 1987). They are also more likely in adult life to show aggression towards others within intimate relationships. This research, however, documents the connection between the quality of the early attachment relationship (rather than a specific abusive act) and the child's predisposition towards continuing both the victim and the victimizer roles within relationships. Findings of this kind have implications for early preventive intervention. They are relevant to the prevention of abuse in further generations and link with evidence from other literature that disturbed peer relationships in childhood are one of the most powerful predictors of pathology in adulthood (Asher & Coie 1990). Also, if these links over time are examined in relation to the concept of the internal working models, it seems to suggest that a child may re-enact not only the model of self, but also the part of the parent in the relationship model.

Although the study described above included some abused and neglected children, the child participants were selected on the basis of the Strange Situation rather than on a history of maltreatment. Another study specifically traced the relationship patterns of children coming from maltreating homes. Egeland and Erickson (1993) identified 80 preschool children from the longitudinal study of 267 high-risk children, whose caretaking experience fitted into four different patterns of child maltreatment. The four maltreatment groups were divided into groups characterized by parenting behaviour histories of physical abuse, hostility or verbal abuse, psychological unavailability and physical neglect. A control group of children and mothers who provided adequate care were selected from the remaining high-risk sample. The two groups were assessed in order to compare the children's developmental pathways and behavioural patterns during the first five years of life.

In general, the insecurely attached children from maltreated groups were characterized by patterns of diminishing IQ scores, increasingly hostile and negative affect and interactional patterns, a lack of self-esteem, poor concentration, creativity and self control in comparison to their non-maltreated securely attached peers. The authors found significant differences between the patterns of response, depending upon the type of maltreatment to which the children were subjected. Nonetheless, the most striking generalizable consequence of maltreatment was the ongoing declining level of cognitive and social functioning displayed by all the groups of abused and neglected children over time.

Egeland et al (1990) documented another stage in the Minnesota longitudinal study. Their analyses sought to determine which symptoms and behaviours seen in high-risk preschool children were predictive of later behaviour in the early school years. They followed 96 of the preschool children on whom data had already been collected since birth and continued to assess them yearly through until the third grade (age eight years). They found a high degree of continuity between the children's preschool behaviour and that seen in the first three years of school. Insecurely attached children who had demonstrated relationship problems in preschool were likely to also have relationship problems in primary school, and children who were socially and academically competent in preschool were also found to be competent in their school years. In fact, more than three-quarters of the children identified as insecurely attached and aggressive in preschool were also identified as aggressive towards their peers in two out of their three years of elementary school. Similarly, over two-thirds of the youngsters labelled as withdrawn in preschool were also judged to be withdrawn in primary school. Furthermore, the children who were classified as aggressive or withdrawn at four years of age scored significantly below the academic achievement levels of the competent children.

Although continuity of behaviour is evident in this study (Egeland et al 1990), the discontinuities are also of interest. There were a number of intervening factors associated with a decrease in behavioural problems. Improvements in behaviour, and movement from an insecure attachment category to a secure one, were linked with a lessening of maternal depression, a reduction in the number of stressful family life events and an increase in the quality of stimulation in the child's home environment. As found in a range of other studies, the severity of maternal depression directly appeared to affect the quality of the relationship between the mother and her child while indirectly impacting on the quality and organization of the home environment (Murray & Cooper 1997, Murray et al 1999).

Based on the Minnesota study, Sroufe (1991) summarized the alternate developmental and relational pathways taken by the insecurely attached children. Data were derived from parent–child observation sessions; preschool observations, the first three years in grade school and a summer camp experience in their tenth and eleventh years of age. Sroufe concluded that the relational and developmental patterns that each group followed reflected their internal representations of self and of self in relation to others. He concluded that children who displayed secure attachment during the 18 month Strange Situation assessment tended to continue to exhibit higher functioning and healthier relationship patterns during the subsequent ten years of study. As preschoolers, they were characterized by greater confidence, resourcefulness, self-direction, enthusiasm, positive affect and problem-solving ability than their insecurely attached peers. They were also likely to be more curious, resourceful and forceful in pursuing tasks and goals.

In the preschool and school years, the secure children were less likely to sit beside the teacher, more likely to initiate positive contact with their peers and more likely to greet their teachers and peers. When confronted with rejection from peers, they were more likely to reframe it positively and to continue to seek contact with other children. As 10- and 11-year-olds, these securely attached children were more likely than their insecure peers to be confident and flexible, and were better able to manage their impulses and feelings. As in the earlier years, these preteens were more likely to display positive affect in all relations with others; they came across as more socially competent and better able to establish and maintain deeper relationships and their interaction with peers was generally characterized by reciprocity and fairness.

The contrasting description of the insecurely attached children was consistent throughout the study. They were characterized as being more aggressive, avoidant and sensitive to rebuff at all stages of development. As early as the preschool years, children who had been insecurely attached as infants showed decreased confidence and less curiosity, and were either unable or unwilling to engage in challenging tasks. Although they were more likely to cling to teachers, they were also less likely to ask a school counsellor or teacher for assistance when experiencing difficulty. In the pre-adolescent years, the insecure children's peer relationships were more often marked by hostility and a lack of commitment. They tended to choose friends who were also insecurely attached and within those friendships, often played either the victim or victimizer role. The interactions tended to be characterized by hostility, teasing, rejection and exploitative behaviour. The type of play observed was also distinctive at each age. As early as the preschool years, the play lacked the fantasy and complexity of securely attached children. When make-believe themes did occur in later years, conflict or problems more often tended to move towards unsuccessful or negative resolution. However, though the profile of the insecurely attached child is certainly discouraging, Sroufe concluded that:

This strong data on the continuity of adaptation over time should not lead to pessimism concerning change. The organizational perspective (on the self) is also useful for conceptualising intervention and change. The inner organization of self is a derivative of organised vital relationships and, as such most likely will undergo change in the context of other significant relationships.

Sroufe 1991, p. 303

While early insecure attachment relationships may be associated with later difficulties there is not an absolute inevitability about the consequences of these. The question is asked – Why is it that some children arrive at adaptive outcomes despite the risk they experience? Protective factors such as an easy temperament, particular skills or abilities, positive relationships with siblings or grandparents may moderate the effects of difficult beginnings (Garmezy & Masten 1991, Horowitz 1987). While some children are clearly more vulnerable than others, and suffer from multiple disadvantage, often in the form of chains of events (Rutter & Rutter 1993), later outcomes for some children can show surprising evidence of change and adjustment often associated with choice of partner, take up of educational opportunities and delay in having children. In a study of young African-American boys born to single teenage parents this kind of point was clearly illustrated with positive parent–child relationships, parental values, community input and relatively long inter-birth intervals before the next child having an effect (Apfel & Seitz 1997).

With concerns about the long term psychosocial consequences of inadequate parenting, a key question is to ask if and how individuals' early parenting might influence how they parent their own children in turn. With the goal of exploring this question, Main and colleagues developed the Adult Attachment Interview (AAI) (Main & Goldwyn 1985). This instrument, in conjunction with the Strange Situation procedure, has allowed researchers to examine the relationship between adults' resolution of attachment experiences and their own ability to parent their child with the sensitivity and consistency necessary to foster secure attachment and consequently a healthier developmental trajectory. The AAI reflects Sroufe's

and others' belief that adult attachment represents more than the individual's early experiences. It allows for the influence of a variety of close relationships in the individual's life in addition to those associated with early care-giving.

This interview, for which intensive training is required, has been used in a variety of studies to assess parents' working models in clinical and non-clinical populations and been useful in exploring how parenting styles and attachment patterns may be linked with those of the next generation. What is important is to consider how such a mechanism might work and particularly how aberrant parenting, such as that involving abuse and neglect, may be transmitted across generations. The next section will examine some research relating to these questions.

INTERGENERATIONAL LINKS

In today's Western society of working couples and isolated nuclear families, many new parents approach the complex task of parenting with little experience. Some aspects of parenting skills are acquired by trial and error 'on the job', however, parenting style and the degree of responsiveness are also powerfully influenced by factors that present long before the infant's birth. A number of family research teams have concluded that fathers' and mothers' psychological adaptation and the relationship between them before the birth of the first child predicts the quality of parenting during the early years (Belsky et al 1985, Lewis & Feiring 1989). Another body of attachment research emphasizes that the parents' role in parent–child interaction reflects relationship patterns that have developed from, and been influenced by, a wide variety of experiences and insights learned within intimate relationships over time (Colin 1996; Kaufman & Ziegler 1987) (Figure 2.1).

Many studies have focused on the transmission of parenting attitudes, models and behaviours across generations. The earlier research developed out of the child maltreatment literature in which the tendency for individuals who were abused as children to have a higher likelihood of abusing their own children has been described (Belsky & Pensky 1988, Herrenkohl & Herrenkohl 1983,

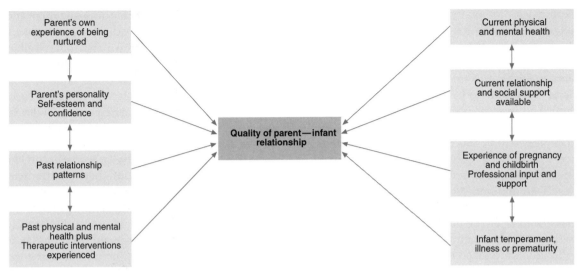

Figure 2.1 Some pathways influencing attachment

Kaufman & Ziegler 1987, Ney 1988, Zeanah & Zeanah 1989). The intergenerational association of parenting behaviours is not restricted to those who maltreat their children. Caspi and Elder (1988) concluded that parental characteristics and experiences are related to parenting style and child behaviour. They found that unstable, irritable, conflicted parents who experienced marital discord are more likely to produce irritable, explosive children. If, however, parents were able to transcend their own marital problems enough to provide positive parenting, children showed little negative behaviour. The presence of a positive sibling relationship has also been found to be protective where marital relationships are antagonistic (Jenkins & Smith 1990).

In relation to the theory of adult attachment, it is thought that parenting behaviour and sensitivity has its roots in parents' own experience of being parented. This early experience leads to internal representational models that influence the degree and manner of responsiveness they will be able to show their children (Bowlby 1988, Main et al 1985). Parents who were raised with sensitivity as infants are more likely to be open and responsive to their infant's needs than abused, rejected or insensitively reared parents (Colin 1996). More recent work suggests, however, that these early models may also be modified during or after childhood through prolonged experience with another attachment figure or a supportive

partner, or within a therapeutic relationship (Colin 1996, Egeland et al 1988, Fonagy et al 1994, Werner 1989).

This section describes a number of studies that have contributed to our understanding of both transgenerational cycles of parenting and those factors that may interrupt the transmission of negative or insecure internal representational models across generations. The AAI (Main & Goldwyn 1984) is commonly used in many of these studies. The adult attachment paradigm presents a unique way of looking at the intergenerational links and associations. Rather than supposing that a parent's own childhood experience functions as a model and translates literally into a childrearing style, the theoretical approach is based upon the belief that it is the *currently held* internal representation, and therefore the current interpretation of the past, that affects the quality of parenting. The previously held more simplistic assumption that insensitively raised, abused or neglected parents automatically repeat the experience with their own children is, within this paradigm, replaced by a more dynamic interpretation in which change through insight, external factors and significant other relationships can facilitate a conscious reworking and alteration of early experience.

The AAI assesses the adult's 'state of mind' with respect to attachment relationships, rather than directly focusing on the individual's past experience. Although this instrument requires extensive training for the actual classification of the participants, the concepts and approach taken in the interview may be useful for health professionals wishing to understand individuals' reactions to parenthood. For this reason, it will be described in some detail.

AAI participants are asked a series of questions and probes designed to elicit as full a history as possible of their childhood attachment experiences. The manner in which these experiences are described and understood, rather than the nature of the experiences themselves, leads to an overall classification of the adult's *current* state of mind with respect to attachment. During the interview, individuals are asked to describe childhood experiences with their own parents and how they feel the experiences affected their adult personality and their current behaviour with their children. On the basis of the experiences described, and the ways in which the participant reflects on them and derives meaning, the adult is classified into one of the three groups – secure/autonomous, insecure/dismissing and insecure/preoccupied – that most accurately characterizes his or her state of mind regarding attachment relationships (Main & Goldwyn 1984).

A significant association has been demonstrated between the mother's classification in the AAI and the observed behaviours of her infant in Ainsworth et al's (1978) Strange Situation. Main et al (1985) demonstrated that mothers of securely attached children, in describing their childhood experiences, share the common characteristic of having achieved some integration between current feeling and past experiences relevant to attachment, unlike the parents of insecurely attached children. Securely attached mothers are more objective and show balance in their evaluation of childhood experiences in much the same way that securely attached children steer a middle course between attachment behaviours and autonomous exploration in the Strange Situation. The mother's insight in relation to her experience is thought to leave her free to respond sensitively to her child's needs instead of being entangled in her own. Dismissing (insecure) adults on the other hand share in common a history of some rejection and an organization of thought that permits attachment to be relatively deactivated or avoided through

self-deception (leading to high idealization and poor recall), grandiosity (leading to a derogatory attitude) or denial (leading to a view of the self as unaffected by adverse experiences). They are cut off from attachments in much the same way as insecurely attached infants ignore caregiver cues.

Van Ijzendoorn (1992) carried out a review of the literature related to the intergenerational transmission of parenting in non-clinical populations. Reviewing four studies using the AAI, he reported a strong concordance between the parent's view of his or her attachment biography and his or her attachment relationship to the infant. An example is found in Main et al's (1985) study of 40 mothers and their 6-year-old children. These children had been assessed as infants using the Strange Situation at 12 and 18 months of age. At the six year follow-up, the parents completed the AAI. The correspondence between the mother's state of mind with respect to attachment and her infant's attachment classification from the Strange Situation procedure 5 years earlier was 75%. Similarly, in their European study, Grossman and Fremer-Bombik (1988) found an 88% agreement between the parent's AAI classification and her behaviour toward the infant as well as the infant's patterns of attachment to her using the Strange Situation procedure. The authors concluded that it was not just the mother's experience as a child that was important, but also the parent's conscious awareness and insight into her own experience of being parented. Mothers who had received inadequate parenting but as an adult had a clear image of how they were treated by their parent, and were able to discuss its impact, were able to relate to their infants in a sensitive way that promoted attachment security. They concluded that:

> . . . a mother who remembers well how she felt when something bad happened to her and how her parents responded to comfort her, will listen empathically to her infant's distress signals. A mother who cannot remember much of her childhood distress, or remembers only in a distorted form, seems less able to listen openly and feel sympathetic with her infant. She may push aside memories of her own distress by ignoring her infant's distress.
>
> Grossman & Fremer-Bombik 1988, p. 255

In carrying out research on 'problematic populations', Ainsworth and Eichberg (1991) found a high level of agreement between mother and infant classification when studying infants and their mothers who had experienced loss and were in the process of mourning. A number of other, often small scale studies, are of value in understanding some of the factors involved in the transmission of aberrant parenting behaviours. De Lozier (1982) assessed adult attachment using a questionnaire rather than an interview, in addition to a separation anxiety test. Her sample consisted of 18 mothers who were known to have abused their children, and 18 matched controls. In comparing the participants' childhood experiences, she found significant differences between the groups. Abusive mothers were found to have experienced a greater incidence of threat of separation or withdrawal of care-giving during childhood than were the controls. Such threats included ones of abandonment, harsh punishment and being sent away. There was also the perception by the maltreating mothers that they, as children, were expected to care for their caregivers. In adulthood, these women saw significant others as being essentially unavailable. The quality of support around the birth of the maltreated child was also a distinguishing factor. The abusing mothers reported feeling fearful, alone, unsafe and dissatisfied with the availability and support of significant others.

The Minnesota longitudinal study (Egeland et al 1988; Weinfield et al 2000) also provides useful insights into the transmission of maltreatment as well as the factors related to its repetition or interruption. Of the 267 high-risk families involved in this research, 47 of the mothers were classified as having been abused as children. During the first 5 years of the study, 18 (38%) of these mothers were found to maltreat their own children. Twelve (25%) were reported as giving clearly adequate care to their children. The remaining 17 could not be definitively classified into either category. The research team examined the factors differentiating the two 'classifiable' groups. The results of the analyses showed that mothers who broke the abusive cycle were more likely to have received emotional support from a non-abusive parent or other close adult during childhood, participated in individual or group therapy for at least a year,

and had a stable emotionally supportive relationship with a partner.

In another study by Ney (1988) 154 families were followed, 21% of which were known to have abused their children, in order to try and identify those factors which could distinguish abusive from non-abusive parents. He found that women who suffered domestic violence from their partners were more likely to abuse their children. He also found a relationship between mothers who as children were physically or sexually abused and those who verbally abused their own children.

In summary, the research described shows that parenting, like any important relationship, is influenced by a myriad of factors, many of which are present long before conception. The mother's relationship history is of particular importance in influencing the sensitivity and ease with which she nurtures her infant. This relationship history includes her own experience of being parented, her relationship with other important adults in her life and her adult relationship history. Of special relevance is her ongoing relationship with her partner. The adult attachment paradigm stresses that the level of insight that a parent has into his or her own experience of being parented must be assessed in attempting to anticipate the quality of parenting he or she will provide to their infant. Given the key role of insight in modifying parenting patterns, it is not surprising that a parent's participation in therapy is influential in determining his or her ability to interrupt the cycle of insensitive or hurtful parenting.

INFANT FACTORS AND ATTACHMENT SECURITY

Infants are active participants in the initiation and development of their relationships. In examining the development of attachment and the nature of early parent–infant relationships it is critical to consider not only what the parent contributes, but also what the infant brings to the situation. Babies differ in many respects and individual differences can play a substantial part in affecting how new parents respond and cope. One of the ways in which newborn and infants differ is in temperament, often thought of as the precursor of later child and adult personality (Buss 1995, Prior 1992).

A newborn infant is a product of his or her genes as well as nine months in experience and development in the intrauterine environment.

Some babies are easy to respond to in a positive way: they are strong, healthy, cuddly, clear in their demands and easy to comfort and settle. Parents can react to these infants with sensitivity and consequently feel competent as a parent. Many otherwise healthy, full-term babies may be experienced as difficult to nurture and parent, either because of their low level of adaptability or relative lack of cuddliness, or because of an unusual level of hypersensitivity to stimuli. These infants require a greater level of parental skill, creativity and commitment in order for them to settle and feel consistently nurtured and contained. Because of their unique nature or physiology, hypersensitive babies may send confusing signals of rejection to their parents. Without support, parents may feel inadequate and discouraged in the task of parenting these infants. A number of clinicians and theorists have examined the impact of and continuity in infant temperament and its relationship to the child's developmental trajectory (Kagan 1997, Prior 1992, Thomas & Chess 1997). The work most directly useful to health professionals working with healthy and sick newborns and their families, is that of Brazelton and colleagues (Brazelton 1979, 1981, 1984, Brazelton & Nugent 1995).

The Neonatal Behavioural Assessment Scale (NBAS), first published in 1973 aimed to help both professionals and parents to gain a better understanding of newborn behaviour. The emphasis was and continues to be on identifying individual differences and variations in the newborn's behavioural responses to the environment in which he finds himself. The stimuli used to assess the baby are largely the same ones that parents use in interacting with their infant. During the assessment, the baby is evaluated while being held, talked to, touched, rocked and cuddled (midwives and other health professionals can now be trained with the UK Brazelton Centre: www.brazelton.co.uk). The newborn's responsiveness to a range of stimuli, as well as irritability and 'soothability', is assessed and scored. A profile of the infant, as well as ways of supporting, soothing and containing him or her, results from the information collected in the course of each assessment. Several sequential NBAS assessments, even of normal full-term infants, are advised where possible, as points of similarity and difference can show, for example, an infant's recovery from a difficult labour and delivery, the effect of analgesics given to his or her mother in labour, or improvements in alertness as jaundice levels decline. Babies who may have been born preterm, growth-retarded or with medical problems are also likely to behave differently at this time and to present novice and experienced parents with a range of challenges as a consequence of these differences (Brazelton & Nugent 1995, Meier et al 2004).

Some researchers had hoped to find links and continuities between early indices of an infant's temperament in the responses to items on the NBAS and later infant and child behaviour. However, cumulative data mostly show only weak relationships between NBAS scores and later behaviour (Brazelton & Cramer 1990). This is not surprising given the multiplicity of factors at work that may influence newborn behaviour (some of which were mentioned above), but which are probably not directly related to temperamental trait differences between individuals (Buss 1995).

The NBAS has been used in clinical and research contexts as a way of exploring the newborn's early capability for interaction with a caregiver (Brazelton & Nugent 1995, Gutbrod 2004, Meier et al 2004). The infants' behaviour and responses to the handling that occurs in using the scale can help parents understand the unique and sometimes unexpected needs and responses of their infant. The assessment facilitates a discussion of their baby's strengths and difficulties and utilizes parents' own observations. Not only is it important for them to learn about how to meet the needs of their baby, but this kind of assessment, carried out in a standard way also helps them understand infant behaviour without misinterpretation. For example, it is easy for parents to interpret the behaviour of a stiff, non-cuddly baby who is easily upset and hard to settle as being rejecting or critical of them as parents. If parents are not able to respond and cope with the individual differences and needs of a temperamentally difficult baby, it is likely to be more difficult to build a positive relationship and to feel competent in their role. Infants may experience parental confusion as non-support and insensitivity and it is possible that insecure attachments may result.

Some developmental psychologists have questioned the relationship between infant temperament, parental sensitivity and later attachment behaviour (Belsky & Rovine 1988, Kagan 1982). They hypothesized that attachment security was influenced by the infant's innate temperamental characteristics rather than the caregiver's level of sensitivity or responsiveness. A variety of research has, however, demonstrated that attachment security tends to show greater stability than does infant temperamental classification (Colin 1996). In her research, Colin found that even characteristics such as cuddliness and adaptability were to some extent dependent upon, and varied according to which parent or caregiver was handling or interacting with the baby.

In a meta-analysis based on a variety of studies that compared the impact of infant temperament and maternal sensitivity on determining infant attachment patterns, Goldsmith and Alansky (1987) concluded that it was the mother's sensitive responsiveness rather than infant measures that predicted attachment security. Van Ijzendoorn (1992) came to similar conclusions in another meta-analysis of more than thirty clinical studies. He concluded that when maternal problems (such as a history of abuse, mental illness or poor social support) were present in a study group, there was an increase in insecure attachment in the infant. In contrast, there were few demonstrated effects of a child-related factor (e.g. prematurity, developmental disability or illness) on the attachment distribution. He summarized:

> Our data suggest that if mothers suffer from mental illness or engage in disturbed caregiving behaviour (e.g. maltreatment) their children cannot compensate for the resulting lack of maternal responsiveness and are vulnerable to insecure forms of attachment. However when children are impaired (physically or mentally in various degrees) their mothers are generally capable of compensating for this potential handicap in the dyadic relationship.
>
> Van Ijzendoorn 1992, p. 90

However, other researchers have emphasized the role of contextual factors such as those related to stress and social support as also having an impact on the way that parents are able to respond to their infants. For example, Crockenberg (1981) used the NBAS to study 46 mother–infant pairs. The infants were assessed for irritability on the fifth and tenth days of life. A 4-hour home visit was made when the babies were 3 months old, when the mother was assessed for maternal responsiveness. During the same visit, mothers were interviewed in relation to their sources of support and the levels of stress in their life. The babies were later assessed for attachment security at 12 months of life. High infant irritability, as measured by the NBAS, was only associated with an increased incidence of insecure attachment when the mother also experienced poor social support and high stress. The authors concluded that when the infants were relatively undemanding and easy to comfort, the mother could provide responsive care even in the absence of good social support. If the baby was difficult, emotional and material support from others could make a critical difference in the mother's ability to provide responsive care (van den Boom & Hoeksma 1994). Vaughn et al (1992) concluded that attachment and temperament could be more usefully conceptualized as overlapping domains because child behaviour and affect regulation occur and are inevitably measured in a social context. In her review Colin (1996) concludes that the emerging consensus is as follows:

> Infants differ from each other at birth and in the early weeks because of genetic and prenatal factors. Differences such as irritability, sociability, fearfulness, proneness-to-distress, and being 'easy' or 'difficult' may certainly affect the tone of parent–infant interactions. Such differences are subject to change with maturation and social experience and are unlikely in themselves to determine the security of the infant's emerging attachment. However, in interaction with other factors, such as the parent's responsiveness and the social support available to the parent, congenital differences in temperament may influence attachment.
>
> Colin 1996, p. 114

The 'goodness of fit' between a baby or young child and his environment is critical. Individual and contextual factors interact. As Horowitz (1987, 1990) argues, a resilient child may do well in a poor environment and take full advantage of the opportunities available, whereas a child with more vulnerabilities will not do so well. In a similar way an irritable or difficult newborn or young baby who is cared for in a facilitative, stimulating and accepting environment is likely to have a better outcome than one reared in an environment that is poorer in practical and social terms (Belsky 1984, Mangelsdorf et al 1990, Thomas & Chess 1977).

In focusing on the vulnerabilities and protective factors present in an individual newborn the assessment of a newborn's characteristics, for example, adaptability, soothability and response to social and more aversive stimuli, could be an important part of postpartum care in addition to responding to a mother's history and details of the pregnancy and birth. It would allow the midwife, and in some instances the health visitor, to focus on the salient issues of the moment for parents, particularly those of the mother and to individualize the teaching of infant care to the needs of specific mothers and babies. This may be particularly helpful in relation to feeding and the associated problems that some mothers and babies experience. If, in the course of an assessment, a baby is found to be difficult in a number of respects, in addition to vulnerabilities resulting from the mother's history, environment and psychological resources, additional support, advice and contacts may be needed.

THERAPEUTIC INTERVENTIONS

A variety of therapeutic intervention programmes have aimed to address the issue of the link between insecure parent–infant attachment and an increased risk of malfunctioning in the emotional–social domain in the longer term. The majority of these programmes have been aimed at either enhancing parental sensitivity to infant cues or supporting maternal representational models. Some of the studies relevant to midwives will be reviewed below.

Two categories of research have addressed this issue: the first being more behavioural, and the second aimed at the mother's internal representa-

tional models of attachment. The first type of study reviewed will be of those attempting to influence parental sensitivity to infant cues. These are based on previously described hypotheses that parental responsiveness and sensitivity are key factors in the development of secure attachment in the infant (Ainsworth et al 1978). Ainsfeld et al (1990) designed a behavioural approach. They hypothesized that a mother's sensitivity to her infant would be enhanced quite easily by increased physical contact with her infant. They assumed that greater sensitivity would lead to secure attachment. They divided 49 mothers of low socioeconomic status between an experimental and a control group. Upon discharge from hospital, mothers in the experimental group were given soft infant carriers and encouraged to use them daily with their infants. Those in the control group were given plastic infant seats. At 3.5 months, the mothers and infants were visited in their home, and the mothers were rated on their sensitivity of response to their infants. Additionally, the Strange Situation procedure was used at 13 months to assess the quality of infant–mother attachment. Although slightly equivocal results were obtained in relation to sensitivity, the difference in infant attachment was marked between the groups. In the experimental group (using the soft infant carriers), 83% of the infants appeared to be securely attached, whereas only 38% of the control group were secure. The authors concluded that the infant's experience of being carried close to the mother seemed to have affected the infant's attachment security to a degree far beyond that attributable to increased maternal sensitivity.

A small-scale preventive intervention study was designed by Lyons-Ruth et al (1990) to determine whether a year of a trustworthy, accepting, professional relationship during the infant's first year of life could counteract the impact of poverty, maternal depression and an inadequate caregiving history. The intervention group of 10 high-risk families received weekly home visits designed to support the mother and provide modelling and reinforcement of developmentally appropriate exchanges between mother and infant. A secondary goal was to decrease social isolation. At 18 months of age, scores of maternal sensitivity, covert hostility and flatness of affect in the mothers, and from the Strange Situation procedure in the infants, were compared with those of a matched control group. Although the study found no significant effects of treatment on maternal sensitivity, again there was a marked difference in attachment security of the infants.

Van Ijzendoorn et al (1995) reviewed a number of studies from the Netherlands. One by van den Boom (1994) is of particular interest to this review. One hundred highly irritable infants from lower-class families were selected for the evaluation of a short-term intervention for enhancing maternal sensitivity to difficult infants. Interveners visited the control mothers three times at home between the infant's sixth and ninth month of life. The intervener assisted the mothers in adjusting to the infants' unique cues, particularly negative signals such as crying. The mothers were rated on maternal sensitivity pre- and post-test using a number of instruments. The quality of the infant–mother attachment was also evaluated at 12 months of age using the Strange Situation procedure. Mothers who received coaching were found to be significantly more responsive to their infants on the post-test than were the control mothers. In addition, 68% of the experimental group infants were found to be securely attached at 12 months compared with only 28% of the control group.

Van Ijzendoorn et al (1995) also conducted a meta-analysis of 12 different intervention studies designed to influence both maternal sensitivity and the security of infant attachment. The analysis involved a total of 900 mother–infant dyads using a variety of modes of intervention. Overall, the authors concluded that the families profited by the intervention, the greatest impact being in the form of increased maternal sensitivity to the infants' needs and cues. A highly significant combined effect size for maternal sensitivity was reported, though the combined effect size for infant attachment was not significant. The authors attribute the discrepancy in the combined effect sizes to the immediacy of the intervention impact. They hypothesize that the interventions for enhancing maternal sensitivity are inevitably more successful as the goal is more proximal and more easily achieved. The impact on infant security is, however, more complex and may require more time to measure change.

Other more recent and ongoing intervention studies in the UK (Cooper et al 2003, Murray et al

2003) have focused on using therapeutic and clinically based methods to try and intervene in relation to postnatal depression, in attempting to improve maternal sensitivity and the psychosocial environment for the infant and young child. A review of randomized trials by Lumley et al (2004) also focuses on interventions aimed at reducing postnatal depression (PND). Although there is particular concern about PND, there is wider concern about the quality of parenting infants receive and providing support for the developing parent–infant relationship, especially in groups considered to be at risk in some way. In a recent Sure Start project, Svanberg (2004) and health visitor colleagues, in a controlled study using video-recordings of mother–infant interactions and support from psychologists, have focused on increasing parental sensitivity and responsiveness and have so far shown effects on parent and infant behaviour, as well as parental wellbeing in the intervention group.

ASSESSMENT AND INTERVENTION DURING THE PERINATAL PERIOD

So far in this chapter, we have reviewed attachment-related theory and research with the purpose of establishing a conceptual and research base from which to examine the midwife's role in informal screening, promotion and possible intervention in the early parent–infant relationship. The research to date has made a credible link between:

- a mother's attachment security and that of her infant;
- the quality of the early parent–infant relationship and the later security of the infant's attachment to the mother;
- insecure attachment in the infant and suboptimal developmental and relational patterns in the child.

The literature also suggests focal points and time periods for assessment and potential intervention. This section will begin by discussing the factors shown to influence the quality and sensitivity with which a mother relates to her infant. Particular emphasis will be placed upon observations and information that could be gained in the course of the midwife's interaction with the mother.

ASSESSMENT IN THE PRENATAL PERIOD

The assessment of a mother's psychological well-being and her attitude to the pregnancy should begin early on. Midwives and other health professionals need to be alert to the symptoms or signs of maternal alcohol and substance abuse, domestic violence and postnatal depression (Department of Health 2004, 2005, National Institute for Clinical Excellence 2003) and for antenatal depression for which screening may become routine in the future (National Institute for Clinical Excellence 2004). It may also be possible for midwives to assess women's own experience of parenting. The aim would be to 'screen' for insecurely attached mothers who may be unable to meet their infants' needs with sensitivity and consistency as a result of their own negative experience of being parented. In addition, it would also be relevant to document the presence of environmental factors such as high levels of stress, social isolation and a lack of social support systems that could compound a mother's ability to respond to her infant's psychological and other needs. Boxes 2.1 and 2.2. summarize the historical and current risk factors and Box 2.3 lists the factors that are thought to have the potential to counteract the influence of early abuse or insensitive parenting on the mother's ability to respond with sensitivity to her infant. The literature indicates that the mother's own early care-giving experience can have a profound impact upon her ability to parent her child. Her early experience of being parented provides the foundation of her long-term relationship patterns. However, as Sroufe (1996) emphasizes, these patterns are not laid in stone. There are a variety of relational, cognitive and therapeutic experiences that can serve to modify a parent's attitudes, insight and internal representational models with respect to attachment experiences (Box 2.3). Understanding a woman's internal representational models, and therefore her insight into her relational history and patterns, is complex and likely to take time. Thus considering such issues relatively early in pregnancy is preferable.

Box 2.1 Checklist of mother's childhood 'historical' risk factors

Relationship history

- Physical, sexual or emotional abuse by the caregiver.
- Physical or emotional neglect.
- Death of parent or abandonment by parent or primary caregiver.
- Loss of parent through abandonment or apprehension.
- Frequent changes of primary caregivers (relatives, nannies, foster parents).
- Prevalent parental inconsistency or unavailability.
- Parental mental illness that prevented parent from nurturing.
- Parental alcoholism or drug abuse that interfered with availability or consistent care.

Box 2.2 Checklist of current risk factors

Past relationship factors

- Current memory distortions of childhood attachment.
- Inability to remember significant periods of childhood.
- General or global memory of parenting contradicts specific memories.
- Obsessed with childhood memories.
- No insight into impact of negative parenting on self. Unable to imagine parenting role with child or unable to imagine parenting differently. No goals for child's wellbeing.

Current relationship factors

- Abusive partner.
- Highly conflictual or unsupportive relationship with partner.
- Single parent with minimal support from family or friends.
- Other risk factors.
- Social isolation of mother or family.
- Significant environmental or economic stressors.
- Substance abuse by mother or partner.
- Psychiatric diagnosis in mother or partner that interferes with relationships.

Although the AAI (Main & Goldwyn 1984) is a tool that requires specific training and experience, the approach it embodies provides a format and philosophy that could be used for health professionals such as midwives in 'screening' for unresolved attachment problems and parenting issues. The goal of this type of assessment at this time would be to identify mothers who might need referral for counselling, therapy or for extra nurturance and support during pregnancy and the early postpartum period.

As the evidence discussed in previous sections suggests, when a woman's childhood experiences are ones of abuse, neglect or parental insensitivity and unavailability, and she does not have insight into their impact upon her, she may be at risk of repeating the same mistakes with her own child. If a mother is so preoccupied with her own treatment as a child that it is difficult to talk about her infant or gain insight into how she wants to parent differently, her infant may also be at risk. A preoccupied parent can be so wrapped up in her own needs that she may resent her infant for demanding her attention.

It may be possible for a midwife who regularly sees a pregnant woman to talk about the woman's experiences as a child and young person in the context of her upbringing and also current stressors or relationship patterns. Listening to what the woman has to say and how she reflects on these experiences may help to identify some of the key risk and moderating factors that present in her life

that may impact on the relationship to her new baby (see checklists in Box 2.1, 2.2, 2.3).

If a midwife begins working with a mother early in pregnancy, this professional relationship has the potential to provide, at least in part, a form of interaction that may help the mother and influence the sensitivity of care that she shows her infant. The year that a midwife spends with a set of parents, including both the prenatal and the postpartum period, has the potential to contribute to the development of more effective internal working models of a mother or couple. If, however, a mother has a difficult attachment history and many risk factors, without evidence of resolution or insight, it may be advisable to refer her for counselling or an appropriate form of therapy. Effective communication with the GP and health visitor caring for the woman and her baby will facilitate appropriate support and care after her baby is born.

Labour and delivery, as well as the immediate postpartum period, are a time during which the midwife can make a profound difference. Sensitive support and care of a mother and father during the perinatal period can lead to a greater responsiveness, willingness and ability to care for their infant. Allowing for peaceful, undisturbed time for parents and infants to get to know each other during the immediate postpartum period provides a unique opportunity for an optimal start to the parent–infant relationship. Assessing an infant's social behaviour, cuddliness, soothability and temperament takes additional skill and knowledge on the part of the midwife but very little additional time. With training, an experienced midwife can begin to identify those infants likely to be more difficult to parent, to nurse or to soothe, at least in the short-term (Brazelton & Nugent 1995). By being aware of how much what seems like a temperamentally difficult infant can influence the quality of parental comfort and commitment, the midwife can learn to give a higher priority to such mother–infant pairs. Much of the task of promoting parent–infant attachment is a matter of insight, and sensitivity on the part of the professional and the benefits for women and their families can be substantial.

Of course, a midwife cannot be expected to be all things to all parents and their infants. However, an awareness of the importance of the early parent–infant relationship for the long-term health of the individual and of society will enable her, in her interaction with the family, to be alert for those families and their babies who may need additional support and possibly intervention. This unique opportunity to potentially influence the long-term physical and emotional health of the individual is something that midwives caring for women and their families value enormously. The motivation resulting from feeling that you can make a difference at such a critical time is an important aspect of job satisfaction in this area of work. However, there are also training and professional development issues here: support mechanisms and arrangements for supervision of midwives need to be clear if they in turn are to be able to support women and their families with a wide range of experiences, at this time.

IMPLICATIONS FOR THE MIDWIFE

The need to change and further develop the roles of health professionals working with children, women and their families has been widely recognized. A review summarizing the evidence in relation to home visiting in the antenatal and postnatal periods by a range of professionals, including midwives was published by the Health Development Agency (Bull et al 2004) and the National Service Framework for Children, Young People and Maternity Services (Department of Health 2004) clearly envisages the role of the midwife as a multifaceted one in which the emotional, psychological and health needs of women and their babies, in the UK at least, will be addressed for as long as several months after the birth if necessary, depending on individual need.

THE RELATIONSHIP BETWEEN MIDWIVES, WOMEN AND FAMILIES

Midwives work with women at a critical point in the development of this most fundamental relationship, the initiation and growth of the love between the mother, the father and their child. Parents bring to pregnancy and the birth of their child the history of their own relationships, life circumstances and mind set. This history is the

most powerful determinant of the relationship trajectory between parents and child. Nevertheless, the actual pregnancy and birth of the baby is the birth of the family. The woman's care and her experience may have significant effects on her relationship with her baby. It is important for midwives to be aware of both the opportunity to support the growth of this relationship and the possibility of disturbing it. A positive and rewarding relationship at this stage is likely to be a foundation for the enduring commitment that helps parents to make the necessary efforts and adjustments to provide physical and emotional care, guidance and support until their child reaches independence. The commitment embodied in this early relationship and love and affection, becomes the root of a child's sense of self and a pattern by which his or her future relationships may be shaped.

The literature reviewed in this chapter makes clear the importance of secure attachments to the future survival and wellbeing of children and their development to become competent and happy adults. There are a number of important lessons for midwives. Understanding the processes involved in the development of secure and insecure attachments and the implications of these in terms of development and future relationships is key if midwives are to care for women appropriately and effectively. It is recognized that many of the patterns for parenting were laid down long before the mother became pregnant and before the midwife met the parents. Nevertheless, because of the dynamic nature of the development of maternal or paternal sensitivity, there are still opportunities for the midwife to influence the development of family relationships in a number of ways. These include nurturing and supporting the mother through the pregnancy and birth, 'screening' for families who have the potential for greater problems than others, assessing the behaviour of the newborn and working with parents on the basis of this assessment, and providing extra support for and referral of high-risk families.

DEVELOPING SENSITIVE SYSTEMS

However, utilizing this knowledge and the research evidence summarized above, requires appropriate organizations and cultures of care. Unfortunately, many systems of care work against such individual sensitivity and responsiveness. Most babies in the industrialized world are born in hospital. As Klaus and Kennell note:

> ... crucial life events surrounding the development of both attachment and detachment have been removed from the home and brought into the hospital over the past 60 years. The hospital now determines the procedures involved in birth and death. The experiences surrounding these two events in the life of an individual have been stripped of the long established traditions and support systems built up over centuries to help families through these highly meaningful transitions.
>
> Klaus & Kennell 1976, p. 2

It is all too easy, in busy hospital systems, to forget the significance of birth as a transition and to lose sight of the individuals who are in our care (see Chapter 3). Where care is fragmented between many different caregivers, there is no one professional who gets to know the woman and her family as individuals. Care is likely to become routine and the individual needs of women and their families be unknown or ignored.

Despite the heightened awareness of the importance of the development of attachment between mother, father and baby, problems that may disturb or distort the development of attachment persist in many hospitals. The physical environment, aspects of clinical care and the quality and type of information provided contribute to an experience that is not always positive. Antenatal clinics are not always well thought out in terms of processes and design; some provide very little privacy for discussing important issues and professionals do not always appreciate what is important to pregnant women. Labour and delivery rooms are often like intensive care units, engendering a high level of anxiety. Some women and their partners are left alone in labour (Garcia et al 1998) and then, after the birth, there is sometimes a rush to transfer the mother and baby to a postnatal ward, giving the new mother and father little chance to enjoy and get to know their baby in those first irreplaceable moments. In Britain particularly, there is an acknowledged and wide-spread problem in postnatal wards, where many mothers and babies spend the first two days of family life. New mothers have reported what amounts to a sense of neglect (Garcia et al 1998, McCourt & Page 1996) at a vulnerable time when they deserve to be, and would benefit from, being cherished.

Over recent decades, we have seen the beginning of two important changes that are directly or indirectly related to an awareness of the need to support the development of the early parent–child relationship and the process of attachment. These deserve further consideration because they may be the most important basis on which midwives will be able to alter the structure and approach of their practice, particularly within the hospital setting.

INTERVENTIONS TO SUPPORT EARLY PARENT–INFANT RELATIONSHIPS

The first of these changes is the increased awareness, which became apparent in the 1960s, that hospital routines may be interfering with and having negative effects on the experience of families and the early relationship with their baby. It was common during that time for the mother and baby to be separated, often for some days after birth (Klaus & Kennell 1976). Barrera and Rosenbaum (1992), in their overview of randomized controlled trials, describe the enormous popularity in the late 1960s of the concepts of 'bonding' and 'attachment'. Although these words are often used interchangeably, they are usually used to refer to slightly different concepts:

> Bonding has usually referred to the affectional tie between a mother and her infant believed to occur immediately after birth, perhaps to a sensitive or critical period. As such, bonding was conceived as a rapid, mainly unidirectional, process, facilitated by skin to skin contact.
>
> Klaus & Kennel 1976, p. 221

However, there is little or no evidence for a sensitive or critical period, as in the animal model, and the establishment of a mother or parent–child relationship is currently conceptualized as occurring over a much longer period of time and as being subject to considerable individual variation. Mode of delivery, maternal and infant health problems and the availability of appropriate facilities for care can mean that mothers and babies are not together or in contact in the period immediately after birth. On balance there is more evidence for recovery from more difficult beginnings associated with, for example, caesarean section delivery or preterm birth than of later negative effects, unless of course there are other factors at work, such as health problems for the mother or baby, a lack of social support, antenatal or previous periods of depression as listed in Box 2.2.

Nevertheless a range of studies have shown some benefits of early contact for mothers of full-term infants and those who have been born too soon or too small (Conde-Agudelo et al 2003, Feldman et al 1999, 2002), though further well-designed randomized controlled trials and other studies may help to tease out some of the direct and indirect effects of such early contact. Relationships begin early, both sides of the parent–infant partnership benefit from learning about each other and causal attribution in these circumstances is difficult. Care must also be taken in focusing on just the mother–infant dyad, for it can be argued that multiple attachments to more than one caregiver are now seen as the norm Schaffer (1996).

The overview of randomized controlled trials of interventions aiming to support parents and promote attachment describes the evaluation of a number of approaches. Much of the early work on 'bonding', stimulated by Klaus and Kennell, explored the broad question, 'Does early contact of mother with newborn infant enhance bonding, and lead to measurable changes in maternal attitude and behaviours?' (Barrera & Rosenbaum 1992, p. 222). These research studies looked at a range of early interventions:

- increased mother–newborn contact in the immediate postnatal period;
- extended early mother–infant contact;
- increased father–infant contact;
- educational and supportive interventions prior to hospital discharge;
- supportive interventions during the transition from hospital to home;
- centre-based and home-based parental support.

Many of the evaluations assumed a linear cause-and-effect process and did not take into account the dynamic nature of the process, which is multifactorial. Many were restricted to the hospital, although some extended to the community. While recognizing the limitations of the research reviewed, in terms of methods, small sample size and different outcome measures, Barrera and Rosenbaum (1992) value the increasing recognition that multiple factors contribute to the development, continuity, nature and strength of later attachment between parent and child. This is certainly reflected in the studies described earlier in this chapter and in those currently being carried out and is an important consideration for midwives in their thinking and their practice. In aiming to support parents, it is necessary to take this complexity into account.

Of great importance is the issue of consistency among studies regarding the positive effect of supportive intervention on socio-economically disadvantaged families or less experienced parents. Where there is a question of the equitable use of resources, midwives would do well to offer extra support to parents in these groups. Barrera and Rosenbaum comment that:

> . . . despite the multitude of studies on maternal 'bonding' and 'attachment', and intervention studies to promote development and to support families, there is a paucity of intervention literature describing the actual promotion of attachment between mother/father and child.
>
> Barrera & Rosenbaum 1992, p. 241

In moving into our general vocabulary, 'bonding' has been understood by some to be an instantaneous event with the implication that if the chance of bonding at birth is lost, it will not be regained. Though the research evidence is lacking, there has been concern expressed about the guilt feelings aroused in mothers if they do not relate instantly to their baby (Littlewood & McHugh 1997). Inevitably perhaps, because of the hospital context in which parents and babies first get to know each other, 'bonding' and the provision of 'bonding time' have become another procedure for the mother to follow and the midwife to observe. Such an approach denies its complexity, the diversity of factors that affect it and the lengthy nature of the subsequent development of attachment between parents and child. Of course, as Niven recommends (in Littlewood & McHugh 1997), the woman's contact with her baby should be determined by her needs. A mother exhausted by a long and difficult labour may well not want to look at, let alone hold, her baby for a while. But while we ensure that procedures for supporting this early relationship are not imposed on the mother and baby against the mother's needs, we make sure that the experience of receiving the baby directly into her arms and against her heart is not denied to those many women who want it. The enlarging time frame for midwives in the UK to support and intervene right across the perinatal period and during the early months provides even greater opportunities for their input and for multi-disciplinary working with families to support parent–child relationships (Department of Health 2004).

DEVELOPING SUPPORTIVE, WOMAN-CENTRED CARE

The second change we have witnessed over the past twenty years is a more general change to systems of care that will provide more individually sensitive and supportive care. These alternative systems have included the provision of a known and named midwife to care for individual women and their families throughout the system of care (continuity of carer), and birthing centres. Although the goals of such schemes have not always been explicitly or solely concentrated on support for establishing a enjoyable relationship between parents and baby, they have included a number of aspects that are likely to contribute positively. For example, some schemes include an element of extra social support by midwives, visits to the woman and family in their home, a community presence and a known and trusted midwife for care during labour and birth (McCourt & Page 1996).

Some of the evaluations have included indicators of positive responses of the mother to her experience of care, as well as to pregnancy and birth, and to her baby. These indicators are in part related to the nature of the relationship, at an early stage, between the mother and her baby. For example, one study undertaken in London evaluated an innovation in which the key component was the provision of a One-to-One named midwife who cared for individual women through the whole of pregnancy, labour and birth and the early weeks of the life of the baby (see Chapter 7). This evaluation of women's experience of the new form of care consisted of a controlled study with women ($N = 728$) in the intervention group who received the new service and women in the control group, who received conventional care ($N = 675$).

The new service was set up in a neighbourhood that was the most deprived area served by the local maternity service (Page et al 1999, 2001). More women in the study group were in low social and occupational classes and were living in rented rather than privately owned accommodation. They were less likely to have the support of a partner and less likely to be white and English speaking. However, a clinical audit revealed no significant differences between the groups in terms of parity or risk status. The study used a wide range of methods, including quantitative and qualitative, to ensure participation by a wide cross-section of women.

Questionnaires included standard measures to assess any possible impact on women's psychological wellbeing and feelings of confidence and preparedness for giving birth and caring for the baby. Intervention group women were more likely to feel 'very well prepared for the birth' (18%) than control group women (12%). Feelings of preparedness for the birth were matched by feelings of confidence and preparedness for motherhood. They were also more likely to be very confident (51%) than control group women (39%) even though they were less likely to have a planned pregnancy.

Such systems of care are likely to allow more sensitive and personal assessments than would be possible in one-off visits in a hospital setting. Earlier, it was proposed that the assessment of a mother's 'state of mind' in relation to attachment should begin early in pregnancy. It was also suggested that if a midwife begins working with a mother early in pregnancy, the quality of this professional relationship has the potential of providing, at least in part, an alternative model of nurturing that the mother may be able to internalize to influence the sensitivity of care that she shows her infant.

It is difficult to imagine how this kind of proposal can be implemented if care is fragmented. Getting to know the woman over time, making visits in her own home and developing a relationship of trust are a pre-requisite to this approach. However, although such alternative systems of care may be necessary for screening for and assessing factors that are likely to support the relationship between parents and baby, they may not be sufficient in themselves. Midwives practising in such new systems may well have come from settings that do not recognize the importance of issues such as the quality of parent–child relationships and attachment. They may need further education to develop a theoretical basis and the degree of personal sensitivity and wisdom to undertake the assessment, interpret the findings and provide support.

Many midwives who continue to practise in more conventional settings in which fragmented care is the norm will find that the extent of their ability to assess and support developing parent–infant relationships is limited. Nevertheless, they will find opportunities to make some assessments and supportive interventions. Importantly, an awareness of the importance and power of a secure attachment, and the negative effect of an insecure attachment, is necessary to midwives whatever their style of practice or working environment. Such an awareness should, given the possibility of facilitating the development of these important relationships, remind them to act with respect in all of their contacts with mothers, fathers and babies.

CONCLUSION

This chapter provides an extensive review of the literature that acts as a theoretical basis for understanding the growth of love and the development of attachment between parents and their baby. The nature of understanding over years of painstaking research has evolved to show that the development of attachment is complex and interactional.

Cycles of abuse and neglect have been acknowledged over recent years. However, the recently discovered indication that the lack of a secure attachment in itself may be associated with more negative relationship patterns over many years, and also with victimization and aggression may have important and profound consequences not only for individuals, but also for society at large.

Although the early experiences of the parents in their own primary relationships are the most powerful predictor of the quality of their maternal and paternal sensitivity and relationship with their own children, it is now known that other factors may ameliorate earlier negative influences. This is an important piece of information for midwives, who may otherwise believe that there is little they can do to support parents in getting to know their baby and establishing this first relationship.

A number of specific approaches to the assessment of families and to supporting the early relationship and contact between parents and babies have been proposed for midwives to integrate into their practice. Some may be reluctant to become involved in such approaches, being fearful of interfering in the private domain of family relationships and of labelling parents from an early stage, yet the importance of supporting parent–child relationships and laying down a secure attachment should make such an approach as important as is the assessment of parents with high-risk pregnancies, for example. It should be remembered that this is a unique opportunity, and may be the only opportunity, to identify parents who may need extra support.

Many midwives practise in institutions that are dominated by technology, strict medical protocols, routines and a lack of time to do those things which matter in a human sense. It may be difficult in such situations to remember that the way in which we treat women and their partners, and their babies when they are born, may have profound and long-lasting consequences. However, the power of the first relationship between the parents and their baby, the growing attachment and the need for enduring commitment for survival and wellbeing, are fundamental to the birth of the family.

The midwife may, through the sensitivity of her care particularly, influence the mother, and perhaps also the father, aiding the development of the parental responsiveness and sensitivity that is fundamental to the future of the baby.

POINTERS FOR PRACTICE

- 'Screening' to identify families who may need extra support or referral includes the assessment of a number of factors, including the history of the parents' own experience, moderating factors in a high-risk history, present life circumstances, the newborn's behaviour and specific clinical and experiential aspects of the pregnancy and birth.
- In her provision of sensitive care and working with the mother from early in pregnancy, the midwife may, through the quality of this relationship, provide a model of care that the mother may internalize to influence the sensitivity of care she shows her infant.
- It is important to remember that the nature and behaviour of the baby will be a factor in the development of attachment. The use of a newborn behavioural assessment scale and its interpretation to the parents may help them to appreciate their baby's strengths and to prevent the parents feeling rejected by their baby.
- It is important to bear in mind the effect of depression in the postnatal period on the mother's ability to respond to the needs of her new baby, and if she has them, other children too.

References

Ainsfield E, Casper V, Nozyce M, Cunningham N 1990 Does infant carrying promote attachment: an experimental study of the effects of increased physical contact on the development of attachment. Child Development 61: 1617–1627

Ainsworth M D 1967 Infancy in Uganda. Johns Hopkins Press, Baltimore

Ainsworth M D 1973 The development of infant–mother attachment. In: Caldwell B M, Ricciuti N (eds) Review of child development research, vol. 3. University of Chicago Press, Chicago

Ainsworth M D, Blehar M C, Water E, Wall S 1978 Patterns of attachment: a psychological study of the strange situation. Lawrence Erlbaum, Hillsdale, NJ

Ainsworth M D, Eichberg C 1991 Effects on infant–mother attachment of mother's unresolved loss of an attachment figure. In: Parkes C M, Stevenson-Hinde J, Marris P (eds) Attachment across the life cycle. Routledge, London

Apfel N, Seitz V 1997 The firstborn sons of African American teenage mothers: perspectives on risk and resilience. In: Luthar S, Burack J, Cicchetti D, Weisz J (eds) Developmental psychopathology: perspectives on adjustment, risk and disorder. CUP, Cambridge

Asher S, Coie J 1990 Peer rejection in childhood. CUP, New York

Barrera M E, Rosenbaum P L 1992 Supporting parents and promoting attachment. In: Sinclair J C, Bracken M B (eds) Effective care of the newborn infant. Oxford University Press, Oxford

Belsky J 1984 The determinants of parenting: a process model. Child Development 55: 83–96

Belsky J 2001 Developmental risks (Still) associated with early child care. Journal of Child Psychology and Psychiatry 42: 845–859

Belsky J, Lang M, Rovine M 1985 Stability and change in marriage across the transition to parenthood: a second study. Journal of Marriage and the Family 47: 855–865

Belsky J, Pensky E 1988 Developmental history personality and family relationships: toward an emergent family system. In: Hinde R A, Stevenson-Hinde J (eds) Relationships within families: mutual influences. Oxford University Press, New York

Belsky J, Rovine M J 1988 Nonmaternal care in the first year of life and security of infant–parent attachment. Child Development 59: 157–167

Bowlby J 1969 Attachment and loss, vol. 1. Basic Books, New York

Bowlby J 1973 Attachment and loss, vol. II. Basic Books, New York

Bowlby J 1980 Attachment and loss, vol. III. Basic Books, New York

Bowlby J 1988 A secure base. Basic Books, New York

Bowlby J 1991 Ethological light on the psychoanalytical problems. In: Bateson P (ed.) Development and integration of behaviour. Cambridge University Press, Cambridge

Brazelton T B 1973 Neonatal behavioral assessment scale. Clinics in Developmental Medicine No. 50 Spastics International Medical Publications, London

Brazelton T B 1979 Behavioural competence of the newborn infant. Seminars in Perinatology 3: 35–44

Brazelton T B 1981 On becoming a family. Delacorte, New York

Brazelton T B 1984 Neonatal behavioural assessment scale. Lippincott, Philadelphia

Brazelton T B, Cramer B C 1990 The earliest relationship: parents, infants and the drama of early attachment. Addison-Wesley, Reading, MA

Brazelton T B, Yogman M W 1986 Affective development in infancy. Ablex, New Jersey

Brazelton T B, Nugent J K 1995 Neonatal behavioral assessment scale. 3rd edn. Mackeith, London

Bretherton I 1985 Attachment theory: retrospect and prospect. Monographs of the Society for Research in Child Development 50 (1–2, No. 209)

Bull J, McCormick G, Swann C, Mulvihill C 2004 Ante- and post-natal home visiting programmes: a review of reviews, evidence briefing. Health Development Agency. Online. Available: www.hda.nhs.uk/evidence

Buss A 1995 Personality: temperament, social behaviours and the self. Allyn and Bacon, Boston

Caspi A, Elder G H 1988 Emergent family patterns: the intergenerational construction of problem behaviour and relationships. In: Hinde R, Stevenson-Hinde J (eds) Relationships within families: mutual influences. Clarendon Press, Oxford

Colin V L 1996 Human attachment. Temple University Press, Philadelphia

Conde-Agudelo A, Diaz-Rossello J, Belizan J 2003 Kangaroo mother care to reduce mortality and morbidity in low birthweight infants. Cochrane Database Systematic Review Update (2) CD002771

Condon J T 1993 The assessment of antenatal emotional attachment. British Journal of Medical Psychology 66: 167–183

Connell D B 1976 Individual difference in attachment: an investigation into stability, implications and relationships to structure in early language development. Unpublished doctoral dissertation, Syracuse University, Syracuse

Cooper P J, Murray L, Wilson A, Romaniuk H 2003 Controlled trial of the short- and long-term effect of psychological treatment of post-partum depression. 1. Impact on maternal mood. British Journal of Psychiatry 182: 412–419

Crockenberg S B 1981 Infant irritability, mother responsiveness, and social support influences on the security of infant–mother attachment. Child Development 57: 857–869

de Chateau P, Wiberg B 1984 The long-term effect on mother-infant behaviour of extra contact during the first hour post-partum. III. Follow-up at one year. Scandinavian Journal Social Medicine 12: 91–103

DeLozier P 1982 Attachment theory and child abuse. In: Parkes C M, Stevenson-Hinde J (eds) The place of attachment in human relationships. Basic Books, New York

Department of Health 2004 National service framework for children, young people and maternity services. Department of Health, London

Department of Health 2005 Domestic violence resource manual, 2nd edn. Department of Health, London

Dunn J 1993 Young children's close relationships: beyond attachment. Sage, Thousand Oaks, CA

Egeland B 1993 A history of abuse is a major risk factor for abusing in the next generation. In: Gelles R, Loseke D R (eds) Current controversies on family violence. Sage, Newbury Park, CA, pp 197–208

Egeland B, Erickson M F 1993 Attachment theory and findings: implications for prevention and intervention. In: Kramer S, Parens H (eds) Prevention in mental health: now, tomorrow and ever? Jaon Aronson, Northvale, NJ

Egeland B, Jacobvitz D K, Sroufe L A 1988 Breaking the cycle of abuse. Child Development 59: 1071–1088

Egeland B, Kalkoske M, Gottesman N, Erickson M F 1990 Preschool behavior problems: stability and factors accounting for change. Journal of Child Psychology and Psychiatry 31(6): 891–910

Feldman R, Eidelman A, Sirota L, Weller A 2002 Comparison of skin-to-skin (kangaroo) and traditional care: parenting outcomes and preterm development. Pediatrics 110: 16–26

Feldman R, Weller A, Leckman J, Kuint J, Eidelman A 1999 The nature of the mother's tie to her infant: maternal bonding under conditions of proximity, separation and potential loss. Journal of Child Psychology and Psychiatry 40: 929–939

Fonagy P, Leigh L, Steele M, Steele H, Kennedy R, Mattoon G, Target M, Gerber A 1996 The relation of attachment status, psychiatric classification, and response to psychotherapy. Journal of Consulting and Clinical Psychology 64: 22–31

Fonagy P, Steele H, Steele M 1991 Maternal respresentations of attachment during pregnancy predict the organization of mother–infant attachment at one year of age. Child Development 62: 891–905

Fonagy P, Steele H, Steele M 1994 The Emanual Miller Memorial Lecture 1992. The theory and practice of resilience. Journal of Child Psychology and Psychiatry 35: 231–257

Fraiberg S 1980 Clinical studies in infant mental health: the first year of life. Basic Books, New York

Fraiberg S, Adelson E, Shapiro V 1975 Ghosts in the nursery: a psychoanalytic approach to the problem of impaired infant–mother relationships. Journal of the American Academy of Child Psychiatry 14: 387–423

Garcia J, Redshaw M, Fitzsimons B, Keene J 1998 First class delivery: a national survey of women's views of maternity care. Audit Commission and the National Perinatal Epidemiology Unit, London

Garmezy N, Masten A 1991 The protective role of competence indicators in children at risk. In: Cummings E, Greene A, Harrekere K(eds) Lifespan developmental psychology: perspectives on stress and coping. Lawrence Erlbaum, Hillsdale, NJ

George C, Kaplan N, Main M 1985 The adult attachment interview. Unpublished manuscript. Department of Psychology, University of California, Berkely

Goldsmith H H, Alansky J A 1987 Maternal and infant temperamental predictors of attachment: a meta-analytic review. Journal of Consulting and Clinical Psychology: 805–816

Grossman K, Fremer-Bombik E 1988 Maternal attachment representation as related to patterns of mother–infant attachment and maternal care during the first years of life. In: Hinde R, Stevenson-Hindle J (eds) Relationship within families: mutual influences. Clarendon, New York

Gutbrod T, Wolke D, Soehne B, Ohrt B, Riegel K 2004 The effect of gestation and birthweight on the growth and development of very low birthweight small for gestational age infants: a matched group comparison. Archives of Disease in Childhood Fetal Neonatal edn. 82(3): F208–214.

Hazan C, Shaver P R 1987 Romantic love conceptualized as an attachment process. Journal of Personality and Social Psychology 5: 511–524

Hazan C, Shaver P R 1994 Attachment as an organizational framework for research on close relationships. Psychological Inquiry 5: 1–22

Herrenkhol E C, Herrenkhol R C 1983 Perspectives on the intergenerational transmission of abuse. In: Finkelhor D (ed) The dark side of families. Sage, New York

Hodnett E D, Gates S, Hofmeyr G J, Sakala C 2003 Continuous support for women during childbirth. The Cochrane Database of Systematic Reviews, Issue 3. Art. No.: CD003766

Horowitz F 1987 Exploring developmental theories: towards a structural behavioral model of development. Lawrence Erlbaum, New Jersey

Horowitz F 1990 Developmental models of individual differences. In: Colombo J, Fagen J (eds) Individual differences in infancy: reliability, stability, predication. Lawrence Erlbaum, Hillsdale, NJ

Jenkins J, Smith M 1990 Factors protecting children living in disharmonious homes: Maternal Reports, Journal of the American Academy of Child and Adolescent Psychiatry 29: 60–69

Kagan J 1982 Psychological research on the human infant: an evaluative summary. WT Grant Foundation, New York

Kagan J 1997 Temperament and reactions to unfamiliarity. Child Development 68: 139–143

Kaufman J, Ziegler E 1987 Do abused children become abusive parents? American Journal of Orthopsychiatry 57(2): 186–191

Klaus M H, Kennell J H 1976 Maternal–infant bonding. Mosby, St Louis

Klaus M H, Kennell J H 1982 Parent–infant bonding. Mosby, St Louis

Klaus M H, Kennell J H, Klaus P H 1995 Bonding: building the foundations of secure attachment and dependence. Addison-Wesley, New York

Lewis M, Feiring C 1989 Infant, mother and mother–infant interaction, behaviour and subsequent attachment. Child Development 60: 831–837

Littlewood J, McHugh N 1997 Maternal distress and postnatal depression: the myth of Madonna. Macmillan, Basingstoke

Lumley J, Austin M P, Mitchell C 2004 Intervening to reduce depression after birth: a systematic review of the randomized trials. International Journal of Technology and Assessment of Health Care 20(2): 128–144

Lyons-Ruth K, Connell D B, Gruenbaum H U, Botein S 1990 Infants at social risk: maternal depression and family support services as mediators of infant development and security of attachment. Child Development 37: 671–674

Main M, Goldwyn R 1984 Predicting rejection of her infant from mother's representation of her own experience: implications for the abused-abusing cycle. Child Abuse and Neglect 8: 203–217

Main M, Goldwyn R 1985 Adult attachment classification rating system. Unpublished manuscript, University of California, Berkely

Main M, Kaplan N, Cassidy J 1985 Security in infancy, childhood and adulthood: a move to the levels of representation. In: Bretherton I, Waters E (eds) Growing points in attachment theory and research. Monographs of the Society for Research in Child Development 50: 66–104

Main M, Weston D 1981 The quality of the toddler's relationship to mother and father: related to conflict behaviour and readiness to establish relationships. Child Development 52: 932–940

Mangelsdorf S, Gunnar M, Kestenbaum R, Lang S, Andreas D 1990 Infant proneness-to-distress, maternal personality and mother-infant attachment associations and goodness of fit. Child Development 61, 820–831

McCourt C, Page L A 1996 Report on the evaluation of One-to-One midwifery practice. TVU, London

Meier P, Wolke D, Gutbrod T, Rust L (in submission). The influence of infant irritability on maternal sensitivity in a sample of very premature infants: Term to 3 months post-term age. Infant Behavior and Development

Murray L, Cooper P J 1997 Effects of postnatal depression on infant development. Archives of Disease in Childhood 77: 99–101

Murray L, Cooper P J, Wilson A, Romauniuk H 2003 Controlled trial of the short- and long-term effect of psychological treatment of post-partum depression. 2. Impact on the mother–child relationship and child outcome. British Journal of Psychiatry 182: 420–427

Murray M, Sinclair D, Cooper P, Ducournau P, Turner P, Stein A 1999 The socioemotional development of 5-year-old children of postnatally depressed mothers. Journal of Child Psychology and Psychiatry 40: 1259–1271

National Institute for Clinical Excellence 2003 Antenatal care: routine care for the healthy pregnant woman. Clinical guideline. RCOG, London

National Institute for Clinical Excellence 2004 Puerperal/perinatal mental health scope. NICE, London

Ney B G (1988) Transgenerational abuse. Child Psychiatry and Human Development 18 (3): 151–168

Oppenheim D, Sagi A, Lamb M, 1988 Infant-adult attachment on the Kibbutz and their relation to socioemotional development four years later. Developmental Psychology 24: 427–433

Page L A, McCourt C, Beake S, Hewison J, Vail A 1999 Clinical interventions and outcomes of one-to-one midwifery practice. Journal of Public Health Medicine 21: 243–248

Page L, Beake S, Vail A, McCourt C, Hewison J 2001 Clinical outcomes of one-to-one midwifery practice. British Journal of Midwifery 9: 700–706

Prior M 1992 Childhood temperament. Journal Child Psychology and Psychiatry 33: 249–279

Rutter M 1981 Maternal deprivation reassessed. 2nd edn. Penguin, Harmondsworth

Rutter M 1995 Clinical implications of attachment concepts: retrospect and prospect. Journal of Child Psychology and Psychiatry 36: 549–571

Rutter M, Rutter M 1993 Developing minds: challenge and continuity across the lifespan. Penguin, Harmondsworth

Schaffer R 1996 Social Development. Blackwells, Oxford

Shaver P, Collins N, Clark C 1996 Attachment styles and internal working models of self and relationship partners. In: Fletcher G J O, Fitness J (eds) Knowledge structures in close relationships: a social psychological approach. Erlbaum, New Jersey

Sroufe L A 1991 An organizational perspective on the self. In: Cicchetti D, Beeghly M (eds) The self in transition. University of Chicago Press, Chicago

Sroufe L A 1996 Emotional development: the organization of emotional life in the early years. Cambridge University Press, Cambridge

Stern D 1977 The first relationship. Harvard University Press, Harvard

Svanberg P 2004 Early screening and primary prevention; a brief introduction to the Sunderland Infant Programme. Enriching early parent–infant relationships. UK Brazelton Centre Conference, London

Tessier R, Cristo M, Velez S, Giron M, Ruiz-Palaez J, Charpak Y, Charpak N 1998 Kangaroo mother care and the bonding hypothesis. Pediatrics 102: 17–26

Thomas A, Chess S 1977 Temperament and development. Bruner-Mazel, New York

Troy M, Sroufe L A 1987 Victimisation among preschoolers: role of attachment relationship history. Journal of American Academy of Child and Adolescent Psychiatry. 26: 166–172

van den Boom D (1994) The influence of temperament and mothering on attachment and exploration: An experimental manipulation of sensitive responsiveness among lower class mothers with irritable infants. Child Development 65: 1457–1477

van den Boom D, Hoeksma J 1994 The effect of infant irritability on mother-infant interaction: A growth-curve analysis. Developmental Psychology 30: 581–590

Van Ijzendoorn M H 1992 Intergenerational transmission of parenting: a review of studies of nonclinical populations. Developmental Review 12: 76–92

Van Ijzendoorn M H, Femmie J, Duyvesteyn G C 1995 Breaking the intergenerational cycle of insecure attachment: a review of attachment based interventions on maternal sensitivity and infant security. Child Development 63: 463–73

Vaughn B E, Stevenson-Hinde J, Waters E et al 1992 Attachment security and temperament in infancy and early childhood. Developmental Psychology 28: 463–473

Waters E 1978 The reliability and stability of individual differences in infant-mother attachment. Child Development 49: 483–494

Waters E, Hamilton C, Weinfield N 2000 The stability of attachment security from infancy to adolescence and early adulthood. Child Development 71: 678–683

Weinfield N S, Sroufe L A, Egeland B 2000 Attachment from infancy to young adulthood in a high-risk sample: continuity, discontinuity and their correlates. Child Development 71(3): 695–702

Werner E 1989 High risk children in young adulthood: a longitudinal study from birth to 32

years of life. In: Hinde R, Stevenson-Hinde J (eds) Relationships within families: mutual influences. Clarendon Press, New York

Whitelaw A, Heisterkampf G, Sleath K, Acolet D, Richards M 1988 Skin to skin contact for very low birthweight infants and their mothers. Archives of Disease in Childhood 63: 1377–1381

Winnicott D W 1987 The child, the family and the outside world. Addison-Wesley, Reading, MA

Zeanah C, Emde R 1994 Attachment disorders in infancy and childhood. In: Rutter M, Taylor E, Hersov L (eds) Child and adolescent psychiatry: modern approaches. 3rd edn. Blackwell, Oxford

Zeanah C H, Zeanah P D 1989 Intergenerational transmission of maltreatment: insights from attachment theory and research. Psychiatry 52: 177–198

Zeanah C H 1993 Handbook of infant mental health. Guildford Press, London

Chapter 3

Becoming a parent

Christine McCourt

INTRODUCTION

Childbirth is always a social and cultural event as well as a personal matter. As well as bringing a new life into the world, it creates new or changed relationships and roles. It has significance for the woman and her partner, the family and the wider society. From the woman's viewpoint birth is not so much a medical event as a major transition in her life, a transition which implies major changes in personal and social identity and roles (Kitzinger 1989). The meaning of pregnancy and birth is broad and complex, and takes its form within a web of cultural and social influences and within a life history.

As a result, becoming a parent has been described both as a major life transition and a major life crisis, a time of crucial psychological and social adjustment. Becoming parents requires a couple to make major adjustments as they alter their lifestyle and relationships to accommodate a new family member. New behaviour patterns are necessary as soon as the birth occurs. The weeks and months after the birth have been identified as a time of considerable stress as well as a time of considerable pleasure. On a scale of major life events and their associated stress, the arrival of a new family member has been rated in the first twenty (Holmes & Rahe 1967). A further survey of 2500 adults found that childbirth was the sixth most stressful life event of the 102 events that were noted (Dohrenwend et al 1978).

This chapter focuses on the midwife's role in relation to transition to parenthood, in providing appropriate care and support to the new mother, her partner and family, to contribute to the adjustment process. Topics covered include the everyday role changes associated with parenthood; the mothering role as it is constructed in modern post-industrialized societies; social support during pregnancy, birth and early parenthood and women's emotional wellbeing after the birth. It reviews relevant evidence from psychological, social and cultural as well as midwifery research to support practice. It aims to provide a grounding in knowledge relevant to the transition to parenthood, plus ideas and directions for further study, and to encourage reflection, learning from experience and learning from mothers, their partners and families about the meaning and importance of this period and how midwives can help.

Although some of the changes described in this chapter apply particularly to first-time parents, the parents of subsequent babies also face enormous changes in demands and family relationships as they adjust to the presence of a second, third or subsequent child. Moreover, midwives may expect more experienced parents to need very little support when in fact they often also feel uncertain, overwhelmed and exhausted. It is important, therefore, for midwives to consider the adjustment and change issues for all women and families they care for.

EARLY RESEARCH ON TRANSITION TO PARENTHOOD

The following quotes, from a 14th century English woman and an 18th century 'man-midwife' illustrate that the theme of difficulty and anxiety in the transition to parenthood is not merely a modern one. In different cultural and historical settings, pregnancy and childbirth have often been seen as times of vulnerability, owing to the great personal, spiritual, social and physiological changes involved.

> When this creature was twenty years of age, or somewhat more, she was married to a worshipful burgess and was with child within a short time, as nature would have it. And after she had conceived, she was troubled with severe attacks of sickness until the child was born. And then, what with the labour pains she had in childbirth and the sickness that had gone before, she despaired of her life.
>
> Kempe 1985, p. 41

> The patient's imagination must not be disturbed by the news of any extraordinary accident which may have happened to her family or friends; such information hath been known to carry off the labour-pains entirely, after they were begun, and the woman has sunk under her dejection of spirits: and even after delivery.
>
> Smellie 1756, pp 395–396

Most of the early sociological research about becoming a parent used either a 'crisis' or a 'transition-to-parenthood' framework and was based mainly on the experiences of middle-class, first-time parents in the USA and UK. As with any research, the degree of stress or change may well have been underestimated given the problem of respondents making socially desirable responses. Likewise, thinking may well have been generalized from the reports of some families to all, despite the diversity of people midwives work with. We cannot assume that experiences and needs of all families are similar, even though the most fundamental transitions of childbirth are universal.

The crisis framework was largely based on Hill's (1949) suggestion that adding a family member constituted a crisis for married couples. Hill defined crisis as:

> Any sharp or decisive change for which old patterns are inadequate. A crisis is a situation in which the usual behaviour patterns are found to be unrewarding and new ones are called for immediately.

These early studies found that most couples experienced a degree of crisis that was extensive or severe (LeMasters 1957). These couples appeared to have completely romanticized their view of parenthood. They felt that they had little if any preparation for parental roles, some couples stating that while 'they knew where babies came from', most of them 'didn't know what they were like'. More recent research indicates that many parents in the early twenty-first century feel very much the same: just as unprepared, just as confused and just as 'taken in' by the many romantic myths about being a parent.

Dyer's (1963) findings largely supported those of LeMasters (1957). Women reported feelings of anticlimax or 'being let down' by the mothering experience, of being tied down and having constantly interrupted rest and sleep, as well as decreased house-keeping standards. The men mentioned the necessity of sharing with relatives, the worry of a decreased income and the general adjustments required given the unexpected demands of parenthood. Later research using more representative samples reported a lesser degree of crisis than that found by LeMasters and Dyer (Elliott et al 1985, Hobbs 1968, Russell 1974).

The term 'transition to parenthood' was introduced by Rossi (1968) to signify the various changes and adjustments involved in moving from a childless state to parenthood. Using a transition-to-parenthood framework, the sociological literature on first-time parenthood has progressed somewhat from a focus on crisis to a more balanced assessment of the major adjustments required when a dyad is transformed into a triad. Research from a transition framework has included investigations of the family dynamics associated with parenthood, for example changes in marital satisfaction, the household division of labour and social network structures.

Most of these early researchers found that satisfaction with the marriage declines following the birth of the infant (Belsky et al 1985, Blum 1981, Boles 1985, Tomlinson 1987). Of importance is the finding that average crisis scores were significantly higher for women than men in most of the early crisis research. Moreover, in some transition-to-parenthood studies, women experienced a greater decline in marital satisfaction following the birth of the infant. As well as a decline in marital satisfaction, another consistent finding in both the early and the more recent research is the more traditional household division of labour which occurs after the birth of the first child. New parents shift away from a view of male and female roles as being equally shared (Ozaki 1986, Tomlinson 1987). This suggests that although traditional gender divisions have declined in Western societies in recent decades, becoming a parent often triggers a return to more divided gender roles, which are no longer so 'in line' with common social expectations.

As noted, much of this early research made assumptions about the 'normal' family, which tended to apply more to white, middle class parents and to Western countries. In reality, and in other settings, the family is more varied, and so the precise nature of the changes and adjustments may differ. This is increasingly being recognized by professionals as the multi-cultural nature of society, and rapid changes in family life and gender roles are acknowledged.

Nonetheless, the themes of transition found in earlier work have endured, although later work has shown them to be more complex (Tomlinson 1996). Studies from the 1990s onwards (some of which are discussed below) have similar themes of difficulties, or at least challenges in adjustment, with parents feeling caught between romanticized and idealized notions of parenthood, and everyday experiences of tiredness, postnatal health problems and the challenges of learning to juggle new roles and responsibilities, often with very little hands-on support.

MATERNAL ADJUSTMENT

Women have described the early months after the birth as a stressful time of adjustment, when they experience an intense change of self (Barclay et al 1997, Mercer 1986, Ruchala & Halstead 1994, Sethi

1995), a time characterized by considerable physical, emotional and social change (Gjerdingen & Fontaine 1991, Percival 1990). Almost half of the women in Tulman and Fawcett's (1991) study found that the first 6 months after the birth were more difficult than expected. Some women had not fully recovered from the birth by 6 months in that they had not resumed some of their usual prebirth activities, household tasks, physical exercise and usual occupational activities.

There are several reasons why this time is so stressful for women. After the birth, the average new mother must cope with the needs of a new infant as she recovers her own physical and emotional equilibrium. Researchers have found high levels of postnatal ill health including physical and psychological symptoms, many of which have not been reported or identified in postnatal care (Bick & MacArthur 1995, Glazener et al 1995, MacArthur et al 2003). For women, pregnancy, childbirth and parenting are commonly described as events that stimulate identity adaptations, induce the reorganization of interpersonal relations and promote personal maturation (Rubin 1967a, 1967b, 1975). The developmental changes necessary in adapting to first-time or subsequent parenthood require a modification of everyday patterns of functioning. These changes require a great deal of energy and a large investment of time (Belsky & Rovine 1990, Mercer 1986).

The new mother must undertake many new role behaviours as she adjusts to her new role and establishes a relationship with her infant. Such behaviours include learning to care for the infant and the development of a sensitive awareness of the infant's needs and patterns of expressing these needs. There must also be an alteration of lifestyles and relationships to accommodate a new family member (Mercer 1986, Walker et al 1986). There are important adjustments for the father and other family members too. For example, fathers may feel their relationship with their partner has changed, as she focuses more on care for their child, and older children may feel overlooked or resentful of having to share parental attention and resources with a new infant.

Rubin (1967a, 1967b) first used the concept of maternal role attainment to describe and explain the psychological processes that occur during pregnancy and after birth as the mother becomes competent and integrates the maternal role into her current role to achieve maternal identity. Oakley (1980) referred to this as adjustment to motherhood. Rubin (1967a, 1967b) identified four developmental tasks necessary for maternal adaptation. The first task is seeking and ensuring a safe passage for the mother and her infant during pregnancy and childbirth. The second is the acceptance and support of her baby by significant others. The third is binding in to the infant, and the last giving of herself to her infant.

Mercer (1981) built on Rubin's early work, describing maternal role attainment as a process that had four stages of development: anticipatory, formal, informal and personal. As the mother travels through these stages, she progresses from learning the expectations of the role, to following the directions of others and coping with other role models, to developing her own individual behaviour and finally to gaining confidence and competence in her performance. During the formal stage, the mother relies on others, for example health professionals such as midwives and significant others, to guide her behaviours and expectations. As we have noted, much of this work was based on samples of women which did not necessarily reflect the social and cultural diversity of mothers today. While these stages are likely to be shared, the details of who women rely on, and how far they use formal or informal support is likely to vary. This was reflected in Hodinott and Pill's study of working class mothers and breastfeeding, where informal and family sources of support were far more important than professional ones (Hodinott & Pill 1999).

THEORETICAL VIEWS OF ADJUSTMENT

Researchers have undertaken research on adjustment to motherhood from different theoretical perspectives. Overall, those which emphasize the individual, for example psychoanalytic theory, tend to look at internal attributes as causes of dissatisfaction or lack of adjustment. Conversely, a social perspective focuses on the structure of society and the difficulties associated with the mothering role within this context.

INDIVIDUAL APPROACHES

Psychoanalytic theory is individualistic in that it emphasizes the personality of each woman. It is rooted in the early and widely influential work of Freud, who saw the person's conflicts, anxieties and resentments, particularly as established in infant and early childhood relationships, as accounting for her experience. While this school of thought does focus on the mother's social situation and relationships, it considers this to be of secondary importance to the mother's internal characteristics in deciding her adaptation. It was also strongly influenced by the work of Jung who took a broader, more cultural view than Freud. Traditional psychoanalytic theorists tended to see motherhood as being essential for the fulfilment of women; women who experienced dissatisfaction with or problems in adjusting to the maternal role were seen as having problems with their psychosexual development (Benedeck 1959, Deutsch 1944).

Some researchers within the psychoanalytic tradition have emphasized the importance of recognizing pregnancy and new parenthood as major developmental milestones and opportunities for growth (Chodorow 1978, Osofsky & Osofsky 1983). Within this framework, even women who are psychologically well adjusted who want a child may experience considerable psychological upheavals during pregnancy and the adjustment to a new baby. However, women must be able to integrate the maturational changes and adjustments that accompany this period if they are to achieve a new equilibrium. For some women, the adaptation process may result in an opportunity for further growth. For others, the experience may lead to long-term difficulties or poor adjustment.

Later theories have also focused on the intergenerational implications of the mothers' wellbeing for her infant. In particular, attachment theory established the importance of early maternal-infant (or carer–infant) interaction to the subsequent development and security of individuals, and showed how poor health and difficult experiences in the mother might negatively affect her capacity to respond to her infant. The effects of early experiences on the child have been shown to be potentially life-long, including, in turn, the way she or he copes with parenthood. Good support from others, though, has been shown to make a difference to how women who themselves have had difficult early experiences cope with others, and so the midwife's role has a real potential to be helpful in the long term. These issues are discussed in depth in Chapter 2 and are also noted below, in discussing postnatal depression.

SOCIAL APPROACHES

Inherent in socially based theories of motherhood is the belief that the quality of the mother's experience of motherhood is dependent upon the way in which the role is institutionalized and evaluated within the society. Within a sociological framework, society is seen as shaping and influencing the woman's experience as a mother. In more recent years, there has been an increased emphasis by sociologists and social anthropologists on the experience of motherhood, particularly following Oakley's work in the late 1970s and 1980s (Oakley 1979, 1980). Before this time, most of the research on mothers and children focused almost exclusively on the child, the woman's experience being considered almost coincidentally, or as a matter of concern since it affected the health and wellbeing of the child. Mothers were the 'producers' of the next generation (Lewis 1990). During the past two decades, the values of social researchers who have omitted the woman's experience of motherhood have been questioned. In addition, although psychoanalysis is certainly individualistic, some later psychoanalytic theorists have attempted to respond to these criticisms and integrate their work with more socially orientated approaches, while sociologists have also begun to take more account of the agency of individual women within society.

In their early analysis of parenthood from a conflict framework, LaRossa and LaRossa (1981) concluded that mistaking social problems for individual troubles not only impedes the discovery of solutions, but may also in fact add to the social problem itself. It may, however, seem easier to treat the individual mother with therapy or medication than it is to address the socio-cultural issues surrounding the social role of mother (Oakley 1980).

These shifts in thinking – from individual problems to socially situated ones – are reflected in UK health policy of the early 21st century. From the 1990s, policy documents acknowledged the importance of seeking structural as well as individual solutions to health and social problems, particularly through working in and with local communities. The UK Department of Health's National Service Framework for Children, Young People and Maternity Services (Department of Health 2004) for example, emphasizes the need for maternity services to develop more pro-active roles in providing or facilitating support to women, and in providing appropriate care for groups of women who may have particular difficulties in the transition to parenthood. Some of these policies are described below, in the section on social capital.

CHILDBIRTH AS SOCIAL AND CULTURAL TRANSITION

CULTURAL APPROACHES

The above overview of research on transition and adjustment to parenthood supports the view that the transition to parenthood is a challenging time for the mother and the wider family. The period of transition for the mother has meaning in terms of her entire life experience, family roles and history. For example, as we have discussed, early childhood experiences may have an impact on a woman's adjustment to mothering. In many societies, the birth of a first child marks a point of transition to full adult status and brings with it differing social roles and responsibilities beyond the immediate physical and emotional demands of infant care. The birth of subsequent children prompts further changes to family roles and structures.

Theorists of life changes (Marris 1974, Murray-Parkes 1971) have argued that even positive life changes, such as the birth of a child or a new home, may lead to a sense of loss and grief. In order to cope with change positively and without experiencing undue distress, people need opportunities to make sense of what is happening and to integrate new identities and experiences with previous ones so as to maintain a sense of order in their lives.

Anthropologists have discussed in detail the role of ritual in creating or maintaining such a sense of order within social and cultural groups. Interestingly, the term 'ritual' is often used in a derogatory tone in critical texts in the health services to refer to practices that, in biomedical terms, are felt to be empty and meaningless because they have no direct or apparent curative or caring function. An anthropological perspective, however, suggests that ritual activity is highly meaningful, but on a primarily symbolic level where meaning is complex and often multivocal (it can be expressed and interpreted in many ways). Anthropologists in the UK between the 1950s and 1970s argued strongly for the functional value of much ritual activity in maintaining a sense or feeling of order and control within change situations (Douglas 1966, Gluckman 1962).

As early as the 1930s, the anthropologist Gennep coined the term 'rites of passage' (from the French *rites de passage*; Gennep 1960) to describe a clear pattern of ritual activity that is found in a wide range of cultures and social contexts to accompany and manage life changes. The classical rite of passage was particularly associated with puberty and transition to adulthood.

Rites of passage surrounding the transition to parenthood are of major importance in many cultures (see Kitzinger 1989, Vincent-Priya 1992). The classical structure of a rite of passage as outlined by Gennep has been remarkably durable and was even strikingly echoed in the accounts of American sociologists in the 1950s of rites of entry to hospitals, prisons and other 'total institutions' (Goffman 1968) as well as in the analysis of the 'sick role' (Parsons 1951).

The rite is marked by three phases: separation, liminality and reincorporation. Liminality is derived from the Latin word *limen* (threshold) and conveys well the state of being in transition, betwixt and between two states. Typically, initiates in such rites are separated from ordinary social existence, roles and responsibilities. They may be physically or geographically separated or secluded from everyday social activity, or the separation may be symbolic, as in the removal of hair or everyday clothes. The liminal phase is seen as outside culture and society, and thus fraught with danger.

Rites of passage are found in traditional cultural rituals surrounding pregnancy, childbirth and the puerperium but they are also found in Western hospital childbirth practices (Davis-Floyd 1994, Jordan 1993, Kitzinger 1989). In modern hospital birth, a woman is separated from her ordinary social world, with activities such as the removal of ordinary clothes, admission traces and the withholding of food and drink, transferred to a labour ward for delivery and thence moved to a postnatal ward, where flowers and visitors are received. This parallels neatly the three phases of the traditional rite of passage, but the needs being served here are not necessarily those of the parents so much as the needs of the institution and its smooth running; needs such as the staffing of wards and areas, keeping a throughput of beds by moving women quickly through the system, maintaining a sense of order through hierarchy and 'going with the flow' (Hunt & Symonds 1995, Kirkham 1989). This means that rather than the potentially very supportive aspects of the rituals being to the fore – to help families in coping with transition – their needs are secondary to those of the institution. This is reflected in the research on women's experiences of birth and postnatal care in hospital, which often leave them feeling relatively unsupported, even frightened, and far less satisfied than they are with domiciliary care (Garcia et al 1998, McCourt & Pearce 2000, McCourt et al 1998).

The time period of this transition ritual is short, and increasingly so, the overwhelming interest of obstetrics being in active labour and the delivery of the baby. This is a transition period that bears a closer relationship to the concerns and interests of maternity professionals than to the significance of the transition in the woman's life, which is seen in a much longer time frame. The character of such rituals appears to reflect more closely the needs of the institution and of health professionals for a sense of order and control in a situation characterized by uncertainty, rather than the needs of the woman and her family in this transition. Recent changes in the character and provision of postnatal hospital care bring out this difference particularly clearly, since the significance and meaning of the drama and journey of birth are barely acknowledged in the task-centred and limited character of postnatal hospital care (Ball 1994, McCourt et al 1998, Simkin 1991).

Sociological research has also indicated that such attitudes towards the transition of birth are permeating cultural expectations, the implication being that women should make a rapid recovery and return to ordinary life, as though life has not changed. In a study of the postnatal recovery of women in a US setting, where postnatal home care is not routinely provided as in the UK. Ruchala and Halstead (1994) found that women were responding to strong expectations that they should be functioning normally within a short period of birth. A news report in a US paper in 2004 commented on this trend, citing research that professional women in particular in the US are increasingly anxious about being able to return to their previous life, range of activities and body image, as though becoming a parent should not change their lives at all (Abraham 2004). Such reports suggest the cultural pressures on women becoming mothers are not diminishing.

The term 'back to normal' seems in itself to deny that a fundamental adjustment in roles and relationships is taking place. An examination of historical and cross-cultural texts, despite the fact that written sources are limited, consistently shows a distinct but different pattern of ritual surrounding birth, with a longer time span and a much greater focus on the period following birth. The title 'monthly nurse' or 'monthly' was still commonly used in the UK early in the 20th century, referring to the practice of midwives, nurses or handywomen providing care within the home for a month following birth, and cross-culturally prescribed periods or rest and seclusion following birth have ranged from about 10 to 40 days (Towler & Bramall 1986). The historian Wilson describes how, from the 17th century in England, ways of managing birth were challenged and changed, with doctors criticizing the traditional practices of midwives and 'gossips' to care for and protect the mother and infant following birth (Wilson 1995). Even so, a 'lying-in' period of 10 days was written into the 1902 Midwives Act in the UK, and carried over into the tradition of midwife visits for 10 days following birth.

A recent study by Newell (2004) on the 'churching' of women in Christian societies, reflects on the ways in which this ritual provided a kind of protected time and space for women, as well as marking the 'reincorporation' into the ordinary social world which is a feature of rites of passage. Although it partly reflected the traditional ideas that women were ritually vulnerable and polluted following childbirth, it ensured a valuable period of rest and seclusion from ordinary social duties, that can weigh heavily on new mothers.

'Traditions' are also found today and may vary across different cultures. The customs and practices of medically-oriented hospital units have already been mentioned. In Islamic societies, the importance of birth as a transition is marked by the whispering of verses from the Quran into the infant's ear. The baby is entering a social world. In many societies, giving birth and becoming a mother mark the attainment of a full adult woman's role, and results in important, positive changes in dynamics and status within the wider family. Some writers have argued that women in modern, or post-modern culture experience difficulties compounded by very ambivalent attitudes towards parenthood – seen alternatively as important and as socially devalued, particularly in comparison to paid work outside the home (Barclay et al 1997). Whereas women in some cultures gain greater power through becoming a mother – such as by greater authority in the extended family – in others they may feel their power is reduced.

CHANGING GENDER ROLES

Both parents, then, face many challenges during the transition to parenthood as they adjust to their new roles. However, although men and women face the same event, their experiences of the event are unlikely to be comparable. The fathering role varies considerably in different societies. This role has also changed historically and continues to evolve as the roles of men and women change (Edgar 1993, Marks & Lovestone 1995). These changing roles may be a source of stress, confusion and uncertainty for men as they undertake the transition to first-time (and subsequent) parenthood and define their own sense of self as father, within a context of wide social changes.

However, women must also face the birth. In addition, in most modern post-industrialized societies, many women also leave the workforce (at the very least for a short time) and undertake a new full-time role (Terry 1991). Regardless of recent role shifts (although there are some exceptions), women usually assume the role of primary carer for the new baby. Moreover, most women assume this new role almost immediately after the birth. They no longer have the luxury of being cared for as they recover from the birth, as they would have been earlier in the century; instead, they must become the carers.

The life change that the woman undergoes during the transition to parenthood may be accentuated because it is now usual for her to work until just before the birth of the first child. Fifty years ago, most middle-class women in the UK gave up paid work on marriage. In addition, in countries such as the UK, USA, Canada and Australia, a number of broader cultural factors can make life more difficult for both parents, particularly the mother. The way in which the role of mother is constructed in most modern post-industrialized societies makes enormous demands on women and creates difficulties for both parents. Also, the romanticized images that surround the mothering role suggest that it is instinctive and effortless. Moreover, the low status of mothering in society does little for women's self-esteem; many give up 'important' paid work to start their new job and then often feel the need to apologize because they are 'just' a mother (Oakley 1979, 1980).

WOMEN, SOCIETY OR BOTH

Within the psychoanalytic traditions, then, it was largely assumed that 'normal' women adapt to and 'cope' with motherhood. Without doubt, the personal attributes that a mother brings to her new role are important in her adaptation. Of enormous importance, however, is the social situation in which she plays out her role. Based on their interviews with women themselves, researchers have concluded that an easy adaptation to first-time motherhood in modern post-industrialized societies is unusual: most women are likely to experience problems (Crouch & Manderson 1993, Oakley 1980). Miller, in her study of adaptation to motherhood in Britain commented on the contradictions we have cited above: women felt enormous differences between the rhetoric or ideal images of motherhood and their own experience, and were reluctant to voice their difficulties for

fear of being seen as a bad mother. These fears meant that professionals, friends and family may not be fully aware of the degree of difficulty which women (and their partners) commonly experience. Few felt prepared for the personal and social changes first-time motherhood would make to their lives, and the length of time and energy adaptation demanded (Miller 2002).

Many factors affect the adaptation of women to the maternal role, and research has been undertaken from differing theoretical perspectives. The following are found in many studies:

- higher levels of social support have been shown to be related to easier adjustment to the maternal role (see the section on social support below);
- the amount of life change, life stress and events: women considered to be most at risk are those with high amounts of life stress and low levels of social support (Grace 1993, Mercer 1986, Terry 1991);
- maternal health status (Mercer 1981, Russell 1974);
- maternal age: older women show a lower level of gratification in the maternal role (Blum 1981, Brown et al 1994, Grace 1993, Mercer 1986); however, younger women were found to have fewer psychosocial skills to cope with the maternal role, while older women demonstrated more nurturing behaviours towards their infants (Mercer 1986);
- higher levels of maternal education, which are associated with more difficult adjustment (Grace 1993, Mercer 1981, Younger 1991);
- the process of adaptation to the maternal role may be more difficult for career-orientated women (Alexander & Higgins 1993, Levy-Shiff 1994, MacDermid et al 1990);
- personality characteristics such as self-concept, self-esteem, ego strength, self efficacy and individual coping style (Demyttenaere et al 1995, Mercer 1986, Younger 1991);
- the woman's early relations with her own mother (Benedeck 1959, Deutsch 1944), including separation before the age of 11 years (Frommer & O'Shea 1973);
- the woman's relationship with her mother during pregnancy: the more positive this relationship was, the more the woman reported

possessing the characteristics necessary for mothering and the more self-confidence she felt in herself as a mother (Deutsch et al 1988);

- the birth experience (Green & Baston 2003, Green et al 1998, Halman et al 1995);
- infant behaviour (Brazleton 1962, Deutsch et al 1988);
- previous experience with children (Berry 1988, Younger 1991).

MIDWIVES SUPPORTING PARENTS

Given these many stressors, it is not surprising that the weeks and months after the birth have been identified as a time when the support needs of parents, particularly mothers, are high (Barclay et al 1997, Rubin 1967a, Ruchala & Halstead 1994, Sethi 1995). As we discuss below, this needed support may be available either from informal networks of family or friends, or from formal sources. The formal support available to women and men at this time includes that given by midwives and health visitors (community/child health/public health nurses) and in some places by maternity care aides or assistants. During the antenatal, birth and postnatal period, midwives and health visitors are in an ideal position to provide support to influence all the factors shown by the literature to be important during the transition to parenthood. These include acquiring new skills and incorporating new tasks, acquiring a new self-concept and adapting to changing roles.

There are a number of different ways in which midwives can support or care for women, and these have been discussed throughout the book. In this chapter, we concentrate on the positive ways in which midwives can assist parents to adjust to their new roles. Although adequate research is available that emphasizes the enormous role change occurring at this time, very little of this practical and accurate information actually reaches parents. Instead, they receive a constant barrage of information from the media that emphasizes only the ease, joy and wonder of parenting, or overly dramatizes ordinary problems, while information from professionals in pregnancy tends to focus on the pregnancy and birth, rather than living with a new baby. In countries such as the UK, USA, Canada and Australia, despite an increase in antenatal education, many parents simply do not recognize how much a baby will change their lives (Barclay et al 1997, Brown et al 1994, Miller 2002, Ruchala & Halstead 1994, Sethi 1995).

Childbirth preparation courses are typically available in most communities, but very few programmes address the mental health and shifting emotional strains of expectant parents. While preparation for the birth itself is essential, Nolan (1997) concluded that the courses available do not give attention to the social and psychological preparation for parenthood that the significance of this major life event merits. Certainly, the emotional aspects of the birth itself have recently been paid more attention, given the importance of the actual experience of birth to many women. It is now fair to say that, in most developed countries, in one sense physical outcomes for mothers and their babies are usually positive, in that it is unusual for women to die during and after childbirth, although there is a very high rate of surgical intervention which may lead to problems related to unnecessary medical treatment. However, some women feel so depressed after the birth of their beautiful and healthy baby that they would, at times, like to die. As many as 1 in 5 women experience severe and disabling postnatal depression, which in many cases lasts months and even years.

Worryingly, the 2004 CEMACH report in the UK on Why Mothers Die indicated that a significant proportion of maternal deaths are related to social and psychological problems, in pregnancy and postnatally. The leading cause of maternal death was suicide and other key risk factors included social disadvantage, living in poor communities, ethnic minority status, domestic violence and substance abuse. Social disadvantage was particularly related to women without partners and women and partners being unemployed. Many of these deaths are preventable, and midwifery, with its focus on 'being with the woman' should be well placed to make a difference (CEMACH 2004). The findings suggest, however, that maternity services need to re-orient themselves more to focus on the social and psychological needs of women and dealing with the effects of disadvantage where possible. It contradicts the common professional assumption that physical care is basic while social and psychological aspects of care are 'extras' or even 'luxuries', or that they are only of concern to more privileged women. There has been relatively little research on the experiences and views of socially disadvantaged women, or minority ethnic communities. Two linked studies of minority ethnic women receiving conventional or caseload maternity care found that the women generally wanted and valued similar things to the majority – particularly to feel cared for, supported and safe with maternity care providers, but in practice they rarely found this in conventional care. Some found the experience – in a fragmented and highly medicalized service – alienating and frightening, and staff often uncaring. They were particularly likely to value caseload midwifery since they could get to know the midwife, feel that she was 'there for you' and could guide and support you through the experience (Harper-Bulman & McCourt 2002, McCourt & Pearce 2000). It is ironic, then, that responses to new developments following Changing Childbirth have sometimes been dismissed as inequitable, although a number of recent developments, such as Sure Start midwifery group practices have provided more continuity of support to women living in socially disadvantaged areas. The focus of the Department of Health's National Service Framework for Children (Department of Health 2004) recognizes this and advocates changes in services and practice better support all women, and reach out to women with the greatest needs for care and support, who often are not receiving the best quality of care.

The real challenge for midwives is to give the same attention to preparing parents for the overall period of transition as they have given to the labour and birth process. This transition may in reality last months and even years rather than the few weeks allocated by many health professionals. The remainder of this chapter looks at areas and ways in which midwives can help parents to experience a more positive period of transition. Midwives do not work alone, and should never expect to carry the burden of care for such a fundamental social transition, so these sections also discuss other types of help, through from the everyday help of family, friends and community, to other agencies and professionals.

SOCIAL SUPPORT

Since birth takes place in a social context and, as anthropologists have emphasized, is a social as well as physiological transition, social support has been an important aspect of pregnancy and birth care historically and in most, if not all, cultures (Jordan 1993, Kitzinger 1989, Towler & Bramall 1986). Medicine in European and North American societies (which social scientists refer to as biomedicine) is unusual in the degree to which such aspects of care have been overlooked in its development. For example, Kitzinger points out that although in most societies, women kin and neighbours have important roles in supporting women giving birth, with the development of obstetrics, lay women were gradually excluded from birthing environments. She notes that, as recently as 1975, popular obstetric texts advised against the presence of birth companions, suggesting that 'old wives' tales' and stories would frighten women giving birth (Kitzinger 1989 referring to Bourne 1975). This approach is linked to the mind/body dichotomy in biomedical thinking and practice (Helman 1994), where instead of being seen as part of life, childbirth in the modern obstetric unit is set apart from the context of the woman's life. When such a view of birth prevails, understanding of social or cultural issues, if sought at all, is often geared to understanding the way beliefs, attitudes and behaviour may impede the practise of medical care.

Midwifery philosophy does not split the medical and the social body in the same way and much attention has been given to the importance of social support for mothers and families, and the roles of midwives and others in either providing, or encouraging this (McCourt 2003). The old English meaning of midwife – mid wif, meaning 'with woman' – is seen as a fundamental root of midwifery practice. However, much of the midwifery literature in recent decades has reflected concerns about the withdrawal of much of this supporting and 'presencing' role (Mander 2001) as services became increasingly organized around a fragmented, production-line model of hospital-centred care.

WHAT IS SOCIAL SUPPORT?

The meaning of social support is so broad and diffuse, that it may seem impossible to define and study. Nonetheless, there is considerable research evidence that levels of social support have a major impact on health in general and the health of mothers in particular, and there are a number of theories and mechanisms that have been put forward to explain this (McCourt 2003). In order to measure its effect, researchers have tended to break the concept down into meaningful components. The following aspects reflect a wide span of studies, and people's perceptions of what social support is:

- *Emotional support*: this is probably the aspect most commonly recognized. The term implies a warm or caring relationship, and one which conveys esteem, but emotional support may be as simple as presence or companionship and willingness to listen.
- *Informational support*: being given good information and advice is widely perceived as being supportive. It underlies ability to make positive choices, increases confidence and sense of security. It may also help by increasing personal sense of control.
- *Practical or tangible support*: types of practical support may vary widely but its importance should not be underestimated. It may include measures as varied as financial support for a pregnant woman, physical comfort measures during labour and birth, or practical support for breastfeeding.

Social support also has objective and subjective aspects – it is possible to define an activity, relationship or intervention as support, but its effectiveness is always dependent on whether it is experienced as supportive by the person receiving it. Support which is given but not perceived as such may be ineffective, or even unhelpful, if it undermines the person's own coping resources, self-esteem or sense of control. This is often explored by psychologists in terms of the concept of person/environment fit (Cohen & McKay 1983). Perceptions of support may also be enhanced by clarifying what support is expected or available, since difference between expectation and experi-

ence are likely to be unhelpful (Levitt et al 1993). Social ties or relationships cannot simply be assumed to be beneficial and Oakley (1992) highlights the possibility of health professionals offering support or care which is not helpful. This is important to bear in mind when considering the roles of maternity services – and their limitations – in offering social support.

Studies of women's experiences and perceptions of pregnancy and birth have consistently shown that women across a wide span of time and place see supportive maternity care as including good communication – not only being given information but also being listened to and able to discuss their concerns and options; being treated as individuals; having a sense of choice and control over what happens to them as well as trust and confidence in the competence of professionals (Garcia et al 1998, Green et al 1998, McCourt et al 1998, Reid & Garcia 1989, Wilkins 2000). Studies of women in different social class and ethnic groups (Handler et al 1996, Harper-Bulman & McCourt 2002, Hirst et al 1998, Laslett et al 1997, McCourt & Pearce 2000, MORI 1993) suggest that such core principles are relevant to a wide range of women, rather than confined to an articulate minority. Women's specific concerns about support do vary, however, as do their specific experiences of health care, with many women in minority groups, for example, experiencing poorer access to supportive care.

SOCIAL CAPITAL

Sources of social support can be divided into two main categories: *formal* – professionals, paid helpers – and *informal* – family, friends, neighbours, community groups and so on. It is important to remember that professionals are not the main source of social support, except for very isolated people and this is reflected in the different findings of some recent studies on social support for women becoming mothers. On the whole, studies which specifically targeted *extra* support on women who lacked good levels of informal support, or who had particular needs for support, have tended to show greater positive impact. Some of these studies are outlined in sections to follow.

The evidence that different social settings or communities may have very different levels and types of resources for social support is reflected in the term *social capital* which is being used increasingly in social policy. It refers to the kinds of resources that are essential underpinnings of social and community life, which could be as broad as community organizations, public facilities and viable social networks. The use of the word capital draws on the notion that social relationships can be regarded as a kind of resource, without which people and communities are unable to function effectively and achieve wellbeing. It can be said to represent an attempt to move away from more individualized to more socially-based approaches to health. As the importance of social capital for wellbeing has been acknowledged, health policies have begun to take account of the need to build or support resources more effectively within communities. This can be found in the Sure Start programme developed in the UK in the 1990s, which aimed to tackle the roots of life-long inequalities by working with new parents. Sure Start schemes, which are mainly located in areas of social deprivation but available to all families within them, focus on the transition to parenthood with antenatal and postnatal support groups, activities and resources of various types. Their philosophies tend to integrate the psychological, the social and the cultural aspects of becoming parents, using a broadly health promotional approach. Typically schemes may include 'parent to be' clubs, which emphasize the transition aspects of pregnancy and birth, and take a broader view than the hospital based antenatal education which tends to focus on the birth, rather than parenthood, and on skills and knowledge, rather than on feelings and experience. They also include a range of schemes to promote social links and health, such as 'weaning clubs', 'breastfeeding cafes', and 'baby talk' groups. Projects of this type also offer opportunities for midwives to return to working in a more community-based context, and in a more inter-disciplinary approach, with others such as maternity support workers, health visitors, psychologists, social workers and nursery workers.

ANTENATAL PREPARATION FOR PARENTHOOD

In traditional societies, preparation for parenthood was managed less formally, with most women receiving information, advice and help from female kin and neighbours, but as social ties have become more diffuse, women increasingly need to rely on midwives and other professionals for such preparation. Additionally, as family sizes have become smaller, many women have less experiential knowledge, and come to rely instead on more theoretical forms, whether these are obtained from informal sources such as the media or formal ones such as professionals and antenatal classes. In the early 20th century in the UK and in many other societies, midwives roles were mainly focused on birth and postnatal care. Antenatal care and provision of classes were developed in response to public concerns about the 'quality' of the population, suggesting that right from the start antenatal education may have been influenced by public health concerns, rather than the concerns of women themselves, as they approached motherhood. Nolan argues that

> ... because the antenatal education most women receive is a product of the system which effectively deprived women of freedom and choice in childbirth, its agenda has generally been narrow, conformist, patronizing and disempowering. There have been many studies of its effectiveness, but few which have been able to report positively on its outcomes.
>
> Nolan 1997, p. 1200

Nolan argues that this lack of effectiveness stems from its history as an artificial construct, attempting to replace the information and emotional insights traditionally passed on informally. She also notes that attendance at antenatal classes is largely confined to middle class, ethnic majority women in the UK, who may be more at ease with professional advice.

Several commentators have also pointed out that risk assessment in pregnancy has relied overwhelmingly on biomedical indicators, which are largely untested, and give little or no weight to psycho-social risk factors (Lane 1995, Oakley

1992). In antenatal care generally, it seems that there is a lack of clarity regarding the purpose of care, the care provided varies greatly between different countries and some researchers have questioned the value of the standard regime of care in the UK (Hall et al 1980). Sikorski and colleagues' subsequent study of a reduced schedule of antenatal care showed that although clinical safety was not compromised, satisfaction with care was decreased, suggesting that many women are seeking more from maternity care than birth safety alone (Sikorski et al 1996). Hirst and colleagues (1998) argue that reassurance is a major attribute which women seek from maternity care; a need which is not always met, since health checks can cause anxiety as well as reassurance and the content of care, for example, communication or support versus routine checks, has not been given sufficient consideration.

In an early overview of trials of social support during pregnancy, Elbourne and colleagues (Elbourne et al 1989) found that provision of additional support by maternity services generally reduced anxiety, psychological and physical morbidity and, in most cases, increased satisfaction with care. The fourteen trials included social and psychological support as the main focus or as one objective. They involved a range of forms of support, from provision of information to more comprehensive support packages including home visits. The interventions were also applied to a range of women, including minority ethnic women, socially disadvantaged women and women with high obstetric risk status. The overview concluded that social support may have a range of positive effects, which cluster around feelings (for example, confidence, nervousness, fear or positive feelings regarding birth), communication, satisfaction with care and sense of control.

A later systematic review of trials of social support in high-risk pregnancies (Hodnett & Fredericks 2004) indicates that clinical benefits found in such trials have been marginal, apart from a reduced risk of caesarean section, but that women may have reduced anxiety, be better able to access other support at home and feel better about their care. The reviewers point out that such interventions may not be adequate to counter the

well researched effects of poverty and social disadvantage, but they recommend that further research be conducted on the psychosocial effects since trials which have shown benefits of antenatal support have been those which look at outcomes such as psychological health or satisfaction of the mother, or less easily measurable aspects of infant health. Studies have included a range of types and levels of support, offered by different people, some focusing only on particular aspects of support, such as information, while others are broader. Bearing in mind the distinction drawn between perceived and received support, trials have not always sought the perceptions of the mothers involved about whether the care or intervention offered was considered as supportive. This is particularly the case where trials involve educational interventions, which may be perceived as supportive by professionals but not by service users themselves.

Educational interventions vary widely in approach and it has been suggested that they are often about educating women to accept services rather than 'empowering' or supporting them (Gagnon 2004). The heavy reliance on educational programmes in some trials which showed little effect of social support indicate the importance of clarifying what is being offered to participants in a study. On the whole, then, although there are good reasons to expect that antenatal preparation should be beneficial for women, there is little direct research evidence to show whether it is effective in practice. Studies can be difficult to interpret, since often women with fewer problems have been the most likely to attend such classes, and women who need the most help may find that antenatal preparation is difficult to access, or does not meet their needs. The amount and type of preparation available also varies widely across different societies and some forms of preparation may be far more effective than others.

It can be difficult to unpick from different studies which aspects of support or care are beneficial, and for whom. Nonetheless, at a time when many midwives do not have the time and resources they would like to devote to supporting women, it is important to weigh up what is most likely to be effective, using research evidence and taking into account the nature and needs of their local communities. In a recent systematic review of antenatal preparation for the Cochrane Library, only five trials were found which met the Cochrane quality criteria and these gave varied findings (Gagnon 2004). The studies were small, and the type of education, the settings, the focus (for example, on birth per se or more broadly on becoming a parent) and outcomes measured varied widely. Very little evidence of impact was found overall. One reason for the difficulty in conducting randomized controlled trials in this area, however, was lack of willingness to be randomized, since most women who are contacted do not wish to be denied access to antenatal preparation. Pregnant women perceive a need for antenatal preparation, even if that need is not always met effectively.

Some non-experimental studies of alternative approaches to preparation have shown more positive results. These tend to emphasize parental participation, using less didactic educational approaches, and to include social and psychological aspects of the transition (Parr 1998, Renkert & Nutbeam 2001, Schmied et al 2002).

A POSITIVE EXPERIENCE OF BIRTH

Support during labour and birth is not just about helping women to cope well with birth itself, since there is good evidence that women's experience of birth may affect her emotional wellbeing and how she copes with the wider transition of becoming a parent (Percival 1990). Green et al's large scale psychological studies, for example, have shown that women having a sense of control and feeling they had a say in what happens to them, are likely to cope better, even if they need medical interventions (Green & Baston 2003). Factors such as high levels of intervention during labour, assisted delivery and caesarean birth have been associated with postnatal depression, as have dissatisfaction with labour and birth, having no say in decisions and the presence of unwanted people at the birth (Brown et al 1994). It may well be that it is not the type of birth but how the woman feels about such issues and how much of a say she has in controlling her environment and experience that are the critical factors. In a US study of women's views about nursing support during labour, the most helpful behaviours identified included: feeling

cared about as an individual and treated with respect, praise, staff appearing calm and confident and assistance with breathing and relaxing. The study used an instrument listing 25 potentially supportive behaviours, which a group of four nurse-midwives were asked to categorize as emotional, information or tangible support (Bryanton et al 1994). The women regarded all the categories as important but behaviours categorized as emotional support were perceived as the most helpful by the women. The authors note that these findings were highly consistent with those of previous studies of women's views of support, even when different methods, samples and terminology were used.

A series of trials systematically reviewed by Hodnett and colleagues, showed that the continuing presence of a support person, normally female, lay or professional, could make significant differences not only to labour interventions and outcomes, but also to postnatal wellbeing (Hodnett 2004). Such differences were most marked for women who lacked such support – either personally or owing to the nature of the birth environment. They were also found in studies where the main support person was not a professional – usually a 'doula', a lay women with personal experience of birth and only basic training. The results of the trials lend support to the many smaller and qualitative studies which have explored women's experiences of childbirth, what they find helpful and why. Overall, there is very strong evidence to support the widespread view in midwifery that the nature and quality of support given to birthing women is important – and as we have discussed, the concept of 'being with' the birthing women, and her family, is at the heart of midwifery.

POSTNATAL CARE AND SUPPORT

Postnatal care has been described as the 'Cinderella' of maternity services (Glazener et al 1995). As with antenatal care, what support is offered does vary widely between different countries and there is evidence to suggest not all forms of support are effective in making a positive difference to women and families (Morrell et al 2000). Informal sources of support – from family and community may not be available for new parents and with decreasing family sizes they also lack experiential knowledge and confidence in parenting. Before regulated midwifery or state maternity systems, most cultures had some form of customary post-natal support – often from a midwife, 'handy-woman' or 'monthly nurse' (Wilson 1995). This form of traditional support has continued in the Netherlands, where home birth remains common, with the provision of maternity aides who offer practical support free for one week for families in their home (De Vries et al 2001).

Recent developments in maternity services, despite policies to promote women-centred care, have tended to reduce the levels of postnatal care available to women in the UK. This section dis-cusses the evidence on reducing length of hospital stay, the introduction of selective postnatal home visiting by midwives, as well as the evidence on the quality of care that is given by midwives, in hospital and at home.

The biomedical approach to birth, and a ten-dency to view the needs or interests of mother and infant as separate has been reflected in increasing investment in technologies of pregnancy and birth and a reduction in hospital provision for postnatal care of mothers and babies. In a study of the support needs of 347 mothers, from 36 weeks of pregnancy to 6 weeks postnatally, Ball (1994) noted the historical role of midwives as female companions to mothers, but emphasized that maternity services have the capacity to undermine as well as to enhance support. For example, the experience of hospitalization, in itself, may be stressful to women 'as it causes them to relinquish control of their patterns of daily living' (Ball 1994, p. 2) so that it is important for service providers to avoid creating additional stress. The study looked at the impact of hospital practices on mothers' experiences, noting that they often worked against the provision of social support. For example, practices and routines which led to unnecessary separation of mother and baby soon after birth. Ironically, now that maternal–infant bonding has been recognized as an issue by health professionals, these have often been replaced by a practice of 'rooming in' coupled with loss of prac-tical support. She noted fragmentation of care, task rather than person based work and routines, didactic style when giving help or advice, care focused mainly on physical examination of the mother and feeding of the baby, and observed inadequacies in support for feeding as common aspects of maternity care which are not sup-portive for women. She also noted a mismatch between midwives' summing up of women's emotional states and their more specific com-ments, for example, on the numbers of women who had been crying or showing sleep or appetite disturbances – suggesting that they either see this as 'normal' or give low priority to emotional states.

Factor analysis in her study showed that emo-tional wellbeing and satisfaction with mother-hood were associated with antecedent factors (such as aspects of the woman's experience, per-sonality and background), other stress factors and self-confidence on return home. Women's experi-ences of other stress factors were strongly influ-enced by postnatal care practices, the key factors being feelings at the time of birth, self-image in feeding the baby in hospital and conflicting advice or lack of rest in hospital. A later national survey by the Audit Commission (Garcia at al 1998) con-firmed the lack of postnatal support felt by some women. Within a context of generally quite high levels of expressed satisfaction with maternity services, women were least likely to be satisfied with postnatal care. Among the problems noted were lack of rest, inconsistent advice, fragmenta-tion of care and busy, rushed staff. Similarly, in an ethnographic study of support for breastfeeding in the hospital setting in the UK, Dykes found that the help offered to women was limited, and often not experienced as helpful (Dykes 2004). This study also questioned the benefits of the Baby Friendly Initiative in a Western setting where rooming-in and short hospital stay was already the norm. It appeared from her observations and women's accounts that in an institutional environ-ment, the letter rather than the spirit of the initia-tive was being followed, with midwives following a checklist approach in an attempt to meet the 'ten steps' towards Baby Friendly status (UNICEF 1991). For such reasons, a number of researchers have raised the question of whether maternity units should, instead, be focusing on a 'mother friendly' approach (Downe 2002).

With the reduction in postnatal hospital length of stay in recent years, there is some evidence that the expectation of a period of rest and recovery following birth has also declined. In a US study Ruchala and Halstead (1994) found that a predominantly middle class group of white women, with partners, (i.e. not at high risk for lack of social support) were suffering considerable symptoms of fatigue, unhappiness and incongruence of experience with expectations. The mothers described physical, psychological and social difficulties in recovery and adjustment after birth, and these were stronger in first time mothers. Although women were able to call on their mothers and partners for primary sources of support, this was generally for limited periods, and the women were affected by feelings that they should be able to cope normally within a short period after birth. Postnatal home visits by health professionals are not normally provided in the US, in contrast to the UK, where women expect home visits by midwives, and to the Netherlands, where maternity aides are also available to provide practical support. The authors suggest that more postnatal care is needed but point out that much of what the women needed did not require professional support per se, but may not be available from family, friends or community.

In a qualitative study of young, working class mothers experiences of postnatal care and support for feeding, Hodinott and Pill (1999) described the cycle of loss of confidence which often takes place for new mothers. Lack of practical and moral support, or support given in an undermining manner, led to feelings of not coping and loss of confidence, precipitating a change in feeding method. She drew on the anthropological concept of embodied, as opposed to theoretical, knowledge to describe the ways in which social change had made women more vulnerable to inadequacies or inconsistencies in the provision of professional advice or support. Young women with direct personal experience of contact with new born babies held more embodied knowledge and so were less vulnerable to loss of confidence. Similarly, women valued an apprenticeship style of personal support and being given adequate information to help them make their own decisions, rather than direct advice.

In a survey and interview study with women receiving caseload midwifery or conventional care in the UK, women described considerable gaps in support during their postnatal hospital stay, which involved some hospital midwives as being unavailable in a literal sense – too busy – and in a metaphorical sense, of being off-hand or uninterested or unsympathetic, and a tendency when giving help or advice to undermine rather than enhance women's self confidence (Beake et al 2005). Only about half of women reported they had received all the help they needed, or attention from the staff when they needed it and fewer than this felt they had received enough rest. Views of postnatal care at home were more positive, although some women receiving conventional care complained of receiving conflicting advice from different midwives, and a number of women would have preferred visits over a longer period than the 10 day UK norm for postnatal care. Just over half of the women received support at home from their mother, and from 16–25% received support from sisters, friends and/or mothers in law (Beake et al 2001).

As the length of postnatal hospital stay and level of midwife provided postnatal support have declined in the UK in recent years, several trials have examined the effects of maternity support workers, or the provision of additional postnatal support. Such trials are fraught with similar difficulties to those of other forms of support – diversity of intervention and clients, lack of clarity on the nature and quality of the support intervention and lack of data on what the clients perceived as helpful. A study of postnatal support workers by Morrell and colleagues (2000) even found that despite being perceived as helpful, the intervention did not make a difference to women's health and could even undermine women's wellbeing in the longer term. Their discussion suggested that this may occur through delaying or undermining women's utilization of informal sources of support, so that resources are not there when the additional support is withdrawn. Studies which have targeted additional support to women identified as lacking the usual informal sources such as family, and support from partners, have tended to show more positive results.

In a recent trial of a woman-centred model of postnatal care, MacArthur and colleagues (2002) found positive benefits for women, including better postnatal depression screening scores. The positive outcomes found here may perhaps be attributable to a model which enabled midwives to tailor care to the needs of each woman and family, with the potential for extended periods of contact. Similarly, small qualitative studies of postnatal and infant feeding support which is hands-on, geared closely to women's expressed needs, and informed by philosophies of building confidence and building on the woman's background and knowledge, have tended to suggest benefits (Beake et al 2005b, Dykes 2003).

Such approaches have parallels with theories of education which emphasize that the process as well as content of education are important, and that non-didactic, adult centred models are more appropriate for health care (Barrows & Tamblyn 1980). This highlights that what a midwife does is not the only important issue – how she does it is equally so. Busy clinics and rapid postnatal visits, focused on routine checks and getting through the work are not conducive to a learner-centred model of education. There are some excellent case studies of ways in which midwives, often in collaboration with others, such as Sure Start Health Visitors, have been able to develop different models for preparing and supporting women and families. One such is the approach to ante- and postnatal groups of the Albany Midwifery Practice (Sandall et al 2001). Groups facilitated by the midwives are run from the Practice's community base, which is effective in involving women from all sections of a diverse and deprived inner-city community. They actively involve women who have given birth recently, and encourage women to participate, to share experience and to consider and draw on non-professional resources for support. The potential value of such an approach is pointed to by the high rates of breastfeeding found in the Practice.

RECOGNIZING AND RESPONDING TO DISTRESS AND DEPRESSION

Unhappiness, tiredness and feelings of stress or distress are common following childbirth – estimated to affect from about 50% to 80% of women (Dennis & Creedy 2004). A significant minority of women will experience such feelings to a degree which can be categorized as depression, and midwives have an important role in recognizing and responding to this (Wheatley 1998). Whether unhappiness after birth is perceived as normal or

as pathological, it is inherently undesirable for women to suffer such symptoms in response to what they hope will be a happy and fulfilling experience (Miller 2002).

The lower rates of depressive symptoms identified in some maternity intervention studies (Macarthur et al 2002, Wolman et al 1993) show that it is possible for midwives to make a difference. However, in their systematic review of trials of interventions aimed to prevent postnatal depression, Dennis and Creedy (2004) found similarly mixed results to those for overviews of research on ante- and postnatal support. While concluding that 'overall psychosocial interventions do not reduce the numbers of women who develop postpartum depression', they identified that provision of intensive, professionally-based postpartum support can be helpful, based on the trial of a flexible, individualized approach cited above (Macarthur et al 2002).

The causes of postnatal depression are unclear, and debate remains about the relative importance of physical, psychological and social factors, but it is widely agreed that it is complex and multifactorial, so that help with any potential factor may make a difference. Common risk factors include high levels of life stress combined with low levels of support, but depression may also be influenced by early life experiences. This may include women's own experiences of being mothered, an issue which is discussed in more depth in Chapter 2. Women with prior experience of depression, including depression in pregnancy, are also known to be more vulnerable to postnatal depression (Gotlib et al 1991, O'Hara et al 1991, Thorpe et al 1992). Conversely, new mothers with appropriate amounts of situation-specific support are less depressed, anxious, angry and/or fatigued than other mothers (Gottlieb & Mendelsom 1995). Support from the husband or partner is particularly valuable (Demyttenaere et al 1995, Nicholson 1990, Percival 1990, Thorpe et al 1992). Midwives have an important role in identifying problems and referring women for more specialist help when needed. The Edinburgh Postnatal Depression Scale is the most widely validated and used screening tool, and it is used routinely by a number of midwives and health visitors to identify symptoms which may indicate depression. Scores (EPDS) over a certain level should then be followed up by specialist clinical interview (Cox & Holden 1994). The EPDS has been found to be acceptable to women, and it may form a useful prompt for discussion and offering more support to women who may often be reluctant to ask for help (Harrison et al 1995). Miller has argued, however, that some level of postnatal distress is very common, and concerns about being judged as having a mental health problem may deter women with such symptoms from confiding in midwives or health visitors. She recommends that rather than automatically turning to routine screening tools, professionals should explore with women how they are feeling, and reassure them that some level of depressive symptoms is normal (in the sense of being common, rather than unimportant or something to be ignored) (Miller 2002). Various specialist approaches have been found to be helpful for women with depression, including counselling, psychotherapeutic approaches, peer support, and cognitive behavioural therapy (Dennis & Creedy 2004). As noted, the importance of this response has been underlined by the UK's CEMACH reports and National Service Framework for Children. There is also considerable evidence as to the effects of maternal depression on the wellbeing and development of infants, with a large number of studies identifying enduring problems such as impaired cognitive and language development, behavioural problems and insecure attachment (Beck 1995). Liaison with other practitioners, such as health visitors and general practitioners, has also been highlighted as important to ensure women get the support they need.

CONCLUSION

In conclusion, midwives have a major role in empowering parents during the transition to parenthood by making them aware that they are normal people who are going through a time of great change in their lives. Moreover, they need to know that most parents experience the same changes and challenges. Women and men also need to know that it is a positive thing to break the conspiracy of silence that surrounds images of parenthood. Breaking this conspiracy of silence means that parents can talk about the difficulties

they are experiencing; they can talk about their need for extra support; and they do not have to pretend that they are managing alone for fear that others will believe they are a 'bad' or 'abnormal' family. Parents need to be able to ask for help without the spectre of the 'perfect mother' hanging over them. Midwives can tell parents that being able to ask for support from either family, friends or professionals is a positive move, one meaning that they are good parents who want to be even better.

We have discussed the importance of childbirth as a physiological, social and cultural transition, and the need for appropriate care which acknowledges and supports this. Research evidence suggests that good quality, responsive midwifery care is highly valued by women, and if designed and targeted appropriately around women's, families' and communities' needs, can make a positive difference. We have also discussed, however, how not all forms of care are perceived by women or demonstrated by research to be helpful. Unfortunately, despite many positive developments in maternity care, much of existing care, particularly postnatal care provided from a hospital base, has been found to be less than satisfactory. Midwives, therefore, need to work towards changes in the system of care provision which would facilitate them in providing care which is satisfying for themselves and the women and communities they care for. This time of transition is an important point of contact, when women are experiencing enormous changes, and keen to receive support and information in order to manage it well, but it is still a limited time within the life course, and there will always be limitations to what midwives can achieve. While midwives cannot change the world, or indeed change women's life circumstances and history, they are working with women at what in many ways can be a turning point. One woman, speaking about the value of support from 'her midwife' simply said: 'you had that person you knew you could turn to all the time' (McCourt & Pearce 2000).

POINTERS FOR PRACTICE

Becoming a parent:

- Childbirth is always a social and cultural event as well as a personal matter.

- It is a time of transition to the new roles and responsibility of parenting and professionals may support or disturb this transition.
- Parenting is often romanticized and it is important to break the conspiracy that supports unrealistic views of parenting.

- Biomedical and fragmented production line approaches of hospital-based care are harmful and alternative approaches are required.
- Parents need to be supported in order to be effective.

References

Abraham L 2004 The perfect little bump. New York Times. Online. Available: http://www.newyorkmetro.com/nymetro/health/features/9909/ accessed December 2005

Alexander M, Higgins T 1993 Emotional trade-offs of becoming a parent: how social roles influence self-discrepancy effects. Journal of Personality and Social Psychology 65(6): 1259–1269

Ball J 1994 Reactions to motherhood: the role of postnatal care. Cambridge University Press, Cambridge

Barclay L, Everitt L, Rogan F, Schmied V, Wyllie A 1997 Becoming a mother – an analysis of women's experience of early motherhood. Journal of Advanced Nursing 25: 719–728

Barrows H, Tamblyn R 1980 Problem Based Learning: an approach to Medical Education. Springer, New York

Beake S, McCourt C, Bick D E 2005a Women's views of hospital and community-based postnatal care: the good, the bad and the indifferent. Evidence-based Midwifery 3(2): 80–86

Beake S, McCourt C, Rowan C 2005b Evaluation of the role of an infant feeding support worker in the community to support breastfeeding in disadvantaged women. Maternal & Child Nutrition 1(1): 32–43

Beake S, Page L, McCourt C 2001 Report on the follow-up evaluation of one-to-one midwifery. TVU, London

Beck C T 1995 The effects of postpartum depression on maternal–infant interaction: a meta-analysis. Nursing Research 44(5): 298–304

Belsky J, Lang M E, Rovine M 1985 Stability and change in marriage across the transition to parenthood – a second study. Journal of Marriage and the Family 47(4): 855–865

Belsky J, Rovine M 1990 Patterns of marital change across the transition to parenthood: pregnancy to three years postpartum. Journal of Marriage and the Family 52: 5–19

Benedeck T 1959 Parenthood as a developmental phase. Journal of the American Psychoanalytic Association 7: 389–417

Berry S J 1988 The role of maternal expectations and infant characteristics in the transition to parenthood. Dissertation Abstracts International 48(12-B, Part 1): 3669

Bick D E, MacArthur C 1995 The extent, severity and effect of health problems after childbirth. British Journal of Midwifery 3(27):31

Blum M E 1981 The relationship of marital satisfaction, sex role attitudes, and psychological intervention in prepared delivery classes to the transition to parenthood: a short term longitudinal study of middle-income couples. Dissertation Abstracts International 42(5-B): 2094–2095

Boles A J 1985 Predictors and correlates of marital satisfaction during the transition to parenthood. Dissertation Abstracts International 46(2-B): 634

Brazelton T B 1962 Crying in infancy. Pediatrics 29: 579–588

Brown S, Lumley J, Small R, Astbury J 1994 Missing voices: the experience of motherhood. Oxford University Press, Oxford

Bryanton J, Fraser-Davey H, Sullivan P 1994 Women's perceptions of nursing support during labor. Journal of Obstetric, Gynecologic, and Neonatal Nursing 23(8):638–644

CEMACH 2004 Why mothers die. Confidential enquiry into maternal and child health. RCOG, London

Chodorow N 1978 The reproduction of mothering: psychoanalysis and the sociology of gender. University of California Press, London

Cohen S, McKay G 1983 Social support, stress and the buffering hypothesis: A theoretical analysis. In: Baum A, Singer J E, Taylor S (eds) Handbook of psychology and health, Volume 4. Erlbaum, Hillsdale, NJ

Cox J, Holden J (eds) 1994 Perinatal psychiatry. Use and misuse of the Edinburgh postnatal depression scale. Gaskell (Royal College of Psychiatrists), London

Crouch M, Manderson L 1993 New motherhood. Cultural and personal transitions. Gordon & Breach, Camberwell, Australia

Davis-Floyd R 1994 The ritual of hospital birth in America. In: Spradley J P, McCurdey D W Conformity and conflict. Readings in cultural anthropology. Harper-Collins, New York

Demyttenaere K, Lenaerts H, Nijs P, Van Assche F A 1995 Individual coping style and psychological attitudes during pregnancy predict depression levels during pregnancy and during postpartum. Acta Psychiatrica Scandinavica 91: 95–102

Dennis C L, Creedy D 2004 Psychosocial and psychological interventions for preventing postpartum depression. The Cochrane Database of Systematic Reviews 2004, Issue 4. Art. No.: CD001134.pub2. DOI: 10.1002/14651858.CD001134.pub2

Department of Health. National service framework for children, young people and maternity services 2004. Online. Access: http://www.dh.gov.uk/PublicationsAndStatistics/Publications/PublicationsPolicyAndGuidance/PublicationsPolicyAndGuidanceArticle/fs/en?CONTENT_ID=4089113&chk=OK6NXz accessed May 2005

Deutsch F M, Ruble D N, Fleming A, Brooks-Gunn J 1988 Information-seeking and maternal self-definition during the transition to motherhood. Journal of Personality and Social Psychology 55(3): 420–431

Deutsch H 1944 The psychology of women, vol. 1. Grune & Stratton, New York

DeVries R, Benoit C, Teijlingen van E, Wrede S (eds) 2001 Birth by design: pregnancy, midwifery care and midwifery in North America and Europe. Routledge, New York

Dohrenwend B, Krasnoff L, Askenasy A, Dohrenwend B 1978 Exemplification of a method for scaling life events. Journal of Health and Social Behavior 19: 205–229

Douglas M 1966 Purity and danger: an analysis of concepts of pollution and taboo. Routledge & Kegan Paul, London

Downe S 2002 First normal birth research conference, post conference report. University of Central Lancashire, Preston, Lancs.

Dyer E D 1963 Parenthood as crisis: a restudy. Marriage and Family Living 25: 196–201

Dykes F 2003 Infant feeding initiative. A report evaluating the breastfeeding practice projects 1999–2002. Department of Health, London. Online. Available: www.doh.gov.uk/infantfeeding accessed May 2005

Dykes F 2004 Feeling the pressure – coping with chaos: breastfeeding at the end of the medical production line. PhD, University of Sheffield

Edgar D 1993 Parents at the core of family life. Family Matters 36: 2–3

Elbourne D, Oakley A, Chalmers I 1989 Social and psychological support during pregnancy. In: Chalmers I, Enkin M, Keirse M, (eds) Effective care in pregnancy and childbirth. Oxford University Press, Oxford, p 221–235

Elliott S A, Watson J P, Brough D I 1985 Transition to parenthood by British couples. Journal of Reproductive and Infant Psychology 3(1): 28–39

Frommer E A, O'Shea G 1973 The importance of childhood experience in relation to problems of marriage and family building. British Journal of Psychiatry 123: 157

Gagnon, A J Individual or group antenatal education for childbirth/parenthood. [Systematic Review] Cochrane Pregnancy and Childbirth Group Cochrane Database of Systematic Reviews. 4, 2004

Garcia J, Redshaw M, Fitzsimons B, Keene J 1998 First class delivery: a national survey of women's views of maternity care. Abingdon, Oxon, Audit Commission/National Perinatal Epidemiology Unit

Gennep A Van 1960 The rites of passage. Routledge & Kegan Paul, London

Gjerdingen D K, Fontaine P 1991 Family-centered postpartum care. Family Medicine 23: 189–193

Glazener C, Abdalla M, Stroud P, Templeton A, Russell I, 1995 Postnatal maternal morbidity: extent, causes, prevention and treatment. British Journal of Obstetrics and Gynaecology 102:282–287

Gluckman M (ed.) 1962 Essays on the ritual of social relations. Manchester University Press, Manchester

Goffman E 1968 Asylums. Essays on the social situation of mental patients and other inmates. Penguin, Harmondsworth

Gotlib I, Whiffen V, Wallace P, Mount J 1991 A prospective investigation of postpartum depression: factors involved in onset and recovery. Journal of Abnormal Psychology 100: 122–132

Gottlieb L N, Mendelsom M J 1995 Mothers' moods and social support when a second child is born. Maternal–Child Nursing Journal 23(1): 3–14

Grace J T 1993 Mothers' self-reports of parenthood across the first 6 months postpartum. Research in Nursing and Health 16(6): 431–439

Green J M, Baston H A, 2003 Feeling in control during labour: concepts, correlates and consequences. Birth 30(4): 235–247

Green J M, Coupland V A Kitzinger J V 1998 Great expectations: a prospective study of women's expectations and experiences of childbirth. 2nd edn. Books for Midwives, Hale, Cheshire

Hall M, Chng P, McGillivray I 1980 Is routine antenatal care worthwhile? Lancet ii:78–80

Halman L J, Oakley D, Lederman R 1995 Adaptation to pregnancy and motherhood among subfecund and fecund primiparous women. Maternal–Child Nursing Journal 23(3): 90–100

Handler H, Raube K et al 1996 Women's satisfaction with prenatal care settings: a focus group study. Birth 23(1): 31–37

Harper-Bulman K, McCourt C 2002 Somali refugee women's views and experiences of maternity care in west London. Critical Public Health 12(4): 365–380

Harrison M J, Neufeld A, Kushner K 1995 Women in transition: access and barriers to social support. Journal of Advanced Nursing 21(5): 858–864

Helman C 1994 Culture, health and illness. Butterworth-Heinemann, Oxford

Hill R 1949 Families under stress. Harper, New York

Hirst J, Hewison J, Dowswell T, Baslington H, Warrilow J 1998 Antenatal care: what do women want? In: Clement S (ed.) Psychological perspectives on pregnancy and childbirth. Churchill Livingstone, Edinburgh

Hobbs D F 1968 Transition to parenthood: a replication and an extension. Journal of Marriage and the Family 30(3): 413–417

Hodinott P, Pill R 1999 Qualitative study of decisions about infant feeding among women in east end of London. BMJ, Jan 318: 30–34

Hodnett E D 2004 Caregiver support for women during childbirth. [Systematic Review] Cochrane Pregnancy and Childbirth Group Cochrane Database of Systematic Reviews. 4, 2004

Hodnett E D, Fredericks S 2004 Support during pregnancy for women at increased risk of low birthweight babies. [Systematic Review] Cochrane Pregnancy and Childbirth Group Cochrane Database of Systematic Reviews. 4, 2004

Holmes T, Rahe R H 1967 The social readjustment rating scale. Journal of Psychosomatic Research 11: 213–218

Hunt S, Symonds S 1995 The social meanings of midwifery. Journal of Advanced Nursing 23(1): 70–75

Jordan B 1993 Birth in four cultures. A crosscultural investigation of childbirth in Yucatan, Holland, Sweden and the United States. Waveland Press, Illinois

Kempe M 1985 The book of Margery Kempe. Translated by BA Windeatt. Penguin Classics, Harmondsworth. Original manuscript 15th century

Kirkham M 1989 Midwives and information-giving in labour. In: Robinson S, Thomson A, (eds) Midwives, research and childbirth. Chapman & Hall, London

Kitzinger S 1989 Childbirth and society. In: Chalmers I, Enkin M, Keirse M (eds) Effective care in pregnancy and childbirth. Oxford University Press, Oxford

Lane K 1995 The medical model of the body as a site of risk. In: Gabe J. (ed.) Medicine, health and risk. Sociological approaches. Blackwell, Oxford

LaRossa R, LaRossa M M 1981 Transition to parenthood: how infants change families. Sage, Beverley Hills

Laslett A, Brown S, Lumley J 1997 Women's views of different models of antenatal care in Victoria, Australia. Birth 24(2):81–89

LeMasters E 1957 Parenthood as crisis. Marriage and Family Living 19: 352–355

Levitt M, Coffman S, Guacci-Franco N, Loveless S 1993 Social support and relationship change after childbirth: an expectancy model. Health Care Women Int. 14(6):503–512

Levy-Shiff R 1994 Individual and contextual correlates of marital change across the transition to parenthood. Developmental Psychology 30(4): 591–601

Lewis J 1990 Mothers and maternity policies in the twentieth century. In: Garcia J et al (eds) The politics of maternity care. Clarendon Press, Oxford

MacArthur C, Winter H R, Bick D E et al 2003 Effects of redesigned community postnatal care on womens' health 4 months after birth: a cluster randomised controlled trial. Lancet 359: 378–385

MacDermid S, Huston T, McHale S 1990 Changes in marriage associated with the transition to parenthood: individual differences as a function of sex role attitudes and changes in the division of household labor. Journal of Marriage and the Family 52: 475–486

Mander R 2001 Supportive care and midwifery. Blackwell, Oxford

Marks M, Lovestone S 1995 The role of the father in parental postnatal mental health. British Journal of Medical Psychology 68: 157–168

Marris P 1974 Loss and change. Routledge & Kegan Paul, London

McCourt C 2003 Social support. In: Squire C (ed.) The social context of midwifery. Radcliffe Medical, Oxford

McCourt C, Page L, Hewison J, Vail A 1998 Evaluation of One-to-One midwifery: women's responses to care. Birth 25(2): 73–80

McCourt C, Pearce A 2000 Does continuity of carer matter to women from minority ethnic groups? Midwifery 16:145–154

Mercer R T 1981 Factors impacting on the maternal role: the first year of motherhood. In: Lederman R P (ed.) Perinatal parental behavior: nursing research and implications for newborn health. Alan R Liss, New York

Mercer R T 1986 Predictors of maternal role attainment at one year postbirth. Western Journal of Nursing Research 8(1): 9–32

Miller T 2002 Adapting to motherhood: care in the postnatal period. Community Practitioner 75(1): 16–18

MORI 1993 A survey of women's views of the maternity services. Maternity services research study. Department of Health, London

Morrell C J, Spiby H, Stewart P, Walters S 2000 Costs and benefits of community postnatal support workers: a randomised controlled trial. (HTA) Health Technology Assessment Programme, Department of Health, UK) 4 (6)

Murray-Parkes C 1971 Psycho-social transitions. A field for study. Social Science and Medicine 5: 101–115

Newell R 2004 The thanksgiving of women after childbirth. A blessing in disguise? Unpublished PhD, University of Dundee

Nicolson P 1990 Understanding postnatal depression: a mother-centred approach. Journal of Advanced Nursing 15: 689–695

Nolan M 1997 Antenatal education – where next? Journal Of Advanced Nursing 25(6): 1198–1204

O'Hara M, Schlechte J, Lewis D, Varner M 1991 Controlled prospective study of postpartum mood disorders: psychological, environmental, and hormonal variables. Journal of Abnormal Psychology 100: 63–73

Oakley A 1979 From here to maternity: becoming a mother. Penguin, Harmondsworth

Oakley A 1980 Women confined: towards a sociology of childbirth. Martin Robertson, Oxford

Oakley A 1992 Social support and motherhood. The natural history of a research project. Blackwell, Oxford

Osofsky H J, Osofsky J D 1983 Adaptation to pregnancy and new parenthood. In: Dennerstein L, Burrows G D (eds) Handbook of psychosomatic obstetrics and gynecology. Elsevier Biomedical, Amsterdam

Ozaki M M 1986 Marital role performance during the transition to parenthood. Dissertation Abstracts International 47(2-B): 801

Parr M 1998 Parent education. A new approach to parent education. [Journal Article. Research] British Journal of Midwifery 6(3): 160–165

Parsons T 1951 The social system. Free Press, New York

Percival P 1990 The relationship between perceived nursing care and maternal adjustment for primiparae during the transition to motherhood. Unpublished Doctoral dissertation, Curtin University of Technology, Western Australia

Reid M, Garcia J 1989 Women's views of care during pregnancy and childbirth. In: Chalmers I, Enkin M, Keirse M (eds) Effective care in pregnancy and childbirth. Open University Press, Oxford

Renkert S, Nutbeam D 2001 Opportunities to improve maternal health literacy through antenatal education: an exploratory study. Health Promotion International 16(4): 381–388

Rossi A S 1968 Transition to parenthood. Journal of Marriage and the Family 30(1): 26–29

Rubin R 1967a Attainment of the maternal role. Part 1: Processes. Nursing Research 16(3): 237–245

Rubin R 1967b Attainment of the maternal role. Part 2: Models and referents. Nursing Research 16(3): 342–346

Rubin R 1975 Maternal tasks in pregnancy. Maternal–Child Nursing Journal 4(3): 143–153

Ruchala P L, Halstead L 1994 The postpartum experience of low-risk women: a time of adjustment and change. Maternal–Child Nursing Journal 22(3): 83–89

Russell C S 1974 Transition to parenthood: problems and gratifications. Journal of Marriage and the Family 36(2): 294–301

Sandall J, Davies J, Warwick C 2001 Evaluation of the Albany Midwifery Practice. Kings College, London

Schmied V, Myors K, Wills J, Cooke M 2002 Preparing expectant couples for new-parent experiences: a comparison of two models of antenatal education. [Journal Article. Questionnaire/Scale. Research. Tables/Charts] Journal of Perinatal Education. 11(3):20–27

Sethi S 1995 The dialectic in becoming a mother: experiencing a postpartum phenomenon. Scandinavian Journal of Caring Science 9: 235–244

Sikorski J, Wilson J, Clements S, Das S, Smeeton N 1996 The antenatal care project: a randomised controlled trial comparing two schedules of antenatal visits. British Medical Journal 312:546–553

Simkin P 1991 Just another day in a woman's life: women's long term perceptions of their first birth experience. Birth 18(1): 203–210

Smellie W 1756 A treatise on the theory and practice of midwifery. Vol 1. 3rd edn. Wilson and Durham, London. Quoted in Marland H 2004 Dangerous motherhood. Insanity and childbirth in Victoriam Britain. Palgrave Macmillan, Basingstoke

Terry D 1991 Stress, coping and adaptation to new parenthood. Journal of Social and Personal Relationships 8: 527–547

Thorpe K J, Dragonas T, Golding J 1992 The effects of psychosocial factors on the mother's emotional well-being during early parenthood: a cross-cultural study of Britain and Greece. Journal of Reproductive and Infant Psychology 10: 205–217

Tomlinson P S 1987 Spousal differences in marital satisfaction during transition to parenthood. Nursing Research 36(4): 239–243

Tomlinson P S 1996 Marital relationship change in the transition to parenthood: a re-examination as interpreted through transition theory. Journal of Family Nursing 2(3):286–305

Towler J, Bramall J 1986 Midwives in history and society. Croom Helm, Beckenham

Tulman L, Fawcett J 1991 Recovery from childbirth: looking back 6 months after delivery. Health Care for Women International 12: 341–350

UNICEF 1991 Baby Friendly Hospital Initiative. Online. Available: http://www.unicef.org/programme/breastfeeding/baby.htm accessed May 2005

Vincent-Priya J 1992 Birth traditions and modern pregnancy care. Element Books, Dorset

Walker L O, Crain H, Thompson E 1986 Maternal role attainment and identity in the postpartum period: stability and change. Nursing Research 35(2): 68–71

Wheatley S 1998 Psychosocial support in pregnancy. In: Clement S (ed.) Psychological perspectives on pregnancy and childbirth. Edinburgh: Churchill Livingstone

Wilkins R 2000 Poor relations: the paucity of the professional paradigm. In: Kirkham M (ed.) The Midwife–Mother Relationship. Macmillan, Basingstoke

Wilson A 1995 The making of man-midwifery: childbirth in England 1660–1770. Harvard University Press, Massachussets

Wolman W L, Chalmers B, Hofmeyr J, Nikodem V C 1993 Postpartum depressions and companionship in the clinical birth environment: A randomised, controlled study. American Journal of Obstetrics and Gynecology 168(5): 1388–1393

Younger J B 1991 A model of parenting stress. Research in Nursing and Health 14(3): 197–120

Chapter 4

Midwifery partnership: working 'with' women

Sally Pairman

INTRODUCTION

'Midwifery is the partnership between the woman and the midwife' (Guilliland & Pairman, 1994, p. 6). Karen Guilliland and I made this claim in 1994 as we attempted to explore and describe key aspects of relationships between women and midwives that were evolving in the changing context of midwifery practice in New Zealand in the early 1990s. This change in context for midwifery practice resulted from legislation passed in 1990 that reinstated midwifery autonomy and enabled midwives to once again provide care to women throughout the childbirth continuum on their own responsibility. Over the next 15 years the New Zealand maternity system was reshaped to one that is now both woman-centred and midwife-led (Pairman & Guilliland 2003). One result of these changes is that midwives have become more aware of the importance of their relationships with women and have begun to articulate what this means to midwifery practice. New Zealand midwifery has defined the midwife–woman relationship as one of partnership, and further claims that midwifery itself is this partnership relationship (Guilliland & Pairman 1995, New Zealand College of Midwives 1993, 2005). It is relationships between midwives and women that provide the medium for midwifery care and where these relationships are equal and negotiated partnerships there is increased possibility for the empowerment and strengthening of both women and midwives (Guilliland & Pairman 1995, Kirkham 2000a, Pairman 1998).

That midwifery is a relationship between a childbearing woman and a midwife seems obvious. Indeed midwives around the world have always embraced the concept of 'with woman' (that is the meaning of the Anglo Saxon word 'midwyf') to define their role as midwives, and many midwives have for some years now identified the importance and centrality of the midwife–woman relationship to midwifery practice (Donley 1989, Flint 1986, Hunt & Symonds 1995, Kirkham 1996, McCrae & Crute 1991, Page 1993, Pelvin 1990, 1992, Powell Kennedy 1995, Sandall 1995).

Internationally then, the midwife–woman relationship has begun to be recognized as different to the more traditional hierarchical relationships between health professionals and clients where health professionals are seen as 'expert' and clients frequently lack power and control over their care. Midwives have actively worked to equalize relationships between themselves and the women they work with and to shift power to those women so that they can control their own childbirth experiences.

In New Zealand this has led to a new definition of midwifery professionalism – midwifery partnership, that now underpins all aspects of midwifery at the political level, within the professional organization, within midwifery regulation, within midwifery education and, most importantly, within the day-to-day practice of midwives (Guilliland & Pairman 1995, Pairman 1998). In the New Zealand midwifery professional framework 'Partnership' is a philosophical stance, an ethical stance, a standard for practice, a competency for entry to the Register of Midwives and a central component in the definition of the Midwifery Scope of Practice (Midwifery Council of New Zealand 2004, New Zealand College of Midwives 2005).

To work with women in an equal relationship such as partnership, requires more than just the will to do this, although that is the first step. Like any human relationship the development of partnership between a midwife and a childbearing woman is a complex process requiring self-knowledge, well-developed communication skills, willingness, honesty, trust, generosity and time. Mavis Kirkham's book The Midwife–Mother Relationship brings together varying perspectives from a number of midwives in Britain and elsewhere who are attempting to work with women in more equal relationships and there is much to learn from their experiences (Kirkham 2000a).

This chapter provides some guidance from the New Zealand perspective where radical changes to the way that maternity services are delivered has meant that the majority of women now receive care from a known midwife in a one-to-one caseload model. This context for practice has enabled midwives and women to explore their relationships and to identify those elements that characterize many midwife–woman relationships. From these explorations a theoretical framework, the Midwifery Partnership Model, has been developed that can be used to guide midwives and students in their learning and thinking about how to work 'with women' during the childbirth experience (Guilliland & Pairman 1995; Pairman 1998). This chapter will provide an overview of the development of the Midwifery Partnership Model, examine the model and its refinements and discuss the implementation of the model, both in practice and in the profession of midwifery in New Zealand. It will also explore the potential for application of this model in countries other than New Zealand.

OVERVIEW OF DEVELOPMENT OF MIDWIFERY PARTNERSHIP IN NEW ZEALAND

New Zealand is a small and relatively isolated country. Located in the South Pacific it has a popu-

lation of only 4 million people, and a birth rate of approximately 56,000 per annum. New Zealand's nearest neighbour is Australia, three hours away by air. New Zealand's indigenous people, Maori, have lived in New Zealand for about a thousand years. Maori have deep cultural and spiritual connections to the land that, amongst other things, carries with it a sense of joint ownership that embraces family, tribal groups and ancestors across time. British settlers began immigrating to New Zealand from the early 1800s to establish farming, to search for gold and to establish a new colony for Britain. They also brought different cultural values and understandings about, for example, notions of ownership, individualism and the meaning of land. In order to live alongside each other Maori and British settlers had to recognize and acknowledge their differences and negotiate relationships acceptable to both. This recognition and respect of differences and negotiation of relationships continues today, but it was first formalized through the Treaty of Waitangi in 1840.

TREATY OF WAITANGI

The Treaty of Waitangi is a '... formal agreement between Maori hapu and the British Crown [that] took the form of a treaty written in both Maori and English which was signed initially at Waitangi ... in 1840.' (Ramsden 2002, p. 74). Its purpose was to establish a constitutional framework within which both Maori and Pakeha (non-Maori) were assured a rightful place for each in New Zealand. The Treaty recognizes the unique place and status of Maori as Tangata Whenua (people of the land) and guarantees Crown protection of Maori taonga (treasures), Maori control over Maori resources, and the same rights and privileges as those enjoyed by the British settlers (Ramsden 2002). The Treaty governs the relationship between Maori and the Crown and inherent in the Treaty are the principles of partnership, participation, protection and equity. Partnership is understood to be mutually defined and negotiated on an equal basis, with full participation of both partners and ensuring the protection of each (Ramsden 1990).

Due in part to ongoing disputes between Maori and the Crown in relation to ownership of land

and access to resources and the meaning of the Treaty in relation to these disputes, the concept of partnership is now culturally embedded in New Zealand society (Guilliland & Pairman 1995). 'Partnership' is part of everyday language in New Zealand and is used to describe a variety of social, political, cultural and economic relationships. Increasingly it is used to describe relationships in which imbalances in power and status are recognized and attempts are made to redress these imbalances through negotiation between both partners.

MIDWIFERY PARTNERSHIP AND THE TREATY

In New Zealand as in many parts of the world, women frequently experience a maternity service where power and control rests with doctors, midwives and other health professionals, and women's knowledges of childbirth are undermined and unacknowledged. This is particularly so when women birth in hospitals and the power of institutions is imposed on women's childbirth experiences through routine care, protocols and hierarchical systems of care.

New Zealand's maternity services have benefited from the political activities of several maternity consumer organizations that have raised issues and worked to bring about changes since the 1930s (Parkes 1993). During the latter part of the twentieth century these maternity consumer groups were influenced and strengthened by the political agenda of the international women's health movement that swept the western world in the 1970s and 1980s. A strong political agenda recognizing women's rights led to a variety of legislative changes to raise the status of women. A landmark inquiry into the denial of women's rights to informed consent at National Women's Hospital led to widespread acceptance of entitlement for all consumers of healthcare to principles such as self-determination, patient centred care, cultural sensitivity and health provider accountability (Cartwright 1988, Ministry of Women's Affairs 1989). In New Zealand these decades also saw increasing societal awareness of the Treaty of Waitangi and its principles, and so it was not surprising that when maternity consumers demanded

a certain kind of midwife they demanded midwives who could work in partnership with them (Dobbie 1990, Strid 1987).

Midwives too, were influenced by the concept of Cultural Safety developed by Irihapeti Ramsden in 1990 and introduced as part of midwifery and nursing education in New Zealand from 1992 (Ramsden 1990). Using the Treaty of Waitangi as a foundation Cultural Safety focused on the power relationships that existed in healthcare delivery and required nurses and midwives to recognize themselves as '. . . powerful bearers of their own life experience and realities and the impact this may have on others' (Ramsden 2000, p. 117). The model of Cultural Safety was further developed from 1990 onwards, and as will be discussed later, it fits closely with the model of Midwifery Partnership, because both models are about individual relationships in which power imbalances are recognized and addressed.

For New Zealand midwifery, therefore, 'Midwifery Partnership' evolved from New Zealand's unique cultural, social and political context in which the Treaty of Waitangi has a central place. While this unique context was the springboard for Midwifery Partnership, this does not mean that the model is not relevant to other countries. Midwifery Partnership is about relationships between midwives and childbearing women. In all parts of the world women and midwives experience these relationships every day as together they share the experiences of childbirth. The New Zealand model offers one way to explore these relationships and in particular to explore the role of the midwife in working 'with women'.

NEW ZEALAND'S MATERNITY SERVICE

The development of New Zealand's maternity services in the late 19th and early 20th centuries was strongly influenced by the British system, as most of the early European settlers came from Britain and the few trained midwives available had mostly trained in Britain. Midwives were regulated from 1904 when the Midwives Act established registration for midwives and marked the beginning of midwifery training in New Zealand. Women received maternity care in their own homes from midwives and doctors or through the state-run St Helen's maternity hospitals that were established in all the main centres and were run by midwives. From 1938 maternity care was free to all women and it remains so today, with private obstetricians the only group who are entitled to charge women on top of the government subsidy.

In the early part of the 20th century midwifery in New Zealand was a strong and autonomous profession. However, this changed rapidly from the 1920s onwards as government policies, implemented to reduce the infant mortality rate, and demand for 'pain free childbirth' by women, led to increased medical intervention in childbirth and increased hospitalization. The role of the midwife was reduced from autonomous practitioner to doctor assistant. This changed scope of practice was reflected in legislative changes that first combined midwifery with nursing and then in 1971, removed the word 'midwife' from the legislation altogether so that midwives were now defined as nurses and were required to work under medical supervision. Throughout these years midwives almost lost their identity as midwives and their sense of themselves as 'guardians' of the normal birth process. Women experiencing childbirth in this highly fragmented, medicalized and hospital-based maternity service also lost their faith in their abilities to give birth without intervention. By the early 1970s midwifery was at its lowest point and facing near extinction.

It was this near decline of midwifery that led to its re-emergence. Through the 1980s midwives regrouped through political activity to reclaim their identity as separate to nursing and to regain control over their future. During the same years maternity consumer activists were demanding the return of autonomous midwifery, as they believed that only midwives working autonomously would be able to assist them to regain control over their birth experiences. Midwives and women recognized their common goals and, in partnership, embarked on a well thought out political strategy from 1987 onwards to bring about changes in legislation to restore midwifery autonomy. This succeeded in 1990 with the Nurses Amendment Act, which allowed midwives to once again provide care to women throughout the childbirth experience on their own responsibility and gave pregnant women a choice in caregivers of midwives, doctors or both.

This legislation signalled the beginning of a more than a decade of change in New Zealand's maternity service. The service was restructured to ensure that each woman had a choice of caregiver to coordinate or personally provide all care throughout the entire childbirth experience from early pregnancy to six weeks postpartum – a Lead Maternity Carer (LMC). Increasingly the LMCs chosen by women have been midwives and in 2002 some 73% of women had a midwife LMC (New Zealand Health Information Service 2004).

LMC midwives can be self employed, based in the community and paid directly by government or they can be employed by hospitals. In either case they mostly work in pairs or in small groups of three. Often several midwife-pairs will join together to establish a larger group practice, providing more flexibility for unexpected cover such as illness. Now, no matter whether a woman chooses to birth at home, in a birthing unit or in a large maternity hospital, she receives individualized care from her LMC midwife (and her midwife partner) throughout the entire childbirth experience.

This one-to-one caseload model of midwifery practice is now the cornerstone of the New Zealand maternity service. Larger maternity hospitals still require midwives to work on shifts and these midwives, known as core midwives, work alongside and support the LMC midwives when they come into the units with their clients. Core midwives may also provide care themselves to women who have serious complications and require in-patient care or for those women who, for whatever reason, do not have a midwife LMC.

THE NOTION OF PARTNERSHIP

Midwifery autonomy regained in 1990 enabled midwives to work in a new way with women. Previously only the few homebirth midwives who practised in New Zealand prior to 1990 had been able to work one-to-one with a woman throughout pregnancy, labour, birth and the postnatal period. After 1990 this opportunity was available to any midwife who wanted to take it up and New Zealand midwives have embraced the opportunity. In 2002 some 40% of midwives reported working primarily in caseload midwifery while

53% reported working primarily in core facility midwifery. The remaining 7% were primarily in administration and management, education, professional advice/policy development or in research, and many of these midwives also provided care (in a caseload model) to a small number of women each year (Nursing Council of New Zealand 2004).

With the opportunity for midwives and women to form relationships over a nine to ten month period came new understandings of the nature of these relationships. That midwives and women, as groups, had a relationship of partnership was recognized in 1989 when the New Zealand College of Midwives was formed as the professional organization for midwives. The political partnership of midwives and women that succeeded in bringing about the 1990 Nurses Amendment Act led to recognition of the interdependence of midwives and women. To achieve their different but related goals, politically active midwives and women's groups had worked together to bring about midwifery autonomy. Through this process midwifery was able to separate from nursing and re-establish itself as a profession in its own right. Similarly women achieved their goals of midwifery autonomy and direct entry education that they expected would bring a new kind of midwife – one who recognized their right to be in control of their own birthing experiences. Reflection on this collaborative political activity saw the New Zealand College of Midwives define the relationship between the midwifery profession and maternity consumer groups as 'partnership' and the slogan 'women need midwives and midwives need women' was coined. In recognition of this partnership the constitution of the New Zealand College of Midwives established consumer representation at every level and consumers are involved in all College processes including decision-making and policy development (Donley 1989, Guilliland 1989, Pairman 1998).

From here it was only a small step for midwives to recognize that their individual relationships with women were also partnerships, or that they should be. In identifying partnership as a central concept from the inception of the College in 1989, New Zealand midwifery was actively working to redefine traditional notions of the professional as 'expert', to a definition of professionalism as 'partnership' whereby both the midwife and the woman make an equally important contribution and power differentials are recognized and equalized (Tully 1999).

Although New Zealand midwives embraced the notion of partnership, it was not until 1994 that any work was done to try and explore what midwifery partnership might mean in practice. In 1994 Karen Guilliland and I wrote The Midwifery Partnership: A Model for Practice that was published as a monograph in 1995 (Guilliland & Pairman 1995). This model was an attempt to tease out the components of midwife–woman relationships and to explore the notion of midwifery as a partnership. Through reflection on our own experiences as midwife practitioners, as midwife teachers and as midwife politicians, as well as our discussions and observations of many other midwives and women over many years, we developed a theoretical model to describe Midwifery Partnership (Guilliland & Pairman 1995). The model appears to have struck a chord with many midwives. It has become a required text in all New Zealand midwifery schools and several overseas. It underpins midwifery education curriculum development in New Zealand as well as some programmes in Australia. The monograph has been reprinted a number of times and seems to be in constant demand from midwives around the world.

In 1996/7 I undertook master's level research to further explore the midwife–woman relationship. Six independent (case loading and self-employed) midwives and six of their clients were individually interviewed and also participated in two focus group meetings. The participants were actively involved in analysis of the data and identification of the emerging themes. At the final stage participants compared the findings of the study with the model of Midwifery Partnership as developed by Karen and myself. Refinements were suggested and the participants teased out midwifery partnership to also mean 'professional friendship' (Pairman 1998, 2000). The next section provides an overview of Midwifery Partnership and discusses the original concepts as well as those modifications suggested later as a result of the study described above (Pairman 1998).

THE MIDWIFERY PARTNERSHIP: A MODEL FOR PRACTICE

Midwifery partnership is defined as:

> A relationship of 'sharing' between the woman and the midwife. Involving trust, shared control and responsibility and shared meaning through mutual understanding.
> Guilliland & Pairman 1995, p. 7

This relationship constitutes midwifery because it is the medium through which midwives provide midwifery care to women within the Midwifery Scope of Practice. The Midwifery Scope of Practice spans the life experiences of pregnancy, labour, birth and new mothering/parenthood to six weeks postpartum and sets the boundaries within which midwifery practice takes place (Midwifery Council of New Zealand 2004). Midwifery Partnership distinguishes midwifery from other professions involved in provision of maternity care, such as nurses and doctors, and it identifies the unique contribution that midwives have to offer women during the childbirth experience.

Although a single diagrammatic representation of Midwifery Partnership is presented, this is not to imply that all relationships between midwives and women are the same or that all women want the same things from midwives or that all midwives work in the same way. Rather, Midwifery Partnership recognizes the individuality of each partner, their differences as people, their different needs and priorities, their different experiences. Because each midwife and each woman brings different dimensions to their relationship, each partnership will be different. A partnership requires both partners to define their relationship, to negotiate how they will work with each other and to define their expectations of the relationship. This negotiation is overt and requires active participation by both partners and clear communication. The negotiated outcomes of each partnership will be different to accommodate the needs of both partners and therefore few partnership relationships will look the same. Because it is a professional relationship it is the midwife's responsibility to initiate the partnership and to work with each woman to achieve this. The model of Midwifery Partnership offers a framework for

these different relationships that identifies the characteristics and principles of partnership and can guide midwives in working with women in a more equal and shared way.

THE PARTNERS

The two partners in a Midwifery Partnership are a midwife and a woman. They enter into a relationship for the purpose of receiving and giving midwifery care and together they share the woman's experiences of pregnancy, labour and birth and the postnatal period. This nine to ten month experience reflects the Midwifery Scope of Practice and sets the boundaries of midwifery care (Midwifery Council of New Zealand 2004). Through this timeframe a woman and a midwife are able to get to know each other intimately in a way that makes their relationship distinctly different from usual health professional/client relationships.

Both partners in a Midwifery Partnership exist within their own social context. As indicated in Figure 4.1 below, each woman is part of her family (as defined by her) and she will be influenced by the beliefs and values of this group. The baby is depicted within the woman to symbolize the connection between mother and baby. During pregnancy a mother and baby are physically one. After birth the baby exists separately but its mother is recognized as the person who ultimately makes decisions for the baby. For midwifery, the needs of mother and baby are always seen as an integrated whole, 'where the needs of one will be the needs of the other' (Guilliland & Pairman 1995, p. 42).

Each midwife too, is part of her social group, but because it is her professional role that enables her to be in a relationship with each of her women clients, the midwife is depicted within the professional framework of midwifery. Her practice will be guided by the philosophy, standards and ethics of the midwifery profession to which she belongs.

Gender, class, history, culture and society shape both partners. As discussed earlier, the Treaty of Waitangi is a unique aspect of New Zealand society. In other countries there will be other societal influences to consider when applying the model. In the revised model another circle surrounding both partners was added to depict the impact that the maternity system, including the place of birth, the wider health system and societal beliefs about childbirth, will have on women and midwives during their experiences of childbirth. In New Zealand and most Western countries, medicalization is still the dominant ideology of childbirth. Midwifery Partnership attempts to challenge this dominance by offering women and midwives an alternative model for midwifery practice, 'which is emancipatory and equalises power relationships within maternity services' (Guilliland & Pairman 1995, p. 9).

Figure 4.1 below depicts the partnership between the woman and the midwife as two equal and intertwined circles. The equal size of the circles represents the equal status of each woman and each midwife that must be recognized by both partners if a true partnership is to develop. Both partners have acknowledged expertise and make equally valuable contributions; the midwife contributes her midwifery knowledge and experiences and professional framework and the woman contributes her self-knowledge, experiences and needs and desires for this birth. Both partners need the other's contribution to ensure a positive and safe birth experience. The intertwined

section depicts the shared experience of pregnancy, labour, birth and the postpartum period that makes up the Midwifery Scope of Practice. The woman symbol in this section indicates the woman-centred focus of the relationship. The principles identified within this intertwined section are important if the relationship is to be a partnership, and provide guidance for how a midwife and a woman can work together.

In the 1998 revision of the model detail was also added to describe more fully the characteristics of each partner and what they contributed to the relationship (Pairman 1998). The women in my study had certain expectations of midwives and the type of care they were seeking. These women wanted midwifery care based on trust, respect, equality and openness. They wanted to be actively involved in their care, to take responsibility for themselves and to be in control of their childbirth experiences. They also wanted to have this intimate midwife–woman relationship with another woman. As Bizz (one of the women in the study) said:

> I wanted someone that I could initially build a trust in and get to know leading right up to the birth. Just that more personal and

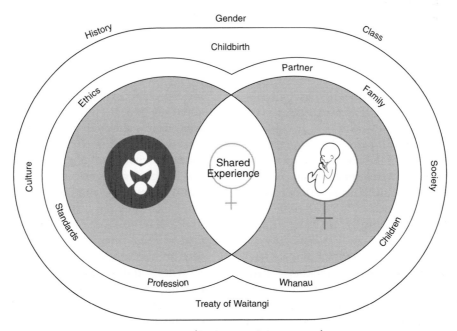

Figure 4.1 The Midwifery Partnership: The partners (Guilliland & Pairman 1995)

trusting relationship. And hearing the same things from the same person . . . it was important that it was someone I could talk to quite confidently, someone approachable . . . it was important too that she was a woman . . . to have an equal relationship.

BF in Pairman 1998, p. 75

Another woman, Dianne, wanted midwifery care because her previous experiences with doctors meant she did not believe she would get the information she needed to feel safe during her pregnancy.

It was a really important event for me, and there were a lot of questions I wanted answered and I suppose from some of my other experiences doctors just don't release the information and sometimes I feel they think its not to be released. . . . (In my childhood) we went to see the doctor and he knew everything, so there's still that sort of feeling when you go to a doctor. I go into the surgery and I sit in the chair and he asks 'how are you' – 'I've got this problem'. Whereas you should be able to say you've got a problem and talk to them normally, but you still feel like he's sitting in a big chair and you're sitting in a little wee small chair, going 'yeak' and squeaking, thinking 'am I allowed to say what I've got wrong?' Which is not the sort of experience that I want when you're having a baby. You really need to know what's going on and have answers. It's not an illness . . . you've got to know all the answers. They're dealing with another human being.

D McD in Pairman 1998, p. 81

Dianne's description of visiting her doctor illustrates her perception of the doctor as 'expert' and her own sense of powerlessness in the doctor–patient relationships she has experienced. She indicates that she wants a different type of relationship with her caregivers during pregnancy.

In the woman circle of the refined model I have added the concepts of 'seeking professional care', 'seeking active participation, self-responsibility and control', 'seeking trust, respect, equality and openness' and 'being female' to indicate that women actively choose midwifery care because they are looking for a specific type of professional relationship in which they will have power and control over their birthing experiences.

To some extent the characteristics that women seek from midwives were also mirrored in the concepts that were added to the midwife circle in the refined model. To work with women in a partnership relationship requires a midwife to have certain qualities that become evident through the way the midwife works 'with' each woman. These qualities include the way in which a midwife utilizes her knowledge and skill and 'self' in her practice; the way in which she is accessible to women, provides emotional support to women and builds their confidence; and the way she brings herself as a woman to the relationship.

As Bizz said:

I trusted her professionalism and all her knowledge, but I felt very equal with her. I needed her expertise and I was very confident in it, but I suppose her confidence built my confidence.

BF in Pairman 1998, p. 117

Sarah, too, talked about the importance of getting to know the midwife as a person and how this led to individualized care that met her needs.

MW and I just seemed to click so we get on really well, we talk about lots of different things . . . there were a lot of other things to talk about rather than just the appointment for me to have a baby. I found that I learnt things about MW as she learnt things about me. She didn't expect me to do all the talking about me and my life and how things were going here – she'd tell me how Matthew (her son) was doing and he came with her on a couple of visits. So I got an insight into MW and her family as well . . . so I don't think she learnt all about me and I learnt nothing about her . . . its probably only natural that she finds out more about me, because she's got to deal with me through the nine months, and then through the labour and knowing how I'll react and different things – how my past pregnancy had been – just to find out so she knows so she can do more either actively or by changing the way she might word things. If I was a morning person she'd come in the morning . . . just different things like that would probably change her . . . I think the more you can help them and be honest about it the better it'll be for you in the end.

SC in Pairman 1998, p. 119

Amy confirmed this individual approach to each woman when she said:

I think MW's guideline was made by each individual she came across – everybody lives differently so we all have to have a different set of rules.

AA in Pairman 1998, p. 99

The midwives recognized the active role inherent in being 'with women'. As Chris said about working with women in labour:

I take great delight in supporting. I used to do all the back rubbing and getting this and getting that and now I take real delight in working for them, helping them to work together because it's their birth and I work quite a bit now at not being intrusive and supporting the husband to support the wife rather than just directly supporting the woman. I guess I do that as well but it's using her support people to do the work to provide the support to make her feel cared for and loved and supported and everything else so that you're in the background rather than the foreground.

CS in Pairman 1998, p. 101

When working 'with' women the midwives deliberately used their knowledge, skills, and 'self' to form trusting relationships with women and help women to build and draw on their own resources of support, control and initiative. The midwives were actively present with the women in both a physical and emotional sense, critically reflecting on their practice as a way of developing and trusting practice wisdom. For these midwives, practising in New Zealand in the early 1990s meant that they had to work out what it meant to be independent practitioners, able to care for women on their own responsibility. With this professional autonomy came responsibility and accountability

and recognition that 'independence' is an active midwifery role that says more about how the midwife practises than it does about how she is employed or the model of care in which she works. As Kay said:

I see what I do now as a complete job not part of it or bits of it or half of it, because what you and the woman decide antenatally impacts on what happens postnatally . . . it's given me freedom in that I am my own boss and I will make decisions with the woman about what happens.

KF in Pairman 1998, p. 73

And Kate:

I'd like to think that if I went back into the hospital situation, that my whole feeling of practising as a midwife would be different from what it was when I was there . . . I guess before the Nurses Amendment Act I felt like I was employed and doing a job, and to me now, caring for women and being an independent midwife has got a totally different feel about it than being a midwife working in a hospital . . . it's a sense of . . . it's a whole lot more commitment – it's a life commitment rather than a job I guess, that's the difference.

KS in Pairman 1998, p. 74

Thus, to the midwife circle I have added the concepts of 'being female', 'giving support', 'being accessible', 'using knowledge, skill and self in practice', 'being with', 'developing practice wisdom' and 'practising independently' to further describe what a midwife brings to her midwifery practice (see Fig. 4.2).

Midwifery practice is active in that a midwife utilizes her knowledge, skills and experiences thoughtfully and with regard to the specific needs of each woman she works with. Even when she appears to be doing little a midwife is observing, analysing and thinking about what is happening and how she can support and enhance what is happening for the woman.

As Chris said:

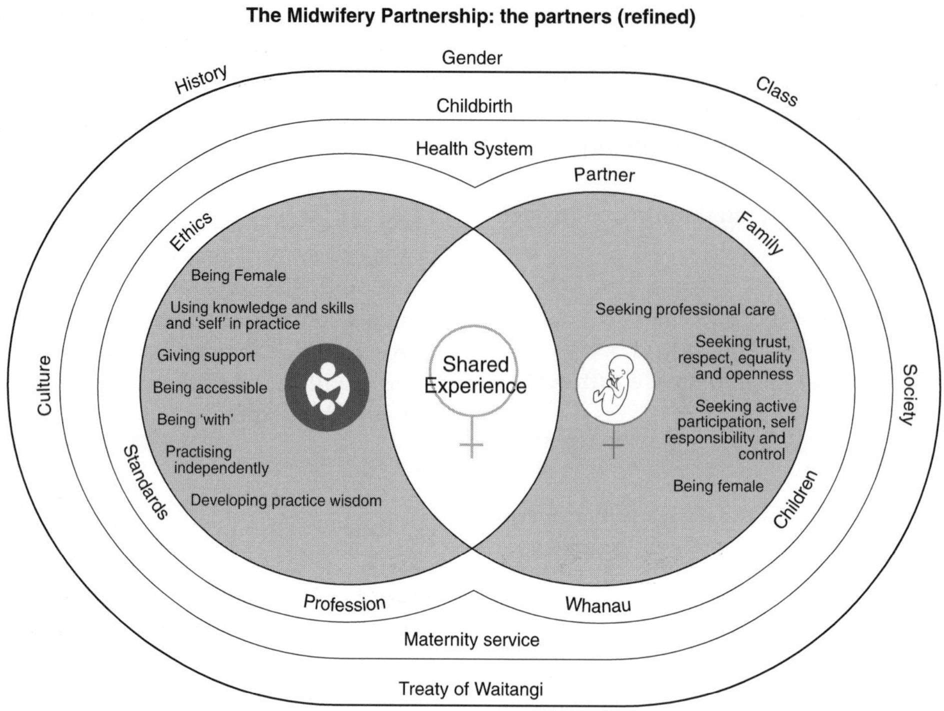

The Midwifery Partnership: the partners (refined)

Figure 4.2   The Midwifery Partnership: the partners (refined) (Pairman 1998, p. 188)

I think that in midwifery caring for the pregnancy is a small part of actually caring for the woman. I think that's where a lot of GPs miss out, they care for the pregnancy, the physical part and perhaps some of the emotional part, but whether they actually support the woman with what's going on in her life and the changes she needs to make . . . if you don't give them the time then they don't get a chance to explore those things.

CS in Pairman 1998, p. 99

Kate, another midwife, talked of the importance of understanding her own beliefs and attitudes as well as the woman's context in order to provide appropriate midwifery care:

It's the whole family dynamics; it's the people that are close to her. It's not just the woman,

it's everyone that affects her, and everything that affects her . . . the more I practise, the more I think where the caregivers and support people are that affects what happens with a woman . . . I think where the midwife is coming from is really important.

KS in Pairman 1998, p. 99

CULTURAL SAFETY

The importance of midwives understanding their own attitudes and value systems and recognizing the power inherent in their professional roles and how these factors can all impact on each woman they work with is a key principle in another New Zealand theory for practice, Cultural Safety. Developed by Maori nurse educator Irihapeti Ramsden in the 1980s, Cultural Safety is defined as:

The effective nursing or midwifery practice of a person or family from another culture and is determined by that person or family. Culture includes, but is not restricted to, age or generation; gender; sexual orientation; occupation and socio-economic status; ethnic origin or migrant experience; religious or spiritual belief and disability. The nurse or midwife delivering the nursing or midwifery service will have undertaken a process of reflection on his or her own cultural identity and will recognize the impact that his or her personal culture has on his or her professional practice. Unsafe cultural practice comprises any action which diminishes, demeans or disempowers the cultural identity and wellbeing of an individual.

Nursing Council of New Zealand 2002, p. 7

For midwives who are part of the dominant culture such as white, heterosexual and middle class, and in relation to their professional role, have status and power as midwives within a powerful health system, understanding the principles of Cultural Safety can be uncomfortable and challenging. Members of the dominant culture are not taught to recognize their privilege but learn to think of their lives as 'morally neutral, normative and average' (McIntosh 1988, p. 16). In other words members of a dominant culture believe that the realities of society are natural and normal, and are the same for everyone. This notion that everyone should be treated the same is implicit in Transcultural Nursing theory (Leininger 1991) in which midwives (and nurses) were taught the concepts of cultural awareness (becoming aware of difference) and cultural sensitivity (acknowledgement of the legitimacy of difference) from the perspective of the midwife. Such an approach placed power with the midwife to identify the needs of people from other cultural groups and did not require self-knowledge or change in attitude. It also led to development of cultural stereotypes and cultural checklists for care and ignored the existence of power relationships in the delivery of health care (Ramsden 2000). Transcultural Nursing theory places the nurse (midwife) in the position of 'external observer' for the purpose of providing culturally specific care, while Cultural Safety addresses the issue of power between the client

(woman) and the nurse (midwife) along with interpreting culture in the broadest possible sense (Ramsden 2002).

> Leininger's culturally congruent care model is different from Cultural Safety in that nurses and midwives need to move from treating people regardless (my emphasis) of colour or creed towards a model of care that is regardful of all those things that make them unique.
>
> Ramsden 1993, p. 5

Cultural Safety begins with self-reflection and attitude change through a process that requires midwives to recognize themselves as '. . . powerful bearers of their own life experience and realities' and to understand the impact this may have on others (Ramsden 2000 p. 117). The midwife is challenged to recognize her personal power and the power of her professional role and the institutions in which she works (Richardson 2000). Cultural Safety makes visible the invisible structures of power (including our own) and attempts to transform anything that creates inequality. Cultural Safety shifts power from the provider (midwife) to the recipient (woman) by requiring the woman and her family to decide whether the midwife's care is safe for them (Ramsden 2002). 'Safety' in this context includes not only physical safety but also a sense of emotional, psychological and spiritual safety.

Cultural Safety is primarily about establishing trust, gaining a shared meaning about vulnerability and power and carefully working through the legitimacy of difference (Ramsden 2000). It requires midwives to examine their own realities and attitudes they bring to practice and to understand how historical, political and social processes impact on people's health.

In a midwife/woman partnership relationship the differences between both partners are identified, respected and negotiated. In this way trust is established and relationships are flexible as together midwives and women work with the uncertainty and paradox that difference constantly presents to them (Spence 2004). This takes courage, patience and kindness. Cultural Safety is an instrument that allows a woman and her family to judge if the maternity service and delivery of midwifery care is safe for them (Ramsden 2002).

Although Cultural Safety originated in New Zealand out of a context of biculturalism in which the Treaty of Waitangi was central, it is applicable in other societies and contexts. Indeed as Irihapeti Ramsden said (2002, p. 181):

Cultural Safety was designed as an educational process by Maori and it is given as koha (gift) to all people who are different from service providers, whether by gender, sexual orientation, economic or educational status, age or ethnicity.

Cultural Safety is inherent in Midwifery Partnership as it provides a framework for recognizing cultural 'difference' between a midwife and a woman, the power inherent in the professional role of a midwife and the impact that the culture of the midwife may have on her professional practice. Like Midwifery Partnership, Cultural Safety seeks to shift power from the midwife to the woman by recognizing that it is the childbearing woman and her family, not the midwife, who determine that the midwifery care she receives is effective and 'safe'. Like Midwifery Partnership, Cultural Safety relies on trust. As Irihapeti Ramsden said

Cultural Safety is about the formation of trust and the components of trust becoming

recognisable to patients (women) and nurses (midwives). Only when trust has been established can exotic differences be revealed, discussed and negotiated in the actions of giving and receiving nursing (midwifery) care. This often involves the transfer of power from nurse (midwife) to patient (woman) and the renegotiation of traditionally held positions (Ramsden 2002, http://culturalsafety.massey.ac.nz/chapter eleven. Htm Retrieved 1.5.05).

PHILOSOPHICAL UNDERPINNINGS

The formation of a midwifery partnership relies on the midwife, at least, holding certain philosophical beliefs. The woman may also hold these beliefs. They underpin midwifery partnership because they direct and support the practice of midwifery. These beliefs are: pregnancy and childbirth are normal life events; midwifery is an independent profession; midwifery provides continuity of caregiver; and midwifery is women centered (see Fig. 4.3 below). These philosophical beliefs are shared by midwives around the world and distinguish midwifery from other disciplines involved in the provision of maternity care (Association of Radical Midwives 1986, Australian

Figure 4.3 Supporting Structure for the Midwifery Partnership (Guilliland & Pairman 1995)

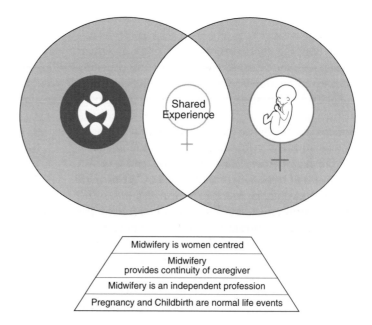

Midwifery is women centred

Midwifery provides continuity of caregiver

Midwifery is an independent profession

Pregnancy and Childbirth are normal life events

Nursing and Midwifery Council 2005, Houd 1993, International Confederation of Midwives 1990, Midwifery Council of New Zealand 2004, Midwives Alliance of North America 1991, Page 1988, 1993). These beliefs were supported by the participants in my study and their insights added depth to our understanding of these aspects of midwifery practice (Pairman 1998).

PREGNANCY AND BIRTH ARE NORMAL LIFE EVENTS

Midwifery knowledge is constructed from the belief that pregnancy and childbirth are normal life events. This understanding directs midwifery practice and defines the role of the midwife as one of Kaitiaki or guardian, to support and protect this unique physiological process and transformative life stage (Donley 1986). The belief in the normalcy of pregnancy and childbirth is one of the main differences between the midwifery and medical models of childbirth. If one believes that childbirth is a physiological process then one's role is to enhance and support that process while still keeping a watching brief to ensure that it stays within normal parameters for each individual woman. If one believes that it is a physiological process that is unreliable, inconsistent and fraught with potential danger then it is necessary to try to control the process to guarantee a good outcome.

At the heart of this is the ability to trust women's bodies and trust physiology. Of course not all births will be straightforward and have a good outcome. However, Western societies have embraced science and technology to such an extent that trust in physiology appears to have been lost. Much research and practice has focused on ways to control childbirth in order to guarantee a healthy baby rather than seeking ways to support and enhance physiology. Childbirth services that have been constructed in Western societies mean that most women birth in hospitals and experience some form of surgical, technological or pharmacological intervention (Crabtree 2004). Western maternity services not only undermine women's confidence, they also undermine midwifery knowledge and confidence, as midwives are increasingly involved in implementing these interventions. As Downe and others have noted, midwifery's claim to be the guardian of normal birth while apparently implementing a variety of interventions during the childbirth process, is paradoxical (Downe 2004, Kirkham 2000b). Even where models of midwifery care support one-to-one care from a midwife, such as in New Zealand, intervention rates in childbirth continue to rise.

Clearly the physiological process of childbirth is finely tuned and requires not only belief but also recognition of the myriad of interacting factors that can enhance or impede it. These factors may include a woman's personal and familial history, the environment in which she labours and gives birth, the ideology that frames the attitude and response of caregivers, the attitude and expectations of her family and friends and her own fears and beliefs (Crabtree 2004, Downe & McCourt 2004).

A significant challenge facing midwifery today is to recognize the complexity and uncertainty of childbirth and to reframe it as 'uniquely normal' rather than expecting pathology (Downe 2004). Foureur and Hunter (in press) propose a 'package' of care to keep childbirth normal involving a close personal and trusting relationship with a midwife in a one-to-one caseload model; a strong belief in childbirth as normal physiology; and a familiar environment for birth that enhances and supports the normalcy of childbirth. Pairman and Guilliland (2003) have suggested that midwives and women need locations for birth that are not dominated by the medical model philosophy of birth within which they can strengthen their understandings of birth as physiology and reduce their reliance on technological interventions for routine screening and pain relief.

Midwifery Partnership recognizes each woman as uniquely normal and when midwives and women work together throughout the childbirth experience and in women's own environments, midwives begin to understand the range of 'normal' that can only be defined individually for each woman (Katz Rothman 1984). When midwives internalize this understanding they begin to challenge their practice and find ways to resist and reframe the dominant medical ideology such that they can once again claim to be the guardians of normal.

MIDWIFERY IS AN INDEPENDENT PROFESSION

Independent midwifery practice involves a midwife practising autonomously from a specific philosophy and body of knowledge without reference to another discipline and taking responsibility for the midwifery judgements made and the actions implemented. Independence is about how a midwife practises and the way she sees her professional role. It is not about her employment status or where the woman gives birth. Independent practice occurs when midwives provide care across the scope of midwifery practice on their own responsibility.

Autonomy is an important aspect of midwifery's professional identity as it provides midwives with the freedom to make decisions with women rather then being constrained by rules or dictates of other disciplines such as medicine or by the protocols of employers or maternity facilities. A midwife's judgements arise instead from professional standards and guidelines and from discussion and negotiation with each woman. Midwifery care will be informed by evidence when possible and often decisions and uncertainties will be discussed with midwifery colleagues or obstetric specialists, as midwives do not work in isolation. However, the key point about professional autonomy and independent practice is that it allows a midwife and a woman to begin to reframe childbirth as normal and unique to each woman. It allows a midwife and a woman to work together in a way that shifts control to the woman, recognizes her active involvement and meets her needs. The woman and the midwife share responsibility for decisions made and the midwife remains professionally accountable for her judgements and actions.

Midwifery Partnership relies on independent midwifery practice so that a midwife can work in partnership with a woman 'to provide the complete service throughout pregnancy, labour, birth and the postnatal period on her own responsibility' (Guilliland & Pairman 1995, p. 37). When midwives practise independently and in partnership with women they are no longer seen as 'experts' with power 'over' woman as in 'old' notions of professionalism. Instead Midwifery Partnership provides an example of 'new' professionalism whereby both midwives and women have recog-

nized authority and the midwife's role moves from 'expert' to 'reflective practitioner' whose task is to support, guide and accompany a woman within a more equitable, interdependent and empowering relationship (Pairman 2005, Tully 1999). By articulating midwifery as a partnership New Zealand midwives have redefined traditional notions of professionalism. However, midwives need to understand this definition and midwifery needs to reinforce the implications of this 'new' style of professionalism to midwifery practice so that midwives do not abuse their power and authority.

> Instead of seeking to control childbirth, midwifery seeks to control midwifery, in order that women can control childbirth. Midwifery must maintain its women-centered philosophy to ensure that its control of midwifery never leads to control of childbirth.
> Guilliland & Pairman 1995, p. 49

MIDWIFERY PROVIDES CONTINUITY OF CAREGIVER

Midwifery is the only profession involved in the care of women through the childbearing cycle that provides continuity of caregiver and it is essential that it continues to find ways to do so. Continuity of caregiver enables midwives to work in their full scope of practice and it provides time for midwives and women to get to know each other, to build trust and to build partnerships. When midwife–woman relationships span pregnancy, birth and beyond there is time to work with each woman to discuss her wishes and her fears for birth and motherhood and to build her self-confidence. There is time to work with families to uncover their fears and misconceptions and to build their confidence. Decisions can be thought through over time as information and options are explored. There is time to talk about what labour might be like, or how each woman might respond to pain; to discuss the impact of the environment; to talk about uncertainty and complexity so that ideally by the time a woman begins labour she is willing and confident to 'let go' and trust her body to give birth.

Continuity of caregiver means 'one midwife (and her backup colleague) providing midwifery care throughout the entire childbirth experience' (Guilliland & Pairman 1995, p.39). Midwives working outside this continuity model (core midwives) provide the essential link and support for the caseloading midwife and the woman to maternity facilities if the woman is birthing in hospital and to obstetric services if the woman requires extra care. As the 'wise women' of the institutions core midwives facilitate the experience of caseloading midwives and their clients, providing practical help and support as required. A partnership relationship between core midwives and caseloading midwives means that women can be assured of a smooth transition between primary and secondary services if necessary and the midwife–woman partnership is supported and protected even as other professionals such as the obstetric team become involved.

Continuity of care is explored elsewhere in this book (see Chapter 7). Despite the increasing evidence that demonstrates the benefits of continuity of care and one-to-one support in labour to women there are few maternity services outside of New Zealand that have enabled and supported midwives to develop and maintain one-to-one caseloading models of care. However, for Midwifery Partnership they are essential. While midwives have effective and positive relationships with women in other models of practice, it is the time and consistency that come with continuity of caregiver that is so important to the development and practice of partnership.

MIDWIFERY IS WOMEN CENTERED

'Women centeredness' gives primacy to the woman who is the recipient of midwifery care. It acknowledges that midwifery only exists to 'facilitate the optimal experience of birth for pregnant women and their families' (Guilliland & Pairman 1995, p. 41). It recognizes that it is the woman who is the focus of all midwifery care, acknowledging each woman's individuality and encouraging midwives to work with each woman in whichever way she wants in order to meet her individual needs.

Women centeredness does not deny the important role of the woman's family or deny the importance of caring for the baby. Rather, a woman-centered philosophy recognizes each

woman's connection and integration with her family and baby and recognizes that each woman will decide how she wants the midwife to interact with and involve her family. Women centeredness recognizes that a midwife's primary relationship is with each woman she cares for and that this care must be provided in such a way that the woman's individual context is respected. As Bizz explained:

> The midwife spoke about my pregnancy and a whole thing with me, Eric and the baby, rather than just my body and my baby inside it.
>
> BF in Pairman 1998, p. 183

THEORETICAL CONCEPTS

The philosophical beliefs outlined above provide the conditions within which Midwifery Partnership can form. However, there are also certain principles that must be integrated in the relationship if partnership is to be successfully implemented and maintained. These concepts are individual negotiation, equality, shared responsibility and empowerment and informed choice and consent (Guilliland & Pairman 1995). These were refined and made more explicit to describe how midwives and women work together. In the refined model the following concepts were identified; being equal, sharing common interests, involving the family, building trust, reciprocity, taking time and sharing power and control. Empowerment, emancipation, developing midwifery knowledge and challenging the medical model of childbirth were identified as potential outcomes of a partnership relationship between a midwife and a woman (see Fig. 4.4).

The concepts discussed below are key principles from both models that exemplify the way in which Midwifery Partnership is enacted. In many ways these concepts overlap in their meaning and it is the integration of these concepts that characterize Midwifery Partnerships.

NEGOTIATION

Both partners must participate and contribute if the partnership is to work. Negotiation is the process through which a midwife and a woman work through issues such as mutual rights and

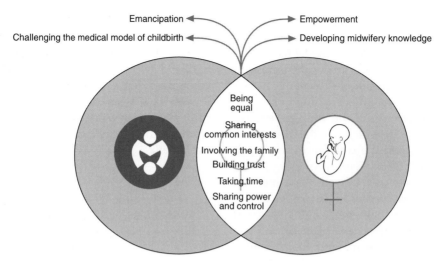

Emancipation ← → Empowerment
Challenging the medical model of childbirth ← → Developing midwifery knowledge

Being equal
Sharing common interests
Involving the family
Building trust
Taking time
Sharing power and control

Figure 4.4   Principles inherent within the partnership model and outcomes of midwifery partnership (refined) (Pairman 1998)

responsibilities, the balance of power and decision-making. 'The underlying premise of the partnership is that it is individually negotiated, recognising the essential contribution of each' (Guilliland & Pairman 1995, p. 44). Negotiation is a process for working things through and coming to mutual understandings and agreements. It relies on open and effective communication and a positive sense of self. Because both partners are different the way in which their relationship is negotiated will be different and each partnership will be unique.

EQUALITY AND RECIPROCITY

While differences between partners are recognized and respected, each must feel equal to the other if a partnership is to work. The midwife carries with her the power associated with her professional role and if she is to provide care that the woman finds to be culturally safe the midwife must have examined how this professional power could impact on her midwifery practice. The midwife needs to understand that her professional knowledge and authority can have limited effect if the woman does not contribute her knowledge of herself and her wishes or does not maintain her health or does not work with the midwife. It is important that the midwife recognizes and

respects the woman as having equal status with an equally valuable contribution. There may be many differences between them but the midwife must take responsibility for acknowledging and respecting those differences.

When a midwife and a woman begin their relationship from a position of mutual respect and equity, their understanding of each other will deepen as they get to know each other. Their relationship is reciprocal in that there is two-way sharing and mutual exchange that creates shared meaning and is beneficial to both.

TRUST AND TIME

Trust develops between a midwife and a woman as they get to know each other over time. Trust is essential in any healthy human relationship and in Midwifery Partnership trust underpins information sharing, decision-making, power sharing and empowerment. Trust between two people helps them feel safe with each other and willing to expose their vulnerabilities because they know these will be respected. Faced with the uncertainty of childbirth midwives and women need to trust each other as they also have to trust themselves and trust the process of birth.

> . . . She knew that I was scared, she knew how I was feeling. Because we discussed

Lauren's birth in detail, and so she knew where I was coming from and I felt very comfortable with her . . . I trusted her totally.

LF in Pairman 1998, p. 121

Trust develops over time and therefore continuity of caregiver enhances the development of trust. So too does visiting women in their own homes where they are comfortable and in control and the midwife can get to know the woman in her own context. As Barrington said:

Continuous care, involving generous commitments of time, allows a midwife to gather a store of impressions that will substantiate future intuitions and actions. Her familiarity with the norms of mother and babe enables her to notice deviations from these norms immediately.

Barrington 1985, p. 19

Midwives not only make generous commitments of time through providing continuity of care but also in giving each visit the time necessary for full discussion and being flexible with appointments so as to meet the woman's needs. Midwives are also accessible to women as required and while women respect midwive's time off it is important that they can access help and advice as necessary. The timing of visits, the place of visits and who to contact for help if the midwife is having time off or is sick are all aspects of the partnership that can be negotiated to suit both partners.

SHARING POWER AND RESPONSIBILITY

In Midwifery Partnerships both partners exercise power and the balance of power is negotiated and mutually agreed. Power is shared through information sharing; through decision-making and through recognizing and enhancing each woman's sense of control. Feeling in control during childbirth leads to a sense of satisfaction, fulfilment and positive well being (Green et al 1990). The exercise of power and personal control is dependent upon having resources and options that enable choice, having sufficient information about choices, being able to make decisions and being able to implement those decisions once they are made (Walker et al 1995).

Midwifery Partnership provides a framework within which a woman can achieve a sense of personal control. In equal and negotiated relationships where both partners trust each other and feel safe midwives can actively support women to exercise their power and make decisions without the midwife imposing her own beliefs. As Dianne described:

It was at the back of my mind that she must have her own feelings about what should be done but it never came through. That's what I found really amazing about her, that I never felt in any way that whatever she carried with her (because I believe that anyone who makes a decision – there's a whole lot of other things as to why they make that decision), and I never felt she brought any of that into the situation . . . she was there but she never moved in.

D McD in Pairman 1998, p. 134

Along with the power to make decisions and be in control comes responsibility for those decisions. While midwives are always professionally accountable for their midwifery judgements and actions, in Midwifery Partnership women also share responsibility for the outcomes of decisions jointly made. As Dianne described taking responsibility and making decisions can be an empowering process:

You've got to take responsibility and I think once you take responsibility for your life you can do so much more. It's tied up in a circle – you can evolve much beyond that. It's like taking hold of your life. If you take responsibility then if you get a bad thing out of it then you learn from your mistake. If you get a good thing out of it then you get a real buzz. It's not anyone else's – they might have contributed to it, but it's like 'yeah, I did that and I can take the credit for it' . . . even today I look at Jessica and I find it really amazing that she grew up in me. I ate really healthy and I felt whatever I did would be reflected in Jessica and I wanted a really good healthy baby . . . then at the end we got this fantastic little baby who was really alert from day one. Even now she's raring to go. I take a wee credit for that.

D McD in Pairman 1998, p. 168

EMPOWERMENT AND EMANCIPATION

'For it is in the relationship between women and midwives as they go through the child-bearing process together that the message of value and worth is given. It cannot be given by strangers mouthing words – it is given by the midwife's commitment to the woman and the process she is involved in.'
Pelvin 1990 cited in Guilliland &
Pairman 1995, p. 48

As this quote from New Zealand midwife Bronwen Pelvin exemplifies, Midwifery Partnership can provide the context for both women and midwives to be empowered. Midwifery aims to enable women to recognize their personal power and strengths and to increase women's sense of autonomy and confidence as mothers and women. Because pregnancy and birth are such life changing events they often cause women to ask questions about themselves and their lives and seek to make changes. As Nicky Leap (2000, p. 5) said:

The question marks of pregnancy are the beginning of a process of grappling with the uncertainty and decision-making that will persist throughout the experience of raising a child.

Midwives can work with women in ways that facilitate empowerment for women and this in turn can be empowering for midwives. Key facilitation skills for midwives are believing in women and inspiring confidence, and knowing when to intervene and when to withdraw (Leap 2000). Taking control of their birth experiences may be the first time a woman has controlled anything in her life, and the sense of satisfaction she feels from this may lead to further changes in her life. As Kate commented:

It's a nice feeling to see a woman go from thinking that everyone else owns, or has a right to dictate, to deciding – and to see it spill over into other areas is really neat . . . and start questioning other areas and other things in her life . . . that's a major plus I think to work with a woman over a longer time.

KS in Pairman 1998, p. 166

Although midwives share significant life events with women they are involved in women's lives for only short periods of time in a lifespan. Their involvement with women can be empowering if they work to facilitate independence and self-determination rather than dependence. One way to do this is to encourage women to build their own networks of support rather than relying on midwives who will not be there for the long-term. As Chris explained:

I like to think that the focus is that they're developing their own independence and their own networks to support them, because when you move towards leaving them at six weeks postpartum or whenever, I usually find, not quite that you're rejected, but that you're not needed anymore. By the time you finish they're competent, confident and managing and have set up networks to keep going.

CS in Pairman 1998, p. 150

Midwifery Partnership can be empowering for both women and midwives. As midwives work with women through an equal and negotiated relationship their beliefs about birth and about midwifery are reinforced and strengthened. Observing the uniqueness of each woman's birth experience builds midwives' confidence about the ranges of 'normal' that are possible and builds trust in women's bodies. Sharing and negotiating power and decision-making and being able to see the outcomes of these decisions strengthens midwives' trust and confidence in women, and in themselves as autonomous practitioners.

Midwifery Partnership also has emancipatory potential. Women who experience Midwifery Partnership often encourage other women to seek this type of care. 'Emancipation is a dynamic state of being in which self-knowledge (enlightenment) and self-advocacy (empowerment) are connected to knowledge and advocacy for others' (Henderson 1995, p. 66). As most systems of maternity care in Western societies are still entrenched in the medical model, there is huge scope for women to persuade other women through the telling of their stories about the normalcy of birth and the benefits of one to one midwifery care. As Liz explained:

Your relationship with your midwife is amazing. Everyone I've spoken to since I've just been raving to about it. Hopefully I'm spreading the word . . . it's a shame some people just don't have the confidence in midwives or themselves or aren't aware of that 'oh no, we must have a doctor scenario' . . . I personally can't see any other option now . . . I just can't see the advantages of doing it in any other way . . . I'm sold, I'm sold.

LG in Pairman 1998, p. 171

New Zealand and Canada provide two examples of where political action by women has led to sig-

nificant structural and philosophical changes in the way that maternity services are delivered and developments of more women-centered models of care.

PROFESSIONAL FRIENDSHIP

The participants in my study teased out Midwifery Partnership to mean 'professional friendship' (Pairman 1998). The term 'professional friend' described for them the friendship aspect of the relationship between women and midwives but also recognized the professional nature of the relationship and its time limited nature. As Bizz explained:

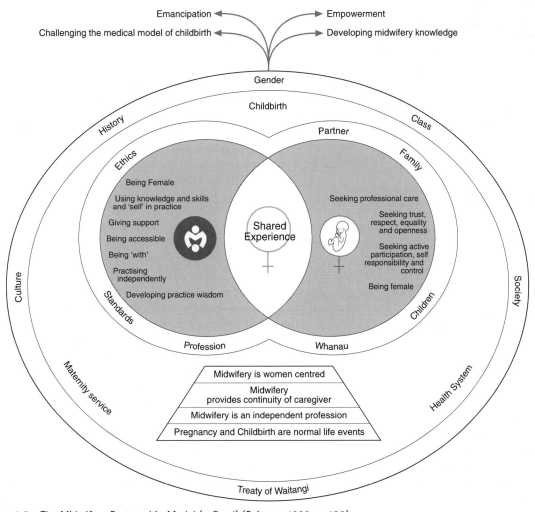

Figure 4.5   The Midwifery Partnership Model (refined) (Pairman 1998, p. 190)

I think we had a really good relationship actually. It was more of a friend relationship, but a friend you could trust in – a professional friend you could rely on.

BF in Pairman 1998, p. 163

The refinements to the partnership model (see Fig. 4.5 below) as suggested from this study provided further depth and understanding of the concepts by exploring how women and midwives experienced midwifery partnerships. Further exploration of the notion of professional friendship will contribute to midwifery's understanding of the practice of partnership.

THE IMPORTANCE OF PARTNERSHIP TO MIDWIFERY

Without partnership midwifery would be just another professional/client relationship where the midwife holds authority as the 'expert' and wields this authority and power through clinical decision-making. The client in this relationship may not disclose her own fears or expectations or ask questions because the power base is such that she may feel intimidated or unwilling to disturb her perception of the correct way to behave to the midwife.

This type of health professional relationship will be familiar to many. Midwives who work in the hospital system of shift work are unlikely to know the women they care for. They are kind and concerned for these women and try their best to provide them with good care. But they don't know the women and women don't know them. If women have birth plans or if they are asked midwives may be aware of some of their wishes for birth. Very often though the routine of the hospital dominates and women receive a similar level of care no matter what their individual needs or wishes.

The context of hospital maternity services very often constrains midwifery care through fragmentation of care, insufficient staffing numbers, hierarchies and organizational control. Such settings can undermine midwifery knowledge, confidence and trust, making it difficult for midwives to support women to take control of their birthing experiences (Kirkham 2000b).

A partnership relationship on the other hand, allows a midwife and a pregnant woman to get to know and trust each other over time. As the midwife and the woman see each other as individuals and understand each others' perspectives they are able to negotiate how they will work together to meet the woman's needs while still respecting the midwife's professional boundaries. Through this negotiation the power balance shifts and equalizes.

To work in this way requires self-knowledge, personal security, integrity and maturity. The midwife can no longer rely on her professional role as 'expert' to guide her practice. Instead she must open herself as a person to each woman she works with and be willing to recognize and embrace each woman as an equal partner as together they explore the physical, emotional, social and spiritual ramifications of childbirth for that woman. The midwife brings her midwifery knowledge and understandings to the relationship, as the woman brings her knowledge and experiences. But rather than directing care the midwife works 'with' the woman to support her to take up her power as a woman and as a mother so that she can direct and control her own birthing experience and feel confident in her new role as a mother.

When midwifery is practised independently and in partnership with women it has potential to not only enhance women's (and midwive's) empowerment and emancipation, but also to contribute to the reframing of childbirth as a normal life event, to build midwifery knowledge and understandings and to challenge the medical dominance of childbirth. By redefining professional relationships from midwife as 'expert' to relationships where women are partners in their care, midwives and women can create contexts in which women-centered care can flourish.

When midwives and women work together in partnerships with a political imperative changes can be made to maternity services and the choices for care that are available to women. Midwifery Partnership provides a model for the development of political partnerships between maternity consumer groups and midwifery professional organizations. As seen in New Zealand these partnerships can be a force for social change. Successful implementation of small changes such as establishing one-to-one care in a single maternity unit can lead to further developments as more women demand this type of care and more midwives demand to work in this way.

However, partnership, like autonomy and independence, also carries responsibility. When New Zealand women took political action to achieve midwifery autonomy they did so because they believed that midwives would provide them with an alternative model of maternity care in which women would be in control as decision makers. Therefore midwives had a moral obligation to provide the kind of care and relationships that women sought.

Partnership also carries a moral obligation for midwives to recognize and respect individual differences in women and to provide care that meets these individual needs.

Midwives in any country and in any cultural context work with childbearing women who are different to them. Midwives need to examine their relationships with childbearing women because these relationships are at the heart of midwifery practice. Midwifery Partnership provides a framework for achieving meaningful relationships between midwives and women whereby women are active agents in their care.

Working in partnership is demanding. It requires self-knowledge, strong and effective communications skills and a secure sense of self on the part of midwives. It takes trust, time and the ability to be reflective. Like any human relationship it will change and evolve and at times both partners may feel uncertain and insecure. Each new relationship with a woman will add to a midwife's understanding of herself and how she works with women if she is willing to examine these.

The model of Midwifery Partnership provides guidance to midwives wanting to develop partnerships with women and the concepts discussed above are a starting place for reflective practice and learning about working in partnership.

CONCLUSION

Midwifery must be concerned with relationships because, unlike any other health profession, mid-

wifery is privileged to have the opportunity to be 'with' women throughout the life experiences of pregnancy, birth and new motherhood. In their professional roles midwives are able to develop relationships with women that last up to 10 months (sometimes longer) and they have the opportunity to work with women in their own homes and communities, away from the influence and control of institutions. In such settings the traditional practitioner/patient relationship where the practitioner is the 'expert' and has the authority to make decisions is clearly inappropriate. Midwives who work in continuity of care models work in contexts in which relationships are valued and where midwifery care such as support, caring and enabling is recognized as skilled midwifery practice. Midwives and childbearing women in these settings need to develop relationships of equity, trust and mutual understanding.

So too do midwives and women working within the constraints of hospital services where the context is generally much more challenging and unsupportive to the development of partnership relationships between midwives and women.

However, the potential for empowerment of women through their childbirth experiences cannot be overlooked. Nor can the need to reframe childbirth away from the medical model perspective to recognition that childbirth is a normal life process that generally requires support rather than intervention. For these important processes to be achieved women must be in control of their own birthing experiences and supported to make decisions for themselves. Women who feel empowered during childbirth will take that confidence with them as new mothers and this in turn will strengthen their families and society. The ripple effects of positive birthing experiences are far reaching and cannot be underestimated.

Midwifery Partnership provides a framework for a new way for midwives and women to work together – one that is meaningful and mutually beneficial to both. Midwifery Partnership challenges professional power structures and medical dominance over childbirth through recognizing birthing women as active partners of equal status in the shared experience of maternity care.

Midwifery Partnership provides a framework for achieving long-lasting social change in developing women-centered and midwife-led maternity services.

POINTERS FOR PRACTICE

- Midwifery is the partnership between the woman and the midwife.
- In New Zealand the shift from 'power over' to one of 'partnership' has led to a new definition of professionalism for midwifery.
- Cultural safety means that it is important for midwives to understand their own attitudes

and value system and how these might impact on others.

- For midwives who are part of the dominant culture such as white, heterosexual and middle class, understanding the principles of cultural safety can be uncomfortable and challenging.
- Midwifery knowledge is constructed from the belief that pregnancy and birth are normal life events.
- Continuity of caregiver is crucial to partnership, and enables midwives to work in their full scope of practice.

References

Association of Radical Midwives 1986 The vision: proposals for the future of the maternity services. ARM, London

Australian Nursing and Midwifery Council 2005 Role, scope of practice and development of national competency standards for midwives. Online. Available: https://www.anmc.org.au/ 31 March 2005

Barrington E 1985 Midwifery is catching. NC Press, Toronto

Cartwright S 1988 Report of the cervical cancer inquiry. Government Printing Office, Auckland

Crabtree S 2004 Midwives constructing normal birth. In: Downe S (ed.) Normal childbirth: evidence and debate. Churchill Livingstone, London

Dobbie M 1990 The trouble with women. The story of Parents Centre New Zealand. Cape Cately, Whatamongo Bay

Donley J 1986 Save the midwife. New Women's Press, Auckland

Donley J 1989 Professionalism. The importance of consumer control over childbirth. New Zealand College of Midwives Journal, September, 6–7

Downe S 2004 Aspects of a controversy: summary and debate. In: Downe S (ed.) Normal childbirth: evidence and debate. Churchill Livingstone, London

Downe S, McCourt C 2004 From being to becoming: reconstructing childbirth knowledges. In: Downe S (ed.) Normal childbirth: evidence and debate. Churchill Livingstone, London

Flint C 1986 Sensitive midwifery. Heinemann Midwifery, London

Foureur M, Hunter M (in press) The place of birth. In: Pairman S, Pincombe J, Thorogood C, Tracy S (eds) Midwifery: preparation for practice. Elsevier, Sydney

Green J, Coupland V, Kitzinger J 1990 Expectations, experiences and psychological outcomes of childbirth: a prospective study of 825 women. Birth 17: 15–24

Guilliland K 1989 Maintaining the links – a history of the formation of the NZCOM. New Zealand College of Midwives Journal September, pp 14–15

Guilliland K, Pairman S 1994 The midwifery partnership – a model for practice. New Zealand College of Midwives Journal 11: October, pp 5–9

Guilliland K, Pairman S 1995 The midwifery partnership: a model for practice. Monograph series: 95/1. Department of Nursing and Midwifery, Victoria University of Wellington, New Zealand

Henderson D 1995 Consciousness raising in participatory research: method and methodology for emancipatory inquiry. Advanced Nursing Science 17(30): 58–69

Houd S 1993 The spirit of midwifery. Keynote address, proceedings of the International Confederation of Midwives, 23rd International Congress, Vancouver, May, 75–86

Hunt S, Symonds A 1995 The social meaning of midwifery. MacMillan, London

International Confederation of Midwives 1990 Definition of a midwife. Position Statement 90/1. ICM, London

Katz Rothman B 1984 Childbirth management and medical monopoly: midwifery as (almost) a profession. Journal of Nurse–Midwifery 29(5): 300–306

Kirkham M (ed.) 2000a The midwife–mother relationship. Macmillan, London

Kirkham M 1996 Professionalisation past and present: with women or with the powers that be? In: Kroll D (ed.) Midwifery care for the future.

Meeting the challenge. Bailliere Tindall, London, 164–201

Kirkham M 2000b How can we relate? In: Kirkham M (ed.) The midwife-mother relationship, Macmillan, London

Leap N 2000 The less we do the more we give. In: Kirkham M (ed.) The midwife–mother relationship. Macmillan, London, 1–17

Leininger M 1991 Culture care diversity and universality: a theory of nursing. National League for Nursing, New York

McCrea H, Crute V 1991 Midwife/client relationships: midwives' perspectives. Midwifery 7: 183–192

McIntosh P 1988 White privilege: unpacking the invisible knapsack. Online. Available: http:// www.utoronto.ca/acc/events/peggy1. Retrieved 8/8/2004

Midwifery Council of New Zealand 2004 Midwifery scope of practice. Online. Available: http://www.midwiferycouncil.org.nz/main/ Scope/ 31 March 2005

Midwives Alliance of North America 1991 MANA core competencies for basic midwifery practice. MANA, Bristol, VA

Ministry of Women's Affairs 1989 Women's health: what needs to change. Ministry of Women's Affairs, New Zealand Government, Wellington

New Zealand College of Midwives 1993 Midwives handbook for practice. NZCOM, Christchurch

New Zealand College of Midwives 2002 Midwives handbook for practice. NZCOM, Christchurch

New Zealand College of Midwives 2005 Midwives handbook for practice. NZCOM, Christchurch

New Zealand Health Information Service 2004 Report on maternity 2002. Maternal and newborn information. Ministry of Health, Wellington

Nursing Council of New Zealand 2002 Guidelines for Cultural Safety, the Treaty of Waitangi, and Maori health in nursing and midwifery education and practice. NCNZ, Wellington

Nursing Council of New Zealand 2004 New Zealand registered nurses, midwives and enrolled nurses. Workforce statistics 2002. NCNZ, Wellington

Page L 1993 Redefining the midwife's role: changes needed in practice. British Journal of Midwifery, May, (1): 21–24

Page L A 1998 The midwife's role in modern healthcare. In: Kitzinger S (ed.) The midwife challenge. Pandora, London

Pairman S 1998 The midwifery partnership: an exploration of the midwife/woman relationship. Unpublished masters thesis, Victoria University of Wellington, Wellington

Pairman S 2000 Women-centred midwifery: partnerships or professional friendships? In: Kirkham M (ed.) The midwife–mother relationship. Macmillan, London, pp 207–226

Pairman S 2005 Workforce to profession: an exploration of New Zealand Midwifery's professionalising strategies from 1986 to 2005. Unpublished doctoral thesis. University of Technology Sydney.

Pairman S, Guilliland K 2003 Developing a midwife-led maternity service: the New Zealand experience. In: Kirkham M (ed.) Birth centres: a social model for maternity care. Books for Midwives, London

Parkes C 1993 The impact of medicalisation of New Zealand's maternity services on women's experience of childbirth 1904 – 1937. In: Bryder L (ed.) A healthy country. Essays on the social history of medicine in New Zealand. Bridget Williams, Auckland

Pelvin B 1990 Midwifery: the feminist profession. Proceedings of New Zealand College of Midwives first national conference. Dunedin, August

Pelvin B 1992 Current ethical considerations. New Zealand College of Midwives Journal, December, 6–9

Powell Kennedy H 1995 The essence of nurse-midwifery care: the woman's story. Journal of Nurse–Midwifery 40(5): 410–417

Ramsden I 1990 Kawa Whakaruruhau: cultural safety in nursing education in Aotearoa. Ministry of Education, Wellington

Ramsden I 1993 Kawa whakaruruhau: cultural safety in nursing education in Aotearoa (New Zealand). Nursing Praxis in New Zealand 8(3): 4–10

Ramsden I 2000 Cultural safety / Kawa whakaruruhau ten years on: a personal overview. Nursing Praxis in New Zealand 15(1): 4–12

Ramsden I 2002 Cultural safety and nursing education in Aotearoa and Te Waipounamu. Unpublished PhD thesis. Victoria University of Wellington, Wellington

Richardson F 2000 What is it like to teach cultural safety in a New Zealand nursing education programme? Unpublished thesis presented in partial fulfilment of the requirements for the Degree of Masters of Arts. Massey University, Palmerston North

Sandall J 1995 Choice, continuity and control: changing midwifery towards a sociological perspective. Midwifery 11: 201–209

Spence D 2004 Prejudice, paradox and possibility: the experience of nursing people from cultures other than one's own. In: Kavanagh K H, Knowlden V (eds) Many voices, toward caring culture in

healthcare and healing. The University of
Wisconsin Press, Wisconsin, pp 140–180

Strid J 1987 Maternity in revolt. Broadsheet 153:
14–17

Tully E 1999 Doing professionalism differently:
negotiating midwifery autonomy in Aotearoa/New
Zealand. Unpublished doctoral thesis. University
of Canterbury, New Zealand

Walker J, Hall S, Thomas M 1995 The experience
of labour: a perspective from those receiving
care in a midwife-led unit. Midwifery 11:
120–129

Chapter **5**

The politics of involving women in decision making

Nicky Leap and Nadine Edwards

> *We need to develop a more nuanced view of choice, one that recognises how historical and present patterns of oppression construct and constrain women's choices, but also acknowledges women's agency and capacity for self-determination.*
>
> Gregg 1995, p. 144

INTRODUCTION

We both embraced with enthusiasm the opportunity to write a chapter together about involving women in decisions about their care. We share similar passions about the subject and, as a midwife and childbirth activist, we will be drawing on our combined 60 years of experience of engaging with women and midwives who are facing decision making around childbirth.

Although our lives have taken different paths, our motivation to write about birth issues stems from a similar well of experience and understanding that stretches back to when we first gave birth (Nicky in 1968 and Nadine in 1976). Having received positive messages from our mothers about birth, we were both politicized by the struggles we had in trying to give birth to our babies at home. These experiences were the beginning of a profound understanding of, and respect for, women's power and vulnerability during pregnancy, labour and birth. This led us to address the crucial roles that autonomy, ethics, feminism and

midwives play in women's decision making about birth and motherhood and the barriers that contrive to undermine and restrict these decision-making processes. For both of us, this has meant engaging with individual women and institutions, running antenatal groups, and being involved in collective action in order to achieve changes to the way maternity care is provided.

Along the way, we have learnt more about the deep attachment between women and their babies, which enables them to go to extraordinary lengths to do what they feel is right for them, their babies and their families. We have also seen the positive impact when women are wholeheartedly supported to do what they believe is best – even if plans change as events unfold. Many people have inspired us, including courageous women, and courageous midwives and obstetricians who support women who want to exert their autonomy in ways that are unacceptable to our society. This has taught us to understand more fully the nuanced difference between choice and autonomy and the complexities of how women's and midwives' autonomy can be supported, rather than undermined, in maternity service provision.

We share the same values and bring feminist perspectives to our awareness of the potential for birth to have long-term emancipatory consequences for women, their families and communities. Our experience, mainly in the UK and Australia, has taught us that, although this potential can manifest as empowerment, often the vulnerabilities and upheavals of pregnancy and childbirth in the face of a system that is unlikely to understand and support individual needs, can leave women feeling fragile, angry, traumatized and disempowered. In order to develop strategies that maximize the potential for empowerment it is necessary to critique systems that perpetuate fragmented care and devalue and discourage women's and midwives' knowledge and expertise.

We do not think we can talk about 'involving women in decisions about their care' without talking about the relationship that they have with their carers. We recognize that in some circumstances this relationship might be built during pregnancy with an obstetrician or GP. However, for the purposes of this chapter, we will concentrate on the most common care experienced by childbearing women, that is, care provided by midwives.

In our exploration of how this relationship can affect decision making we will draw on examples where the building of mutual trust between women and their midwives is made possible, ideally through continuity of carer that occurs in community settings (Edwards 2000, Leap 2000, Wilkins 2000). Given that this is the ideal and not the dominant model of midwifery care in Western countries, we will also discuss how midwives can make a difference to women's sense of control and independence in situations where they are unable to get to know each other well. Throughout the chapter, we have given fictional examples to illustrate communication that potentially aids or hampers decision making. We have constructed them so that they apply to situations where fragmented care is the norm.[1]

The voices of women who have contributed to our understanding will be used to illuminate the issues. In particular we will use quotations, in italics, from the 30 women who contributed to Nadine's study on women's experiences of planning to give birth at home (Edwards 2001, 2005).

---

1 While research shows that continuity of carer holds clear benefits for women and midwives, we know that many midwives are providing the best care they can in services that fragment their care. We therefore wanted to include midwives working in a variety of settings.

WHY DOES DECISION MAKING MATTER TO WOMEN?

Birth is not only about making babies. Birth is also about making mothers – strong, competent, capable mothers who trust themselves and know their inner strength (Katz-Rothman 1996, p. 254).

The following quotation describes one woman's experience of pregnancy and birth and captures the essence of what we see as the goal of involving women in decision making about their care.

I still have the confidence of that whole period. And I think that will stay with me for the rest of my life. Definitely a great sense of triumph really. It's incredible.

The midwife's ability to involve women in decision making can have far reaching consequences beyond a midwife's interaction with a woman. Becoming and being a mother is a life-long process of weighing up factors in order to make decisions. We would argue that the midwife's role, responsibility and skill is to enable situations in which women have a chance to develop their confidence in their capacities, shoring them up for the challenges of new motherhood. This is described by this woman, who had a supportive and known midwife:

If I have a crisis of confidence, I think back to the birth and it's a very good anchor for me. You know it makes me believe in my ability to make good choices and things like that and I think it's made a tremendous impact on how I can make decisions. It just feels pivotal – a pivotal part of my politics really. It's almost like it drew together lots of sides that I had already and made them more cohesive as part of my life.

Women have identified that how they feel as new mothers is directly related to how much control and involvement they felt they had at every stage of pregnancy, labour and new motherhood (Green et al 1988, Green & Curtis et al 1998, Green, Renfrew & Curtis 2000). Making decisions is about autonomy and autonomy cannot be separated from identity (Griffiths 1995, Mackenzie & Stoljar 2000). Threatening or undermining choice threatens a person's identity. In other words, '. . . we cannot simply choose to abandon our cares or give up what matters to us. Or rather, we cannot do so without forfeit or loss' (Mackenzie 2000, p. 135). Women talk about birth being 'formative', with long-term repercussions in terms of how women feel about themselves when they feel disempowered by the experience (Edwards 2005):

> It's left me with a feeling that I didn't handle the situation very well and feeling that I should have really handled the situation better. I should have been stronger you know. I should have sort of held out. I should not have given in. I should have been strong and sort of said, 'no I don't want to be induced'. Why didn't I? Why wasn't I strong? I could have avoided all that. And I mean, I know why I didn't. But I didn't and I just sort of feel I probably made the wrong decision – although it's understandable why I made it. But you know it wasn't a good choice I made.

In contrast, where midwives facilitate situations in which women are able to make decisions that are relevant to their lives, there is evidence that both short and long term improvements to health outcomes and social wellbeing may result (Ickovics et al 2003, Oakley et al 1996, Sandall et al 2001).

CONSTRAINTS TO DECISION MAKING

THE PROBLEMATIC NOTION OF 'INFORMED CHOICE'

Patients' autonomy is generally reduced to the exercise of 'informed choice' in which the information provided is restricted to that deemed relevant by the health-care provider. Even in 'ideal' cases in which patients have strong autonomy skills and full access to all the available information, it is important to recognize the influence that oppression may have on the information base and, thereby, on the meaningful options available to patients (McLeod Sherwin 2000, p. 267).

While there is general recognition that women should have choice and control in childbirth (Department of Health 1993), an understanding that these concepts are complex and problematic is essential if practitioners are to engage with women in a way that enables empowerment. The contemporary notion of 'informed choice' places the onus of control on the individual, with little

recognition that social inequalities, in particular poverty, play a major role in restricting the ability of women to make changes in their lives, or even to engage in a process of making choices.

Women make choices that are already limited by intersections of ideology, resources, class, race and other factors, to a predetermined, medically-oriented menu, over which they have little control to define or change (Browner & Press 1997, Cartwright & Thomas 2001, Kirkham 2004, Kitzinger 1990, Lazarus 1997, Mander 1993, 1997, Mason 1998, Wagner 1994). Not only are choices limited by obstetric regimens, but also making choices about these is largely meaningless when women are likely to have little understanding about, or control over, the value systems on which such regimens are based. The assumption by liberal feminists that increasing choice is good for women and enhances their perception of control is not necessarily the case. Radical and socialist feminists see choice for what it is: 'a social construction that makes people feel free, even in the context of oppression, and supports the status quo' (Gregg 1995, p. 27).

Power imbalances ensure that in most situations, the person who does the 'informing' influences the decisions that individual women will make. Mavis Kirkham's book, Informed Choice in Maternity Care (2004) shows very clearly that in mainstream services, women are sometimes offered limited choices about aspects of care – but they are not *involved* in decision making. They are 'helped' to make choices that practitioners feel comfortable with rather than exploring decisions that feel right for them. Where there are points of conflict, it seems that women have to be confident, articulate, assertive, knowledgeable, and determined to make their own decisions. Alternatively they have to seek out independent care or disengage from mainstream maternity services.

Cross-cultural analyses have demonstrated particularly clearly that similar women apparently make different choices in different areas or hospitals (Davis-Floyd & Sargent 1997, DeVries et al 2001). From this it seems that choices are constructed in line with what others want and expect women to choose (Green et al 1988, Green & Coupland et al 1998). The issue of place of birth is a vivid example of this. In some cultures, home birth is an almost impossible 'choice', whereas in others it is almost impossible to 'choose' anything else. There are striking variations even within Britain depending on how available an option it is seen to be and how far it is supported by midwives and other practitioners. Many practitioners claim that women in their area do not want home births or births in midwifery-led birth centres, but in areas where these choices are supported, the home birth rates increase dramatically and women want and will opt to access birth centre care. (Leyshon 2004, Sandall et al 2001, Shallow 2003, Smethurst 1997). (See also Chapter 1.)

Part of the explanation as to why informed choice is problematic is that even when women are well informed and know their rights, most women will not make 'choices' that antagonize their carers. In addition, even when practitioners are committed to information giving and choice, women are usually encouraged to make their own decisions until there is a decision to be reached about which the practitioners feel strongly (Kirkham 2004). Indeed:

> No choice is a free choice when others have feelings, beliefs and values about the choice that is made. The choice becomes much more than, 'Will I do this or that?' It is about, 'Will doing this bring other consequences with it, will it harm a relationship, will it offend, will it create barriers to on-going help?'
> Smythe 1998, p. 232

This is a very different reading to standard political interpretations of 'choice', which have been inappropriately applied to maternity care. In standard interpretations, rationality and equality are assumed to exist unproblematically and uniformly, and power differentials remain unacknowledged within the narrow boundaries of the woman's encounters with practitioners (Shildrick 1997). At its worst, it seems that coercion is seen as simply a necessity as this comment with an obstetrician makes clear:

> I think that as obstetricians what we need to learn is to start being very manipulative with women because they are being very manipulative with us. Our only defence is going to be manipulative back because our normal standard approach, which is using logical, factual information and sense isn't working.
> Simpson 2004, p. 228

Such patriarchal assumptions about control and the stereotype of 'high control women' attempting to 'dictate' have been refuted by Green and Coupland et al (1998). On the contrary, their research showed:

> . . . a picture of women who are relatively active rather than passive, who see the birth as their responsibility as well as the staff's, who have a fairly clear idea of the sort of delivery they want and who see involvement in decision making as a necessary prerequisite for achieving this.
> Green et al 1998a, p. 152

This description is more akin to feminist debates about decision making (Belenky et al 1986, Gilligan 1985), which suggest that women place emphasis on relational ways of information gathering and discussion based on mutuality rather than control. This is why an approach that encompasses the Five Steps to Evidence-based Midwifery (see Chapter 17) is so important. Since there is no strong evidence to guide individual decision making in the majority of situations involving health (Sackett et al 1997), there is an imperative for midwives to learn to engage with women in ways that recognize the pitfalls of standard interpretations of 'informed choice' and prioritize mutual discussion and information sharing.

THE PROBLEMATIC NOTION OF CONTROL

While choice is clearly problematic, the notion that it leads to control is equally fraught with problems. Over the second half of the twentieth century, the notion of 'control' has encompassed fragmented meanings with a number of components (Green & Coupland et al 1998, Kitzinger 1990). These can broadly be defined in two categories: internal selfcontrol and external control of the environment.

The notion of self-control arises in part from the cultural fear of disorderly bodies. In the 1960s this led to the development of psychoprophylactic techniques, which ensured compliance. The emphasis was on women controlling themselves and their bodies, so that they could be docile and follow practitioners' instructions and accept their practices. Later, this approach was transformed by natural birth discourses which espoused a more complex version of self-control through attunement with bodily processes: following one's instincts and simultaneously letting go in culturally acceptable ways (Cosslett 1994). External control over what is done by others to the self (Green & Coupland et al 1998) and the environment was also seen as crucial: 'le controle sur mon environment, ca permet d'etre plus secure' (Lemay 1997, pp. 92–93).[2]

Such approaches do not necessarily take into account the development of political understandings of power and control. Wendy Trevathan (1997) sounds a note of caution about the meaning of control and how free women are to exert it. She suggests that social norms will usually decide where and how the woman gives birth, what 'artefacts' will be used, how she behaves and who receives the baby: '. . . only in rare circumstances can a woman act and behave exactly as she wishes during the birth process' (Trevathan 1997, p. 80).

When control is as infused with the values of dominant ideologies as it is today, women must attempt to take control from a position of subordination and relative powerlessness (Murphy-Lawless, 1998). Curious sequelae ensue. For example, Jo Green, Vanessa Coupland and colleagues (1998) found that women wanted to be active decision-makers and wanted control over what was done to them (Green & Coupland et al 1998, pp. 64–65). They identified that 'feeling in control was central to their experiences' (Green & Coupland et al 1998, p. 160). At the same time, the researchers noted stereotypical views of, and hostility towards, women wishing to have natural births (Green & Coupland et al 1998, p. 19), which reconstructed the usually positively viewed well-educated, well-informed woman, as problematic (Green & Coupland et al 1998, p. 24). Acts of control by professionals were particularly noticeable towards women who were deemed to have the strongest views: they were most likely to receive the opposite of what they wanted. The researchers suggested that 'The extreme [sic] views of these women were seen as irrational by staff and provoked an anti-reaction' (Green & Coupland et al 1998, p. 128).

Diana Scully's (1994) research demonstrated that doctors expect to be in control in maternity care settings. Furthermore, they like compliant

women who share their backgrounds and values and dislike women who they experience as non-compliant, questioning or 'difficult' (Scully 1994, pp. 91–93). As Scully observed, this affected the treatment of the women in their care: those who were seen as difficult tended to be ignored or even cruelly treated (Scully 1994, pp. 130–136). More recently, Julia Simpson's (2004) ethnographic study in a large obstetric unit suggests that:

> [Doctors have] . . . very low opinions of their obstetric clients. Rather than being perceived as knowledgeable, able, well-informed and able to make their own choices, pregnant women's preferences are trivialised by the registrar who suggests that 'they' want what is fashionable at the time'. Furthermore, the pregnant woman's desire for information is defensively perceived by the consultant obstetrician as a desire to blame someone . . . The consequences of these medical perspectives are twofold: either women's preferences and requests will not be taken seriously, or they will be dealt with by the obstetricians in such a way that they are ignored or not heard.
>
> Simpson 2004, p. 224

Such findings about the way women can be treated hint at the deeper structures of violence in which the status quo of the 'technocratic' culture of maternity services is maintained (Davis-Floyd 1994, 2001, Kitzinger 2000, Murphy-Lawless 1998).

NOTIONS OF 'SAFETY' AND 'RISK' IN THE TECHNOCRATIC CULTURE OF MATERNITY CARE

The word 'technocratic' is used to imply systems of maternity care in industrialized countries that are driven by the ideology and values of obstetrics, which in turn are based on the technological beliefs and values of the wider society. The use of 'technocratic' rather than 'medicalized' is an attempt to avoid the binary opposition of obstetrics versus midwifery that potentially detracts from understandings of the pervasive power of such systems and their disempowering effect on women (Davis-Floyd 2001). Whatever women had

---

2 Control over my environment allows me to be safer.

wanted prior to labour, medicalization is usually irresistible once women are in a technocratic environment (Green & Coupland et al 1998, Machin & Scamell 1997, Shapiro et al 1983).

The technocratic culture of childbirth maintains that decision making should be based on its assessment of 'safety' and 'risk'. It could be argued that all decisions are to do with safety – but that safety may have different meanings (Edwards & Murphy-Lawless, forthcoming). Technocratic meanings and interpretations of risk and safety dominate birth practices and procedures and have the potential to constrain women's and midwives' autonomy and decision making. Given that meanings flow from cultural values rather than existing in isolation, obstetric decision making may occlude social considerations in a technocratic society. The obstetric definition of safety means that while minor choices exist, conceptual choices cannot. As Shelly Romalis (1985) points out:

> The 'final say' clause in the doctor–patient contract is negotiated relatively early in the pregnancy relationship. 'You can have your baby any way you like as long as you understand that I must step in when the safety of you and the baby is involved.'
>
> Romalis 1985, p. 190

Women's views of safety are often broader than those espoused within the technocratic model of birthing. The decision-making processes women engage with around birth are to do with safeguarding and promoting wellbeing as well as avoiding harm. In considering safety, women are concerned not only about physical damage to their bodies and babies but also about the possibility of emotional harm to themselves and their families. The risk to personal integrity underpins their discussions about risk and safety (Edwards 2005). Thus, a woman who has been traumatized by a previous birth or by sexual abuse may decide to plan a caesarean section or to have a home birth with a trusted midwife. Occasionally, she may even decide to give birth on her own in order to avoid potentially harmful intrusion.

A good example of these broader views of safety occurs in remote indigenous communities in countries like Canada and Australia. In these contexts women are often expected to leave their families when they are 38 weeks pregnant to await birth in far away tertiary referral hospitals. Women often feel that it is more dangerous to them to have to be removed from their kith and kin than it is to give birth in their local communities (Kaufert & O'Neil 1993, Kildea et al 2004). Consequently some women decide not to leave even when they know that there are no immediate caesarean section facilities. In the Northern Territory of Australia up to 20% of women who are flown out of their remote communities in late pregnancy to await birth in a tertiary referral hospital, manage to hitch a lift back home before giving birth (Kildea 1999). For these indigenous women, issues of 'safety' may include having their babies in their communities, according to customary law, surrounded by women they know, who speak their language and uphold customs that are seen to make babies strong (Kaufert & O'Neil 1993, Kildea 2003; Mills & Roberts 1997). In many societies, particularly in rural areas, for women who are expected to leave home to wait to give birth in distant maternity units, thinking about 'safety' may also involve having to protect their other children and their homes from potential harm during their absence.

THE INSTITUTIONALIZATION OF BIRTH

Part of the risk of being in an institutionalized environment is the effect it has on the individual in terms of compliance and the difficulty of resisting others' expectations and 'rules' (Edwards 2005). Being in an institution involves the risk of: not being oneself; not being able to stand up for oneself; becoming 'infantilized'; of being exposed to the greater coerciveness of an ideology in its own setting and to our socialized and gender-learnt responses to institutional power (Belenky et al 1986). As Morwenna Griffiths (1995) observed, exposure to these risks can form the basis of lowered self-esteem.

The quotation from Kirsi Viisainen's (2000) study below exemplifies how women's autonomy, and thus integrity, may be at risk in an institutionalized setting:

> I do not want to go into hospital because of what happens to me there. I am such a good person. I do what they ask me to. And they will ask a lot. 'Let's have an enema, let's examine, all right lady, let's stay still, we'll listen to the baby's heartbeat, we'll put this

strap here and this string here, and let's break the membranes'. I do not want that. I want my birth to progress in peace on its own . . . I have to relax and concentrate: I cannot fight with them at the same time.

Viisainen 2000, p. 805

A technocratic institutional birth environment and lack of relationship with known caregivers can render women feeling powerless to 'choose' anything other than the choices available:

Once you go into hospital it's like, forget everything that you've learnt or put in your birth plan. (Sighing) I kept hoping that it wasn't the case, but it was very much the case. And eventually you get so fed up that it's just like, oh do anything, you know, to end this pain. So (sighs) you are then asking for whatever it is that they're going to do, when if they had been in tune with you from the beginning it might not have been necessary to do what ends up happening. If people would be much more involved with you – mobilizing you and trying to help you cope without diamorphine – then it might not get to that, where you're just, get this over with. 'Cos that is how I felt at the end. It was just, okay, yes, let's just get this over with, however it has to be done. You have no choice, you haven't really got any choice. The choice that I made was, let's get this finished and over with or do what I had been doing for the past four hours, for another couple of hours. So okay, let's get this over with.

Women describe how they might be less able to exert their autonomy and keep their concerns in the foreground if their agendas and that of the institution diverge, because institutionalization requires professional allegiance to itself and its ideology, rather than to those it serves:

I definitely think that people working within a hospital environment, especially where there's a lot of teaching going on, have a completely different attitude towards you, that you're somebody that they're learning off, or that they're teaching off or whatever. So in a hospital it wouldn't matter if I was assertive or not, the hospital couldn't change their procedure just to suit me.

Recognition of the difficulties for women in exerting control in hospital settings has led to theories

suggesting that the different basis of the relationship between woman and carer enables her to be more in control at home:

> It is this external sense of control which is most likely to be experienced as lost immediately a woman enters the hospital institution. Hence, for some women maintaining control may mean having their babies at home.
>
> Green et al 1998a, p. 19

> The social relationships between the child-bearing woman and her carers are different when the birth occurs in the woman's home, where she is in control and her carers are guests.
>
> Campbell & Macfarlane 1994, p. 4

> When women give birth at home they own the whole shop and can be in charge of the whole enterprise.
>
> Martin 1987, p. 43

However, women may suggest a more complex relationship between internal and external control, and that the control assumed at home is relative rather than absolute. As Maggie Banks observes, women may indeed only be 'truly autonomous' at home, but 'when one hears [home birth] women talk of "I had to . . ." or "they made me . . ." this is clearly not the case' (Banks 2000, pp. 214–215). The assumption that venue alone impacts on decision making is flawed. However, it can begin to make a difference because the environment inevitably has some impact on both practice and ideology (Kirkham 2003).

Moving beyond current polarized debates which dichotomize home and hospital birth is key to unblocking dichotomous discourse and practice. Placing hospital and home birth at the centre of the divide between technocratic and social meanings of birth, in situations where technocratic meanings take precedence, obstructs this. However, the attempt to fuse these meanings through the rhetoric of choice, communication, and control may result in the hospital being brought into community settings. The overall goal has to be that women are enabled to make decisions that make them feel powerful, wherever they are and with whoever attends them when they give birth. They can only feel safe, secure and protected if they know that their concerns will be respected and that their integrity and autonomy will be preserved.

THE STRUGGLE TO PRIORITIZE 'RELATIONSHIP' IN A TECHNOCRATIC BIRTH CULTURE

The relationship between a woman and a known midwife can ameliorate the impact of a technocratic birth culture (Berg et al 1996, Fleming 1994, 1998, Halldorsdottir 1996, Kirkham 2000, Pairman 2000, Smythe 1998, van Olphen Fehr 1999). Ideally, the midwife becomes a professional friend (Pairman 2000, Wilkins 2000), supporting women to give birth in the way they believe to be right for them and their babies. This relationship includes an emotional engagement, each party placing the other within a personal and biographical context (Wilkins 2000).

However, the fact that the development of relationship, trust and confidence might be important is not a concept that can easily surface in a technocratic model of birth. The randomized controlled trials whose results inform the standards and policies for practice tend to define birth as essentially mechanistic, rather than a complex interplay between body, mind, and spirit in a social context. Essentially, a mechanistic view of birth cannot facilitate decision making that includes social and spiritual dimensions because technical competence, rather than engagement, becomes the main definition of a good practitioner.

In her research into the mother-community midwife relationship, Ruth Wilkins (1993) suggests that professionalism can also be a major barrier to the emotional engagement necessary for such relationships to work well. Wilkins defines how the professionalism paradigm situates midwives and the women they attend in different social dimensions. For a midwife, the danger is that her biographical, social and psychological self is excluded from her professional practice. Instead she operates with her focus on a discreet body of professional knowledge, divorced from her social and relational context of individual interactions with women. The current conceptualization of professionalism manifests ways of knowing and practising that are based on dualistic patterns of thinking that make it 'conceptually blind' to rela-

tionships (Wilkins 2000). When this happens, professionalism exists to assert its own authoritative knowledge, which denies other ways of knowing: in her words, 'professional practice is the application of professional knowledge in an object-orientated relationship of domination and control, whether of a body, a mind or a situation' (Wilkins 2000, p. 30). This necessarily excludes relationships based on mutuality and subjectivity (partnership); thus, clinical assessment, monitoring and giving of advice take precedence over caring (Wilkins 2000, p. 34).

In its most extreme presentation 'detachment and indifference', become all but synonymous with professionalism (Smythe 1998, p. 268). According to Mary Cronk (2000), professional status is associated with a perception, reinforced by both the public and the professions themselves, that 'the expert knows best'. Cronk draws on transactional analysis theory to identify how this power imbalance directly reinforces a parent–child relationship between so-called experts and parents, one that discourages parents from taking responsibility for decision making.

In this view, the professional 'biographies' – personal histories, experiences and experiential knowledge described by Carolyn Weiner and colleagues (Weiner et al 1997) – which professionals necessarily embody, are at odds with the concept of professional knowledge. By denying other epistemological spaces, professionalism cannot comprehend midwives' or childbearing women's knowledges. Women's and midwives' knowledges, which are outside scientific evidence, are packaged into the supposedly mysterious and untrustworthy anathema to science – intuition. Feminists have made an appeal for the ongoing exploration and exposition of what women's subjective knowledge might encompass:

> [We have] learned a great deal about the development of autonomy and independence, abstract critical thought and the unfolding of a morality of rights and justice in both men and women. We have learned less about the development of interdependency, intimacy, nurturance and contextual thought.
>
> Belenky et al 1986, pp. 6–7

All that we have described above about the complexities and barriers to women's and midwives' autonomy means that one of the major problems facing women and midwives is:

> ... the difficulty of contesting the scientific approach, for it is a deeply privileged one, deeply embedded in our culture. Therefore to stand outside that rational order may be a virtual impossibility. On the other hand, it is important to try to identify the sites where women can work to develop alternative definitions.
>
> Murphy-Lawless 1998, p. 45

Alternative approaches that identify ways of addressing the constraints to women's decision making tend to lack visibility, coherence and authority. Making decisions that challenge the dominant culture of technocratic ideology depends on there being the skills, knowledge and support in this other paradigm. The rest of this chapter discusses some ways in which this can happen.

ENGAGING WITH WOMEN AROUND DECISION MAKING

BUILDING TRUST AND A SENSE OF 'SAFETY'

> If a relationship is such that the practitioner does not listen, does not come to know the hopes and fears of the woman, does not respond to her anxieties, then the mode of care can only ... be based on the semblance of what the practitioner thinks should be happening. It lacks attention to the things that are 'mattering'. It traps the woman into a passive role of accepting inappropriate, unsafe care, rather than freeing her to involve herself in the accomplishment of personalised care that promotes all that is safe.
>
> Smythe 1998, p. 202

The ability to build a trusting relationship is at the very heart of engaging with women in decision making and enabling situations in which they feel safe. Even in situations where this relationship has to be built in a hurry because the midwife and woman do not know each other, the midwife can engender a sense of 'safety' that could be described as 'midwifery watchfulness'. This approach neither looks for, nor denies, danger, but attempts to be open to recognizing it as and when it arises. This is the procedural, circumstantial approach described by Smythe (1998). It rests on the premise that while we cannot erase uncertainty, we can develop responses to meet its challenge and create safety.

Engaging with women around uncertainty is not straightforward. It requires awareness on the part of the midwife of the potential for power imbalance within the midwife–woman relationship (Fleming 1994, 1998, Guilliland & Pairman 1995, Smythe 1998). As Smythe identified, 'the practitioner woman relationship is very open to the tentative hopes of the women being overridden by the practitioner' (Smythe 1998, p. 174). This applies particularly when responding to women's requests for information. We both have experience of running workshops in which midwives identify that it is much easier to present information than to ask questions and listen to women. The culture in which midwives learn and practise may tend to indoctrinate a way of behaving that reinforces the midwife as expert whose mission is to 'educate' women. The following fictional cameos illustrate these differences in approach: (Box 5.1 and 5.2).

As identified in these cameos, even in a situation in which there is little chance of women experiencing continuity of carer by meeting the same midwife again, subtle differences in approach and language can help women build confidence in their abilities to negotiate maternity systems. The challenge to midwives who do not work in ways that mean that they can get to know women is to see their interaction with each individual woman as part of an ongoing dynamic process for the woman during this life-changing event.

Throughout the course of a woman's maternity care, decisions may overlap and change, and may need to be re-visited time and again. Formulaic tick lists covering 'discussion points' in women's maternity notes are often used and tend to reinforce a linear process where packages of information are provided at designated times. This may be at odds with the woman's need to engage in a dynamic and dialogic process that embraces complexity and uncertainty (Downe & McCourt 2004). (Box 5.2).

In Julianna van Olphen Fehr's (1999) discussion on caring relationships, and in the extensive review and theory development on caring

> **Box 5.1** Alternative responses to requests for information
>
> 1. *Mary*: I'd like to be able to move around during labour . . . I wasn't allowed to last time at St Somewhere. Will there be a problem with this here?
>   *Midwife Millicent Meanswell*: Well here at St Elsewhere we encourage all of that. You can swing from the chandeliers if you want! That's as long as everything is progressing normally of course. There's plenty of evidence from research to show that it makes sense. It can make your labour shorter because gravity helps to bring the baby down. So it's written into our protocols that we must allow women the choice to move around. So don't worry Mary, you'll be able to do whatever you want if labour's going well.
> 2. *Mary*: I'd like to be able to move around during labour . . . I wasn't allowed to last time at St Somewhere. Will there be a problem with this here?
>   *Midwife Felicity Facilitator*: Was there a reason why you were unable to move around last time Mary? (Mary tells the story of her last labour and explains why this issue is important to her – she was strapped to a fetal heart monitor because the midwife kept leaving the room. She 'desperately wanted to get off the bed but wasn't "allowed" to'). That must have been hard for you Mary. Look, most of the midwives here at St Elsewhere will encourage you to respond to whatever your body is telling you to do in labour, but I'll make a note of our discussion here to make it clear what you want and so that you don't have to keep going over the same thing with different people.

> **Box 5.1** Alternative responses to requests for information
>
> *Midwife Millicent Meanswell*: I see here that you have already decided about Vitamin K. Right, that's fine, we don't need to waste any time talking about that again. So what have you decided to do about feeding your baby? Breast or bottle?
> *Midwife Felicity Facilitator*: I see here that you have decided to give your baby Vitamin K orally. Do you still feel comfortable with that decision? Is there anything you'd like to talk further about that before we explore some other decisions you'll be making for your baby after you've given birth?

carried out by Sigridur Halldorsdottir (1996), it was evident that, while there were different meanings and roles located within caring, both connection and trust seem to form the essence of these encounters. The development of effective relationships was based on increasing reciprocity, mutuality, personal disclosure and decreasing anonymity and stereotyping. In addition, while some of the qualities attributed to caring encounters were located in the individual carer, some – such as trust, respect, and seeing the whole person – could only easily develop within the context of a relationship involving continuity of care (van Olphen Fehr 1999, pp. 138–139).

CONTINUITY OF CARER: WHAT DOES IT MEAN FOR WOMEN?

> *Like I said to you before, all that time you spend with them and yet what do you do? You chat about the same things with each of them that comes. You never really scratch the surface. I think it would have been better if you'd known who you were going to get and I know that's really difficult, but at least you could have said, right, well, that's who I'm going to get. Let me try and knock her into some sort of shape before the event. Whereas you can't try and knock six of them into shape by meeting them all once each.*

It is because of the need for ongoing dialogue that decision making happens more easily in the context of relationships involving continuity. Having experienced continuity of carer, women tell us in a myriad of ways that relationships with midwives matter a great deal. Relationships are experienced as being able to provide the engagement, trust and nurturing needed for women to feel safe enough to move through birth to motherhood:

What you want is a mother probably, to be mothered when you're just becoming a mother yourself.[3]

Decisions about such important life events as birth ideally should come at the end of a long process of consideration about what matters for an individual woman. In order to know what *really* matters to a woman, her hopes and her fears, the midwife needs to engage with the woman in a way that makes her feel as though she – the woman – is leading an exciting process of discovery:

I think that she [the midwife] made me more and more confident to explore areas. It was important for me that I did what I wanted, and when I found that my midwife was really interested in the way that I thought, it made me feel more confident. I just felt like she was saying, whatever you do, it's fine by me and of course it's my space. But it helped me to enjoy planning it knowing that she was enjoying some of the things that I had in my mind. I think that did help me to grow because I thought that she trusted my ideas and she found them interesting. It made me follow through instead of just wishing. I got more and more confident about getting exactly what I wanted.

Anecdotal evidence suggests that a reluctance to provide midwifery continuity of care often stems from a fear of 'burn out' and a fundamental misunderstanding of Jane Sandall's (1997) study, which suggested that 'burn out' can be *avoided* where midwives:

- are able to develop meaningful relationships with women;
- have occupational autonomy;
- have good support at home and at work, including meeting together frequently to negotiate flexible time 'off call'.

The justification for not providing an intrapartum component to continuity of care is based on the suggestion that women have stated retrospectively that they did not mind having a midwife they did not know in labour as long as she was kind and competent (Green & Curtis et al 1998a, Lee 1997). However, in-depth studies that have evaluated

women's (and midwives') experiences of continuity of carer have shown both quantitative and qualitative benefits (Flint 1991, McCourt & Page 1997, McCourt et al 1998, Sandall 1997, Sandall et al 2001, Stevens & McCourt 2002, van Olphen Fehr 1999). In these studies women expressed their appreciation of 'knowing' the midwife or midwives who would be there at the birth.

A wistful articulation of how women can feel when they are not able to develop a knowing relationship is articulated here:

If I'd had one midwife who I really respected and had built a relationship with over a lot of weeks or months then maybe I would have been able to talk to her about the kind of emotional difficulties that I had around not being able to talk about the value level and things. It would have depended on what midwife I got obviously, but had it been somebody who I developed a rapport with, a lot of those difficulties could have been a lot less, just from knowing somebody and knowing where they're coming from. Even just having longer to work out how it is that I can say things that otherwise would feel difficult because that's another way round having to be bluntly assertive – working out, well, how do you say this in a way that can be heard. You know, for me it can take quite a long time of negotiating around with somebody to find out what they can hear and what they respond well to and what I wouldn't be able to say or whatever.

MIDWIVES TRUSTING WOMEN

As Gay Lee (1997) has pointed out, it is simplistic to think that continuity of carer in itself is the answer to responding to women's needs. The attitudes of individual midwives and the way in which they engage with women is what matters to women:

She [the midwife] is different from the other midwives and she's quite kind of, I don't know, doing her own thing or something. And I think in a way I maybe got more of a chance with her just because when she came she said that the head was still high and I said, well, where you're pushing, you're having to push much harder to feel where his head is than the other midwives did. And she went, oh, right, right, right. Well since you think he's

---

3 By mothering we mean nurturing rather than (s)mothering.

moving down, when I come back we'll sort of see how things are going. So I don't know if any of the other midwives would have done that. But I just felt that she did really trust. She sort of seemed to say, well, you'll know, and I did know.

Clear messages to women that the midwife trusts their ability to make decisions, and to monitor their baby's wellbeing during pregnancy and after birth go a long way to building up women's confidence in their ability to be experts about their own bodies and babies and to cope with looking after their children (Leap 2000). These messages can be given regardless of whether the interaction is with a woman the midwife knows (Box 5.3).

Similarly in the early postnatal period, asking women about how their baby is instead of performing routine head-to-toe 'strip searches' which involve the midwife physically examining the baby, will go a long way to making a woman feel that the midwife trusts her ability to monitor her baby's wellbeing.

Box 5.3 Trusting women's expertise to monitor their baby's well being in pregnancy

Midwife Millicent Meanswell: OK Mary, I'm just going to listen to the baby's heart using the Doppler. Yes it's very reassuring to hear it isn't it? Women love to hear their baby's heartbeat. Ticking away beautifully, nice and steady, 130 beats a minute. That's excellent, well within the range of normal.

Midwife Felicity Facilitator: So tell me about how your baby is moving Mary. Is it the same sort of pattern as usual? Felicity Facilitator and Mary then discuss how her baby's been moving and after that, Felicity suggests . . . We can listen in with the Doppler if you want, but it's not going to tell us anything new about how your baby's getting along. As you know, you're the most important monitor of that Mary, and it's great that you're so in tune with how and when your baby moves.

FACILITATING DECISIONS ABOUT PLACE OF BIRTH

An individual midwife's attitudes will also have a profound effect on how, and when, a woman decides about where to give birth. This following cameo captures the sort of interaction that may underpin the discrepancies in home birth rates between localities and the apparently different decisions women make (Box 5.4).

There are times when midwives are challenged by the decisions that women make and find it hard to support their choices. This situation can arise particularly where there has to be a weighing up of 'risks' (see Chapter 11). As discussed earlier, this can be complex for women who live in rural and remote areas. The following cameo addresses two approaches to this situation (Box 5.5).

How people make decisions is grounded in their individual embodiment of who they are, where they have come from and what concerns they bring to any life event. Decisions arise from ongoing experiences in childhood through to adulthood (Cronk 2000). For example, there is some evidence that women who plan to give birth at home have previously been exposed to home birth, whereas those planning hospital births have had little or no contact with anyone giving birth at home (Madi & Crow 2003).

Recognition of this has led some midwives to adopt a 'wait and see' approach to the place of birth. The South East London Midwifery Group Practice, now the Albany Midwifery Practice (Sandall et al 2001), have been particular exponents of this approach. Throughout pregnancy, women and their support people are encouraged to adopt a flexible approach to where birth will take place.

The midwives will say something like this: 'We'll visit you at home in labour and we carry all the equipment that's needed for a safe birth. If labour is progressing well, it's very safe for you and the baby if we stay at home. Women who avoid being disturbed by being in a strange place labour really well. If you need help, then we'll go to hospital'. When offered this sort of option, many women who would never have thought about choosing a home birth – particularly where their families would frown on such a decision –

Box 5.4

1. *Mary*: I saw this woman on 'William and Mary'* have her baby at home last week. It looked nice. I thought I'd quite like that.

   Midwife Millicent Meanswell: We tend to discourage you from having your first baby at home Mary. You see, there's a 50% transfer rate into the hospital for 'primips' because so many women having first babies have posterior labours – where the baby is lying on his back. You get very long, stop/start labours and when this happens, you need a bit of help. We tickle up the contractions with a drip and get things moving. It's all a bit of an unknown factor with an untried pelvis. So generally we like to have you in here already, just in case, but we could book you for the Birth Centre so that you can have a home-like environment, but with all the things needed for a safe birth close by. I think that makes sense, don't you? But if everything goes well this time, you'll have no trouble booking a home birth next time.

2. *Mary*: I saw this woman on 'William and Mary' have her baby at home last week. It looked nice. I thought I'd quite like that.

   Midwife Felicity Facilitator: Yes, I saw that episode last week too. It was a beautiful birth wasn't it? That programme is certainly opening people's eyes to some of the possibilities around birth. Do you know anyone who has given birth at home Mary? . . . No? OK, let's explore some of the issues. Would you like to begin by telling me why it appeals to you?

* 'William and Mary' was a television comedy-drama series set in England and first broadcast in 2004. The main characters were William, an undertaker, and his partner Mary, a midwife.

Box 5.5 Weighing up 'risks'

Mary lives in a remote rural area and the local hospital does not have the facilities to carry out caesarean sections.

1. *Mary*: I don't want to get flown out at 38 weeks this time . . . I want to have the baby here.

   Midwife Millicent Meanswell: I can understand how hard it is for you to leave your children and family Mary, but we just don't have the facilities in the local hospital to deal with sudden emergencies. If the baby needed to be born in a hurry, there's no way we can do a caesarean here. I know it's hard but it's about safety . . .

2. *Mary*: I don't want to get flown out at 38 weeks this time . . . I'd like to have the baby here.

   Midwife Felicity Facilitator: You must have thought a lot about this Mary. It's a big decision isn't it? As you know, some people will find it hard to accept. We'll need to think about some practical things we can do to ensure that everything is in place to support you in giving birth here safely. But first, do you want to tell me why you've decided to stay here?

are able to make a safe decision in labour and give birth in the comfort and security of their own homes. Hospital becomes a positive place to go to 'if you need help' and no one has to hold out at home, trying to avoid the disappointment of a 'failed home birth'. Given the good outcomes demonstrated by the Albany midwives in a community of extreme socio-economic disadvantage (Sandall et al 2001) and the fact that over 50% of women currently give birth at home (personal correspondence, 2005) this approach could be seen as an important way to involve women in maximising their chances of having a normal birth.

Any woman who considers a home birth might be discouraged from doing so, but it is often assumed without question that women facing socio-economic challenges do not want and should not have them. Judging by the ongoing experience of the Albany Midwifery Practice, it would seem that, where decisions are made within the context of an ongoing relationship, one that promotes women's confidence in their ability to give birth and nurture their baby, women tend to make decisions that are right for them.

VISITING WOMEN AT HOME IN LATE PREGNANCY

The approach of the Albany midwives includes a visit to each woman in her home when she is around 36 weeks pregnant by the midwife/midwives who are working with her. The 36-week home visit provides an opportunity for the woman's supporters (family/friends) to meet the midwives/midwife and be reassured that they are not going to have to advocate on the woman's behalf against them. At this point in pregnancy it is particularly relevant to discuss labour and birth and to talk enthusiastically about the safety of home birth. There is also the opportunity to discuss how best to support the woman in labour and the early postnatal period (Kemp 2003, Reed 2002a, 2002b). The midwives explain practical arrangements for who will be on call and confirm that whoever ends up attending the labour will have the same philosophy and approach.

A range of other issues are discussed at this visit including:

- approaches to being with women in pain in labour without rushing to take away pain and to ensure that physiology is promoted;
- use of photographs to encourage discussion about normal birth and any particular wishes the woman has for labour and birth;
- making sure that everyone understands how best to conserve energy if the woman's labour takes a long time to get established, including information to reduce premature admission to hospital;
- what to do if the baby is born before the midwife arrives;
- childcare for other children;
- everybody's role during labour;
- practical suggestions for support following birth (Leap 2000, pp. 14–15).

These are all strategies to involve the woman and her family/social support in decision making that enhances a sense of independence and control (Kemp 2003). The mustering of support from within the woman's own family/social support plays an important role in creating situations where she can feel emotionally, as well as physically 'safe'. In her study of midwives', women's and their partners' experience of the 36 week home visit, Joy Kemp (2003) describes the initiative as:

> ... an alternative model of authoritative knowledge, one which acknowledged a role for intervention and technology but placed as central a philosophy of birth as a physiological, transformational and socio-cultural event.
>
> Kemp 2003, p. 4

Kemp's (2003) study portrayed the 36 week birth discussion as an integral part of the ongoing dialogue and relationship of mutual trust that occurs between a woman and her midwife, throughout pregnancy, where the same midwife or midwives are going to be with the woman during labour.

ENGAGING WITH WOMEN AROUND UNCERTAINTY

> Collaboration and planning for their births with their midwives seemed to be a cornerstone of the overall experience and created the rapport and trust that women needed to feel the safety to experience childbirth in their own unique way.
>
> van Olphen Fehr 1999, p. 106

Midwifery is not mechanistic. It is not possible to separate out the social, emotional and physiological understandings of any woman's situation. Engaging with women starts with the midwife asking open questions and listening to the woman's account of how she sees and feels about the overlapping interfaces of all aspects of what is happening in her life as she approaches new motherhood. The ongoing process of interaction depends on the midwife's self-awareness, particularly of the effect this is having on the woman.

If we acknowledge the importance of engagement in relationships, the process of decision making becomes less about presenting a range of options as if they were all equal and much more about listening to women and helping them to mesh decisions with their lifestyles, beliefs and backgrounds.

The drive to give women certainty underpins the obstetric ideology of decision making in pregnancy, in particular around screening and investigations. The processes of offering these tests and following up on results have opened up a whole new arena of discussion, the initiation of which is generally seen as the midwife's role. The complexity of engaging with women around the decisions they make regarding screening encompasses an exploration of values, beliefs and attitudes, beginning with the fraught areas of disability and termination of pregnancy. In busy antenatal clinics, there is rarely time to explore how these issues fit with individual women's lives. Even discussions about so-called 'routine scans' can take a lot of time and it is easy to forget that the offering of ultrasound scans should be seen as a complex choice (Box 5.6).

Interactions before routine ultrasound scans in pregnancy involve more than discussions about the known 'safety' of the procedure. The woman's fundamental feelings about how she approaches motherhood can be at stake in discussions that centre on disability and the potential choice to end the pregnancy or plan for fetal medicine/surgery. On top of this, the midwife needs to decide whether it is appropriate to temper the women's expectation of reassurance with a caution that the discovery of 'variations of normal' – for example: 'a low lying placenta', 'cysts in the baby's brain', 'dilated ureters', 'placental lakes' – are not uncommon. The identification of any of these factors can make the rest of the woman's pregnancy an extremely anxious time, and involve her in further

---

Box 5.6   Offering 'routine scans'

1. *Midwife Millicent Meanswell*: Right Mary, here's your form for the 20-week scan. You might like to take your husband with you because seeing the baby really helps men to bond with the baby. They will give you a photo of the baby for a small fee. You also need to decide before you go if you want to know the sex of the baby and tell them before they start.

2. *Midwife Felicity Facilitator*: Mary, have you thought about whether you want to have the scan at 20 weeks? It's rare these days, but some women do decide not to. Shall we talk through why you might want to have one and why you might decide to give it a miss?

---

tests – usually for no valid reason (Katz-Rothman 2001).

ENGAGING WITH WOMEN AROUND FEAR AND PAIN

It may be that the most important area in which midwives need to trust women is in their ability to cope with pain in labour. Anxiety about pain has been shown to be a strong predictor of negative experiences during labour, lack of satisfaction with birth, and poor emotional wellbeing postnatally (Green et al 2003). Increasingly we are seeing a culture where women want to avoid pain in labour: a number of women are so scared of labour that they opt to by-pass it all together by planning an elective caesarean section (Silverton 2001). In many industrialized countries the elective caesarean section is being seen as a choice that should not be challenged. However, there is some evidence that where women are given increased time during pregnancy to discuss their fears, many of them will end up changing their mind about elective caesarean section (Bewley & Cockburn 2004). Midwives often feel unable to discuss the idea with women that pain has a purpose in case this is interpreted as 'persuasion' – the notion of choice is respected to the extent that the elective epidural or even caesarean is seen as a woman's right. Counteracting this conditioning takes courage on the part of midwives.

Support by midwives for helping them find ways to cope with pain in labour is important to women (Chamberlain et al 1993, Lundgren & Dahlberg 1998, Smith et al 2003). The ways in which information and support are given around pain are significant in terms of how women feel about themselves and their experiences of childbirth (Halldorsdottir & Karlsdottir 1996, Hodnett 2002, Lundgren & Dahlberg 1998). Caregivers therefore need to provide women with accurate information about the effects of coping strategies and to be alert to aspects of care that may disrupt women's ability to use these (Spiby et al 2003).

Engaging with women around labour pain requires extreme sensitivity on the part of the midwife. This includes an awareness that variations in the use of obstetric analgesia often appear to be related to institutional or professional opinion factors rather than population factors or individual women's choices (Hodnett 2002).

In discussing labour pain with women, it is important for midwives to remember – and to tell women – that there is no correlation between effective forms of pain relief and greater satisfaction with the experience of birth (Heinz & Sleigh 2003, Hodnett 2002, Morgan et al 1982). In fact, studies have suggested that women who have had epidurals are often less satisfied than those who experience pain (Chamberlain et al 1993, Green et al 2003, Halldorsdottir & Karlsdottir 1996). We also know that analgesia and anaesthesia for pain relief increases the likelihood of interventions and that women who have the least interventions are most likely to be satisfied about their experiences, even if they had wanted interventions prior to labour and birth (Green et al 2003). This may be because the experience of overcoming a huge physical and emotional challenge during labour leaves women with a sense of triumph and confidence associated with empowerment and a rite of passage (Leap & Anderson 2004).

In recent years, the offering of the 'menu' of various methods of 'pain relief' (Leap 1997) has been associated with the notion of a woman's right to make 'informed choices' about all aspects of her care (Department of Health 1993, NHMRC 1996). When adopting this approach, practitioners systematically explain the advantages and disadvantages of each method 'on the menu' so that the woman may make appropriate choices, usually in advance of labour. This is a hierarchical menu, starting with the non-pharmacological methods that midwives tend to feel all right about, such as water and aromatherapy, and ending with the epidural at the bottom of the list. This offering of 'the menu' in itself creates a culture where both women and their attendants end up seeing some form of 'pain relief', however seemingly innocuous, as a necessary part of the process of giving birth. A different approach is to talk to women about their ability to be able to cope with the pain of an uncomplicated labour. This involves explaining about the role of endogenous opioids. These two approaches are seen in the following cameo (Box 5.7).

The concept of 'working with pain' (Leap 1997) and enabling the woman to release her body's own endogenous opioids demands a midwifery

---

Box 5.7 'Choosing' pain relief in labour

1. *Mary*: I have a low pain threshold so I'm wondering what my options are for pain relief?

   Midwife Millicent Meanswell: Well Mary, we have a range of options you can choose from to help you cope with pain. I'll run through them if you like and we can explore the advantages and disadvantages of each method so that you can start to think about the choices you might like to make. But let's start with the non-pharmacological methods because these are the ones without any side effects. The longer you can go just using these, the better for you and the baby.

2. *Mary*: I have a low pain threshold so I'm wondering what my options are for pain relief?

   Midwife Felicity Facilitator: The first thing to say Mary is that labour pain is quite different from other pain – say the pain of injury – and how women react to it doesn't seem to be related to how high or low their pain threshold is. Maybe this is because when you're getting good strong contractions and your baby is lying in a helpful position, the pain of labour triggers your body into making it's own internal painkillers – some people call these 'endorphins'. Has anyone told you about this? OK, well would you like me to explain some more about it?

---

approach that many women and midwives understand and covet. It is an approach that prioritizes enabling situations in which women can build their confidence in their ability to give birth, one that aims to override the negative conditioning that women receive about pain in society. The second midwife in the cameo above is attempting to counteract the notion of the stereotype of a woman with a 'low pain threshold'.

The experiences that women and midwives share around pain in labour arguably form a body of knowledge that is an important key to the concept of 'keeping birth normal'. In turn, this notion is directly linked to enabling situations where childbearing women are able to take power and become confident mothers.

FACILITATING RATHER THAN STEERING DECISIONS

Decisions are always limited by a host of complex factors. However, there are also enabling factors, in particular, the initiation of discussion that can turn apparently limited options into expansive decision-making processes for women. This is particularly challenging, and rewarding for all involved, where midwives are working with women who are unused to, or have been prevented from, exerting autonomy in their lives or where women want to make certain decisions but find they have little support for these.

Testimony from women makes an important contribution to challenging the perception that many women want the practitioner to decide for them. The idea that women do not, will not or cannot make decisions is reinforced every time a woman asks the midwife what she thinks she should do, or what she would do (or did do) herself. There may be all sorts of underlying meanings underpinning such questions and these often get misinterpreted. For example, for the woman, asking her midwife what she thinks she ought to do could be:

- a rhetorical question that needs no immediate response;
- a way of attempting to engage on a personal level;
- a lack of confidence to say what she is really thinking;
- a standard response because in her life she is used to doing, or is expected to do, what others say (especially professionals – because 'they know best');
- a way of checking whether there is a 'right' answer.

When a woman seems to be asking a professional to decide for her, this rarely means that she has no opinions, that she does not mind what happens or that she does not want to be involved in decisions, at least to some extent. It is important that midwives do not make the assumption that women do not want to make decisions when they ask questions like, 'What would you do?' or, 'I don't know, you decide . . .' (Box 5.8).

Box 5.8   Avoiding assumptions

1. *Mary*: Well, what would you do if you were me?

   Midwife Millicent Meanswell: I'm afraid I can't decide for you Mary. It has to be your choice. I can give you all the information about this but you have to weigh it up and decide for yourself.

2. *Mary*: Well, what would you do if you were me?

   Midwife Millicent Meanswell: Well if I were you I'd do . . .

3. *Mary*: Well, what would you do if you were me?

   Midwife Felicity Facilitator: I don't know. It's a difficult one, isn't it? It's not straightforward. We probably should set aside some time to explore it all a bit more so that you can work out how you feel about it.

Rather than assuming, as the midwife in the first and second examples did that the woman does not want to, cannot, or will not make a decision, the midwife in the third example acknowledged the complexity of the situation. She interpreted the question as a need for more dialogue and possibly more information. The opportunity to do this is often limited. In such situations, many women attempt to negotiate with maternity services by making a birth plan in order to make their individual needs and aspirations known.

BIRTH PLANS

The birth plan, initially developed in the 1980s by birth activists, was a response to women's unsatisfactory experiences of birth, where lack of continuity meant that women were unable to discuss their views with professionals beforehand. This was an attempt to regain some control over decision making in the light of potentially harmful routine practices and procedures. Birth plans were promoted to support women's desires to have intervention free births, whilst recognizing the need for some authoritative mechanism for communication in contexts where sustaining relationships were not being developed.

Although the design and use of birth plans were to be placed in the hands of women, most hospitals responded by producing their own limited 'tick box' birth plans. Once again this allowed the institutions to regain control over choice. The menu from which choices could be made was restricted to coincide with localized practices and policies. Contrary to enabling more choice for women, there is evidence that using birth plans incites hostility from healthcare professionals, increasing the likelihood of interventions (Jones et al 1998).

In an area health service in Sydney, Australia, an attempt to revolutionize the birth plan was initiated in 2005 by a group of midwives and women whose task was to design a set of woman friendly maternity notes. The group recognized that the culture of including a birth plan in maternity notes was too entrenched to attempt its removal. Users of maternity services identified that they saw it as an important tool in systems where they are not necessarily able to know the midwife who will be with them in labour. The women argued that it should be accessible to all pregnant women within the records that they will carry with them whenever they see practitioners during pregnancy.

In the latest draft of these records,[4] the birth plan was turned on its head and used as an education tool and mandate for practitioners as well as a public message of reassurance to women. The section about preparation for labour and birth states (Box 5.9):

ENGAGING WITH WOMEN SENSITIVELY: SELF-AWARENESS

We just slowly discussed how we both felt about the birth environment, and as we concurred on that, I didn't need to set the tone really. It just became . . . sort of seamless. It just seemed to gel together. So in that way it was more of a discussion. We would have discussions about things that would come up. There would be a programme

---

4 South Eastern Sydney Area Health Service, Draft Woman Held Antenatal Record of Care. This maternity record is still in draft form at the time of publication. Women's and practitioners' views of the record, including the use of the birth plan will be evaluated once they are in circulation.

Box 5.9   In preparation for labour and birth

In thinking about plans for your labour, the birth of your baby and the early days following birth, there may be things that are important to you that you would like to discuss with your midwife or doctor. We have a commitment to making sure you are given a safe, supportive service. We will make sure that you are fully involved in any decisions that are made and that you are informed about choices you might like to make at every stage.

During your labour, your midwives will work with you to ensure that your individual needs and wishes are met. If your labour is straightforward, these might include:

- Moving around and finding positions that are comfortable for labour and giving birth.
- Being free to make noise and use water for comfort.
- Having the people you choose with you for support and comfort.
- A range of strategies for coping with pain in labour.
- Gentle birthing of your baby to avoid an episiotomy.
- You being the first person to pick up your baby at birth.
- Skin-to-skin contact to promote early breastfeeding.

If there are any particular wishes you have please discuss them with your midwife or doctor and write them here so that we can be aware of them.

---

on TV about birth, so we'd discuss it a bit. So we found out how each other felt that way rather than having a question and answer sort of dialogue.

Involving women in decision making depends to a large extent on the communication skills of the midwife. Although the relationship the midwife has with a woman – how 'known she is' – is important, the midwife also needs to 'know' herself. For midwives to work in partnership with women, it is necessary for them to develop finely tuned skills in self-awareness. This includes an understanding of the potential effect of the use of self during interactions and an awareness of the significance of informal interactions.

> It actually took me a while to stop asking questions that I didn't even care about that much and I think she helped me to just become more in touch with what I really needed to know or what I really needed to do in the time that we spent together – which wasn't always ask questions. It was sometimes to ask her questions about her life or just chat about something that had been in the news. You know sometimes that was a better use of the time. We wouldn't cover any major ground. And I think that took me a while to swing into that very informal structure, but I began to realize that I was enjoying the times that I spent with her and that I was feeling more and more confident, even when I hadn't cleared up any specific issue.

REAL TALK: REAL COMMUNICATION

The concept of 'real talk' is one of the ingredients for decision making for many women. Many feminists have observed that 'real talk', occurs in informal rather than formal settings and has thus been attached to the private (supposedly) inconsequential world of women and devalued as 'gossip' or 'chat'. However, women confirm that this is the way 'small truths' (Spacks in Belenky et al 1986, p. 116) are exchanged:

> I think I would pick and choose who I spoke to. One or two of them, I would sit and think, 'Na, I'll wait till next week'. But if it was maybe my named midwife or [the midwife present at my last birth] sitting there, I would chat away to them about it. You see, I think so much of it is, you come in, you sit down, they take your blood pressure, whatever. They do all the bits and pieces, but if they don't chat to you about inconsequential, how's your son, bla bla bla, you don't end up saying – they don't learn so much because you just walk out of there and you think, oh I forgot about, or you don't feel comfortable and you think, och, I won't bother, or if they give the impression that you're a bit late for your appointment and there's somebody else sitting there, then you think, och, it can wait. [Midwife at last birth] will chat to you, my named midwife will chat to you, but

> it's the ones that don't. I don't think they get so much and you don't get so much. But I suppose it's just getting to know somebody as well.

Lack of time and of familiarity – for example in most busy antenatal clinics – prevents opportunities for 'real talk'. Where communication is hurried and separated from relationships, women's ways of talking and relating are muted:

> I haven't really talked to her [midwife] at all. She just says things like, plenty of movements then? And I go, yeh. And then afterwards I think, I wonder what plenty of movements means, you know, like, what is plenty 'cos I don't know, and I've never really talked to her about anything. Whereas with the other one [midwife], who I met just once, when she came round, we just found ourselves chatting. And she included my partner as well. She asked us questions that encouraged us to talk 'cos often I don't think of problems or worries. It's just like, here's my blood, and here's my urine and all that, whereas she encouraged me to think about things slightly differently.

While communication in the technocratic model of birth is grounded in the discourses of information, choices, control and rights, communication for the women in the above quotations was based on connection, trust and the sharing of experiences (stories). Unlike the didactic, disengaged, reductionist and coercive nature of most communication within the technocratic model of birth, these structured, purposeful narratives generate as much knowledge about the teller as about the subject matter. Thus, they hold within them possibilities for communication which can destabilize authoritative knowledge and create new epistemological spaces (Code 1998) from which women and midwives can create different meanings about birth.

THE VALUE OF STORY TELLING

As Robbie Pfeufer-Kahn (1995) identifies, the value of personal storytelling is that it creates conditions for knowing that engage the heart and mind in a fluid process that moves beyond the particular. She identifies that this approach may be at odds with ways of communicating that leave ideas 'fastened by stakes, like a circus tent in one small spot' (Pfeufer-Kahn 1995, p. 14). Midwives, as well as women, need to understand the value of story telling in their practice if they are to engage with women in meaningful ways:

> A story tells more than its tale. It speaks of context and of values. Listeners absorb the story through a web of their own view of the world and by links with their own stories . . . Stories reveal important aspects of midwives work and their careful examination may open up new dimensions in which we can usefully be with women.
>
> Kirkham 1997, p. 183

When observing and interviewing midwives in a London birth centre Hannah Williams (2003) identified that almost all midwifery narratives began with, 'I had a lady who . . .'. Williams suggests that this is the midwifery equivalent of 'Once upon a time . . .'. She concluded that midwifery stories play a major role in developing an occupational culture in which the physiology of birth is admired and respected, where women's strength in giving birth is acknowledged and where midwives are encouraged to develop new skills and new ways of interacting with women. This echoes Bridgitte Jordan's work. In Birth in Four Cultures, Jordan (1993) identifies how midwives in some cultures met challenges by discussing stories and applying knowledge from one story to another situation.

The telling of stories enables women and midwives to engage, negotiate their different subject positions and joint meanings of birth, and dialogue in ways that enable more expansive partnerships. So while women need structures and settings in which stories can be told, these are often not provided within the existing, task-oriented framework of care, as identified here:

> There is so much procedure and so many stock tests to be gotten through. By the time you've done that there is no slack in the appointments procedure for any vague chatting, as they would think of it. Which I think needs to change because I think that's more important than anything else. I think it's very important to know what someone's fears are and what they're strengths are. To me that's crucial and I could bet my bottom dollar that there was no question that would ever address that. I couldn't ask questions like that because it

> would be so jarring. It would just be so personal. It would be like I was gushing all over them if I'd said anything like, I need to discuss how I feel about being naked in front of a complete stranger, or I need to discuss how I feel about making noises. It would seem embarrassing. I'm not embarrassed to discuss these things but in the framework of the NHS system it would be very embarrassing to bring that up because all they're asking you is questions about your weight and your bowel movements and your pee. You know within that setting to try and bring up more emotional complex issues would feel quite wrong. You would feel like you crossed the boundary and I'm sure it would be quite embarrassing for a lot of the individuals if you did that. I don't know though. Maybe they would welcome it but I never felt like trying it really.

The task-focused approach described here is in direct opposition to a situation where women can develop an ongoing relationship with their midwives. Ruth Wilkins (2000) has explored how this relationship is best developed where midwives are based in the community.

A SOCIAL MODEL OF MIDWIFERY

> Where you combine continuity of care with social support from other women, you have a powerful recipe for improving physical and psychosocial outcomes during pregnancy and childbirth for women, children and their partners.
>
> Sandall 1996, p. 12

The personal and psychosocial needs of individual women are more easily made visible where midwifery is anchored within the woman's social context. This important element of a midwifery model aims to focus on birth as a social, rather than a technocratic, event (Kitzinger 2000). The benefits appear countless (Rooks 1997). Some of these were identified by Anne Oakley and colleagues (Oakley et al 1990, 1996). Their randomized controlled trial and seven-year follow-up study demonstrated that the effect of midwives making themselves available, in a 'listening ear' capacity, had profound long term consequences on the relationships and social lives of women, their children and families. When compared with women who did not have support from midwives, women continued to show increased confidence, their children developed better relationships at school and their partners were more involved in domestic chores and childcare. The potential of the midwife's role in this capacity is described by Sheila Kitzinger (2000) in terms of midwives being at the intersection of emotional and biological interactions:

> The art of the midwife is in understanding the relationship between psychological and physiological processes in childbirth. Rather than being the provider of a technical service to support a doctor, or someone who scuttles around getting ready for an obstetrician and cleaning away after him, her skills lie at the point at which the emotional and biological touch and interact. She is not the manager of labour and delivery. Rather she is the opener of doors, the one who releases, the nurturer. She is the strong anchor when there is fear and pain; the skilled friend who is in tune with the rhythms of birth, the mountain tops and chasms, the striving and the triumph.
>
> Kitzinger 2000, p. 164

Concentration on the 'Three 'C's: Choice, Control and Continuity' has often deflected attention away from the importance of that other, overarching 'C': Community. Where midwives are based in the community, they can work according to primary health care principles in a role that embraces community development and public health strategies (Kaufmann 2000, 2002). Midwifery education programmes are increasingly making sure that they prepare midwives to work in this way.

The potential contribution of midwives in the community is often under acknowledged. In the UK, this was identified in a parliamentary report addressing public health in primary care:

> It is worth remembering the role of midwives in this respect, who ... work across sectors, visiting mothers and babies at home and providing a flexible antenatal and postnatal service which includes giving health advice, offering tests and screening, and supporting the psychological health of mothers. Midwives are often passed over by public health

strategists because they are usually employed and managed by the acute sector, which is not at the forefront of the public health agenda, but in fact they have an important public health role ... Midwives work in a social model of health ... such as providing emotional and social support for women in pregnancy, which has been shown to be linked to shorter labours, less analgesia and operative delivery and other positive outcomes ... (House of Commons Select Committee on Health Second Report 2001, Section 75).

ANTENATAL GROUPS

A social model of midwifery sees bringing women together as a crucial strategy to promote their wellbeing (Leap 2005). As suggested by Mavis Kirkham, 'linking women with others makes them stronger' (Kirkham 1986, p. 47). One of the most effective ways of involving women in decision making is to organize antenatal groups where they can meet other women, form friendships, learn from each other, and discuss issues together (Armstrong et al (in press), Leap 1991). Where the focus of antenatal groups centres on antenatal care as well as education and support, significant improvements in outcomes has been identified in disadvantaged communities in the USA through the concept named 'CenteringPregnancy' (Ickovics et al 2003, Schindler Rising 1998). Longer pregnancies and better weight gain for preterm infants was demonstrated where women received care throughout pregnancy in Centering groups.

The concept of facilitating and running groups instead of classes is based in a women-centred philosophy. Women set the agenda in the groups. They learn from each other and build their own support network, thus minimizing dependency on health professionals. This process was described by women who attended a group in Deptford, south east London in a video they made with Nicky (Leap 1991):

> I think it's the only place I go where people don't try to **tell** you how you're supposed to feel ... It sort of makes me feel like I'm the one that's got the power and I used to think that everyone else had the power over me. ... It wasn't about 'experts/novices, women/us' ... we were all seen

*as having a valuable contribution to make; we were seen as having our own expertise . . . The group helps you sort out what **you** want to do. It helps you to make your own decisions . . .*

Midwives and others who facilitate such groups learn about the wealth of expertise that women have and their courageous ability to engage in problem solving together. Learning to work in this way is a challenge to the idea that the midwife is the 'expert' whose role is to educate women. Instead of 'classes' where the midwives instruct the women, antenatal groups can be organized so that each week someone comes back to the group to tell their story. This triggers discussion. Women can go to the group as often as they like, starting in early pregnancy, so they will hear lots of different stories. As one of the women in the video says:

> *Because you hear so many different stories from so many women, it's very rich information that you're getting.*

The midwife's role is described by the women in the video as that of a 'facilitator' who makes sure that each week a round of introductions starts the group. The midwife running groups such as these develops listening skills. She needs to know how to ask open-ended questions and how to draw on the expertise of group members. She will make sure that people feel safe to talk or to remain silent and that no one dominates the discussion. She makes sure that newcomers are looked after and understand how the group operates. The midwife needs to judge when it is appropriate to interject with information, when to explain, and most importantly, when to keep quiet. Her skill lies in picking up cues from the group's discussion. One woman describes how this process changes the way women learn:

> *To have the midwife there to provide some real . . . well yes, 'education' as to what it's all about . . . bringing in the pelvis and 'baby' [doll] and actually showing how the baby travels down the birth canal . . . and that coming up in a sort of organic way as a woman was talking about the birth she'd had last week and how the baby had got stuck somewhere, the midwife showed us. It stayed in my head because it was attached to real people. It wasn't abstract information you were*

getting. It was associated with women in the group so it got absorbed differently.

A model of antenatal education and support where women set the agenda (as opposed to being taught what the midwife has decided they should know about) can have far reaching consequences for both women and midwives. Such groups are best situated in the community but have also been run successfully in hospital antenatal clinics as an alternative to classes and on antenatal and postnatal wards for women who are hospitalized.

Women are highly motivated to continue the friendships they have made in the antenatal groups. Postnatal groups can provide a continuity of friendship and support, which women in the video described as 'a life line' in breaking down the isolation of new motherhood:

> *Just being able to ring someone up in the middle of the night . . . just the fact that you've had a conversation with someone means that you're not there as an island trying to cope on your own.*

> *I think they're probably friends that you'll have for life, even though we're all so different. I would have been very isolated otherwise . . . we formed a network of women who met up outside of the group and carried on meeting for years.*

CONCLUDING THOUGHTS

> *There was a kind of silence in the relationship, a stillness which was very important. And we'd done all the talking in the build up. So the talking was done. I felt confident that she [the midwife] knew where I was coming from and vice versa. It was like we'd done all our dress rehearsal – what if, what if. And on the day there was nothing left to say really. So it just felt very calm, and I think that was the most important thing.*

The range of interactions between midwives and women described in this chapter are about inspiring confidence in women through processes involving mutual trust. Often this means addressing the conditioning that women and their families have been exposed to that obscures their abilities to make decisions that might be in their best interests (Leap 1996, 2005). Decisions are heavily influenced by the persuasive elements of the birth culture the woman happens to be in (Davis-Floyd & Sargent 1997). It may be a legitimate part of a midwife's role to counteract the conditioning that women have had that, to use an example, inhibits them choosing to breast feed their baby. Many people will feel uncomfortable about this idea, given the awareness of how women are coerced within the technocratic model of birth through exploitation of power imbalances. In industrialized society, we claim to shy away from the notion of 'persuasion' without recognizing that some element of persuasion underpins all of our day-to-day interactions (Herrick 2001). To imagine that we can give information in an unbiased way without an element of persuasion is naïve.

In many situations, midwives (and others who counteract the technocratic birth imperative and are thus accused of persuading women, are in fact providing the means for resistance and evening up the odds a little. As Iris Marion Young (1990, 1997) discusses, some power imbalances are so marked, we need positive action to promote alternative philosophies and actions. The dominant culture is after all highly pervasive and persuasive, whether or not we see this. Women and midwives who work with uncertainty, potential and possibilities are addressing this conditioning.

We can take heart from studies such as that of Celine Lemay (1997) and Juliana van Olphen Fehr (1999), that observed that although medical knowledge and power can invalidate women, the relationship between women and midwives can have far reaching positive consequences. Women in these studies saw their midwives' knowledge and power as supporting, validating and complementary, to the extent that they developed a joint knowledge, power and confidence. The relationship between them was fundamental to both the women and the midwives feeling confident and secure.

We trust that midwives will continue to work on enabling situations where women can feel more powerful in their lives. We look forward to a time where the notion of 'informed choice' becomes obsolete; where instead, practitioners respond to women's needs and decisions in a dynamic process of creative reciprocity.

POINTERS FOR PRACTICE

- Social inequalities, power relationships and systems make it hard for women to have genuine informed choice.
- Midwives can increase their sensitivity to the way women may feel through engaging in professional development, role play and group discussion.
- Midwives may make a difference by the way they ask questions and being aware of their own background and personal experience and how these affect their interaction with women.
- Midwives may be helped in understanding the effect they have on interaction by gaining feedback about their abilities to provide information.
- Think about women's views and experiences and how you might gain knowledge about these.

- Think about ways of continuing to improve your midwifery knowledge and understanding about the meaning of birth for individual women.

References

Armstrong F, Clayton L, Crewe J, Edwards N, Seekings Norman L, St Clair A, Wickham S (in press) Communities of women. In: Wickham S (ed.) Best practice, 4th Volume. Books for Midwives, Hale, Cheshire

Banks M 2000 Home birth bound: mending the broken weave. Birthspirit Books, New Zealand

Belenky M F, Clinchy B M, Goldberger N R, Tarule J M 1986 Women's ways of knowing: the development of self, voice and mind, Basic Books,

Berg M, Lundgren I, Hermansson E, Wahlberg V 1996 Women's experience of the encounter with the midwife during childbirth. Midwifery 12: 11–15

Bewley S, Cockburn J 2004 Should doctors perform Caesarean for 'informed choice' alone? In: Kirkham M (ed.) 2004 Informed choice in maternity care. Palgrave Macmillan

Browner C H, Press N 1997 The production of authoritative knowledge in American prenatal care. In: Robbie E, Davis-Floyd R (eds) Childbirth and authoritative knowledge: cross-cultural perspectives. University of California Press, Berkeley, pp. 113–131

Campbell R, Macfarlane A 1994 Where to be born? The debate and the evidence. 2nd edn. National Perinatal Epidemiology Unit, Oxford

Cartwright E, Thomas J 2001 Constructing risk. In: DeVries R, Benoit C, van Teijlingen E R, Wrede S (eds) Birth by design: pregnancy, maternity care, and midwifery in North America and Europe. Routledge, London, pp. 218–228

Chamberlain G, Wraight A, Steer P 1993 Pain and its relief in childbirth. Churchill Livingstone, Edinburgh

Code L 1998 Voice and voicelessness: a modest proposal? In: Kourany J A (ed.) Philosophy in a feminist voice: critiques and reconstructions. Princeton University Press, Princeton, New Jersey, pp. 204–230

Cosslett T 1994 Women writing childbirth: modern discourses on motherhood. Manchester University Press, Manchester

Cronk M 2000 The midwife: a professional servant? In: Kirkham M (ed.) The midwife–mother relationship. Macmillan, London

Davis-Floyd R E 1994 The technocratic body: American childbirth as cultural expression. Social Science and Medicine 38: 1125–1140

Davis-Floyd R E 2001 The technocratic, humanistic and holistic paradigms of childbirth. International Journal of Gynaecology Obstetrics 75: S5–S23

Davis-Floyd R E, Sargent C 1997 Childbirth and authoritative knowledge: cross cultural perspectives. University of California Press, Berkeley, CA

Department of Health 1993 Changing childbirth (Cumberledge report). Department of Health. HMSO, London

DeVries R, Benoit C, van Teijlingen E R, Wrede S (eds) 2001 Birth by design: pregnancy, maternity care, and midwifery in North America and Europe. Routledge, London

Downe S, McCourt C 2004 From being to becoming: reconstructing childbirth knowledges. In: Downe S (ed.) Normal childbirth: evidence and debate. Churchill Livingstone, Edinburgh

Edwards N P 2000 Women planning home births: their own views on their relationships with midwives. In: Kirkham M (ed.) The midwife–mother relationship. Macmillan, London pp. 55–91

Edwards N P 2001 Women's experiences of planning home births in Scotland. Unpublished PhD, University of Sheffield, Sheffield

Edwards N P 2005 Birthing autonomy: women's experiences of planning home births. Routledge, London

Edwards N P, Murphy-Lawless J (in press) The instability of risk: women's perspectives on risk and safety in birth. In: Symon A (ed.) Risk and choice in maternity care. Elsevier, Edinburgh

Fleming V E M 1994 Partnership, power and politics: feminist perceptions of midwifery practice. Unpublished PhD thesis. Massey University, New Zealand

Fleming V E M 1998 Women-with midwives-with-women: a model of interdependence. Midwifery 14: 137–143

Flint C 1991 Continuity of care provided by a team of midwives – the know your midwife scheme. In: Robinson S, Thomson A M (eds) Midwives, research and childbirth vol 2. Chapman and Hall, London, pp. 72–103

Gilligan C 1985 In a different voice: psychological theory and women's development. Harvard University Press, Cambridge

Green J M, Coupland V A, Kitzinger J V 1988 Great expectations: a prospective study of women's expectations and experiences. Child Care and Development Group, University of Cambridge, Cambridge

Green J M, Coupland V A, Kitzinger J V 1998 Great expectations: a prospective study of women's expectations and experiences of childbirth. 2nd ed. Books for Midwives, Hale, Cheshire

Green J M, Curtis P, Price H, Renfrew M 1998 Continuing to care. The organisation of midwifery services in the UK: A structured review of the evidence. Books for Midwives, Hale, Cheshire

Green J M, Renfrew M J, Curtis P A 2000 Continuity of carer: what matters to women? A review of the evidence. Midwifery 16: 186–196

Green J, Baston H, Easton E, McCormick F 2003 Greater expectations? Inter-relationships between women's expectations and experiences of decision making, continuity, choice and control in labour, and psychological outcomes: Summary Report. Leeds: Mother and Infant Research Unit. Online. Available: www.leeds.ac.uk/miru/

Gregg R 1995 Pregnancy in a high-tech age: paradoxes of choice. New York University Press, New York

Griffiths M 1995 Feminisms and the self: the web of identity. Routledge, London

Gulliland K, Pairman S 1995 The midwifery partnership: a model for practice. Victoria University of Wellington, New Zealand

Halldorsdottir S 1996 Caring and uncaring encounters in nursing and health care: developing a theory. Department of Caring Sciences, Faculty of Health Sciences, Linkoping University

Halldorsdottir S, Karlsdottir S I 1996 Journeying through labour and delivery: perceptions of women who have given birth. Midwifery 12(2): 48–61

Heinz S D, Sleigh M J 2003 Epidural or no epidural anaesthesia: relationships between beliefs about childbirth and pain control choices. Journal of Reproductive Health and Infant Psychology 21(4): 323–333

Herrick J 2001 The history and theory of rhetoric: an introduction. 2nd edn. Allyn Bacon, Needham Heights, Massachusetts

Hodnett E D 2002 Pain and women's satisfaction with the experience of childbirth: a systematic review. American Journal of Obstetrics and Gynecology 186(5): S160–S172

House of Commons Select Committee on Health Second Report 2001 Public health in primary care. HMSO, London

Ickovics J R, Kershaw, T S, Westdahl C, Rising S, Klima C, Reynolds H et al 2003 Group prenatal care and preterm birth weight: results from a two-site matched cohort study. Obstetrics and Gynecology 102: 1051–1057

Jones M H, Barik S, Mangune H H, Jones P, Gregory S J, Spring J E 1998 Do birth plans adversely affect the outcome of labour? British Journal of Midwifery 6(1): 38–41

Jordan B 1993 Birth in four cultures: a cross-cultural investigation of childbirth in Yucatan, Holland, Sweden and the United States. 4th edn. Waveland, Prospect Heights Illinois

Katz-Rothman B 1996 Women, providers and control. Journal of Obstetrics, Gynaecology and Neonatal Nursing 25(3): 253–256

Katz-Rothman B 2001 Spoiling the pregnancy: prenatal diagnosis in the Netherlands. In: DeVries D, Benoit C, van Teijlingen E R, Wrede S (eds) Birth by design: pregnancy, maternity care, and midwifery in North America and Europe. Routledge, New York, pp. 180–198

Kaufert P, O'Neil J 1993 Analysis of a dialogue on risks in childbirth: clinicians, epidemiologists, and Inuit women. In: Lindenbaum S, Lock M (eds) Knowledge, power and practice, the anthropology of medicine and everyday life. Berkeley, California

Kaufmann T 2000 Public health: the next step in woman-centred care. RCM Midwives Journal 3(1): 26–28

Kaufmann T 2002 Midwifery and public health. MIDIRS Midwifery Digest March (12 Supplement 1): S23–S26

Kemp J 2003 Midwives', women's and their birth partners' experiences of the 36 week birth talk: a qualitative study, Unpublished MSc thesis. The Florence Nightingale School of Nursing and Midwifery, Kings College, London

Kildea S 1999 And the women said. Report on birthing services for Aboriginal women from remote Top End communities. Territory Health Service, Darwin

Kildea S 2003 Risk and childbirth in rural and remote Australia. Paper presented at the 7th National Rural Health Conference, The Art and Science of Healthy Community -Sharing Country Know How, Hobart

Kildea S, Wardaguga M, Dawumal M 2004 Maningrida women. Birthing business in the bush website www.maningrida.com/mac/bwc/birthing/index.html. Retrieved 16.9.04

Kirkham M 1986 A feminist perspective in midwifery. In: Webb C (ed.), Feminist practice in women's health. Wiley, Chichester, pp. 35–49

Kirkham M 1997 Stories and childbirth. In: Kirkham M J, Perkins E R (eds) Reflections on midwifery. Bailliere Tindall, London, pp. 183–204

Kirkham M 2000 The midwife/mother relationship. Macmillan, London

Kirkham M (ed.) 2003 Birth centres: a social model for maternity care. Books for Midwives, Hale, Cheshire

Kirkham M (ed.) 2004 Informed choice in maternity care. Macmillan, London

Kitzinger J 1990 Strategies of the early childbirth movement: a case-study of the National Childbirth Trust. In: Garcia J, Kilpatrick R, Richards M (eds) The politics of maternity care: services for childbearing women in twentieth-century Britain. Clarendon, Oxford, pp. 61–91

Kitzinger S 2000 Rediscovering birth. Little Brown, Boston

Lazarus E 1997 What do women want? Issues of choice, control, and class in American pregnancy and childbirth. In: Davis-Floyd R E, Sargent C F (eds) Childbirth and authoritative knowledge: cross-cultural perspectives. University of California Press, Berkeley, pp. 132–158

Leap N 1991 Helping you to make your own decisions – antenatal and postnatal groups in Deptford SE London. VHS Video. Available from Birth International. Online. Available: www.birthinternational.com.au

Leap N 1996 A midwifery perspective of pain in labour. Unpublished MSc thesis, South Bank University, London

Leap N 2000 The less we do, the more we give. In: Kirkham M (ed.) The midwife/mother relationship. Macmillan, London, pp. 1–18

Leap N 2005 Rhetoric and reality: narrowing the gap in Australian midwifery. Unpublished doctoral thesis. University of Technology, Sydney, Australia

Leap N, Anderson T 2004 The role of pain and the empowerment of women. In: Downe S (ed.), Normal childbirth: evidence and debate. Churchill Livingstone, Edinburgh

Lee G 1997 The concept of 'continuity' – what does it mean? In: Kirkham M (ed.) Reflections on midwifery. Bailliere Tindall, London

Lemay C 1997 L'accouchement a la maison au Quebec: les voix du dedans. M Sc, Universite de Montreal, Montreal

Leyshon L 2004 Integrating caseloads across a whole service: the Torbay model. MIDIRS 14: Sppl 1, S9–S11

Lundgren I, Dahlberg K 1998 Women's experience of pain during childbirth. Midwifery 14(2): 105–110

Machin D, Scamell M 1997 The experience of labour using ethnography to explore the irresistible nature of the bio-medical metaphor during labour. Midwifery 13: 78–84

Mackenzie C 2000 Imagining oneself otherwise. In: Mackenzie C, Stoljar N (eds) Relational autonomy: feminist perspectives on autonomy, agency, and the social self. Oxford University Press, New York, pp. 124–150

Mackenzie C, Stoljar N (eds) 2000 Relational autonomy: feminist perspectives on autonomy, and the social self. Oxford University Press, New York

Madi B C, Crow R 2003 A qualitative study of information about available options for childbirth venue and pregnant women's preference for place of delivery. Midwifery 19(4): 328–336

Mander R 1993 Who chooses the choices? Modern Midwife 3(1): 23–25

Mander R 1997 Choosing the choices in the USA: examples in the maternity area. Journal of Advanced Nursing 25: 1192–1197

Mander R 1998 Pain in childbearing and its control. Blackwell Science, Oxford

Martin E 1987 The woman in the body: a cultural analysis of reproduction. Open University Press, Milton Keynes

Mason M 1998 Hospital-based childbirth education: in whose interests?' In: Kennedy P, Murphy-Lawless J (eds) Returning birth to women: challenging policies and practices. Centre for Women's Studies TCD/WERRC, Dublin, pp. 34–40

McCourt C, Page L 1997 One to one midwifery practice: report on the evaluation of one-to-one midwifery. Thames Valley University and The Hammersmith Hospital NHS Trust, London

McCourt C, Page L, Hewison J 1998 Evaluation of one-to-one midwifery: women's responses to care. Birth 25: 73–80

McLeod C, Sherwin S 2000 Relational autonomy, self-trust, and health care for patients who are oppressed. In: Mackenzie C, Stoljar N (eds) Relational autonomy: feminist perspective on autonomy, agency, and the social self. Oxford University Press, New York, pp. 259–279

Mills K, Roberts J 1997 Remote area birthing discussion paper. Territory Health Services, Darwin

Morgan B M, Bulpitt C J, Clifton P, Lewis P J 1982 Analgesia and satisfaction in childbirth. Lancet ii: 808–810

Murphy-Lawless J 1998 Reading birth and death. Cork University Press, Cork

NHMRC 1996 Options for effective care in childbirth. Australian Government Printing Service, Canberra

Oakley A, Hickey D, Rajan L, Grant A 1996 Social support in pregnancy: does it have long term effects? Journal of Reproductive Health and Infant Psychology 14: 7–22

Oakley A, Rajan L, Grant A 1990 Social support and pregnancy outcome. British Journal of Obstetrics and Gynaecology 97: 155–162

Pairman S 2000 Woman-centred midwifery: partnerships or professional friendships. In: Kirkham M (ed.) The midwife-mother relationship. Macmillan, Basingstoke, pp. 207–226

Pfeufer-Khan R 1995 Bearing meaning: the language of birth. University of Illinois Press, Urbana

Reed B 2002a The Albany midwifery practice (1). MIDIRS Midwifery Digest 12(1): 118–121

Reed B 2002b The Albany midwifery practice (2). MIDIRS Midwifery Digest 12(3): 261–264

Romalis S 1985 Struggle between providers and the recipients: the case of birth practices. In: Lewin E, Olesen V (eds) Women, health and healing: toward a new perspective. Tavistock, London, pp. 174–208

Rooks J 1997 Midwifery and childbirth in America. Temple University Press, Philadelphia

Sackett D, Richardson W, Rosenberg W, Hayes R 1997 Evidence-based medicine: how to practise and teach. Churchill Livingstone, Sydney

Sandall J 1996 Moving towards caseload practice: what evidence do we have? British Journal of Midwifery 4: 12

Sandall J 1997 Midwives' burnout and continuity of care. British Journal of Midwifery 5(2): 106–111

Sandall J, Davies J, Warwick C 2001 Evaluation of the Albany midwifery practice: final report. Nightingale School of Midwifery, Kings College London, London

Schindler Rising S 1998 Centering pregnancy: an interdisciplinary model of empowerment. Journal of Nurse-Midwifery 43(1): 46–54

Scully D 1994 Men who control women's health. Teachers College Press, New York

Shallow H 2003 The birth centre project. In: Kirkham M (ed.) Birth centres: a social model for maternity care. Books for Midwives, Hale, Cheshire, pp. 11–24

Shapiro M C, Najam J M, Chang A, Keeping D, Morrison J, Western J S 1983 Information control and the exercise of power in the obstetrical encounter. Social Science Medicine 17(3): 139–146

Shildrick M 1997 Leaky bodies and boundaries: feminism, postmodernism and (bio)ethics. Routledge, London

Silverton L 2001 Why women choose caesarean section. RCM Midwives Journal 4(10)

Simpson J 2004 Negotiating elective caesarean section: and obstetric team perspective. In: Kirkham M (ed.) Informed choice in maternity care. Macmillan, Palgrave, pp. 211–236

Smethurst G 1997 Extending choices. MIDIRS Midwifery Digest 7(3): 376–377

Smith C A, Collins C T, Cynae A M et al 2003 Complementary and alternative therapies for pain management in labour (Cochrane Review) The Cochrane Library. Oxford: Update Software. Issue 2. Amended 9th January 2003

Smythe E 1998 Being safe in childbirth: a hermeneutic interpretation of the narratives of women and practitioners. Unpublished PhD thesis, Massey University, New Zealand

Spiby H, Slade P, Escott D et al 2003 Selected coping strategies in labour: an investigation of women's experiences. Birth 30(3): 189–194

Stevens T, McCourt C 2002 One-to-one midwifery practice: meaning for midwives. British Journal of Midwifery 10(2): 111–115

Thompson Faye E 2004 Mothers and midwives: the ethical journey. Books for Midwives, Edinburgh

Trevathan W 1997 An evolutionary perspective on authoritative knowledge about birth. In: Davis-Floyd R E, Sargent C F (eds) Childbirth and authoritative knowledge: cross-cultural perspectives. University of California Press, Berkeley, pp. 80–88

van Olphen Fehr J 1999 The lived experience of being in a caring relationship with a midwife during childbirth. Unpublished PhD thesis, George Mason University, USA

Viisainen K 2000 The moral dangers of home birth; parents' perceptions of risks in home birth in Finland. Sociology of Health and Illness 22(6): 792–814

Wagner M 1994 Pursuing the birth machine: the search for appropriate birth technology. Ace Graphics, Camperdown, NSW Australia

Weiner C, Straus A, Fagerhaugh S, Suczek B 1997 Trajectories, biographies, and the evolving medical technology scene. In Straus A, Corbin J (eds) Grounded theory in practice. Sage, Thousand Oaks, London

Wilkins R 1993 Sociological aspects of the mother-community midwife relationship. Unpublished PhD thesis, University of Surrey

Wilkins R 2000 Poor relations: the paucity of the professional paradigm. In: Kirkham M (ed.) The midwife–mother relationship. Macmillan, London

Williams H 2003 Storied births: narrative and organizational culture in a midwife-led birth centre. Kings College London, London

Young I M 1990 Throwing like a girl and other essays in feminist philosophy and social theory. Indiana University Press, Bloomington, Indiana

Young I M 1997 Intersecting voices. Princeton University Press, New Jersey

Chapter 6

Supporting midwives to support women

Ruth Deery and Mavis Kirkham

THE CULTURAL CONTEXT

We hear such horror stories about going to work in hospital . . . and basically you don't get any support.

Community midwife, quoted in Deery 2003

People were so tired and burnt out, they were dreadful to us newly qualified midwives in particular. My confidence declined and I felt that I was not pulling my weight because I was struggling to cope all the time.

Midwife quoted in Ball et al 2002

In a number of research studies, where NHS midwives have been asked to reflect upon their work situation, they have spoken at length about their support needs and their lack of support (Ball et al 2002, Deery 2003, Kirkham & Stapleton 2001, Stapleton et al 1998). While many support needs have been given, it is noteworthy that these have not been marshalled in any study into an order of priorities by NHS midwives, neither have they spoken of strategies for getting their support needs met. In this respect, the data for NHS midwives stands in contrast to that from UK midwives outside the NHS who spoke of how they had developed support networks to meet these needs (Stapleton et al 1998). The data from NHS midwives reads more like a long list of needs, or an incoherent cry for support, rather than a plan, which could be carried out and needs met. This is probably because the culture of NHS midwifery

is a female culture of 'service and sacrifice' where is it seen as 'selfish' to address personal needs (Kirkham 1999). Also, the wider culture of NHS maternity services is one of measurable outcomes where support, whilst essential, carries little status and is effectively invisible. In this context, working relationships are pressurized and fragmented and support is not valued. Indeed, the individual midwife in relationship with women does not receive the maintenance which is seen as essential for the efficiency of a more technological tool. Nor does she receive the training in relationships skills or in the giving and receiving of the trust and support which underpins the development of such skills. Since the creation of the NHS midwifery practice has changed greatly and become increasingly regulated, professionalized, rule-governed and medicalized. All these changes have brought complexities, contradictions and new responsibilities into the working lives of midwives.

The concept of woman-centred care is central to national policy on maternity care (Department of Health 1993a). The childbearing woman is described as the focus of the midwife's work and there is an expectation that a woman is supported emotionally and practically throughout pregnancy, childbirth and the postnatal period. The midwife thereby becomes involved in what could be seen as a one-way process, a relationship where the woman is deemed to be the one in need of support. Yet, very many midwives have acknowledged that getting to know the women they work with is one of the most rewarding aspects of being a midwife. In order to develop good relationships with different women, midwives clearly need to experience relationships which nurture their own growth. However, there is often a gap between rhetoric and reality in maternity care. Care centred upon an individual woman needs a context of developing relationship and trust between midwife and mother so that the midwife can respond to the woman she knows as an individual. But often services are described as 'woman centred', which are run according to an industrialized conveyor-belt model with no continuity of relationship between midwife and mother and midwives are seen as interchangeable workers who must prioritize keeping the system running. In such a context support needs have been largely ignored.

There is now an increasing body of literature acknowledging the importance of support for midwives and how this can enhance working relationships and help midwives cope within increasingly complex clinical situations (Deery 1999, 2003, Kirkham & Stapleton 2000, Mander 2001, Page 1995) (also see Chapter 7.) Yet many policy initiatives (Department of Health 1993a, 1999, 2000), although supporting the development of different ways of working for midwives, have failed to acknowledge the level of support midwives need in order to achieve woman-centred care and thus an omnipresent contradiction becomes apparent. Midwives are being asked to engage in meaningful, supportive relationships with women, when they themselves have impoverished support. It is likely that when midwives feel unsupported they will also feel insecure. So, just as women's ability to give birth without the assistance of medicalization lies in their capacity to access 'strong social support' (Fox & Worts 1999, p. 330) so too, is the parallel for midwives, in that their ability to help women birth in a social context, without having to depend on medicalization, means they must have access to strong midwifery support.

THE IMPACT OF CHANGING WORK PATTERNS

Since Changing Childbirth (Department of Health 1993a) and Making a Difference (Department of Health 1999) the government has set further difficult challenges in the NHS Plan (Department of Health 2000) and the National Service Framework (Department of Health 2004) in order to achieve change in the NHS. Midwives are being urged to extend their roles and take on more responsibility. New working patterns, together with fewer midwives, have resulted in emotional exhaustion and burnout for some midwives (Deery 2003, Royal College of Midwives 1997, Sandall 1999) and there is widespread dissatisfaction with the maternity services amongst those midwives who leave the profession (Ball et al 2002). Strategies that provide effective support were cited by ex-midwives participating in this study as being important to effective re-recruitment and retention of midwives. Interestingly, the targets set out in the NHS Plan (Department of Health 2000) include a commitment to the provision of support for health practitioners, which is interpreted by many midwives as just another example of the gap between rhetoric and reality.

A climate of continual change within the NHS, that has often been initiated at a point of crisis (Menzies 1979), has become a potential health hazard for midwives in terms of stress related disease (Mackin & Sinclair 1998, Sandall 1997, 1998, 1999). This, coupled with the emotional effort required in being in direct contact with women and their families, makes midwives susceptible to burnout syndrome (Maslach & Jackson 1993, Sandall 1995, 1997). Jane Sandall's research identified three key themes relating to sustainable practice, the avoidance of burnout and the provision of woman-centred care; these were occupational autonomy, social support and developing meaningful relationships with women (Sandall 1997, p. 106).

This work clearly linked support for midwives with both their job satisfaction and the quality of care they gave to women. It would therefore seem important that effective support strategies are put into place, yet as midwives, we still work within a culture that does not move beyond acknowledging the existence of stress and burnout. As a result midwives have had to adapt to, and find different ways to cope with, the stressful nature of their work. Unfortunately, some of the ways in which midwives have learned to cope are not always to their benefit and can actually impede their working lives and affect relationships.

WAYS OF COPING

In 1959, Isabel Menzies Lyth wrote a groundbreaking paper using a psychoanalytical perspective to examine hospital nursing and traditional ways of working (Menzies Lyth 1988). Menzies Lyth viewed the system (the NHS in this case) as an organizational defence against stress and anxiety where work that was task-orientated protected nurses from close contact with their patients. Depersonalization and stereotyping of patients meant that relationships were kept unemotional and distant. When nurses detached themselves in this manner they were better able to cope with the demands made by the organization. Strict routines and standard procedures, that often had set time limits, also minimized responsibility and decision-making which in turn protected them from associated stresses (Menzies 1979). In a classic sociological study, Michael Lipsky (1980) described the dilemmas of public service workers who work directly with the public within bureaucracies. He called them 'street-level bureaucrats' in an analysis which certainly fits NHS midwifery.

> Ideally and by training, street-level bureaucrats respond to the individual needs or characteristics of the people they serve or confront ... In practice, they must deal with clients on a mass basis, since work requirements prohibit individualised service. ... At best, street-level bureaucrats invent benign modes of mass processing that more or less permit them to deal with the public fairly, appropriately and successfully. At worst, they give in to favouritism, stereotyping and routinising – all of which serve private or agency purposes.
>
> Lipsky 1980, p. xii

Likewise, Hunt and Symonds (1995) in an ethnographic study of labour ward culture found that midwives often concentrated on the physical aspects of care and used labelling and stereotyping as ways of controlling their interactions with clients. Such conditions tend to create cultures of obedience where workers spend much of their time trying to fit into the organization in order to conform and survive (Dadds 2002, Kirkham 1999). If we are honest with ourselves many of us will admit to working with, or being midwives, that see service needs as a priority rather than the needs of women and colleagues.

THE PRIMARY TASK AND ANTI-TASKS

Looking at staff support systems in 1979 Menzies Lyth (1988) stressed the need to define the primary task 'which the enterprise must perform in order to survive' (p. 222).

Quite simply, unless the members of the institution know what they are supposed to be doing, there is little hope of their doing it effectively and getting adequate psychological satisfactions from this. Lack of such definition is likely to lead to personal confusion in members of the institution, to interpersonal and intergroup conflicts and to other undesirable institutional phenomenon (Menzies Lyth 1988, pp. 222–223).

Vivien Woodward made a similar plea within midwifery.

> A clear sense of professional goals enables a critical evaluation of imposed change and the necessary basis on which to challenge detrimental policy.
>
> Woodward 2000, p. 73

We are sure that all midwives see the achievement of the best possible physical and emotional outcomes for mothers, babies and families as our primary task, with mothers actively defining what they feel is best for their families. But there are many other tasks, which are crucial to the smooth running of the institution or to the meeting of other aims. For example staffing the labour ward in times of staff shortage, may act to the detriment of postnatal care and staff satisfaction. Meeting targets set by the Department of Health may detract from other aspects of care. Effective teaching of students takes time, which might otherwise be spent on clinical care. Covering our backs, in a climate of litigation and defensive care, is likely to detract from our primary aim. Prioritizing amongst the many tasks required of us is very difficult and 'makes it more difficult to sustain adequately the feeling that the total organization is effective and to provide adequate support through job satisfaction for its members, since the level of performance of each task tends to be reduced by the legitimate demands of the others'

(Menzies Lyth 1988, p. 223). Menzies Lyth goes on to describe the 'redefinition of task into anti-task' where the primary task becomes implicitly redefined because of difficulties and competing priorities. Anti-tasks in midwifery are often revealed by research: midwives ensuring that women make the locally defined 'right' choices, or that they 'go with the flow' of the organization (Kirkham & Stapleton 2001) are good examples. It is an interesting marker that we often keep the language, or rhetoric, of the task whilst pursuing the anti-task. In the studies just referred to the midwives spoke of facilitating informed choice whilst ensuring that women made the choices which were acceptable to the organization and of services in a permanent state of 'plugging the gaps' in staffing which is still described as a 'woman-centred' concept. The proliferation of midwifery work can also be seen as anti-task as midwives concentrate on getting through the work rather than on listening to women. For instance in the area of antenatal screening, the increased agenda of screening-related work which the midwife must get through at each antenatal consultation, without increase in the time available, tends to make care routinized and make it more difficult for women's voices to be heard.

COPING MECHANISMS

Raphael-Leff (1991) develops the work of Menzies further, identifying three defence mechanisms used by midwives and the organization within which they work. These are the splitting up of the midwife–patient relationship, denial and detachment of feelings and redistribution of responsibility. A mechanistic approach to midwifery that involved task-orientated care and no continuity of carer served to protect midwives from situations that might provoke anxiety or involve them in the emotional effort of building relationships with women.

Deery (2003) found, in an action research study exploring midwives' support needs, that community midwives tended to put on a front of cohesive group behaviour within their work team when in fact some of the midwives felt peer support was absent. Pseudo-cohesion was a coping mechanism used to deflect the opportunity to address sensitive interpersonal issues within the work team

that would otherwise take up too much time and thus disrupt the status quo. Resistance to change is therefore a key defence mechanism used by midwives to help them cope with the bureaucratic pressures of working within an organization that sees the system as more important than them or their primary caring task. Pretending to be emotionally well equipped to undertake our primary task when this is not the case and resistance to change in many forms are rational responses by overstretched midwives faced with competing demands upon their time. Yet such coping mechanisms are clearly anti-task in that they limit both professional development and the care that can be given to women. Coping mechanisms that spring from the desperate need to get through the work can also damage midwives directly, as when midwives vent their frustration upon colleagues they see as different from themselves and this is manifest in horizontal violence and bullying (Clements 1997, Hastie 1995, Leap 1997, McIver 2002, Roberts 1983, Royal College of Midwives 1996). Thus our efforts to cope by resistance to change and conformity with the anti-tasks generated by the organization can limit our job satisfaction at the least and often prove highly damaging to midwives.

SUPPORT TOWARDS WHAT END?

Isabel Menzies Lyth's (1988) analysis of task and anti-task helps to explain NHS midwives' strong feelings about their lack of support, their somewhat incoherent cries for support and their tendency to heap blame upon those they see as unsupportive. There is ample support, indeed immense pressure for NHS midwives to conform to the needs of the organizations for which they work, even when this compromises their own well being and that of their clients. Research data from midwives often contains references to the need for midwives to 'go with the flow' or be subject to immense difficulties in their work situation (e.g. Kirkham & Stapleton 2001). In Menzies Lyth's (1988) analysis 'the flow', with all its power, can be seen as support for the anti-task: the needs of the organization which must be put before the needs of women and which often prevents those needs from being voiced.

Support can change behaviour and change lives. We all need to feel that others agree with us and back us up. Definitions in the Collins Dictionary include 'to carry the weight of, . . . to speak in favour of, to give aid or courage, to give strength'. All midwives know how their support can give courage and strength to women in labour and how a midwife's lack of support for her can lead a woman to doubt her own ability to give birth. We also know how the support of those around us can be enabling but this depends upon what we are supported to do.

There is ample evidence that midwives want to be midwives and that being a midwife is an important part of our identity for many midwives (e.g. Ball et al 2002). Most midwives who leave the profession do so with reluctance and disappointment at what midwifery has become, not because they do not wish to be midwives (Ball et al 2002). It is therefore hardly surprising if midwives leave, conform or despair when professional support concentrates upon a host of subsidiary tasks, or even anti-tasks, and the primary aim of midwifery practice is lost sight of. The massive proliferation of tasks also limits the possibility of doing all of them correctly and the consequent anxiety produces the sort of 'high-effort/low-reward conditions' (Siegrist 1996) or 'effort-reward imbalance' (Stansfield et al 1999), which are found to be particularly stressful, unrewarding and unhealthy.

This is not to say that modern midwifery can be made simple, but that there is a desperate need for vision and insight into the relationship between our many tasks and awareness of the potential for anti-tasks strongly supported by 'the flow' of organizational practice.

HOW CAN MIDWIVES SUPPORT MIDWIVES?

MANAGEMENT

Menzies Lyth is firmly of the opinion that 'good management must obviously be orientated to sustaining task-orientated elements and discouraging anti-tasks; but management in the humane institutions is in more trouble than in the institutions that process things' (Menzies Lyth 1988, p. 229). She defines humane institutions as 'people-

changing institutions' (p. 223) with awareness of the potential for positive and negative change. In fieldwork with management in humane institutions, she aimed 'at maximum delegation down the hierarchy' which would certainly fit with midwives' need for professional autonomy and provide powerful supportive models for midwives facilitating their clients' choices. The effect upon staff of their relationships with clients and colleagues and the feeling produced by these relationships is of crucial importance.

> The acknowledgement and working through of such feeling is not easy, although it is an important part of staff support and primary task-performance to do so.
> Menzies Lyth 1988, p. 321

This may be done in a number of ways, discussed below, which need to be prioritized and often instigated by managers with an appropriate degree of social awareness and insight. Where such feelings are not worked through and learnt from, institutionalized defences are built and, in Menzies Lyth's view, 'such social defences are inevitably anti-task' (Menzies Lyth 1988, p. 231) and are 'in the end likely to be anti-supportive to staff' (p. 232). This is certainly true in NHS midwifery.

To call for such levels of insight and awareness, as well as strategic planning, from midwifery managers is asking a lot. We are aware that the problems of modern maternity services, exacerbated by staff shortages, have created a system where managers, as well as midwives, are only just coping and in their endeavours to plug the gaps in understaffed services managers can appear to condone bullying and other anti-task elements of the existing culture (Curtis et al 2003). Nevertheless, there is little option but change, even when it appears threatening. Changes in midwifery management which make its service more focused upon the primary task and psychologically healthy can only create a positive precedent for other areas of NHS management.

In Menzies Lyth's view

> The management of an institution requires some measure of ruthlessness, but this concern for task need not and should not

necessarily be linked with lack of concern for people. . . Much of the task-orientated activity is, in fact, directly good for people. For example, striving for adaptive and mature defences rather than primitive and counteracting the development of destructive subcultures are rewarding. Above all, such task-orientated activities facilitate the support given to staff through belonging to an institution that functions well and gives both the rewards for work well done and the rewarding relationships that go with them.

Menzies Lyth 1988, p. 235

This certainly seems true in those maternity units where managers have made determined efforts to stop bullying, though sadly such efforts are rarely published.

In so far as midwives' support comes from achieving clear primary aims within relationships focused upon achieving those aims, management must bear responsibility for it. Other steps can also be taken by managers to increase support for midwives.

One way forward in terms of building support networks for midwives is for managers to place the same emphasis on communication, interpersonal skill building and therapeutic proficiency that they place on mandatory updating that focuses on medical management of care and interventions in midwifery. Mandatory study days could comprise assertiveness workshops, reflective practice groups or action learning groups. Midwifery managers also need to express their approval of such strategies thereby reinforcing the value of this approach. Indeed they could even instigate their own similar mandatory updating thus role modelling and reinforcing the importance of developing more secure, supportive working relationships. Once a higher level of skill in supportive relationships has been developed, this will be paralleled in the midwives' clinical work and, rather than resorting to the horizontal violence that often comes when working within hierarchies such as the NHS, midwives will be able to experience contagious, mutual support from a secure base.

We are aware that such changes would be difficult to achieve, since most updating requirements for midwives currently are laid down within the requirements of the Clinical Negligence Scheme for Trusts (NHS Litigation Authority 2002). We are also aware that, just as midwives feel themselves to be 'piggy in the middle' pulled between management and clients, so midwifery managers find themselves pulled between the needs of midwives and the requirements of NHS general management. Nevertheless, it is reasonable to expect organizational change to come from those responsible for the organization of the service. Where managers have funded updating for midwives which focuses upon increasing insight and mutual support, such initiatives have been greatly appreciated by midwives (e.g. Jones 2000, Kirkham 2004). Where this is felt to be impossible, it needs to be openly discussed at a strategic level.

STRUCTURE AND SCALE

Independent midwifery is probably the simplest structure in modern midwifery where a woman engages her midwife who is self employed and solely responsible for her midwifery care, which is usually carried out in the woman's home. At the other extreme are highly centralized maternity services covering large cities. It is interesting that independent midwives have been very active in building their own support structures (Stapleton et al 1998) whereas hospital midwives feel unsupported and are more prone to burnout than community midwives (Mander 2001, p. 143). A Dutch study of community midwives found that the midwife's degree of depersonalization reflected the size of the group practice within which she worked (Bakker et al 1996).

They also found that a high proportion of home births is associated with a lower risk of burnout; the researchers suggest that this finding is likely to be mediated by greater job satisfaction. The corollary of this observation is that a high proportion of short stay hospital births correlates with more profound emotional tension.

Mander 2002, p. 142

Again, support and job satisfaction are closely linked.

There are examples of excellent staff support within NHS midwifery and these tend to be found in small units such as birth centres or small groups of midwives working together (see Kirkham 2003). This suggests that midwives' ability to give and receive support is linked with the size of their group of immediate colleagues, their close and continuing relationships with clients and the degree of autonomy they exercise in their practice. Close relationships with clients enhance midwives' job satisfaction and the support they feel that they receive from their clients. In large organizations with fragmented care, no one feels really responsible or satisfied with good outcomes. Midwives working in birth centres or conducting home births feel both responsibility and satisfaction for individual clients. The link between autonomy, or the downwards delegation of responsibility, and support and satisfaction is again clear.

Even within large organizations it is possible for small groups of midwives to be responsible for the care of defined groups of women. This tends to be linked with good clinical outcomes and high levels of mutual support as well as the advantages of continuity of care.

CONTINUITY OF CARE

The 'Know Your Midwife' (KYM) scheme (Flint et al 1989) was a randomized controlled trial that aimed to address continuity of care for women within a team of midwives. This study also highlighted how effective support between team members can enhance motivation and commitment to midwifery work. In 1992 the Winterton Report recommended continuity of care, choice of care and place of birth and women's right to control of their bodies (House of Commons 1992). The government response was Changing Childbirth (Department of Health 1993a) which generated further debate about the normality of childbirth and continuity of care and carer. Within an NHS that was already beginning a constant cycle of large-scale change, this different way of working was implemented to varying extents, and many team midwifery schemes were set up across the UK, with varying degrees of continuity for the women and of autonomy for the midwives. At the same time, increasing emphasis was being placed on greater efficiency and economy (Jenkins 1995, Savage 2000) and where there was an increased

focus on cost-effectiveness, evaluation of care and risk management within the NHS (Brooks 2000). This did not bode well for a pattern of working that required time to build relationships with women and other midwives and effective support mechanisms for midwives to help them work differently.

The midwives in the KYM scheme were an already established work team who were known to each other, unlike some of the midwifery teams that were created with no apparent thought being given to the concept of 'team', the nature of team working, group dynamics and different responsibilities that this way of working brought about (Katzenback & Smith 1993). This inevitably caused anxiety for many midwives and they soon began to report feeling stressed, demoralized and demotivated (Deery 2003, Hughes et al 2002, Kirkham 1999, Sandall 1998). The support they were required to offer women was not paralleled in their own work situation where the focus was more on meeting the organizational demands of the maternity services as cheaply as possible (Bower 1993, Tinkler & Quinney 1998).

Other models of small scale maternity care have also highlighted the effectiveness of support in the context of increased continuity of care and support for women, for example, one-to-one midwifery (McCourt et al 1998), midwife-managed care (McGinley et al 1995) and caseload midwifery (Morgan et al 1998). Although undertaken in the same cultural context of the NHS these schemes gave further thought to reciprocity within working relationships. McCourt et al (1998) found that peer support within a one-to-one midwifery scheme resulted in reducing stress and burn-out (see also Chapter 7). The midwives working in these schemes were able to choose their work partners and, more importantly, they were able to establish their own group practices. This probably resulted in groups of midwives working together that held similar philosophies of midwifery and views concerning work-life balance. The high level of support that the women participating in this scheme reported appeared to be mirrored in the midwives' own support network, indicating that trust, autonomy and reciprocity can spread where midwives and women feel secure and satisfied with their situation.

MIDWIFE–LED CARE

Other changes have occurred within the maternity services in an effort to offer more choice to women as well as provide midwives with a working environment that is conducive to their own philosophies of midwifery. The development of midwife-led units and birth centres provide good examples of midwives working together for the benefit of women and where they are able to work in a culture that offers support and an opportunity to practice within an ideology that accords with their personal philosophy of midwifery. However there is a pressure within the current maternity service to maintain the status quo especially where resistance to change is reinforced by economic pressures (Kirkham 2003).

Nevertheless, midwife-led care is being set up in many places and some evaluations are positive in terms of clinical outcomes (Walsh & Downe 2004) and midwives perceived support (Deery & Hughes 2004, Turnbull et al 1995, Walsh 1995). This is likely to be a positive result of increased professional autonomy with due pride in good outcomes. Whether or not midwife-led care provides a smaller scale of working where midwives can develop improved relationships with a small and constant group of colleagues, and whether or not it provides continuity of care to women with the potential for improved relationships with clients over time, depends upon how the project is organized. Such schemes differ greatly and where midwives offer midwife led care on part of a consultant-led labour ward, with the same organization and fragmentation of care, it is unlikely that midwives will feel more supported because no effort has been made to create a situation where support can be developed.

Hughes & Deery (2002) found that there was a considerable amount of audit and/or quantitative research looking at outcomes in terms of neonatal and maternal morbidity and satisfaction within midwife-led units. The research studies examined presented outcome data (e.g. Apgar scores, vaginal birth rates, episiotomy rates) as though they were solely linked to the booking criteria and transfer policies in place, rather than to the care actually received (Law & Lamb 1999, Tucker et al 1996, Woodcock & Baston 1996). Hughes & Deery (2002)

concluded that the 'essence of midwifery' (p. 18) seemed to be missing from most published work on midwife-led care because most research studies concentrated on interpretation and implementation of booking criteria and policies in place rather than the interpersonal contribution of the midwife and how midwifery care can facilitate positive outcomes.

Walsh (1995) identified that a personal relationship between midwife and woman and continuity of carer were essential factors to midwife-led care. In a qualitative study on the experience of labour of women having midwife-led care, Walker and colleagues (1995) describe constant support during labour and midwifery confidence as some of the features that are central to midwife-led care. Although these studies do not identify the processes within midwifery care that helped to achieve this, they do highlight the necessity for a supportive relationship between women and midwives. This will only be achieved if midwives are supported themselves or, as stated earlier, there is a situation created for support to develop.

THE SUPERVISION OF MIDWIVES

The supervision of midwives is a statutory service which applies to all midwives practising in the UK. It exists to support midwives in developing their practice and to police midwifery practice in the public interest (see Stapleton et al 1998).

Considerable effort has been made in recent years to improve the statutory supervision of midwives: the training of supervisors has been reformed, the ratio of supervisors to supervisees has reduced and most midwives now have a choice of supervisor. Olive Jones (2000, p. 153) developed a framework for midwifery supervision, which focused on the primary task whilst developing group reflection and staff support. It is highly successful. It is also noteworthy that in the birth centre of which Olive Jones wrote, midwives experienced considerable job satisfaction and improved their relationships with other professions with the generosity of spirit which is apparent when workers cease to feel threatened (Kirkham 2003). Olive Jones worked with a high level of insight and awareness of group processes, it must also be added that the context was a birth centre where the midwives were working with a small and constant group of colleagues and were geographically distant from both obstetric and general management colleagues so their sense of professional autonomy was high. With all these factors working together,

> In the model of supervision employed, the midwife is empowered, in turn, the woman is empowered, positive feedback from women and families empowers the midwife, endorsement of the approach to practice empowers the supervisor. As long as the cycle of empowerment remains unbroken, it is self-perpetuating.
>
> Jones 2000, p. 167

There also needs to be acknowledgement that such supervision is much more difficult within a large unit organized upon an industrial model; support is perceived differently by individuals and for varying reasons some midwives may not feel supported by the current model of statutory supervision. Therefore, there needs to be alternative support mechanisms available. Clinical supervision can provide such a support mechanism.

CLINICAL SUPERVISION

Midwifery has not embraced clinical supervision as a support mechanism, probably believing statutory supervision of midwives to be the cure of all ills. The differences between statutory supervision of midwives and clinical supervision have been discussed elsewhere (see Deery & Corby 1996, Deery 1999). Where clinical supervision has been implemented within maternity care, the response to the experience has been very positive (Deery 2003, Derbyshire 2000), but where clinical supervision is not part of the culture of the unit, resistance has been experienced (Deery 2003). Frances Derbyshire looked at clinical supervision in a neonatal unit in a hospital where clinical supervision was used in other areas of nursing.

> The demands that clinical supervision makes on the practice setting are considerable. Clinical supervision is particularly time-consuming if it is carried out properly. However, I believe that the Exeter neonatal experience has shown that such difficulties are far outweighed by the extensive benefits gained. The activity of clinical supervision is

a major staff development activity. It enhances patient care, promotes competent, reflective practitioners and reduces stress, staff sickness and litigation. Clinical supervision should be available to all health care workers and there is no reason why midwives should be excluded.

> Derbyshire 2000, p. 176

We can learn much from each other by working and networking across professional boundaries. Some nurses use the process of professional support and learning (Department of Health 1993b) known as clinical supervision. This has been described as having commonalities that include a 'process orientated, interrelational and reflective approach' (Lindahl & Norberg 2002, p. 809) to working with, and supporting, healthcare practitioners. Clinical supervision does not have monitoring or investigation attached to it and is time that is invested in building team work (Bond & Holland 1998). It has been described as:

- supportive and enabling (Faugier 1998, Wilkins 1998),
- concerned with professional development (Faugier 1998, Hawkins & Shohet 1989),
- client-centred (Morris 1995) and
- an investment in staff (Butterworth et al 1997, Hallberg & Norberg 1993).

There are also numerous models of clinical supervision, each with its own philosophical underpinning according to the stance taken by the clinical supervisor and according to the differing needs of nurses and health visitors. This would seem appropriate where there is a diversity of clinical needs within nursing (Butterworth et al 1997). Midwifery would therefore have to adopt a shared philosophy of care if clinical supervision were to be adopted but for the moment conflicting ideologies (Hunter 2002) are a potential hindrance and common goals are not aspired to. A supportive culture where the autonomous behaviour and independent thinking necessary for women-centred care (Department of Health 1993a) thrive then becomes impossible.

As midwifery is essentially about human relationships, the development of interpersonal skills is essential to help midwives cope with the often stressful nature of their work. Clinical supervision can also help midwives 'work with the unknown' and cope with 'not knowing' (Casement 1985). These are important, but often unacknowledged, concepts in midwifery as most midwives face uncertainty everyday of their working lives. Wilkins (1998, p. 189) has written extensively about the benefits of clinical supervision for community psychiatric nurses and states:

> . . . there are many dark, shadowy moments when we lose direction and cannot see what needs to be done. Yet looking where the light shines does not necessarily mean that you will find what you are looking for. In clinical supervision, we need someone to guide us back to the casework moment, as only then can our retrospective darkness be illuminated by the light of insight.

Similarly clinical supervision could offer midwives the opportunity to step backwards and become more self-aware in their interactions with women and other midwives. This is particularly important in the current organizational system that trains midwives to clinically manage and measure aspects of their work rather than providing a space to reflect and develop practice. More importantly, clinical supervision offers *time* for midwives which helps to reduce burnout (Wilkins 1998) although time has also been shown to be a scarce commodity within the NHS (Butterworth et al 1997, Deery 2003), and undoubtedly within other health services.

Midwives often have to keep their 'emotional lids' (Bond & Holland 1998, p. 65) firmly in place because the constraints of working within the NHS does not facilitate a healthy expression of emotions through a medium such as clinical supervision. This means that midwives choose not to leak their feelings because this might diminish them in the eyes of their clients or colleagues. A fear of leaking feelings might also stem from a desire to keep in control of situations. This is an unfortunate situation because emotion work is central to our role as midwives (Deery 2003, Hunter 2002) and should not be marginalized. When midwives do not experience their work as an energizing process, relationships between midwives and women become starved of positive energy, and midwives tend to experience their relationships as 'disconnected' (Deery 2003). The

whole subject of emotion work in midwifery merits further examination and we are currently working on this.

THE FACILITATOR

Butterworth et al (1997) identified that the facilitator of clinical supervision was a key issue identified by the participants in their research study. The participants stated that this person must have training in the skills of clinical supervision and appropriate educational preparation was crucial and involved reflective, challenging and supportive skills. Faugier (1998) provides some guidelines for the supervisory relationship in clinical supervision stating that generosity, reward, openness, a willingness to learn, an expectation to challenge, humaneness, sensitivity, uncompromising and being practical are key characteristics. Faugier (1998) states that the role of the supervisor is,

> . . . to facilitate growth both educationally and personally in the supervisee, whilst providing essential support to their developing clinical autonomy.
>
> Faugier 1998, p. 25

REFLECTION AND REVERIE

Midwives can also find support by reflecting on practice, although it is hard to think beyond the status quo and solitary reflection often takes the form of self-justification. It is, therefore, important that the model of reflection chosen helps midwives to engage in honest interactions with women and each other rather than resorting to 'professional narcissism' (Kirkham 1997, p. 261).

Johns (1993, 1995) suggests a model of guided reflection to help practitioners think critically. This is achieved through the elements of support, learning and self-monitoring of the practitioner's effectiveness. The epistemological basis from Carper's four patterns of knowing are drawn on; aesthetics, personal, ethics and empirics, adding a further pattern called reflexivity (Carper 1978). The reflexive way of knowing encourages practitioners to connect with previous experiences and to consider how these experiences might be handled differently in the future. If an ongoing experience was being reflected upon then the reflexive dimension provides the opportunity to explore how the situation could be taken further. Within midwifery reflexivity could be used to turn information into knowledge and challenge the concepts and theories by which midwives try to make sense of that knowledge.

Jones (2000) writes about a form of guided reflection that takes place in the Edgware Birth Centre and where midwives are facilitated by a supervisor of midwives to 'arouse curiosity and encourage open debate related to care, inspiring midwives to think critically and increase personal effectiveness' (p. 161). Scenarios, or 'casework moments' (Wilkins 1998) are presented at these guided reflection meetings and a process of peer review takes place. It is unlikely that this form of guided refection would be as successful in a large maternity unit with a dominant medical model and where the system was given precedence over the midwives.

Ci Ci Stuart (2001) stresses the care which needs to be taken to prevent structured reflection from turning into a 'moan session'. As with clinical supervision, the quality of facilitation is important because of the cognitive skills required. These skills are identified as those of description, critical analysis, synthesis and evaluation (Atkins & Murphy 1993, Stuart 2003).

Woodward sees the application of appropriate theory and group reflection as important in clarifying the primary task of midwives.

> Theoretical frameworks and group reflection are means to achieve collective and cohesive midwifery practice, and the ability to clearly articulate the profession's goals and contribution to health.
>
> Woodward 2000, p. 74

Bion (1967) described the importance for the infant's development of the mother's capacity for reverie – her ability to take in the child's communications, contain and consider them, with intuition if not conscious thought, and respond to them constructively. When the child feels distress, the mother can then reflect back a more tolerable understanding of the situation. If midwives are to mother the mothers in their care, their role is somewhat similar. Menzies Lyth (1988) saw the function of reverie as important for hospital staff working with children.

It can be reverie in the individual staff members or it can be something analogous to reverie in group situations, staff talking things through in an intuitive way together. Like the ordinary devoted mother (Winnicott 1958) they need themselves to be contained in a system of meaningful attachment. They need firmly bounded situations in which to work and they need the support of being able to talk things through in quieter circumstances (Menzies Lyth 1988, pp. 253–4).

The parallels between the devoted mother and the devoted midwife are obvious, as are the parallels in the support they need. For midwives to have the opportunity and the experience of such reverie would require considerable cultural change in most instances, as well as emotional skill and support. It would be likely to improve both clinical care and job satisfaction.

To foster the practice of reflection and reverie requires considerable development of analytical and emotional skills, which would in turn improve both clinical care and job satisfaction. Support and trust are key constituents of the safe setting needed for such skill development. Beyond that, a positive spiral can be created where the development of analytical and emotional skills fosters further growth in trust and support. There are, however, many dilemmas surrounding how to start this positive process.

INDIVIDUAL SKILLS AND POLITICAL CHANGE

Greater individual skill and self awareness can certainly help midwives to give and receive more support. For instance, the balancing of engagement/detachment is an important coping mechanism where midwives can learn to use different skills on an individual basis with women thus enabling the development of effective, helping relationships with women. This is reinforced by Carmack (1997) who states that:

> People who successfully balance engagement with detachment know what they can and cannot change or control. They are sensitive to their own emotional needs. They choose their level of engagement based on what they know they can handle at a particular time.

People who successfully balance engagement and detachment understand the importance of self-care.

Carmack 1997, p. 142

Yet midwives already cope by controlling the timing of, and duration, of their encounters with women. Deery (2003) found that in order to control the timing of their working day community midwives changed the approach they took to their work according to the nature of their existing workloads and 'framed solutions' accordingly (Lipsky 1980). For example, a community midwife who had numerous postnatal visits to undertake during the morning was unlikely to offer the level of psychological support to women that she would have preferred if she had a busy antenatal clinic in the afternoon. There is reluctance on the part of midwives to open up any interpersonal or psychological agenda concerning the woman's childbearing experience (Stapleton et al 2002) and many women are not offered the opportunity to ask any questions about their childbirth experience and the health of their baby because of shortage of time. As a result, the midwife will receive no feedback from the woman because the woman respects the busyness of the midwife and the organizational constraints placed upon her (Deery 2003, Kirkham et al 2002). Midwives cope therefore by framing solutions (Lipsky 1980) such as adapting their way of working to fit their workload rather than the needs of women. So individual skills are often used to enable the midwife to go with the flow of the power holders in her organization, often without conscious reflection by midwives or managers upon this process. Midwives also choose not to use skills that may be disruptive or make them unpopular in their work setting. Many of us have learnt assertiveness skills, which are rarely exercised.

Higher levels of self-awareness and skills in social analysis would make us more aware of the social processes in which we are involved. It must be acknowledged, however, that the social defence systems prevalent in NHS maternity care usually concern the evasion of relationship. Equipping midwives with skills in self-awareness with regard to our evasion of fruitful relationships with clients and colleagues is only useful where there is a commitment to growth and relationship. As Isabel

Menzies Lyth observed, 'evasion inhibits growth', whereas the support for our primary task fosters professional and personal growth. 'The evasive social defence system actually inhibits the development of the nurse's capacity to deal with her stress and to experience it less acutely' (Menzies Lyth 1988, p. 109). Until we are aware of such evasion, we cannot create strategies which foster, rather than evade, relationship. It is only within relationships that support can be given and received. Since we are dealing with social defence systems, rather than just individual bad habits, as well as gaining insight into the problems we have to change, we need to build working structures to create safe settings within which relationships can grow.

Thus, a balance is needed between equipping midwives with appropriate interpersonal skills, acknowledgement of their existing extensive interpersonal skills which may be focused upon anti-tasks rather than the primary task, and working for political change in the context within which midwives use their skills and in the resources available to them.

The culture and context of midwifery practice needs real political change. As midwives, we need to work towards this at every opportunity locally and nationally. We also need to develop the political skills to analyse our situation and understand the implications of service changes and the arguments to further our ends. Leadership from midwifery organizations is crucial here.

CONCLUSION

There can be no doubt that NHS midwives feel a great need for support in their primary task of caring for childbearing women. The immense organizational support given to getting through the work has led to social structures and individual coping mechanisms that can undermine our primary task. While midwives must balance many pressures upon them, the present situation is unhealthy for all concerned and results in many midwives leaving the profession, which creates further pressures upon those who remain.

Support is of concern to all midwives: clinicians, managers, supervisors and educators.

Support is given by individuals and we can all consciously develop skills and confidence in giving and receiving support. But the reasons that midwives often do not do this, especially in large units, are entirely logical and concerned with social survival where relationships with clients and colleagues are fragmented and there is overwhelming pressure to 'go with the flow' of an industrial model of organization. Political skills are needed in order to change this.

Factors which enhance support for midwives are also factors which enhance support for their clients: small scale organization of care, a degree of geographical separation from the industrial, obstetric model, enhanced professional autonomy and continuity of care. Within such an appropriate context, the skills of support can be developed together with other social and psychological skills, which enhance practice and clinical outcomes. This may be done through guided reflection or clinical supervision. There are many models which can be used to enable us to work through our experience and learn from it so that we work better together in future. This must be done in a safe setting with time specifically allocated, which in itself increases staff's feeling of self-worth since this demonstrates that they are seen as worth such investment of time and resources. This is important, as midwives currently feel undervalued as well as unsupported.

It is crucial that we work in this direction, as individuals and collectively. We owe this to ourselves and to the women in our care. The better our support the better we can learn to support them. Without changes in this direction we will lose more midwives and could also lose midwifery as we know and love it.

POINTERS FOR PRACTICE

1. Preferred strategies for strong midwifery support in clinical practice (e.g. clinical supervision, guided reflection) need to be discussed and decisions made as to how this support can be offered and received.
2. Facilitating such support in a safe setting with time specifically allocated will not only help to retain and re-recruit midwives, it will also increase midwives' feeling of self worth which must underpin practice development.
3. Seizing opportunities to think differently and work across professional boundaries will help midwives to recognize unhelpful defence mechanisms and an over concentration on subsidiary and anti-tasks that are detrimental to clinical practice.
4. Mandatory study days need to incorporate training in relationship skills and the giving and receiving of trust and support which underpin the development of these skills. This will help midwives become more aware of the social processes in which they are involved as well as the necessary political change in their current work context.
5. Specialist training in facilitation and counselling skills should be accessible to those who wish to develop this aspect of their role with colleagues or clients, especially supervisors of midwives.
6. Midwifery leaders need to express their approval of political change and alternative support strategies rather than conforming to an industrial model of organization. Strategic alliances with user groups could strengthen their position in this respect.

References

Atkins S, Murphy K 1993 Reflection: a review of the literature. Journal of Advanced Nursing 18: 1188–1192

Bakker R H C, Groenewegen P P, Jabaaij L et al 1996 Burnout amongst Dutch midwives. Midwifery 12(4): 174–181

Ball L, Curtis P, Kirkham M 2002 Why do midwives leave? Royal College of Midwives, London

Bion WR 1967 Second thoughts. London, Heinemann

Bond M, Holland S 1998 Skills of clinical supervision for nurses: A practical guide for supervisees, clinical supervisors and managers. Open University Press, Buckingham

Bower H 1993 Team midwifery in Oxford. MIDIRS Midwifery Digest 3(2):143–145

Brooks F 2000 Changes in maternity policy – who, what and why? In: Davies C, Finlay L, Bullman A (eds) Changing practice in health and social care. Sage, London, pp. 37–47

Butterworth T, Carson J, White, et al 1997 It is good to talk: An evaluation study in England and Scotland. The University of Manchester, Manchester

Carmack BJ 1997 Balancing engagement and detachment in caregiving. Image: Journal of Nursing Scholarship 29(2): 139–143

Carper B 1978 Fundamental ways of knowing in nursing. Advances in Nursing Science 11: 13–23

Casement P 1985 On learning from the patient. Tavistock, London

Clements S 1997 Horizontal violence. Birth Issues 6(1): 9–14

Curtis P, Ball L, Kirkham M 2003 Why do midwives leave? Talking to managers. Royal College of Midwives, London

Dadds M 2002 Taking curiosity seriously: the role of awe and Wanda in research-based professionalism. Educational Action Research 10(1): 9–26

Deery R 1999 Improving relationships through clinical supervision: 2. British Journal of Midwifery 7(4): 251–254

Deery R 2003 Engaging with clinical supervision in a community midwifery setting: an action research stud., Unpublished PhD Thesis, University of Sheffield, UK

Deery R, Corby D 1996 A case for clinical supervision in midwifery. In: Kirkham M (ed.) Supervision of midwives. Books for Midwives Press, Hale, pp. 203–212

Deery R, Hughes D 2004 Using action research to support midwife-led care: a tale of mess, muddle and birth balls. Evidence Based Midwifery 2(2): 52–58

Department of Health 1993a Changing childbirth, part 1 (report of the Expert Maternity Group). HMSO, London

Department of Health 1993b A vision for the future: the nursing, midwifery and health visiting contribution to health and health care. HMSO, London

Department of Health 1999 Making a difference: strengthening the nursing, midwifery and health visiting contribution to health and healthcare. HMSO, London

Department of Health 2000 The NHS Plan: A plan for investment, a plan for reform. HMSO, London

Department of Health 2004 National service framework for children, young people and maternity services. HMSO, London

Derbyshire F 2000 Clinical supervision within midwifery. In: Kirkham M (ed.) Developments in the supervision of midwives. Books for Midwives, Manchester

Faugier J 1998 The supervisory relationship. In: Butterworth T, Faugier J, Burnard (eds) Clinical supervision and mentorship in nursing. 2nd edn. Nelson Thornes, Cheltenham, pp. 19–36

Flint C, Poulengeris P, Grant A 1989 The 'Know your Midwife Scheme' – a randomised trial of continuity of care by a team of midwives. Midwifery 5(1): 11–16

Fox B, Worts D 1999 Revisiting the critique of medicalised childbirth, a contribution to the sociology of birth. Gender and Society 13(3): 326–346

Hallberg I R, Norberg A 1993 Strain among nurses and their emotional reactions during 1 year of systematic clinical supervision combined with the implementation of individualised care in dementia nursing. Journal of Advanced Nursing 18(2): 1860–1875

Hastie C (1995) Midwives eat their young, don't they? A story of horizontal violence in midwifery. Birth Issues 4 (3): 5–9

Hawkins P, Shohet R 1989 Supervision in the helping professions. Open University Press, Buckingham

House of Commons 1992 The Health Committee second report: maternity services, Vol 1 (Chair, N. Winterton). HMSO, London

Hughes D, Deery R 2002 Where's the midwifery in midwife-led care? The Practising Midwife 5(7): 18–19

Hughes D, Deery R, Lovatt A 2002 A critical ethnographic approach to facilitating cultural shift in midwifery. Midwifery 18: 43–52

Hunt S, Symonds A 1995 The social meaning of midwifery. Macmillan, London

Hunter B 2002 Emotion work in midwifery: An ethnographic study of the emotional work undertaken by a sample of student and qualified midwives in Wales. Unpublished PhD thesis, University of Wales Swansea, Swansea

Jenkins R 1995 Midwifery – a matter of politics. In: Murphy-Black T (ed.) Issues in midwifery. Churchill Livingstone, London, pp. 1–18

Johns C 1993 Professional supervision. Journal of Nursing Management 1: 9–18

Johns C 1995 The value of reflective practice for nursing. Journal of Clinical Nursing 2: 307–312

Jones O 2000 Supervision in a midwife managed birth centre. In: Kirkham M (ed.) Developments in the supervision of midwives. Books for Midwives, Manchester

Katzenback J, Smith D 1993 The wisdom of teams: creating the high performance organization. Harvard Business School Press, Boston

Kirkham M (ed.) 2003 Birth centres. A social model for maternity care. Elsevier Science, Oxford

Kirkham M 1997 Reflection in midwifery: professional narcissism or seeing with women? British Journal of Midwifery 5(5): 259–262

Kirkham M 1999 The culture of midwifery in the NHS in England. Journal of Advanced Nursing 30(3): 732–739

Kirkham M 2004 Midwives: praise and beyond. The Practising Midwife 7(2): 20–21

Kirkham M, Stapleton H (eds) 2001 Informed choice in maternity care: an evaluation of evidence based leaflets. NHS Centre for Reviews and Dissemination, York

Kirkham M, Stapleton H 2000 Midwives' support needs as childbirth changes. Journal of Advanced Nursing 32(2): 465–472

Kirkham M, Stapleton H, Curtis P, Thomas G 2002 Stereotyping as a professional defence mechanism. British Journal of Midwifery 10(9): 549–552

Law Y, Lamb K 1999 A randomised controlled trial comparing midwife managed care and obstetrician managed care for women assessed to be at low risk in the initial intrapartum period. Journal of Obstetrics & Gynaecology Research 25 (2): 107–112

Leap N 1997 Making sense of 'horizontal violence' in midwifery. British Journal of Midwifery 7(3): 160–163

Lindahl B, Norberg A 2002 Clinical group supervision in an intensive care unit: a space for relief, and for sharing emotions and experiences of care. Journal of Clinical Nursing 11: 809–818

Lipsky M 1980 Street-level bureaucracy: dilemmas of the individual in public services. Russell Sage Foundation, New York

Mackin P, Sinclair M 1998 Labour ward midwives' perceptions of stress. Journal of Advanced Nursing 27: 986–991

Mander R 2001 Supportive care and midwifery. Blackwell Science, Oxford.

Maslach C, Jackson SE 1993 Maslach burnout inventory. 7th printing. Consulting Psychologists, Palo Alto, CA 94303

McCourt C, Page L, Hewson J 1998 Evaluation of one-to-one midwifery: women's responses to care. Birth 25(2): 73–80

McGinley M, Turnbull D, Fyvie H et al 1995 Midwifery Development Unit at Glasgow Royal Maternity Hospital. British Journal of Midwifery 3(7): 362–371

McIver F 2002 Providing care under stress: creating risk. 12 midwives' experience of horizontal violence and the effects on the provision of care. Unpublished MA thesis. Massey University, Palmerston North, New Zealand

Menzies I E P 1979 The functioning of social systems as a defence against anxiety. Tavistock Institute of Human Relations, London

Menzies Lyth I 1988 Containing anxiety in institutions. selected essays, Vol 1. Free Association Books, London

Morgan M, Fenwick N, McKenzie C, Wolfe C D A 1998 Quality of midwifery-led care assessing the effects of different models of continuity for women's satisfaction. Quality in Health Care 7(2): 77–82

Morris M 1995 The role of clinical supervision in mental health practice. British Journal of Nursing 4(15): 886–888

NHS Litigation Authority 2002 Clinical negligence scheme for trusts. Clinical risk management standards for maternity services. Willis, London

Page L 1995 Putting principals into practice. In: Page L (ed.). Effective group practice in midwifery: working with women. Blackwell Science, London, pp. 12–17

Raphael-Leff J 1991 Psychological processes of childbearing. Chapman and Hall, London

Roberts S J 1983 Oppressed group behaviour: implications for nursing. Advances in Nursing Science July: 21–30

Royal College of Midwives (1997) Evidence to the Review Body for Nursing Staff, Midwives, Health Visitors and Professionals Allied to Medicine for 1997. Royal College of Midwives, London

Royal College of Midwives 1996 In place of fear: recognizing and confronting the problem of bullying in midwifery. Royal College of Midwives, London

Sandall J 1995 Burnout and midwifery: an occupational hazard? British Journal of Midwifery 3(5): 246–248

Sandall J 1997 Midwives' burnout and continuity of care. British Journal of Midwifery 5(2): 106–111

Sandall J 1998 Occupational burnout in midwives: new ways of working and the relationship between organisational factors and psychological health and well being. Risk Decision and Policy 3(3): 213–232

Sandall J 1999 Team midwifery and burnout in midwives in the UK: practical lessons from a national study. MIDIRS Midwifery Digest 9(2): 147–152

Savage J 2000 The culture of 'culture' in National Health Service policy implementation. Nursing Inquiry 7: 230–238

Siegrist J 1996 Adverse health effects of high-effort/low-reward conditions. Journal of Occupational Health Psychology 1(1): 27–41

Stansfield S A, R Fuhrer, M J Shipley, M G Marmot 1999 Work characteristics predict psychiatric disorder: prospective results from the Whitehall II study. Occupational and Environmental Medicine 56(5): 302–307

Stapleton H, Duerden J, Kirkham M 1998 Evaluation of the impact of the supervision of midwives on professional practice and the quality of midwifery care. English National Board, London

Stapleton H, Kirkham M, Curtis P, Thomas G 2002 Silence and time in antenatal care. British Journal of Midwifery 10(6): 393–396

Stuart CC 2001 The reflective journeys of a midwifery tutor and her students. Reflective Practice 2(2): 171–184

Stuart CC 2003 Assessment, supervision and support in clinical practice. Churchill Livingstone, London

Tinkler A, Quinney D 1998 Team midwifery: the influence of the midwife-women relationship on women's experiences and perceptions of maternity care. Journal of Advanced Nursing 28 (1): 30–35

Tucker JS, Hall M, Howie P 1996 Obstetrician led shared care was not better than care from general practitioner and community midwives in low risk pregnant women. Evidence Based Medicine, September/October: 190–191

Turnbull D, McGinley M, Fyvie H, Johnstone I, Holmes A, Shields N, Cheyne H, MacLennan B

1995 Implementation and evaluation of a midwifery development unit. British Journal of Midwifery 3(9): 465–468

Walker J, Hall S, Thomas M 1995 The experience of labour: a perspective from those receiving care in a midwife-led unit. Midwifery 11: 120–129

Walsh D 1995 The Wistow project and intrapartum continuity of carer. British Journal of Midwifery 3(7): 393–396

Walsh D, Downe S 2004 Outcomes of free-standing, midwife-led birth centres: a structured review. Birth, 31(3): 222–229

Wilkins P 1998 Clinical supervision and community psychiatric nursing. In: Butterworth T, Faugier J, Burnard P (eds) Clinical supervision and mentorship in nursing. 2nd en. Nelson Thornes, Cheltenham, pp. 189–204

Winnicott DW 1958 Collected papers: through paediatrics to psychiatry. Tavistock, London

Woodcock H, Baston H 1996 Midwife-led care: an audit of the home from home scheme at Darley Maternity Centre. MIDIRS Midwifery Digest 6(1): 20–23

Woodward V 2000 Caring for women: the potential contribution of formal theory to midwifery practice. Midwifery 16: 68–75

Chapter 7

Working with women: developing continuity of care in practice

Christine McCourt, Trudy Stevens, Jane Sandall and Pat Brodie

INTRODUCTION

For optimum health and well-being all women require easy access to services, choice and control regarding the care they receive and continuity of support during their pregnancy, childbirth and the postnatal period.

Department of Health 2004, p. 6

This chapter looks at the role of continuity, the relationship with quality of care, what it means (to midwives as well as to women) and how it can be provided and sustained. We explore and review the evidence from research on continuity of care and carer, but our aim here is to capture and present the practical as well as the philosophical lessons for maternity care providers – how to set-up and practise in systems that enable continuous and one-to-one relationships between women and midwives.

For the childbearing woman, there is a world of difference between having a known and trusted midwife who is with her through the whole of pregnancy, birth and the early weeks of newborn life, and being in the care of strangers, no matter how kind. This type of relationship also has great value for midwives themselves. Being with women throughout the process is very different from providing random and fragmented care to a number of women, as so often happens in modern, centralized maternity services. In this chapter we will draw on a range of studies which have analysed the importance of this relationship, and the

systems which help or hinder the provision of continuous care by midwives.

Campbell (1984), in his description of skilled companionship, says that companionship means 'being with', rather than 'doing to'. This implies a sense of personal involvement even with 'unpopular and difficult people'. This idea of companionship is particularly apt for midwives, who are with women as they journey through pregnancy and birth – an important and challenging journey or rite of passage. It is a journey during which physical and psychological growth and development, and growing love for the baby, help the woman and her partner to adapt to the new roles and challenges of mothering and fathering the child. Being with the woman and helping her to discover her own strengths, while offering skilled companionship, is crucial to this journey of adaptation, an adaptation in role to what are the most important and probably the most exacting responsibilities of adult life. Being able to accompany her on all parts of this journey, that is, caring for her during all the phases of pregnancy, labour, birth and the postnatal period, is important in terms of 'being with', rather than 'doing to'.

Concern about continuity of care and carer arose in the maternity services of many countries in the later decades of the 20th century as a result of progressive fragmentation of maternity services throughout that century. As birth moved into hospitals and midwives became employed by them as part of medically led and large multi-professional teams, continuity of care from the midwife's or woman's point of view was disrupted and women often reported feeling lost in a system that didn't seem to care for them as individuals.

In this chapter, we examine changes to the conventional organization of practice, which allow midwives to follow individual women through the entire system of care, including labour and birth. The movement away from fragmented structures in which midwives staff wards or departments rather than care for individual women within their communities, requires both different organization and approaches to practice. We review some of the changes and policies that have supported midwives in the provision of continuous care and offer practical advice on how to set up, and practise within systems that enable one-to-one relationships between childbearing women and midwives. The systems we discuss should also enable professional autonomy and professional growth for midwives. We present them as systems that undoubtedly call for commitment but which are potentially the most enjoyable form of midwifery practice available.

BEING WITH THE WOMAN: ORGANIZING SERVICES FOR CONTINUOUS SENSITIVE CARE

Continuous sensitive care means responding knowledgeably and sensitively to the individual needs of women and their families. This may be hindered or facilitated by different ways of organizing practice, such as caseload practice, or care in small midwifery-led units. We will describe some of these later in this chapter. We suggest that a change in the pattern of practice to allow greater continuity of care and carer is a necessary but not sufficient measure to develop woman-centred care. New patterns of practice are necessary to provide constant support in labour, to provide information and interventions at the right time and in the right place and to respond to women's individual needs. However, sensitive care also requires midwives' skills and positive attitudes. In particular, it demands personal sensitivity, clinical competence, skills, knowledge and professional wisdom.

In most industrialized countries, with a few exceptions such as the Netherlands and more recently New Zealand and Canada, the majority of midwives practise within an institutional setting. Where change is required the development of systems of care that allow midwives to work in a continuous relationship with women and their families throughout the pregnancy and childbearing period requires a radical shift in the way in which these institutions function. Midwives have become so used to what is an industrial model of care that continuity of care is seen as the alternative rather than being the default model of care. Practice has been influenced by a society in which a factory model has affected many forms of work and organizational life. Thus, the most common model of midwifery care over recent decades has been an assembly line approach with the woman progressing along the line at different points in her pregnancy. Industrial society also brought about a clearer separation of personal and professional life than had been known before. Midwives were once part of the communities where they practised; now their home and work lives are usually quite separate. Changes in the organization of practice, such as the development of One-to-One midwifery (McCourt & Page 1996) may recreate a more traditional integration and balancing of personal and professional life which many workers in the 21st century are seeking.

It is possibly because there is such a strong norm towards these industrial systems of care that the creation of continuity of care or carer across whole services has been difficult. In addition, the development of alternatives such as team midwifery, group practice or caseload midwifery create a number of practical organizational challenges and require a huge change in attitudes. It may be these practical difficulties, which have led to the continued debate on, and controversy over, continuity of care and what it means. Some have claimed that women want continuity of care (consistency of policy and approach from a team of care-givers) rather than continuity of carer (the majority of care coming from a named individual midwife supported by a small number of other midwives).

CLARIFYING THE CONCEPTS

New organizations of midwifery, such as the Know Your Midwife practice (Flint et al 1989), One-to-One midwifery practice (McCourt & Page 1996), and the Albany Practice (Sandall et al 2001) were developed for a number of reasons, including to provide more individual care that is responsive to the needs of the individual woman and her family, and to challenge the increasingly medicalized approach to birth. For nearly two decades, there have been attempts by hospitals to provide what has come to be known as 'woman-centred care', that is, care which is intended primarily to meet the individual needs of the woman and her family rather than meeting the needs of the institution. Many of these changes have been successful, but many have not. Confusion seems to surround the ideas or concepts that underlie these changes, and unless they are clearly defined, understood and agreed, no organizational change can succeed.

Effective organizational change requires that the purpose is clear, and such clarity of purpose requires that everyone involved be speaking the same language. Also, these abstract concepts can be different, and have very different effects, when they are applied in practice. Below we offer some definitions of key concepts.

CONTINUITY OF CARE OR CONTINUITY OF CARER?

General reviews of continuity of care have tended to conceptualize continuity in a range of ways (Haggerty et al 2003). All have aimed to develop a common understanding of the concept of continuity in order to understand the impact in different settings. Unless we understand the mechanisms through which care delivered over time improves outcomes, continuity interventions may be misdirected or inappropriately evaluated.

From these various definitions, it appears that continuity can most usefully be defined as a hierarchical concept ranging from the basic availability of information about the woman's past history to a complex interpersonal relationship between provider and woman characterized by trust and a sense of responsibility (Saultz 2003). At the base of this hierarchy is the notion of informational continuity. This concept might be the most important aspect of continuity in preventing medical errors and ensuring safety (Cook et al 2000), but by itself informational continuity might not improve access to, or satisfaction with care. Longitudinal continuity creates a familiar setting in which care can occur and should make it easier for women to access care when needed, but it does not assure a relationship of personal trust between an individual care provider and a recipient of care.

HIERARCHICAL DEFINITION OF CONTINUITY OF CARE

Level of Continuity	Description
1. Informational	An organized collection of medical and social information about each woman is readily available to any healthcare professional caring for her. A systematic process also allows accessing and communicating about this information among those involved in the care.
2. Longitudinal	In addition to informational continuity, each woman has a 'place' where she receives most care, which allows the care to occur in an accessible and familiar environment from an organized team of providers. This team assumes responsibility for coordinating the quality of care, including preventive services.
3. Interpersonal	In addition to longitudinal continuity, an ongoing relationship exists between each woman and a midwife. The woman knows the midwife by name and has come to trust the midwife on a personal basis. The woman uses this personal midwife for basic midwifery care and depends on the midwife to assume personal responsibility for

her overall care. When the personal midwife is not available, coverage arrangement assures that longitudinal continuity occurs.

(Adapted from Saultz 2003)

By arranging these concepts as a hierarchy, it is implied that at least some informational continuity is required for longitudinal continuity to be present and that longitudinal continuity is required for interpersonal continuity to exist in a midwife–woman relationship.

There have been a number of ways of measuring continuity, ie. who usually provides care, and for how long, normally based on the health record (Saultz 2003). However, these do not take into account the content of the visit and the nature of the interaction. Multiple definitions and measures have also made it difficult to generalize about the effect of continuity (Donaldson 2001). Research on whether continuity of care is effective has measured outcomes such as behaviours of recipients and caregivers, adherence to advice, use of services, clinical sequelae, clinician knowledge of patient's conditions, costs, and patient and staff satisfaction. Surveys have shown that patients and staff value continuity and that it is positively associated with staff satisfaction, but the causal direction is unknown.

These reviews of interpersonal continuity raise some interesting questions. Is informational continuity sufficient to assure the kind of care that women expect and deserve, or is the personal connection inherent in interpersonal continuity an essential element? If this interpersonal intimacy is further eroded, will the essence of the relationship be undermined? Can interpersonal intimacy and trust be preserved in a team-based model of care? It is fine to measure patterns and concentrations of visits if we want to understand longitudinal continuity of care, but to examine accurately the outcomes related to interpersonal continuity will require actual measurement of the variable one is trying to study.

Reviews in this area suggests that more research needs to be done on a) the experience of continuity, i.e. longitudinal studies and of women's journeys, and whether it is more important and effective for some groups of women than others,

b) the relationship between processes of care and benefits and disadvantages (apart from satisfaction), and c) how effective continuity can be achieved and what the barriers are (Freeman et al 2001).

Nutting also shows that more vulnerable populations by dint of age or chronic disease or socio-economic status value continuity of care more (Nutting et al 2003). Is valuing continuity of care an outcome in and of itself that validates its importance? Although satisfaction is considered by many as an outcome rather than a process measure, women can be satisfied with care that is of poor quality and not evidence based. In fact, liking or trusting their care provider might well be precisely what makes women feel their care is of high quality even when it is not. One unintended consequence of relational continuity is that consistent contact with a suboptimal health professional will be far from desirable.

In maternity care, there has been debate about two important and subtly different concepts to examine here – 'continuity of care' and 'continuity of carer'. Continuity of care means ensuring that there is a shared philosophy and approach to care that women experience. As we will show, this is often discussed but difficult to achieve in large fragmented systems of care, even where there is a 'team' approach. Continuity of carer means enabling midwives to organize their practice so that they may form a continuing working relationship with women in their care. It means enabling midwives to work with women through the whole of pregnancy, birth and the early weeks of newborn life, so that they may get to know each other and form a relationship that is based on trust between the two. This relationship, of trust and mutual respect, has been fundamental to the development of midwifery knowledge and wisdom.

MODELS OF MIDWIFERY PRACTICE

The development of systems of care that allow midwives to work in relationships with women and to practise autonomously, were influenced by the Know Your Midwife project (Flint et al 1989), a title that is explicit about the relationship between midwife and woman. It introduced midwifery-led care in small teams. These teams of midwives provided care to a group of women throughout pregnancy, birth and the postnatal period. Following this, team midwifery was set up in a number of places. In some settings, these teams moved away from the fundamental idea of having a small number of midwives looking after a small number of women, to much larger teams (Wraight et al 1993). Later, in an attempt to move away from a whole variety of forms of care subsumed under the name of team midwifery, the term 'midwifery group practice' was developed. This implies smaller groups of midwives caring for individual women, and those midwives 'carried a caseload' (Page 1995a). Later, a distinction was made between carrying a team caseload (a team of midwives sharing the care for a large number of women) and carrying a personal caseload (in which an individual midwife takes the responsibility for the care of a caseload of women) but with the support of other midwives in the group. This model was piloted and evaluated in London in the One-to-One midwifery practice scheme (Beake et al 2001, McCourt & Page 1996) and the Albany Project (Sandall et al 2001). In the years following Changing Childbirth (Department of Health 1993) a number of similar schemes were established across the UK in an attempt to implement the principles of choice, continuity and control for women.

Similar developments occurred in other countries. In Australia, women can access continuity of carer within birth centres, for home births and in some mainstream hospital settings through team midwifery (Biro 2000, Homer et al 2001b, Kenny et al 1994, Rowley 1998, Rowley et al 1995). Midwives within a birth centre setting may work within a small team or group, with either a team or personal caseload, and are usually employed by the birth centre or attached hospital. Those independent midwives working within a home birth setting may work alone, or closely with one or two colleagues, to provide continuity of carer and are, in most cases, employed by the pregnant woman. Since the loss of access to affordable professional indemnity insurance many independent midwives in Australia have ceased to practise privately. A small number of pilot projects offering homebirth through public funded services have emerged (Brodie & Leap 2005, Nixon et al 2003, Thorogood et al 2003).

Although progress has been slower than in the UK, a number of innovative programmes were set up during the late 1980s and 1990s within Australian mainstream hospital settings to provide continuity of carer. Published reports of these programmes include those of Aiken (1997), Biro et al (2000), Gumley et al (1997), Homer et al (2001b), Kenny et al (1994), Rowley et al (1995) and Waldenstrom (1996). Throughout Australia a number of other programmes are being planned or have recently commenced (Nixon et al 2003). Such programmes are largely the result of the efforts of midwives and consumers committed to improving maternity care for women. Primary midwifery-led units are beginning to emerge as they have done in the UK largely as a response to threat of closure following withdrawal of medical services (Tracy 2005).

In New Zealand the College of Midwives established the concept of partnership at the core of its model of midwifery practice (Guilliland & Pairman 1995). New Zealand midwives are able to practise autonomously, like independent midwives but contracted in to the public health service. They are paid and insured to practise in a system similar to that for UK General Practitioners and they carry a personal caseload of women.

In Canada, as midwifery has been regulated across different provinces, some Provinces have established a model of care similar to caseload practice. This grew directly out of the working practices of the lay and home-birth midwives who practised in the years before regulation (Sandall et al 2001). In Brazil, the ReHuNa movement is re-establishing autonomous midwifery practice, including the skills and knowledge of traditional birth attendants, humanization of hospital birth environments and establishment of small midwifery-led units.

FROM STAFFING THE SERVICE TO CARING FOR INDIVIDUAL WOMEN AND THEIR FAMILIES

MOVING POLICY INTO PRACTICE

In most parts of the industrialized world, with notable exceptions such as the Netherlands, where a greater proportion of midwives continue to practise in the community, there has been a shift from structures where midwives worked effectively as obstetric nurses, for the most part staffing wards and departments in hospitals, to systems in which the midwife worked with women where and when they were needed. Where midwives staff the service, they may be permanently allocated to one area, for example the delivery suite or the community, or they may rotate around the various areas. Such an approach centres on the needs of the institution rather than the needs of individual women. It is likely, as Brodie (1997) and Kirkham (1996) note, to lead to an allegiance to the institution rather than the woman. Although independent and lay midwives in many parts of the world, particularly Britain, Canada and the USA, had continued to provide essentially women-centred rather than institutionally centred care, this was confined to small numbers of women.

What is significant about this shift in emphasis is that it sought to reach the women who were part of the mainstream maternity service. For example, the Grace Hospital Low Risk Midwifery Project in Vancouver (Weatherston 1985) and the Know Your Midwife project (Flint et al 1989) both provided care for a small number of women and families who were attending hospital for their care. Both involved four midwives getting to know and caring for a small number of women and families, and both projects were based on a high degree of continuity of carer. Moreover, the midwives in both projects saw them as prototypes of systems that they wished to see developed for all women.

Substantial changes have occurred in the majority of maternity services in the UK and in some maternity services in other parts of the world. This change has, however, usually been confined to a portion of the service rather than involving a change to the service overall. The extent of the change is also quite variable, from large teams that are hospital based to caseload midwifery practices. In the UK, between 1987 and 1990, over 100 maternity services had set up some form of team midwifery (Wraight et al 1993) and emphasis has been in transforming the hospital service and moving a substantial amount of care to the community. This has been made possible because, in the main, maternity services have always been formally integrated between the hospital and the community.

Other parts of the world, including some provinces of Canada and New Zealand, have established midwifery as a primary care service and put midwives on a par with medical practitioners, giving women the right to choose between doctor- or midwife-led care (Wrede et al 2001).

POLICY CHANGES

To a large extent, the national policy changes that have occurred in the UK since the 1990s have followed changes that had already started in practice. Nonetheless, the importance of policy changes should not be underestimated. Putting policy into practice, especially with such fundamental change, is never easy. However, having policy backing makes such change easier than it would be without such authority. Therefore publication of government policy that placed at its centre giving women control in the birth of their babies, of having midwives practise their skills fully and of the importance of a known and trusted carer to women and their families, signified a shift in the mainstream of thought about childbirth.

While earlier government policy documents had emphasized the importance of continuity of care to women they also accepted the dogma of the use of inadequately evaluated technology and intervention, such as universal birth in hospital. The Winterton report (House of Commons 1992), was written as the result of the review of maternity services carried out by the Parliamentary Heath Committee and it questioned what had amounted to a faith in the indiscriminate use of technology. As such it marked a watershed in thinking in the UK. It was a broad report dealing with a number of social as well as healthcare issues that affect women's and children's health. The Changing Childbirth report (Department of Health 1993) was the UK government's response to the Winterton report. Focusing only on the maternity services and ignored recommendations in the Winterton Report about tackling inequalities in maternity care. Its recommendations were based on three fundamental principles of care (Department of Health 1993, p. 18):

■ The woman must be the focus of maternity care, able to feel that she is in control of what is happening to her and to make decisions about her care.

- Maternity services must be readily and easily accessible to all.
- They should be sensitive to the needs of the local population and based primarily in the community.

The ten indicators of success specified in the report focused on practice and service issues relevant to these principles. They included indicators of continuity and accessibility, greater choice and control for women and a re-emphasis on the role and responsibilities of midwives in normal, healthy pregnancy and birth.

A number of innovative services were implemented in the decade which followed, some of which were evaluated and are reviewed below. These included team and caseload midwifery schemes, and improved information for women including the use of patient-held records. However, many midwifery schemes were not sustained or remained on a small scale. During the late 1990s, the principles of choice, continuity and control for women were restated in successive government reports culminating in the publication of a National Service Framework for Children, Young People and Maternity Services in 2004.

While the policy frameworks continued to advocate greater continuity of care and carer and more community-based care, they also contained a specific focus on meeting the needs of disadvantaged women. A number of midwifery group and caseload midwifery practices had been developed in collaboration with Sure Start local schemes (http://www.surestart.gov.uk). These were central government funded projects to improve all-round support for families with young children in socially disadvantaged areas. Thus, by 2004, midwifery developments were increasingly integrated into wider social policies to promote health and wellbeing.

In Australia, during the late 1980s and 1990s, a number of maternity care reviews were conducted, which resulted in specific recommendations. However, in many cases, these recommendations lacked timeframes for their implementation as well as adequate indicators to measure success (Commonwealth Department of Health and Aged Care 1999, Ministerial Review of Birthing Services in Victoria 1990, Ministerial Task Force on Obstetrical Services in New South Wales 1989, Ministe-

rial Task Force WA 1990, National Health and Medical Research Council 1996).

In light of the insufficient changes, in 2002 a broad coalition of consumer and midwifery organizations from across Australia proposed a strategy for Federal and State governments to enable universal access to community based midwifery care. The National Maternity Action Plan (Maternity Coalition, 2002) called for substantial change to the way in which maternity services are provided, by making available to all women the choice of having a midwife provide one-on-one primary maternity care through the publicly funded health system (Maternity Coalition, 2002).

Since this time a number of newer state based policy initiatives and further reviews have also called for greater emphasis on introduction of models of midwifery care that enable women to access continuity of midwifery care and choice of place of birth (A C T Health 2004, Department of Health Services 2004, NSW Health Department 2003). This followed a national inquiry that had highlighted the lack of significant progress in the implementation of changes from earlier reviews including those directed at addressing the inadequacies in service provision for Aboriginal women living in remote communities (Kildea 1999).

THE RESEARCH EVIDENCE ON MODELS OF CARE

The majority of maternity services in the UK have now piloted either continuity of care schemes or midwifery-led services. Many of these have not been evaluated (Green et al 1998, Wraight et al 1993) and few studies have looked in depth at their cost effectiveness or at the experiences of midwives themselves. Although this is a lost opportunity, it is not surprising: midwives have had few resources or support to evaluate such innovations. The evaluation of such innovations is technically challenging since entire service-level changes are complex and deeply context dependent and so not necessarily suitable for evaluation by a conventional randomized controlled trial. It is also made more difficult by the challenges of defining and distinguishing different models of care; for example, schemes called team midwifery vary widely in the size and type of team and the conditions of midwives' work.

While a number of evaluations have been undertaken, there is no comprehensive systematic review of all the evidence. A limited structured review was conducted in the late 1990s (Green et al 1998), but a number of evaluations were excluded and there was no account of qualitative research. A number of studies have also been conducted or published since then.

TEAM AND CASELOAD MIDWIFERY

Caseload midwifery is the standard way of organizing midwifery care in parts of Canada and in New Zealand and is becoming more common in the UK and to a lesser extent, Australia. Caseload models are a form of practice in which each midwife is responsible for, and provides most of the midwifery care for a caseload of women throughout pregnancy, birth and the early weeks after the baby is born. Midwives' work centres around women, rather than being attached to particular clinical locations. They can provide care from a range of locations including hospital, birth centres, women's homes and community settings, according to a woman's needs. In this model, the woman and her midwife get to know each other well over the whole maternity experience, building a relationship of trust with each other, sharing information and decision-making and recognizing the active role that both play in the woman's maternity care.

Most full-time midwives carrying a personal caseload are the primary midwife for between 35–40 women a year and second midwife for a similar number. The primary midwife will provide the majority of antenatal and postnatal midwifery care and provides birth care in a range of settings. Midwives carrying a personal caseload usually work in community-based group practices, which either serve women from several GP lists or women living in a geographical patch. Each midwife usually works with a midwife partner in the group practice who provides on-call cover when the midwife is unavailable. In the team midwifery model, a small team of midwives provides antenatal, birth and postnatal care for a defined number of women. A team of 6 midwives may

share a caseload of 300–350 women, however the size of the group practice can vary from 6 to 16 or more midwives.

Current evidence from a Cochrane Review (Hodnett 2003) and additional trials (Biro et al 2000, Homer et al 2001a, 2001b, 2002, Waldenstrom et al 2000) show some clear benefits for women who received care from a team of midwives. Only two studies (Flint et al 1989, Rowley et al 1995) involving 1815 women were included in the Cochrane Review, which is being updated. Generally, there was a consistent impact on reducing antenatal admissions and increasing attendance at antenatal education programmes, reducing some childbirth interventions such as epidural and pharmacological pain relief, electronic fetal monitoring and neonatal resuscitation. In addition women felt well prepared and supported during labour. Women were happier with the care they received although the measurement of this varied widely. However, there was no impact on outcomes such as induction, caesarean, instrumental delivery or breastfeeding rates. Neither was there any impact on neonatal outcomes such as Apgar score, low birth weight or stillbirth and neonatal death, however the studies were too small to detect changes in these rarer outcomes. One large randomized controlled trial in Australia, which was published after the Cochrane review showed a significant difference in the caesarean section rate between women who received standard care, 17.8% (96/539), and those who received continuity of care from a small team of midwives, 13.3% (73/550). This difference was maintained after controlling for known contributing factors to caesarean section (OR = 1.6, 95% CI 1.08–2.38, P = 0.02). There were no other significant differences in the events during labour and birth (Homer et al 2001b). Known as the 'STOMP' model (St George Outreach Maternity Programme), this service provides care for women of all risk through community-based continuity of care by midwives who work collaboratively with obstetricians. This form of care has also shown to be cost effective (Homer et al 2001a).

There have been no trials of caseload midwifery, however non-randomized studies have shown differences in caesarean rates, vaginal delivery rates and other aspects of normal birth (Benjamin et al 2001, North Staffordshire Changing Childbirth Research Team 2000, Page et al 2001, Sandall et al 2001). In addition, women who have received this model prefer it (McCourt & Pearce 2000). Women in labour who had a known carer were considerably more likely to say this was important than women who had not (Garcia et al 1998, Gready et al 1995). Women tend to express a preference for what they have experienced (van Teijlingen et al 2003) but in some qualitative studies, women have been able to compare different models of care for different births and in such cases they tend to prefer care with a known midwife (McCourt & Pearce 2000, Walsh 1999). The building of relationships between midwives and women during pregnancy contributes to many women's sense of security in childbirth and may explain some of these differences. But without well-designed trials of caseload midwifery, it cannot be said for certain that these promising outcomes are due to caseload midwifery and not other factors.

WHAT DO WE NEED TO FIND OUT?

The studies described above sought to examine continuity of care by a team of midwives, some of which have not achieved that objective, and others have not reported it. Non-randomized studies of caseload midwifery have also shown differences in caesarean rates, vaginal delivery rates and other aspects of normal birth (Benjamin et al 2001, Page et al 2001, Sandall et al 2001). Some of these studies used regression modelling to compare outcomes and the models of care achieved greater levels of continuity of carer than the trials included in the Cochrane review. Currently, we don't know whether there is a real effect on vaginal birth rates and if so, why or how this happens.

In addition we need to know more about how women feel about what happens to them during childbirth. Measurement of psychosocial processes and outcomes is varied and limited in the short and long term. It seems that perceptions of control are related to childbirth interventions and how positive women feel about their experience (Homer et al 2002), but there needs to be a review of psychosocial outcome measures for use in maternity care research.

Although team midwifery has an impact on some childbirth interventions, it has had little impact on childbirth outcomes such as vaginal birth rates and caesarean rates. The important and complex questions we should ask include:

- Why does care by a team of midwives seem to have no impact on the normal delivery rate?
- Do differences occur between some of the above trials because midwives are more able to work in a less interventionist way, and develop shared decision-making with women in some units compared to others?
- What are the effects of the various organizational cultures and approaches and the leadership frameworks within which these models have flourished or perished?
- Are differences due to the level of continuity of carer that women received? We don't know whether these outcomes are due to continuity or a more autonomous way of practice drawing on a more holistic philosophy. It is impossible to disentangle effects of continuity of care with care provider and with one-to-one support during birth.

WHY MIGHT CONTINUITY OF CARER BE IMPORTANT TO WOMEN?

The issue of whether or not continuity of carer is important to women and acceptable to midwives has been a matter of major debate in midwifery in much of the industrialized world over the past decade. It may be divisive because the effective provision of continuity of carer requires fundamental change in the way services work, and it profoundly alters the meaning, experience and expectations of midwifery for midwives. In general, it can alter the allegiance of the midwife from being primarily to the institution, to being with the woman (Brodie 1997, Stevens & McCourt 2002c, 2002d). Such a profound change tends to affect individuals and organizations deeply, on a number of levels and in a number of ways, and may provoke great support but also great hostility (Menzies 1970).

The most difficult aspect of continuity of carer to organize is that for labour and birth. This also seems to be the most contentious issue among the critics. Some argue that existing evidence does not support the view that women want continuity of carer in labour (Green et al 1998). However, this review did not include qualitative research (Homer et al 2000, 2002, McCourt & Pearce 2000, McCourt et al 1998, Proctor 1998, Walsh 1999), which might better answer the question of what it is that women value about continuity of care for labour and birth. It also did not differentiate between different levels of continuity.

In general, quantitative research alone is too limited to understand possible links between continuity of carer and particular outcomes, or indeed what issues and outcomes are important to women. The implementation of continuity of carer brings about the introduction of a whole package of care. Indeed, that is the very purpose of these schemes: to change the structure so that other aims, such as constant support in labour, the provision of better information and more sensitive care, may be accomplished. Researchers sometimes see these other factors as confounding variables rather than part of the change. Evaluating a new model of care that entails a different approach does not lend itself to the manipulation of different variables to see what is associated with what, an approach that has been suggested for future research (Green et al 1998). Some schemes have also, in effect, introduced midwifery-led care for low-risk women for the first time, further complicating the picture.

Where evidence does exist, fundamental problems often arise in interpreting the importance of a known carer in labour. It is common sense that having a known carer in labour will not be important if that carer is unskilled or insensitive, yet a number of studies continue to rank women's wants in a way indicating that a known carer in labour is less important than other things, such as safety. Indeed, Green et al (1998) conclude from their review that 'What probably matters most is that she should feel that they are competent and that they care – about her'. Of course, any woman having to choose between a known carer, and kindness, skill and enough information would choose the latter. Their analysis overlooks the problem of caring for the individual woman when the system militates against this, since the approach of the review, and indeed the majority of evaluations it included, did not look in any detail at the organizational aspects of the services being evaluated.

A difficult issue in assessing the importance of a known carer for labour and birth arises from the difficulty of adequately evaluating women's responses to care. Measures of satisfaction are rarely adequate in establishing any answers to such questions. As highlighted in the evaluation of One-to-One practice:

> . . . satisfaction surveys are fraught with difficulties, from defining or deconstructing the concept of satisfaction to deciding how questions should be asked. On the whole, responses to consumer surveys tend to be neutralised by the use of broad satisfaction measures.
>
> McCourt et al 1998, p. 79

The tendency for women to be satisfied with what they expect, that is, what must be best (Porter & Macintyre 1984) may also limit what can be learned from satisfaction surveys. Satisfaction can be difficult to define and measure in a meaningful way. Moreover, many women feel immense obligation to the staff who have cared for them and relief at having a live, healthy baby; these feelings may be expressed in broad terms as satisfaction with the service even when the women have experienced great distress (Jacoby et al 1990, McCourt et al 1998).

For this reason, the Australian trial of team midwifery (Homer et al 2002), focused on women's 'experiences' as the focus of their questionnaires rather than 'satisfaction'. It was also thought possible by these authors that general questions about 'satisfaction' may extract high reported levels of satisfaction with care and could mask important differences in specific aspects of the experience and particular areas of dissatisfaction (Homer et al 2000).

Continuity and knowing one's carers were the most common themes highlighted across both groups in the evaluation of One-to-One midwifery practice. Women in the One-to-One group said that this was something they wanted to keep and advocated extending the service to other areas, while women in the control group highlighted this as an aspect needing change or improvement (Beake et al 2001, McCourt & Pearce 2000, McCourt et al 1998). In general, the evidence from this study was overwhelmingly that women prefer continuity of care and carer where it is possible.

We are now, with the availability of more open-ended qualitative research, beginning to understand what it is that women appreciate about continuity and that it may be valuable in its own right. As one woman, comparing her experience with a previous birth, commented:

> My first delivery was with a selection of different midwives and students who came and went as they pleased which I found very distressing and upsetting. My most recent delivery was totally different. So much different – it was wonderful to have a midwife I had met before and who stayed with me the whole time – I just wish this had been the case the first time as I am sure that it wouldn't have been so horrendous or distressing if this had been the case.
>
> Garcia et al 1998, p. 60

Those women who have had the experience of being cared for in labour by a known midwife tend to rate this as being more important (Green et al 1998, McCourt & Page 1996). Continuity in labour is important for a number of reasons. First, it allows a constant presence in labour, a factor important to both mother and baby (Hodnett 2003). The One-to-One study (McCourt et al 1998), found that the majority of women who had been allocated to One-to-One care had constant support in labour compared with just over half in conventional care. When asked in the antenatal period, 'would you prefer your main carer [midwife] to attend the birth?' few women in either group said that they would rather not know the person (7 women in the conventional care group vs 1 woman in the One-to-One care group). A large majority (84%) of One-to-One women said, 'yes very much'. The views of women who had conventional care were fairly widely spread. Although their most frequent response was that they did not mind whether their main carer was available (27.5%), this was closely followed by 'yes very much' (26.9%). Both mothers who knew and those who did not know about the One-to-One service expressed the belief that labour and delivery would have been much easier if they had known the midwife beforehand.

Proctor (1998), in her study of perceptions of quality in the maternity services, also describes a consistent theme from her antenatal interviews of the importance of familiarity with the midwife. They wanted, she comments, to feel that they would know, or even recognize, the person who would care for them in labour. She comments that, during the process of labour, the significance of continuity of carer seemed to increase in importance from the early hours of labour to during the actual delivery. Interestingly, in the same study, midwives' comments on the perceived importance of continuity for the mother were divided (Proctor 1998).

Morrison et al (1999), in a phenomenological study of families who had experienced birth at home, found that a consistent theme was the midwife knowing the person in labour and a person knowing them and what they wanted. Coyle (1998) undertook a qualitative study of 17 women who gave birth in a birth centre but had previously given birth in a hospital, reporting that women emphasized the importance of cumulative interactions and the opportunity to develop an ongoing relationship with the midwife. These cumulative interactions resulted in women being comfortable with carers and at ease; and women being known by carers.

Both of these studies found that it was particularly important in labour that the midwife knew the women, what they wanted, how they might act, their fears. This concept of 'being known' was also important to women in the One-to-One study (McCourt & Pearce 2000). In Allen et al's (1997) study, the majority of women who had experienced the presence of their named midwife at delivery said that it mattered a lot. In general, they valued the enormous rapport that had been built up and the trust that had been established.

Allen et al's (1998) evaluation of three midwifery group practices and Green et al's (1998) review found that in some schemes, especially with team approaches, continuity of care overall was reduced simply in order to ensure that women saw a 'known face' in labour. In some cases, this meant women meeting larger numbers of midwives than they would in a traditional shared care system in which they would have seen community midwives for most visits. As we shall see below, such schemes could also prove to be more stressful to midwives (Sandall 1997a, 1997b). Additionally it was unclear what 'continuity' or 'knowing the midwife' meant in practice, and in some cases it could be defined as simply having 'met' a midwife once.

Understandably, women do not want continuity enhanced in one area of care to the detriment of continuity in another. In the Audit Commission study of 1998, 23 women commented voluntarily on continuity of care in the antenatal period, although there were no questions related to this in the survey. Quite a few of these comments about continuity referred to the difficulties of having to explain things to different members of staff, as well as to women's worries that clinical care might not be as good when many care-givers were involved (Garcia et al 1998).

In the Australian randomized controlled trial of 'STOMP' team midwifery described earlier, women in the STOMP group reported significantly less time waiting to access care and easier access. STOMP group women also reported a higher perceived 'quality' of antenatal care compared with the control group (Homer et al 2000).

Continuity of caregiver may also improve the amount of information given to women and the way in which it is provided. This was an issue raised by nearly all women in the qualitative evaluation of One-to-One care. Control group women were far more likely to mention information or communication as a problem, and of the ethnic minority women in the control group, only one was happy about the level of information received (McCourt et al 1998, McCourt & Pearce 2000).

A structure that allows continuity of caregiver also allows the development of a special relationship, one that has some qualities of a friendship (Wilkins 2000). Women who value this relationship and the availability of a known trusted midwife emphasize the confidence, support and reassurance that knowing one's midwife provides (McCourt et al 1998, McCourt & Pearce 2000). This finding was supported by comments made by women in Garcia's study; as one woman commented: 'It was wonderful knowing them [a team of midwives]. It gave me a lot more confidence in my care' (Garcia et al 1998, p. 58).

From ethnographic interviews with 10 women who had experienced caseload care, Walsh described a positive impact on women's experience of childbirth (Walsh 1999). The relationship that evolved between women and their midwives was highly valued by women as being of overriding significance and different from earlier childbirth experiences. Women described the experience in terms of friendship with the midwife and expressed their delight and gratitude. Walsh described the women's reflections on care as 'I was' statements, and characteristics were described using the midwives' names. In contrast, previous experiences of birth were a 'powerful negative experience of maternity care in a hospital context with critical, depersonalized "S/he was" and "they were" statements about caregivers' (Walsh 1999, p. 49). These depersonalized statements perhaps reflect the depersonalization of the care experienced. Similar contrasts in terminology were found in the One-to-One study (McCourt & Pearce 2000). Walsh mentions the possible bias of his sample because the majority of women in his study had given birth at home (Walsh 1999). However, his report reflects the experience of other women receiving such highly personal midwifery care in the other schemes evaluated qualitatively, namely. that it is as likely to be the 'relationship' of care as much as the 'setting' that leads to such responses (McCourt & Pearce 2000).

While labour and birth is a critical time for the woman, the postnatal period may also be a distressing time, and supportive care at this stage is also crucial. As Garcia et al (1998) comment, lack of continuity at this time may lead to conflicting advice, something that many parents find very difficult. Postnatal care is an area where many women feel dissatisfied with the support they receive, especially in hospital (Garcia et al 1998) whereas women who have continuity of care from a small team or caseload midwives tend to feel supported throughout (Beake et al In press).

WHY IS CONTINUITY IMPORTANT TO MIDWIVES, AND HOW IS SUCH PRACTICE BEST ORGANIZED?

The commitment of many of the midwives who implemented continuity of carer schemes has come from the direct experience of providing a personal and continuous service to individual women through pregnancy, birth and the weeks thereafter. It is an experience that may transform approaches and attitudes to practice (see, for example, Bissett 1995, Brodie 1997, Couves 1995,

Farmer & Chipperfield 1996, Minns 1995, Page 1995b).

Many midwives who practise in continuity of care schemes apply to do so because of extreme dissatisfaction with the conventional service and because they feel their role to be limited by it. Once in a continuity of care scheme, they usually express a reluctance to return to the conventional service and intense satisfaction when providing continuity of care (Stevens 2003, Stevens & McCourt 2002c). One of the most important aspects of this satisfaction seems to be the possibility of reciprocal relationships with women in their care, a finding confirmed by Sandall (1997a, 1997b). This is referred to by others as a friendship (James 1997, Walsh 1998, Wilkins 2000). Key qualities of an effective relationship between a woman and her midwife are those of mutual respect and reciprocity. Where these are achieved the midwife will work to secure effective access to services, be an advocate for women, prevent women falling through gaps in care, listen and act on women's wishes, offer humane personal care and shift the balance of power towards each individual woman. For the midwife, she will learn more, see the results of her actions, take more responsibility because responsibility for her practice lies with her.

Other commonly encountered themes are the flexibility and autonomy enabled by such schemes, the intense learning that this form of practice provides and encourages, and the perceived ability to identify and meet women's expressed needs.

We have discussed earlier the difficulty and challenges that innovation can present for midwives who are accustomed, and perhaps resigned to, a system where midwives staff services or areas, rather than being able to work around the needs of women they care for.

Institutional needs or long-established precedents have not hampered the development of these innovative practices established in Canada and New Zealand (in the case of Canada, perhaps, because midwives previously worked outside of the healthcare system, more in the manner of traditional midwifery). They are united by a number of principles of care, the most fundamental of which is the importance of the relationship between the childbearing woman and the midwife. In her PhD thesis, James (1997), using a phenom-enological approach unfolds and illuminates the experience of 'being with woman as midwife'. The thesis provides a way of understanding the potential of such relationships, relationships that go far beyond any idea of relationship as simply transactional, to a depth of mutuality, understanding and trust that transforms midwifery. Her study was conducted in Alberta, Canada, among 'lay midwives' and the women they cared for. Such a situation allows for the emergence of a form of practice characterized by close relationships between childbearing women and their midwives. As midwifery became regulated and part of the healthcare system, midwifery remained a primary care service, with midwives directly reimbursed, and required to provide continuity of care with the aim of trying to maintain this form of practice on a larger scale (De Vries et al 2001).

Pairman (1998) undertook an in-depth study of both the nature and understanding of the relationship between midwives and women during pregnancy, labour and birth in New Zealand. She found that both the midwife and the woman contribute equally to the relationship and value what each brings to it. The 'real' continuity that was offered by the midwives in this study, being available and getting to know women over time, allowed this relationship to develop and seemed to be of mutual benefit to both women and midwives. 'Friendship' and 'partnership' are terms used by both the women and the midwives in this study. The midwife–woman relationship is one of equal status and shared power and control. What is striking in the accounts of the relationship in this study is the sense of attention to the experience as well as the physical outcome of birth, and the thoughtful attention to shared decision-making (see also Chapter 4).

Like Walsh (1999), who describes the challenge to traditional professional roles that is represented by personal midwifery practice, James (1997) reminds us that in most professional relationships there is not usually a blending of the personal and the professional roles. This epitomizes the differences, described clearly by Brodie (1997), between loyalty to the institution and loyalty to individual women when we think about 'staffing women' rather than 'staffing wards'. However, this different style of engaging with women also challenges conventional practices and has the potential to set midwives apart from their colleagues. The shift in organizational and professional allegiances and philosophical approaches that result from the midwives' practice of 'being with women', rather than being part of a ward, department or professional group, confronts both the system and the individuals involved. Interactions between team midwives and their colleagues involved a degree of hostility at times that bordered on horizontal violence (Leap 1997b) and hampered working relationships. This left some team midwives feeling sadness or disappointment with their peers and colleagues as highlighted by one midwife:

> I think it's really sad for the other midwives. . . . that they can't see what we are doing and how it benefits women and midwives too. . . . it was terrible to think that they weren't behind me after all the years I had been working with them.
>
> Brodie 1997, p. 54

While the new role was shown to have distinct benefits, it is clear that there are issues of sustainability and a necessary organizational culture change that make the introduction of these models challenging for all concerned (Brodie 1997).

DO MIDWIVES PRACTISING CASELOAD MIDWIFERY SUFFER FROM BURNOUT?

There are consistent findings that midwives working in teams do suffer from higher levels of burnout (Sandall 1998a, 1998b, 1999). This is due to the low levels of control, fragmented relationships with women and the more stressful nature of on-call in team midwifery. However, midwives carrying their own caseload did not seem to suffer in the same way (Sandall 1997a, 1997b). This seemed to be due to increased control over working life, greater levels of social and professional support within the group practice and being able to develop meaningful relationships with women.

One national study did explore the impact of work organization on the health and wellbeing of midwives. Drawing on data from a survey of a 5% random sample of midwives in England (N = 1166), and controlling for a range of factors, it was found that some new organizational structures were associated with higher levels of midwife burnout. They contained factors such as low control over decision-making and work pattern, low occupational grade, and longer working hours. These factors were particularly prevalent in team midwifery (Sandall 1998b). However, there is a lack of national research in this area looking at caseload midwives, and more needs to be done.

Around 50% of the midwifery workforce in the UK work part-time and 70% have children. Midwives who are not working full-time simply carry a proportionally reduced size caseload. One small study found that midwives who carried their own caseload have greater flexibility over how they manage their time, making it easier to balance home and work life (Sandall 1998a, 1998b) as compared to the demands of rigid and shift work systems. However, responsibility for a personal caseload does require out of hours on-call commitment and midwives without childcare support find it difficult. There is a range of ways of organizing on-call, but the key to successful balance is to devolve the organization of working patterns to the midwives.

PRACTICAL ASPECTS OF PROVIDING PERSONAL, CONTINUOUS CARE

In this section we focus on the more practical aspects of implementing caseload midwifery practice, in particular the One-to-One scheme studied by Stevens (Stevens 2003, Stevens & McCourt 2001, 2002a, 2002b), because it is a model of practice that provides a high level of continuity that has been studied in depth and in a range of national and local settings.

HOW TO PROVIDE PERSONAL AND CONTINUOUS CARE

The provision of continuity of carer means having individual midwives planning midwifery care together with women and their families, and providing most of the care, including, whenever possible, care during labour and birth. There are a number of ways of organizing such a system while keeping the principles intact.

In the One-to-One midwifery practice model, one named midwife coordinates and provides most of the care for women on her personal caseload. Midwives are affiliated to GP practices and the majority of the caseload is within a small geographical catchment area. Women may self refer or be referred by the relevant GPs or by the hospital booking clerks, according to their residential postcode. Midwives are encouraged to plan well ahead and to accept women on to their caseload according to the expected date of birth. Planning for four births per month, apart from when time is taken for annual leave, will produce an annual caseload of about 40 births. Women with low-risk pregnancies will usually receive midwife-led care, and most of their antenatal care will take place in their own homes. Women with high-risk pregnancies will receive obstetrician-led care, the obstetrician providing a point of referral and decision-making alongside the named midwife.

The named midwife works with a partner who shares the antenatal care and provides care when the named midwife is unavailable. This usually ensures the presence of a known midwife if the woman goes into labour when the named midwife is not on call. Postnatally, the named midwife will again provide the majority of care, visiting according to the woman's need until transfer to the health visitor. In relevant areas she also co-ordinates closely with Sure Start workers and facilities. The principle, as highlighted, is not for the midwife to attempt to provide exclusive care but to move away from the fragmented system in which women moved between a confusing array of systems and carers, without the benefit of a continuing personal relationship. Getting to know the women can enable the midwife to work with the women's own personal and community networks, as well as other, more formal, sources of support.

Working with a personal or partnership caseload also enables midwives to retain flexibility, by avoiding the need for fixed on-call rotas, clinics and other duties. This is important for sustainability, since midwives who may be called out to care for women in labour need to be able to ensure they can take rest and take breaks at appropriate times.

DEVELOPING THE RELATIONSHIP: BEING WITH THE WOMAN, GETTING A BALANCE

In the UK, caseload midwifery practice was developed explicitly to change both the structure and culture of care. It was intended to allow midwives to develop a relationship with women that enables them to be skilled companions to women on their journey through pregnancy and birth. Lifting the barriers of inflexible shift systems, and allocations to one area of a service, allows the midwife to work with women in this way (Stevens & McCourt 2002a, 2002b). However, the change demands a careful consideration on the part of the midwife of how she will develop appropriate relationships that are sensitive and supportive without developing undue dependency and without removing all boundaries around her work and its demands.

Stevens' ethnographic study showed that midwives who practise in this way can sometimes become overprotective or have unrealistic expectations of what they can achieve (Stevens 2003). For example, it may not be realistic to get long-term problems of housing or substance abuse sorted out within the context of a midwifery relationship; other sources of professional help are required. The midwives, who served a diverse area (including one of the most deprived in the UK), discovered that they had to outline professional boundaries and define their role as midwives, both to themselves and the women they cared for as some found themselves acting as friends, general supporters, counsellors and social workers. Strategies the midwives learnt for handling this are described below.

There is also the potential to meet one's own need to be needed through such work, setting up a relationship of dependency that is helpful to neither the childbearing woman nor the midwife. Stevens reported that learning to develop and manage appropriate boundaries was an important part of the adaptation period for new caseload midwives, which could take from 6–12 months to achieve (Stevens 2003). The concept of 'skilled companionship' has been described by a number of midwives (Cooke & Bewley 1995, Page 1995a, Smith 1991). This term was formulated by Campbell (1984) to describe the relationship between professional carers and those who seek their help. The work was set in the contexts of medicine, nursing and social work, but is applicable to midwifery as it used the imagery of a journey in which companionship arises from a chance meeting and is terminated when the joint purpose that keeps the companions together no longer applies (Campbell 1984, p. 49). Four features of this relationship are outlined:

1. Companionship involves a bodily presence and necessitates sensitivity.
2. Companionship includes the notion of helping another to move onward on the journey with encouragement and hope.
3. Companionship means 'being with' rather than just 'doing to' in the sense of personal involvement, even with 'unpopular' and 'difficult' people.
4. Companionship involves a limited commitment that is for the duration of the journey, recognizing that both companions have their own lives to lead.

This latter point about limits of the commitment is equally important and over-emphasis on the companionship of the midwife has been criticized by others. Leap (1996) argues that rather than acting as companions, midwives should facilitate friendship and support among the woman's community through networking at antenatal and postnatal groups. This was an explicit feature of the Albany Practice (Sandall et al 2001) and was developed over time by midwives in the One-to-One scheme. Leap (1997a) further highlights the potential of creating mutual dependency in continuity schemes if too much emphasis is placed on exclusive special relationships between women and midwives. Although acknowledging the emergence of friendships, and indeed their importance in engaging in joint efforts to improve maternity services, Leap suggests that they should not be the *focus* of care provision.

As we have noted, this theme of dependency is one highlighted in the literature on continuity. Allen et al (1997) found some evidence of it in their study of three midwifery group practices. Downe (1997) warns of the 'culture of dependency' that may result with intense involvement with women, and Sandall (1996) writes of the 'dependency relationship', which may grow from a trusting relationship between woman and midwife. Benner and Wrubel (1988) have highlighted the dangers

of co-dependency in provider–patient relationships and midwives need to be aware of the importance of creating professional and personal boundaries when working in this way with women.

However, it is becoming evident that developing meaningful relationships with women is a protective factor against burn-out (Sandall 1997a, 1997b), while a lack of such relationships may lead to frustration, stress and disillusionment. Clearly, there needs to be a balance. While continuity of carer may provide intense satisfaction for both woman and midwife, it is also important that the midwife establishes parameters for her practice and relationship with her client, enabling the woman to build a sense of personal control over her own pregnancy and childbearing. This also helps to protect the midwife from unreasonable workloads or demands. The relationship between the woman and her midwife is one to which both the woman and the midwife bring particular expertise and knowledge. The woman holds her own personal knowledge of what is best for her and her situation; the midwife brings accumulated knowledge and expertise in childbirth. There is a theoretical basis to midwifery practice, but in this equal sharing of relationship, it is important that, as James (1997, p. 95) comments, 'we find new ways so that the authority of the theory does not become the central focus of our being together'. In this relationship, then, the woman and her needs should determine what happens.

SUSTAINING PRACTICE, AVOIDING BURN-OUT

Observing the principles and key themes of Sandall's work, we will describe how One-to-One midwives managed their personal and professional lives, integrating them and avoiding stress and burn-out.

Occupational autonomy

Many One-to-One midwives moved into caseload midwifery because of frustration with the traditional, fragmented system of practice, where they considered they were expected to work more as machines in the factory system of the maternity service, as 'caring robots' rather than thinking practitioners. With caseload practice, although finding the prospect scary at first, they came to value taking responsibility for their clients. They particularly appreciated knowing that their work would no longer be undermined by the conflicting advice of a colleague: for example, working through breastfeeding difficulties and then a bottle is given during the night shift. Working with like-minded colleagues who they could trust to provide compatible care was essential for them to be able to relax when taking time out.

Moving from the security of a shift system with rostered days off, usually known weeks in advance, to providing 24-hour cover is not easy and is a source of concern to midwives moving into caseload practice (Farmer & Chipperfield 1996). However, the advantage of working flexibly means that midwives are only 'at work' when either clients or colleagues need them. Antenatal and postnatal visits are planned effectively so that midwives maximize the use of their time, travelling at times convenient to them, e.g. to avoid congestion periods and avoiding unnecessary long distances. Some midwives preferred scheduling the bulk of their routine work into a few long days, so the rest of the time they were free apart from labours and 'emergencies'; others worked shorter days, some being 'early birds' while others were late risers. In this manner they were able to organize their lives and work in a harmonious way and 'make the job work for them' (Stevens 2003).

True occupational autonomy means that the caseload midwives are not used as a reserve work force to be called on when the hospital is busy; neither do they cover regular clinics such as GP clinics.

Time off is organized within the partnership so that only one midwife is on call at night or over weekends. The only time rotas are drawn up is over Christmas and New Year, when usually only two or three members of the group practice work, and time off with family and friends can be ensured with a first, second and third on-call system in place. Annual leave is planned well in advance, with, ideally, only two members of the group practice away at any one time.

Being the lead professional for women with low-risk pregnancies, and decision-making in partnership with women, adds to the sense of occupational autonomy. The responsibility and accountability are clearly attractive to One-to-One

midwives and contribute to their own sense of control (Stevens 2003). Knowing each woman and their situation in greater depth means they are able to help her make appropriate decisions, offering greater flexibility over care, yet remain within the boundaries of safe practice. Twenty-four hour referral to an on-call registrar provides support in situations of clinical uncertainty.

Similar flexibility over care was noted in Brodie's (1997) study of team midwifery where team midwives learned that:

> . . . autonomy and decision making was flexible too . . . we could decide how far to take things . . . within the rules still . . . but just individualizing it for the woman . . . we were encouraged to take risks . . . well, safe risks . . . test our boundaries of responsibility . . . trying different things and being supported in doing things differently.
>
> Brodie 1997, p. 74

Fundamental to the sustainability of such models is a managerial philosophy of support rather than control. Rather than imposing particular guidelines or protocols, where these were found to be needed caseload midwives were supported in developing them. Similarly they were supported in identifying and arranging their training needs rather than have these externally defined.

Developing meaningful relationships with women

The opportunity to develop meaningful relationships with women and their families in order to respond more specifically and effectively to their needs is a major source of satisfaction. As Farmer & Chipperfield (1996, p. 20) wrote, 'it is simply much easier and more satisfying to look after someone you know'. Being called to a labour at 2am was reported not as a chore but like getting up for a friend and attending the birth was 'the icing on the cake'. Much of the midwife's work during labour has already been done and so they are able to focus on providing the watchful support that is so fundamental for normal birth. The midwives admitted it was not so much the women as themselves who were upset if they missed it.

Nevertheless, the potential for creating dependency was highlighted in the early days of the scheme when enthusiastic midwives virtually promised women the earth! A psychologist provided a valuable session on developing professional parameters for practice. Practically, the midwives focus on three areas:

1. describing their role as midwives (and what they are not) at the initial booking interview and reinforcing this throughout;
2. educating women in how, why and when they might best contact their midwife;
3. ensuring that the women are aware that their presence at the birth is not guaranteed and that they receive some antenatal care from the named midwife's partner.

Continuity of carer is as important to midwives as it is to women (Stevens 2003). Campbell's (1984) concept of 'reciprocity' within the relationship between client and professional helper may be pertinent. One-to-One midwives clearly valued being recognized as individuals, reporting they no longer felt like a 'cog in a wheel' but a person: 'the midwife, Mary' becomes 'Mary, the midwife'. The importance of this recognition, the affirmation of her role and the reciprocal valuation exchanged between the mother and midwife may be an important contribution to the sustainability of caseload practice.

Social support

In the One-to-One programme, both peer support at work and emotional and social support at home were important for coping with the demands of the work (Stevens 2003). Working predominantly in the community is potentially isolating, and the support of a like-minded midwife-partner and wider group practice was essential. While the first midwives selected to practise within the One-to-One scheme were able to choose their partners, form themselves into group practices of six or eight midwives, and decide on how they would work together, newer members also needed to establish compatible working arrangements. Thus successful partnerships and group formations were seen to change and evolve rather than become established and set in particular patterns of working.

Although fundamental to the success of such practice, similar philosophies of working cannot be taken for granted but need to be worked at. For the One-to-One practice this was established during an initial away-day meeting, which was then repeated once the practices had settled down and new members joined. It was also reaffirmed on a regular basis through weekly group practice meetings held to discuss issues, solve problems, plan ahead and get an overall picture of current workload. When problems arose, the root was often a failure to communicate with the rest of the group in terms of either giving or receiving support. Learning to work through relationship difficulties with colleagues, rather than ignore them, as reportedly experienced in the conventional service, is an important skill that, if not mastered can lead to serious disruptions (Allen et al 1997, Stevens 2003).

Peer review, described in detail by Cooke & Bewley (1995), was also a means of expressing support, usually in terms of a midwife's action or decision, as well as learning. To know that one's colleagues would have made a similar decision in an uncertain situation, or to be challenged constructively and helped to see a different way, can be enormously supportive. It can also be a useful 'safety net' as advice and suggestions from experienced colleagues can help to maintain professional standards.

Monthly whole practice meetings and regular away-days provided 'time out' for One-to-One midwives to meet each other. Social occasions such as birthday celebrations, leaving parties or preparing for the annual hospital Christmas review were important to many of the midwives and provided a focus for fun and relaxation.

Emotional and social support from family and friends and having a life outside work are also important. Not all the partners of the One-to-One midwives understood and appreciated their new flexible working arrangements, although several commented on how much happier their midwife-partners were. Planning holidays well in advance enabled midwives to pursue their own interests, and by 'booking' women to mainly avoid having women due to give birth while her midwife is on holiday can help to minimize disappointments on either side.

Supportive management

As noted previously, managerial support is essential and should be facilitative rather than directive and hierarchical. Direct support, in conjunction with overt encouragement and advocacy from midwifery managers and administrators, assisted midwives to feel supported and trusted by the organization (Brodie 1997).

> . . . There was a feeling of being trusted in what we were doing . . . we were encouraged to learn our way with the role . . . test out our boundaries and limits . . . they supported us in trying out different things . . . it was how we learnt. There was lots of support from above . . . they believed in it more than a lot of midwives . . . they could see the benefits.
>
> Brodie 1997, p. 88

Midwives should also have an infrastructure of support for referrals and clerical work. In Britain, the research of Stapleton et al (1998) in relation to the supervision of midwives included an in-depth account of the culture of midwifery. This culture has not always been a supportive one. The authors explain this with reference to the work of Freire (1972), who described a cycle of oppression in which those who have been oppressed continue to oppress each other. They describe what is called 'horizontal violence' (Leap 1997b), a form of institutional bullying that they see as part of the culture of midwifery. Certainly, in many situations where there has been a new project set up, midwives working in these innovative areas have not always felt supported by their colleagues. Those setting up and those working within the innovations may suffer what Brodie (1997) also calls horizontal violence. Similar lack of supportive work environment and relationships has been cited by many midwives in conventional practice as their main reasons for leaving midwifery (Ball et al 2002). Australian research has revealed that such barriers may inhibit midwives being able to fulfil a legitimate role in maternity service provision (Brodie 2002).

In setting up new projects, it is important to attend to the culture of practice as a whole, making it more positive and supporting and paying attention to all midwives in the service rather than only those taking the innovation forward. However, boundaries and frameworks of expectation are required, so that it is clear that destruction of the innovation by rumours and innuendo will not be sanctioned.

Time management

Midwives moving into One-to-One practice benefit from thinking about, or training in, time management skills. In the hospital system, although midwives may need good time management skills at work, they do not have to self-manage 24-hour time periods in the same way. This is partly because work is contained by the working day and going off duty provides a clear physical break between professional and personal life. In One-to-One practice, midwifery work is embedded in daily life and commitments may easily spread over 24 hours if they are allowed to. However, with good management, a caseload of 40 births a year can be managed in an average week of 37.5 hours (McCourt 1998). Two tools crucial in facilitating this are a mobile telephone or pager, and a good diary system, while setting priorities, making lists and keeping addresses and telephone numbers together is essential.

Flexibility and the ability of an individual midwife to manage her own time are central to allow for both the provision of care that meets the woman's needs, and the midwife's ability to balance personal and professional life. This latter factor is fundamental to a profession that consists mainly of women. To provide such flexibility, it is important that set commitments are kept to a minimum. Midwives working in this way should never be expected to staff wards or clinics. With a caseload of 40, the daily work of a midwife will consist of a small number of antenatal and postnatal visits. If a labouring woman calls her, it is relatively easy for her to cancel such visits or have her partner undertake them so she can attend the birth or take rest as necessary. This would not be the case for midwives running clinics.

In Britain, the development of caseload practice has led to much discussion about how much 'on-call' is best for midwives. With a partnership model, although the midwife may be 'available' to women for half the time, call-outs will be relatively rare. In One-to-One practice, one midwife and her partner are on call for eight births per month, compared with team midwifery where, with a team caseload of 240 births per year, team midwives are each on call for 20 births per month. In addition, communications are simpler, and it is not as complicated to ensure that the woman knows both of the midwives. If, however, a 'team' of six undertakes to do a 1 in 6 rota, the midwife is far more likely to be called out on her night on-call, is more likely to have a number of women in labour at once and has a higher chance of being called for women she does not know well or even at all. Additionally, with a higher chance of being called, teams are likely to need two midwives on call, meaning that the rota may be 1 in 3. The approach of taking 1 week on and 1 week off, makes a great deal of sense for some midwives. The One-to-One midwives arranged their availability time to suit themselves and their partners. They carried out their visits from home and did not need to visit the hospital first. Arranging visits at mutually convenient times with women in their practice means that they could sleep later and work later, or take their children to school or the nursery before starting work.

Time management skills are important to modern-day life whichever walk of life we are in. A time management workshop given 6 months after the One-to-One project had started helped the One-to-One midwives enormously, since by this time they were keenly aware of the need for such skills. The flexibility demanded by caseload practice requires that midwives pace themselves. For example, if it is probable that midwives will be called out at night, they should try to have an easier day. When midwives have been used to going to work and working flat out on a shift such a change in mindset can be difficult; initially the One-to-One midwives reported feeling guilty when not working during the day, and even sought work:

> This week we haven't been busy at all. I just felt bad, bad about the fact that I'm not work-ing . . . that I should be out there doing something. So what I find myself doing is coming to the hospital and looking up their results
>
> Stevens 2003, p. 174

Such need to 'make busy' has also been described in nursing (Menzies 1970). Nevertheless, once

used to this way of working, the midwives reported it to be much easier.

> You actually have to plan better when you are working shifts. [Now] I find I plan on a weekly basis. Whereas before . . . you have to plan three weeks in advance because that is the way the rotas are done
>
> Stevens 2003, p. 280

Some midwives with young children found this way of working was much easier as they had the greater flexibility to be responsive to family needs. However, others, with rigid childcare support arrangements found it more difficult. Thus it can be understood that caseloading is not incom-patible with family life, indeed it might be preferable to shift work, but this is highly depend-ent on an individual's personal situation (Stevens 2003).

Likewise, the ability to adapt and enjoy the flex-ibility offered by this way of working is a very personal characteristic. Some people thrive in the relaxed atmosphere of work being embedded in life in general, others become irritated or frus-trated by the lack of definition, feeling they are constantly 'at work' and so never able to relax. This fundamental difference in attitude needs to be appreciated as the latter is not compatible with caseloading. Such midwives would be ill advised to attempt working this way as their aptitudes are more suited to shift work.

CONCLUSIONS

This chapter has discussed the concepts and models underpinning the provision of continuity of midwifery care, along with the evidence sup-porting their introduction and some of the key practical aspects of providing continuity of carer in practice. We have highlighted that conceptual clarity is important, as without this it is very dif-ficult to gather or interpret evidence on what works, or what women want from maternity care. We have outlined a hierarchical model of continu-ity in healthcare, which included informational and longitudinal continuity as underpinning interpersonal continuity. It is this last level which research evidence suggests is valued most highly by women, although the importance of consistent information and pathways through services should not be underestimated. We found that much of the existing research evidence does not make clear conceptual distinctions between continuity of care and carer, and does not describe clearly the models of practice which are being evaluated.

Models of care are complex packages that are not easy to research. While it is important to distinguish and explore different aspects of a model of care, it is also important to recognise that these may be more than the sum of their parts. Continuity of care or carer may facilitate or enhance other beneficial aspects of midwifery – such as autonomy, confidence, decision-making skills and positive relationships – which are very difficult to maintain in the industrial model of care which prevails in hospital services in many countries. The research we have reviewed suggests that providing continuity of care may have important clinical and psychosocial benefits for women, but the effects are influenced by the environment and context, and models with similar labels may work in different ways. The midwife–woman relationship is central to this, and has value for the midwife as much as the woman in her care. The relationship is one that should be enabling and centred on understanding the woman's needs, not one of creating dependency.

We have also discussed the impact of such models of care on midwives, looking at how job satisfaction may be enhanced and burnout avoided. Although there are real challenges for midwives involved in providing continuity of carer, and this model will not suit all midwives at all stages of their work, there is also evidence of real rewards. Practical aspects of ensuring that the benefits outweigh the costs, and that new practices are sustainable include forms of organisation and management that enable midwives to learn how to make the job work for them. This requires high levels of autonomy as well as responsibility, and flexibility as well as the requirement to manage one's work and time in a flexible way. We have highlighted the importance of leadership and appropriate management and support as well as some organizational and cultural frameworks to achieve this.

At the outset of this chapter we highlighted how recent UK government reports have empha-

sied the need for greater continuity of care for women in maternity services as well as easy access to services, choice and control regarding the care they receive (Department of Health 2004). The evidence we have discussed suggests that these are not separate issues. In modern maternity care, which has suffered from fragmented services and inappropriate medicalization of care for many women across the world, continuity of carer is an important basis for achieving these aims of women- and community-centred care.

In terms of what we still need to find out, we need to clearly state what we mean by continuity in practice and research terms using the hierarchy of continuity outlined in the beginning. We need to understand that much of the debate and confusion around continuity has been due to this lack of clarity. For example, the majority of research findings are based on team midwifery models which provides longitudinal continuity. However, we don't know enough about the effect, experiences or processes involved in continuity of carer, i.e. caseload midwifery, which provides the third relational level of continuity. From other research on provider recipient relationships which engender trust, we can begin to hypothesize about some specific powerful effects. Caseload midwifery can have many benefits for midwives, if set up and run properly, and we should encourage its development and share experiences of how to deliver it. For example, a listserve supports caseload midwives worldwide: http://www.jiscmail.ac.uk/lists/CASELOADMIDWIFERY.html

POINTERS FOR PRACTICE

- Successful caseloading requires the practitioner to develop a radically different orientation to work and life.
- Personal aptitudes and circumstances support or prevent this orientation.
- Responsibility and accountability act as important safety mechanisms.
- Successful case holding requires organizational features that enhance occupational autonomy.
- Successful case holding is not elitist or isolationist but involves team work.
- The essence of case holding is a personal relationship between women and their midwives.

References

A C T Health 2004 A pregnant pause: the future for the maternity services in the A C T report from the Legislative Committee. A C T, Standing Committee on Health, Australia

Aiken N 1997 Team midwifery: a challenge for Australian midwives. Australian College of Midwives Conference Proceedings, 10th Biennial National Conference. ACMI, Melbourne, Australia

Allen I, Bourke Dowling S, Williams S 1997 A leading role for midwives? Evaluation of midwifery group practice development projects. Policy Studies Institute, London

Ball L, Curtis P, Kirkham M 2002 Why do midwives leave? Royal College of Midwives, London

Beake S, McCourt C, Bick D 2005 Women's views of hospital and community-based postnatal care: the good, the bad and the indifferent. Evidence-based Midwifery 3(2): 80–86

Beake S, Page L, McCourt C 2001 Report on the follow-up evaluation of one-to-one midwifery. TVU, London

Benjamin Y, Walsh D, Taub N 2001 A comparison of partnership caseload midwifery care with conventional team midwifery care: labour and birth outcomes. Midwifery 17: 234–240

Benner P. Wrubel J 1988 The primacy of caring: stress and coping in health and illness. Addision Wesley, Menlo Park

Biro M, Waldenstrom U, Pannifex J 2000 Team midwifery care in a tertiary level obstetric service: a randomised controlled trial. Birth 27(3): 168–173

Bissett S 1995 One-to-One midwifery: a personal experience. British Journal of Midwifery 3(3): 142–161

Brodie P 1997 Being with women: the experiences of Australian team midwives. Degree of Masters of Nursing Thesis, University of Technology, Sydney

Brodie P 2002 Addressing the barriers to midwifery – Australian midwives speaking out. Australian College of Midwives Journal 15: 5–14

Brodie P, Leap N 2005 Publicly funded homebirth in NSW – at last! Midwifery Matters Newsletter of the NSW Midwives Association, Vol 22, No 5. Online. Available: www.nswmidwives.com

Campbell A V 1984 Moderated love: a theology of professional care. SPCK, London

Cook R I, Render M, Woods D D 2000 Gaps in the continuity of care and progress on patient safety. British Medical Journal 320: 791–794

Cooke P, Bewley C 1995 Developing scholarship in practice. In: Page L (ed.) Effective group practice in midwifery: working with women. Blackwell Science, Oxford

Couves J 1995 Working in practice. In Page L (ed.) Effective group practice in midwifery: working with women. Blackwell Science, Oxford

Coyle K 1998 Women's perceptions of birth centre care: a qualitative approach. Unpublished thesis, Edith Cowan University, Perth, Western Australia

De Vries R, Benoit C, Van Tiejlingen E, Wrede S 2001 Birth by design: pregnancy, maternity care and midwifery in North America and Europe. Routledge, London

Department of Health 1993 Changing childbirth. Report of the Expert Maternity Group (Cumberlege report). HMSO, London

Department of Health 2004 National service framework for children. HMSO, London

Department of Health Maternity Services 1992 Government response to the second report from the Health Committee Session 1991–92. HMSO, London

Department of Human Services Victoria Australia 2004 Future directions for Victoria's maternity services. Online. Available: ww.health.vic.gov.au/ maternitycare/serv_statement2004.pdf

Donaldson M S 2001. Continuity of care: a reconceptualization. Medical Care Research and Review 58(3): 255–290

Downe S 1997 The less we do, the more we give. British Journal of Midwifery 5(1): 43

Farmer E, Chipperfield C 1996 One-to-One midwifery: problems and solutions. Modern Midwife (Apr): 19–21

Flint C, Poulengeris P, Grant A 1989 The 'Know your midwife' scheme – a randomised trial of continuity of care by a team of midwives. Midwifery 5: 11–16

Freeman G, Shepperd S, Robinson I, Ehrich K, Richards S 2001. Continuity of care: a report of a scoping exercise for the NCCSDO. NCCSDO, London

Freire P 1972 The pedagogy of the oppressed. Penguin, Harmondsworth

Garcia J, Redshaw M, Fitzsimmons B, Keene J 1998 First class delivery: a national survey of woman's views on maternity care. Audit Commission, London

Gready M, Newburn M, DoddsR 1995 Choices- childbirth options. National Childbirth Trust, London

Green J M, Curtis P, Price H, Renfrew M J 1998 Continuing to care. The organization of midwifery services in the UK: a structured review of the evidence. Books for Midwives, Hale

Guilliland K, Pairman K 1995 The midwifery partnership: a model for practice. Victoria University of Wellington, New Zealand

Gumley S, Haines H, Holland J 1997 Midwife care project: a partnership between Wangaratta District Base Hospital and Ovens and King Community Health Service. ACMI Conference Proceedings, 10th Biennial National Conference. ACMI, Melbourne, Australia

Haggerty J L, Reid R J, Freeman G K, et al 2003 Continuity of care: a multidisciplinary review. BMJ 327(7425): 1219–1221

Hodnett E D 2003 Continuity of caregivers for care during pregnancy and childbirth (Cochrane Review). In: The Cochrane Library, Issue 4. Wiley, Chichester. Last amended March 1999.

Homer C S, Davis G K, Brodie P M 2000 What do women feel about community-based antenatal care? Australian and NZ Journal of Public Health 24(5): 590–595

Homer C S, Matha D V, Jordan L G, Wills J, Davis G K 2001a Community-based continuity of midwifery care versus standard hospital care: a cost analysis. Australian Health Review 24(1): 85–93

Homer C S, Davis G K, Brodie P M, Sheehan A, Barclay L M, Wills J, Chapman M G 2001b Collaboration in maternity care: a randomised controlled trial comparing community-based continuity of care with standard hospital care. British Journal of Obstetrics and Gynaecology 108: 16–22

Homer C, Brodie P, Leap N 2001c Establishing new models of midwifery care in Australia: a handbook for midwives and managers. Centre for Family Health & Midwifery, UTS

Homer C S, Davis G K, Cooke M, Barclay L M 2002 Women's experiences of continuity of midwifery care in a randomised controlled trial in Australia. Midwifery 18(2): 102–112

House of Commons 1992 Second report on the maternity services by the Health Services Select Committee (Winterton report). HMSO, London

Jacoby A, Cartwright A 1990 Finding out about the views and experiences of maternity-service users. In: Garcia J, Kilpatrick R, Richards M (eds) The politics of maternity care: services for childbearing women in twentieth-century Britain. Clarendon, Oxford, pp. 238–256

James S G 1997 With woman: the nature of the midwifery relation. Doctor of Philosophy thesis, University of Alberta, Edmonton

Kenny P, Brodie P, Eckermann S, Hall J 1994 Westmead Hospital team midwifery project evaluation. Final Report. Westmead Hospital, Sydney

Kildea S 1999 And the women said. . . Report on birthing services for Aboriginal women from remote Top End communities. Territory Health Service, Darwin, Australia

Kirkham M 1996 Professionalisation past and present: with women or with the powers that be? In: Kroll D (ed.) Midwifery care for the future: meeting the challenge. Balliere-Tindall, London

Leap N 1996 Caseload practice: a recipe for burn-out? British Journal of Midwifery 4(6): 329–330

Leap N 1997a Caseload practice that works. MIDIRS Midwifery Digest 7(4): 416–418

Leap 1997b Making sense of 'horizontal violence' in midwifery. British Journal of Midwifery 5 (11): 689

Maternity Coalition 2002 National Maternity Action Plan for the introduction of Community Midwifery Services in urban and regional Australia. Available from: http://www.communitmidwifery.iinet.net.au/nmap.html

Maternity Services Advisory Committee 1982 First report on maternity care in action. Part 1: Antenatal care. HMSO, London

McCourt C 1998 Working patterns of caseload midwives: a diary analysis. British Journal of Midwifery 6(9): 580–558

McCourt C, Page L 1996 Report on the evaluation of One-to-One midwifery. Thames Valley University, London. On line. Available: www.tvu.ac.uk

McCourt C, Page L, Hewison J, Vail A 1998 Evaluation of One-to-One midwifery: women's responses to care. Birth 25(2): 73–80

McCourt C, Pearce A 2000 Does continuity of carer matter to women in minority ethnic groups. Midwifery 16(2): 145–154

Menzies I E P 1970 The Functioning of Social Systems as a Defence Against Anxiety. Tavistock, London

Ministerial Review of Birthing Services in Victoria 1990 Having a baby in Victoria. Department of Health, Victoria, Australia

Ministerial Task Force on Obstetrical Services in New South Wales 1989 Maternity services in New South Wales. NSW Department of Health, Sydney

Ministerial Task Force WA 1990 Report of the Ministerial Task Force to review obstetric, neonatal and gynaecological services in Western Australia 1990. Health Department, Perth, Western Australia

Minns H 1995 Teaching in practice. In: Page L (ed.) Effective group practice in midwifery: working with women. Blackwell Science, Oxford

Chapter **8**

The birth of twins: a reflection on practice

Paul Lewis

This chapter is a personal reflection on practice, in which I consider my perceptions and involvement in the birth of twins. The events I describe were real and with their permission, I have made no attempt to hide the identities of those involved. I cover the many deep and detailed discussions I had with the mother and her family and which they are happy for me to share. However, as part of the reflective process, it must be kept in mind that my perceptions of what took place are those of a personal lived experience and may differ from the perceptual realities of others.

BACKGROUND TO MY INVOLVEMENT AND CONTEXT OF CARE

The background to my involvement and context of care is somewhat unusual, as the events took place in New Zealand, where I was not licensed to practice as a midwife and Ness, the woman whose pregnancy and birth I describe, is a member of my close family. My decision to get involved arose from Ness and her husband Iain's wish to have me present during the birth of their babies, as well as their concerns over the heightened possibility of unnecessary medical intervention in their birth. Added to this was the fact that their known, independent midwife had withdrawn from care and I had wanted to be of help at such a momentous time in their lives. This said, I did not enter into such involvement lightly and would advise any other midwife in a similar situation to

consider fully their own personal, practical and professional issues.

PERSONAL AND PROFESSIONAL CONSIDERATIONS

While involvement in any birth is always a privilege, when the midwife asked to attend is a close friend or family member, such involvement carries an added responsibility and needs to be carefully considered. From the moment Ness first told me she was pregnant I had wanted to be of help. However, at that time she was supported by an experienced independent midwife who had also been involved in two of her previous pregnancies. As such, I felt my presence was probably unnecessary but the situation changed when her independent midwife withdrew from care.

It is possible that without a system of Statutory Supervision or appropriate support, Ness's midwife might have felt very much on her own. It is easy to become professionally isolated when caring for women with complex, complicated or high risk pregnancies within a system of care that expects women to conform. Similarly, in such circumstances when trying to meet the needs and expectations of a mother, midwives may well find the constant challenge and tensions stressful and difficult; in effect they are 'between a rock and a hard place'. This is especially so, when the culture expects the midwife to obtain the woman's compliance and holds her accountable when she is unwilling to tread this path or the woman, for whatever reason, makes choices which are out of step with professional norms and expectations. This situation is often compounded when choice is more about acquiescence to a dominant medical model of care and where midwives, often against their better judgements, feel helpless to resist and unable to forge an alternative approach.

This chapter is not intended as a judgement on the midwives and doctors involved in Ness's care. It is, however, a reflection both on and in practice, as to how Ness said she felt as a mother, trying to achieve a birth of her choice, against the institutional power of the hospital system and the influence of medical opinion. A situation made more difficult, when much of that medical opinion bore little relevance to the known research evidence that underpinned her understanding and expectations of the management of care that would take place in the birth of her twins.

Against such a background, I committed to becoming involved in Ness's care. But along with this, I also needed to be clear about what the family expected my role to be and what I could realistically provide in a country in which I was not registered to practice. Like many women in pregnancy, Ness wanted to have someone present during her labour that she knew and could trust; who had the knowledge to give advice and hopefully support her in giving birth without needless intervention.

The key word here is 'needless'. Ness was not averse to intervention if there was good evidence or just cause to support such action. Her birth plan, which she finally drafted with my assistance, acknowledged her desire for a normal birth, but sensibly reflected the potential for change and the possibility that intervention might become a necessity (see Appendix 1).

SUPPORTING EXPECTATIONS AND CHOICES

Although supporting women's expectations is an integral part of the midwife's role, it can be challenging. While I consider myself to be informed, reasonably realistic and able to support women in their choices around birth, I was also forced to consider that in such circumstances and many

miles from home, my own presence might raise unrealistic expectations and might even carry potential risks. I had to consider the consequences not only of failure, but also what could happen if for whatever reasons, the social norms, personal boundaries and professional duty of care that would be expected of me, were at any time breeched or broken. As a UK registered midwife, unable to practise in New Zealand, I needed to discuss what the implications of my involvement might be, what role I could and could not undertake and how Ness, Iain and the family would want me to advise and support them.

This is especially important when the context of care, such as with multiple pregnancy and birth is likely to be contentious and conflicting views may well lead to a lack of objectivity that could impact adversely upon the care of both mother and babies. These considerations, when taken into account, gave rise to the realization that in some circumstances, the involvement of close friends and family members might hinder rather than help the process of birth.

Alternatively, my presence or that of any friend or family member might reinforce a social model of birth, in which the provision of care is not only holistic but also life-enhancing, acknowledging the links between health and social structures such as family support (Walsh & Newburn 2002a). Historically, such an approach more readily values the woman's previous, personal experiences of birth. It also operates on the premise that birth is normal and focuses on the needs of the woman and her family within a model in which they are placed firmly at the centre of care. Continuity by a known midwife is paramount in such circumstances and as Walsh and Newburn (2002b, p. 542) assert: 'midwifery care mediated through known midwives is so important to women and birth outcomes that not to implement it is discriminatory to women and an injustice to midwives'.

It was against this background that I travelled to New Zealand to be with the family during the birth of their twins. Ness and Iain were clear about the role I might play and wanted me to be as involved as I could be under the circumstances. They accepted that while I could bring my knowledge and experience as a midwife to inform and assist them, my primary role would be to support Ness, helping her where possible to realize her birth plan and to give advice and assistance when and if any negotiations or challenging situations arose.

It was accepted that I was unlikely to take part in the provision of direct, hands-on midwifery care and instead, would take on the role as Ness and Iain's 'birth support partner'. I would, work with them, as well as with the midwives and medical staff to optimize their birth experience and facilitate, where possible, the kind of care they wanted.

I arrived in New Zealand when Ness was 37 weeks pregnant and planned my stay so that I would be with her over the next 4 weeks. That way I hoped my arrival date would be before Ness had given birth, and that I would be there in the period when she would be likely to have the twins. With hindsight this was at best overly optimistic. Limiting the duration of my stay was in part to do with needing to limit my time away from work, but it effectively placed unnecessary pressure on Ness to birth within a defined timescale, the implications of which will become evident as this story unfolds.

NESS'S BACKGROUND CLINICAL AND SOCIAL HISTORY

Ness was a thirty-six year old, married woman in her fifth pregnancy. As a Registered Nurse working with the mentally ill she held strong views about individuals being in control of their destiny and enabled to make informed choices in their lives. It was such an approach to her professional life, which had a marked influence on how she wished to be involved in her own care.

Physically she was in good health and had no known medical complications. Her prior reproductive history contributed to her need to stay in control of her pregnancy and labour and she was adamant that she wanted to do all she could, to give birth to her twins normally.

As a young mother in her first pregnancy, Ness had gone into labour at 36 weeks gestation. The subsequent care or indeed lack of it had a devastating effect on her perception of how things might have been and what she would try to avoid in the future. In her subsequent pregnancies, she fought hard to ensure that she remained fully

informed and directly involved in any decisions around her care. She was well supported in this not only by her husband Iain, but also by her midwives and her second baby was born within minutes of her going into hospital, while her third, was born at home under the care of an independent midwife.

Ness already had three children, a boy and two girls, all of whom she had breastfed and were in robust health. She managed her very busy household with real skill and was not actively seeking to become pregnant, believing that her family was complete and the chance of any future babies was unlikely. It came as a surprise therefore, when she conceived again but sadly her fourth child miscarried at around eight weeks gestation.

She struggled with the death of this baby and felt she was destined to have no further children even though, like many women, becoming pregnant and then having a miscarriage made her long for at least one further chance of motherhood. It was therefore with a certain degree of trepidation and a lot of excitement that several months later and without any real intent, she found herself pregnant again with twins.

NESS'S ANTENATAL CARE

From a medical perspective, Ness's pregnancy was uneventful, although considered high risk as a multiple pregnancy. Ultrasound had confirmed the presence of twins with two distinguishable placentas and no obvious fetal anomalies. She remained well throughout the pregnancy and both babies were well grown and active as she approached term.

Initially Ness had booked with the independent midwife who had provided her with care in her two previous pregnancies. She recognized that some medical care was likely to be necessary but she did not wish to go down a route that might give rise to unnecessary intervention. Having an experienced and able independent midwife she felt would optimise the chances of this happening.

Consequently, when her midwife withdrew from care, Ness found herself facing an uncertain future. Her fears regarding her pregnancy management, which involved having to accept regular ultrasound scans, the possibility of an induction at 37 weeks and a medically managed labour seemed justified. This understandably, caused her considerable distress and gave rise to the fear that she was destined to repeat a similar experience to that which she had encountered during the birth to her first child.

As a midwife I understand the pressures that women can face as part of the institutional process of birth. A situation made more problematic, when the pregnancy is classified as 'high risk' and the rightful domain of medicine rather than midwifery. Within the hospital walls, midwives more often than not, play a supporting role to the doctor in the care and management of women with multiple pregnancies. Even when all remains normal, the fear of misadventure gives rise to a risk management approach that imposes its own imperatives over those of the mother. This is well articulated by Evans (1997), when she asks the question as to whether a twin birth can ever be a positive experience and writes 'My concerns and frustrations grew as I watched that daunting, but thrilling experience being taken over and medicalised so that it became a nightmare of worry and something to be "put up with" in the cause of being lucky enough to survive and have two healthy babies'.

Within the descriptive account of her personal experiences, her graphic case studies had resonance with my own realities and once again I felt myself indebted to Jane Evans, one of our profession's notable practitioners. The shared stories, experiences and insights of midwives and mothers are invaluable in helping us to learn and develop our art and science in relation to pregnancy and birth. Above all, they provide the conditions that help to forge a partnership between mother and midwife giving strength and support to both, regardless of the circumstances or outcomes.

WORKING IN PARTNERSHIP

In spite of Ness's initial fears, her consultant obstetrician recognized her needs as a mother, to be fully informed and involved in any decisions affecting her care. It was in relation to this that I was to play a useful sounding board helping Ness and Iain to understand the research evidence and

clinical information. This enabled them to make considered judgements about what direction they wished their care to take, and weigh this alongside the social and medical imperatives that arose during the pregnancy and birth.

Informed choice is central to the provision of maternity care and a hallmark of good practice (Department of Health 1993, 2004). Yet within this, mothers, midwives and obstetricians can face competing tensions that impact upon the provision of care and for better or worse, influence the decisions and the dynamics of the birthing process. As clinicians, we have to balance a mother's right to self-determination alongside our obligations as professional practitioners to provide care, which is not only in keeping with the wishes of the woman, but also based upon robust, research evidence (Page 2000).

Yet such care is rarely immune from the influence of the birth environment and established ways of working (Crabtree 2004). While the beneficial effect of continuous support to women in labour is well documented (Hodnett et al 2003), the extent to which this happens when the context of the birth process is contested, is likely to be determined by the knowledge, skills, understanding, confidence and competence of the practitioner.

Likewise the manner in which the midwife, obstetrician or birth partner interact and support the mother and the views she holds with regard to the nature of childbirth, are also likely to have implications for the practicalities, provision and process of the birth itself. This is even more evident when the view of a pregnancy labels the woman as 'high risk' and where the concomitant complexity of knowledge is more likely to be considered the province of an expert (McLaughlin 2001). In such circumstances choice is often diminished and there is little room for any discussion that either challenges or seeks to change the accepted practice of the midwife or obstetrician.

On my arrival in New Zealand, Ness was 37 weeks pregnant and I was to gain some valuable insights, living with a woman and her family in the late stages of pregnancy. It was comforting to see that in spite of her amazing size, she was not only in remarkably good health, but with three children and a husband, was still able to cope with the demands of family life. My presence, I hope, eased some of the burden and above all, added a sense of reassurance to the family that should anything occur, I was available and at hand should the need arise.

As midwives we argue that 'birth is a normal physiological event', while others view it as a 'risky process' that can only be seen as normal in retrospect. Recent debates within our profession however, demonstrate that current concepts of what constitute normality are at best tenuous (Downe 2002, 2004). Today, many interventions have become routine and are accepted as part of normal birth. As midwives we may fail to give due consideration to the physical and emotional consequences of such interventions for the mother, let alone the financial costs to the health service. Within the United Kingdom, the imperatives arising out of the National Service Framework (Department of Health 2004), strongly suggest that such matters can no longer go unchallenged. Midwives are required to reconsider their roles and relationship with other providers of maternity care and rebuild an approach to practice that is consistent with our insights and understanding of what makes birth normal.

Oakley has argued that the notion of normality in childbirth alters over time and what was once considered normal is no longer the case (Oakley 1986). In the 1940s, 1950s and 1960s in the United Kingdom, birth at home, breech birth and twin birth were clearly within the remit and responsibilities of the midwife. They were deemed as part of the rich and varied tapestry of normality. In the 21st century, midwives and mothers are more likely to be locked into a medical model of care that views birth within a construct of 'risk management' that owes much to the fear of litigation and little to the social or cultural imperatives of the woman and her family (Walsh & Newburn 2002a, 2002b).

Yet whatever stance we take as practitioners, established and inflexible positions will often lead to an ideological viewpoint that at best, minimize or ignores the needs of women and at worst, imposes a pernicious approach to care that is at odds with our professional duty and contrary to the clinical evidence that may emerge during the unfolding events of pregnancy and birth. As midwives, our professional duty of care is to the mother and to the best of our ability we should seek to ensure that her experience of birth is not only 'safe' but one which she can look back upon with joy and a sense of achievement.

Page (2000) advocates an approach that seeks to facilitate such a balance. Using a five stepped process, she recommends that midwives find out what is important to the woman and her family. That we obtain information from our clinical examinations and assess this against the available research evidence, so that our professional judgements and any decisions taken in relation to care are informed. Importantly, throughout this process, the midwife must maintain the woman and her family at the centre of care, talking through what is happening and helping women to reflect upon the feelings, outcomes and consequences of any decisions, actions or events.

Such partnership is in my belief, the foundation or at least the framework for a new midwifery, that Page (2002) so ardently and eloquently advocates. My reflection on the birth of Ness and Iain's twins takes such an approach and I trust provides a basis for other midwives and obstetricians to consider how they might provide care, advice and support in similar circumstances.

THE MEDICAL AND SOCIAL IMPERATIVES OF TWIN BIRTH

According to the Canadian twin birth study protocol, twins comprise approximately 2–3% of all births and are at a higher risk of death and neonatal mortality than singletons of the same birth weight. Other studies provide similar, convincing evidence of increased perinatal and infant mortality in twin versus singletons, when the pregnancy is at or near term and when the birth weight is above 2500 grammes (Cheung et al 2000; Joseph et al 2001; Kiely 1990; Smith et al 2002).

Such increased risk is in part, associated with an increased risk of preterm labour, fetal growth restriction, congenital abnormality and complications with the second twin resulting in trauma and asphyxia. However, the belief that obstetric interventions will prevent such events is as yet, not supported by the availability of robust, research evidence. In such circumstances, it is both understandable and reasonable, when women assert their right to make an informed choice with regards to the management and care of their pregnancy and labour.

It is interesting to note that while many women are fearful of the real risks of preterm labour that arise in multiple pregnancy, when a woman reaches term, a second imperative about 'optimal timing' for birth takes over. This is complicated by the fact that for many obstetricians, the definition for both 'term' and 'optimal timing' of birth in a twin pregnancy is 37–38 weeks gestation. This is based on several retrospective studies which have either used multivariate logistic regression (Luke et al 1993) or factor analysis to compare the rate of perinatal mortality in twin pregnancies with singleton pregnancies at a given gestational specific age (Cheung et al 2000, Cincotta et al 2001; Minakami & Sato 1996).

It is therefore not surprising, that for many obstetricians, twin pregnancy beyond 37–38 weeks gestation is treated with trepidation. This is in spite of the fact that in a recent Cochrane review, only one suitable trial was identified that compared the outcomes in mothers and babies who underwent elective delivery from 37 weeks' gestation in a twin pregnancy with outcomes in a control group who were managed expectantly (Dodd & Crowther 2004).

This trial involved a total of 36 women, with 17 randomly allocated to the induction of labour group and 19 to the expectant management group. The primary outcomes between each group with regard to all caesarean births, caesarean births for fetal distress or perinatal mortality, showed no statistically significant differences. Secondary outcomes such as haemorrhage requiring blood transfusion, meconium stained liquor, an Apgar score of less that seven at five minutes and an infant birth weight of less than 2500 grammes also showed no statistically significant difference between the two interventions of induction or expectant management (Suzuki et al 2000).

On the basis of this single randomized control trial, there are insufficient data to support a practice of elective delivery from 37 weeks gestation for women with uncomplicated twin pregnancy at term. As Dodd and Crowther (2004) point out, 'Well designed randomised controlled clinical trials with sufficient power to detect clinically

meaningful difference are required to answer the question of optimal timing of birth for women with otherwise uncomplicated pregnancy at term'. However, until this happens, there is little robust evidence for one group or another to assert that their practice is the only safe and reliable option available to women and consequently, women should be entitled to make an informed and free choice in relation to their care.

In a midwife's provision of care, it is important that she or he seeks to develop a considered and structured approach, while at the same time, tailoring it to the wishes of the mother, her needs and condition. A logical and sequential manner of social engagement, professional assessment that includes history and clinical examination followed by a plan of care, and subsequent evaluation, is a tried and tested approach in both medical and midwifery practice. However, it is often 'done to' rather than 'done with' the mother and may lead to her wishes being sidelined in favour of the organizational or institutional imperatives. In applying the five steps as advocated by Page (2000), both the mother's wishes and needs as well as the available 'best evidence' is central to the process of care and constitutes a more rigorous way to ensure that our practice as midwives is both 'women centred' and 'evidence based'.

Steps 1–4 take us through a logical sequence in which the midwife finds out what is important to the woman and her family. This is followed by a clinical examination and assessment that provides information and data that can then be compared with the available evidence. In steps 1–4 the basis for care is established and the unfolding events lead to reappraisal and reassessment. Importantly, step 5 enables both women and midwives to engage in a considered reflection of not only the decisions, actions and events that take place, but also the feelings that emerge from these. It is a process that I believe, enables the mother to recognize her own strengths and perhaps come to terms with events that did not go according to plan. For the midwife it provides a valuable learning experience that will hopefully give rise to professional growth and lead to improvements in her practice and provision of care to women.

STEP ONE: FINDING OUT WHAT IS IMPORTANT TO THE WOMAN AND HER FAMILY

Within the United Kingdom, the midwife is required to 'recognise and respect the patients and clients role as partners in their care and the contribution they can make to it. This involves identifying their preferences regarding care and respecting these within the limits of professional practice, existing legislation, resources and the goals of the therapeutic relationship' (Nursing and Midwifery Council 2004, 2.1). As previously stated, I spent time discussing with Ness and Iain what they felt was important to them. However, from this process, it was clear that they were not always of the same mind.

There were few issues with regard to the place of birth, as Ness intended to go into hospital. Although she had considered the possibility of a home birth, her decision to go into hospital was in part due to her family circumstances and her acknowledgement that there were likely to be higher risks associated with twins as opposed to singleton birth. Her decision was also influenced by the lack of midwifery support and the weight of medical opinion against twins being born at home. A position, which in New Zealand, might have been accentuated by an Australian study on home birth that found twin pregnancy to be a significant contributor to the perinatal death rate (Bastian et al 1998).

For Ness, the need to stay in control and minimize intervention was essential, but she also had to balance this with the needs of her family. Her husband, Iain, on the other hand, while wanting everything to go well, was not so sure that induction or even caesarean section might provide them with a far neater solution than the waiting game that pervades all pregnancies at term. Within this dynamic, Ness was also seeking to ensure that the needs of her other children were met, and that they were prepared for the birth and arrival of new family members.

Ness's goals for her impending labour was to keep it as normal as was feasible in the circumstances of a twin birth, to stay in control, to be involved in any decision-making and to ensure that the needs of her family were met not only as she prepared for the birth of her twins, but also when she went into hospital.

STEP 2: OBTAIN INFORMATION FROM CLINICAL EXAMINATIONS

Using evidence from clinical examinations was important in helping both Ness and her family to feel confident that her pregnancy was proceeding as it should. The opportunity for me to carry out observations on her pulse and blood pressure, as well as abdominal assessment and auscultation of the fetal hearts was reassuring, and reinforced that all was well. It also enabled the other children to engage with the process of preparing for the birth of the twins.

At 38 weeks gestation, Ness once again met with the consultant obstetrician who had offered her care during her pregnancy. While it had been suggested that induction or even caesarean section was an option at this gestation, her obstetrician was also very accepting that expectant management was a reasonable, alternative approach. This was reassuring at several different levels and Ness, who had been having strong, regular and at times lengthy periods of uterine contractions at home, was convinced that given time, she would go into spontaneous labour. On abdominal palpation, which I had carried out at regular intervals during my stay, both babies felt well grown and presented head down. The fetal heart rates were reassuring and an ultrasound, which was performed after the obstetric consultation, identified liquor volume as normal; and confirmed the clinical findings as described above.

Throughout the following week, Ness's vital signs remained normal, although with the growth of her babies, she increasingly experienced significant oedema of her lower limbs. Added to this was the frustration that the onset of labour, although much anticipated and in spite of the frequency with which Ness's experienced runs of contractions, did not happen. Inevitably, this dampened Ness's morale and confidence, and while she held firm to her views that everything should progress without intervention, my impending departure brought added pressure to her decision-making.

At just over 39 weeks gestation, Ness met with another consultant obstetrician, as her own was unavailable due to planned leave. This provided a different, and at times difficult, set of challenges. Their discussion revolved around Ness's wish to birth her twins normally and the risks that in the obstetrician's opinion, such an approach gave rise to. The obstetrician was reluctant to accept that there was limited evidence to support planned induction, or that Ness could labour without an epidural in situ. The delivery interval between the birth of the first and second twin was also contentious.

This consultation provided little if any, exploration of available choices. The obstetrician's approach was to convince Ness that the birth needed to be medically managed if she and her babies were to remain safe.

This is a scenario that as a midwife, I have seen played out of many occasions and undermines a woman's confidence and self belief rather than creating the essential framework and partnership, in which informed choice can be made. Mothers and even midwives may find it difficult to reject or even rebut medical opinion when, because of the changing nature of events, they might subsequently find themselves reliant upon the experience and expertise of the medical practitioner.

It was apparent that this obstetrician's approach did more to confirm Ness's fears that the consultation was all about managing and controlling her labour and birth rather than offering advice and evidence to enable her to make important and difficult choices. At times, I intervened in order that Ness could state her own views, which given the available evidence or the lack of it, were reasonable and realistic. It was also in part, to try and work with the obstetrician, who had a wealth of practice experience. It was also the case that, given the circumstances, Ness and Iain needed him to be on board with them.

Any woman's choices need to be carefully considered for as Crawford (2005) points out 'choice is not relative but absolute'. This said, she identifies that such choice may become challenging when it is:

Contrary to local or national guidelines; contrary to the advice of caregivers due to evidence and/or personal opinion;

Exposes the woman or baby to increased risk or perceived risk;
Exposes the employer or midwife to increased risk or perceived increased risk of litigation;
Is not accommodated by local service provision or involves care which caregivers do not feel competent to provide.

Crawford 2005

Yet within the United Kingdom, the Nursing and Midwifery Council (NMC) code is unequivocal on the subject of who has the right to decide and states 'you must respect patient's and client's autonomy – their right to decide whether or not to undergo any health intervention – even where a refusal may result in harm or death to themselves or a fetus, unless a court of law orders to the contrary' (Nursing and Midwifery Council 2004, 3.2).

At the end of the consultation a mutual stand off was the only sensible course to take. However, this potentially unhelpful situation was a major reason that Ness's birth plan was written as it was crucial to try to ensure that there would be no doubt or ambiguity over her preferred options for care. The act of writing the plan also demonstrated Ness and Iain's willingness to work with the midwives and doctors involved and to provide them with a clear framework as to what forms of care were preferred or would be considered, dependent upon the changing events at the time.

Ness, conscious of my imminent departure, and having previously wanted to labour spontaneously, gave up on waiting. It is said that it is a woman's prerogative to change her mind, and in many situations for whatever reasons, they may choose to do so. This change of heart is usually a graduated or staged approach that meets a certain need and it is important that caregivers do not take this as a sign that other preferences or choices carry less weight or can be ignored.

Although at odds with her original desire to go into labour spontaneously, Ness explored the possibility with her consultant of taking an active step in getting labour started and asked if he would be willing to carry out a sweep of her membranes. Boulvain et al (2005), describe the sweeping of the membranes at term as a simple and effective method to start a woman in labour.

Nevertheless, they note that it can cause discomfort, some bleeding and irregular contractions. Their review of trials found that it is generally safe where there are no other complications and reduces the need for other methods of labour induction such as oxytocin or prostaglandins.

On this basis, Ness made the choice to have a membrane sweep in the hope that this might 'kick start' her into labour. Both babies remained in a cephalic presentation and a post sweep cardiotocograph (CTG) demonstrated reactive and reassuring fetal heart rate tracings. Ness was invited to return the following day if she had not gone into labour but she chose to wait a further forty-eight hours in the hope that things would get started and her long and tiring wait would be at an end.

STEP 3: ASSESS EVIDENCE OBTAINED FROM CLINICAL EXAMINATION(S) AGAINST THE AVAILABLE RESEARCH EVIDENCE

Throughout Ness's pregnancy, she had actively sought out literature and information that might enable her to make appropriate, informed decisions in relation to her labour and the birth of her twins. My own expertise was of help and enabled me to place in perspective the results of population studies and small scale, retrospective research in relation to Ness's needs. We were able to discuss the limitations of this information all of which, because of methodological weaknesses of the research methods, militated against using these data to make definitive informed decisions. From this, Ness was aware that there was not enough robust evidence to support planned induction, routine epidural anaesthesia, continuous fetal monitoring, or to define what the optimal delivery interval between twins should be; even the place of birth was contentious. However, her own personal preference to avoid intervention, to take into account the needs of her family, and to give birth within a timeframe where I would be available to provide her with support, meant that she was prepared to consider other options and as such, her decision to have a membrane sweep.

STEP 4: TALKING THE ISSUES THROUGH WITH THE WOMAN

Talking the issues through with women is a vital step in reaching a common understanding as to what is happening and how this fits with the needs and choices she has made. In taking this approach, the midwife seeks to ensure that birth is not just safe, but provides the joy, fulfilment and success that optimize a woman's self confidence and belief in herself; this process is circular and continuous and one which the midwife needs to engage with at regular intervals as the events of pregnancy and birth unfold.

Two days after the sweep of her membranes, Ness had not gone into labour and she made the difficult choice that she would go into hospital and have an induction. This decision was supported by Iain and it enabled them to make the necessary arrangements for her other children.

CARE AND MANAGEMENT OF INDUCTION AND LABOUR

The use of vaginal prostaglandins for induction of labour has been reflected by significant improvements in cervical favourability within 24 to 48 hours; and an increase in successful vaginal delivery with no increase in operative delivery rates (Kelly et al 2003). It was with this understanding and the possibility it implied, that Ness decided to go into hospital for an induction of her labour.

On arrival, her birth plan was presented to the team on-duty and we were made to feel welcomed and supported. The midwife allocated to look after Ness, was as chance would have it, an ex-student of my University and familiar with the ethos of woman-centred care. Her professionalism and support, as with all the midwives we encountered over the next two days, demonstrated a real understanding as to what Ness very much wanted to achieve during her labour. It also meant that my involvement and participation in care was greatly facilitated. Although I had no intention of delivering direct, hands-on midwifery care, I was enabled to provide Ness with ongoing support, to monitor her progress and the condition and wellbeing of her babies. This was immensely reassuring to us both and allowed Iain to provide greater support for their other children who waited at home with increasing excitement and anticipation.

After the initial administration of prostaglandin gel, and a short period of CTG monitoring to ensure fetal wellbeing, Ness returned home to rest. Living close to the hospital had definite advantages and I was able to monitor the impact of the induction in an environment where she felt more at ease and in control. Six hours later, with no notable increase in uterine activity, Ness returned to the labour ward for a further assessment and a second dose of prostin gel. On vaginal examination, her cervical os was 2–3 centimetres and the presentation was –2 above the ischial spines. The presenting fetus (twin 1) was cephalic and engaged in the pelvis and both fetal hearts were reactive and reassuring. A second dose of vaginal prostaglandin gel was given in accordance with the hospital protocol. With both twins appearing to be coping with the process, Ness continued to mobilize and await the onset of contractions and the start of her labour.

Ness did not progress to established labour, in spite of the two doses of prostin and the onset of uterine activity. At the handover of shift, both medical and midwifery staff changed and discussions took place with the obstetric consultant and his team with regard to an epidural being sited. Once again Ness came under extreme pressure to have an epidural on the grounds that if any manipulations were necessary, there would be no pain relief and the impact of this could be 'extremely painful and distressing'. Unfortunately the hospital did not provide a 24 hour epidural service and it would appear that in their enthusiasm to convince Ness of the benefits of having an epidural other forms of pain relief, such a puedendal block, were forgotten.

In her birth plan, Ness had been very clear as to what she wanted to avoid and this stated 'If an anaesthetic is required at any time and especially in an emergency, I would want this to be a regional block either by epidural or spinal anaesthesia. I would want to avoid a general anaesthetic unless it was absolutely indicated'. Neither did she wish to have any opiates or an epidural for pain relief. Yet in the antenatal consultation at 39 weeks she had agreed to have an epidural line inserted towards the end of the first stage of her labour, primarily because of the impasse with the obste-

trician at that time who felt this was an absolute necessity, especially with regard to the management of the second twin. However, Ness recognized that there was little evidence to support such an approach and wanting to stay mobile for as long as she could, she reserved her right to make a final decision on this, as and when necessary.

As the day progressed, Ness's uterine activity became more marked. However, this was the result of prostin stimulation rather than established labour as her lack of cervical dilatation demonstrated. During a long spell of fetal monitoring, it became difficult to differentiate between the two fetal hearts and a mobile ultrasound scan confirmed that the second twin, who had previously been head down, was now presenting by the breech.

This did not come as a surprise to Ness who had felt the baby turn while she was in a recumbent position during an assessment by the obstetrician. It did, however, cause her to reappraise what might now happen with regard to the management of the birth and the potential for both operative delivery and/or increased manoeuvres to manipulate the second twin in order to facilitate his birth.

In my preparation to be with Ness during her labour, I had also carried out an extensive review of the available literature. One interesting and helpful study by Roberts et al (2003) provided an invaluable insight into the management of twin births in Australia and New Zealand. Out of the practising obstetricians she surveyed as part of this study, the method of delivery for an otherwise uncomplicated twin pregnancy varied according to the presentation of the fetuses and their gestational age. Although planned vaginal birth increased with increasing gestational age regardless of fetal presentation, 6% of obstetricians recommended caesarean section for all twin births (Roberts et al 2003). Yet in a systematic review by Hogle et al (2003), although planned caesarean section might reduce the risk of a low 5-minute Apgar score when the first twin was presenting by the breech, there was no conclusive evidence to support planned caesarean section for twins. In contrast, caesarean section for the birth of a second twin not presenting head down was associated with increased maternal febrile morbidity with, as yet, no identified improvement in neonatal outcome. The author states unequivocally that this policy should not be adopted except within the context of further controlled trials (Crowther 1996). It would appear on the limited evidence available, that 'vaginal birth versus caesarean section when the second twin is non-cephalic, does not demonstrate any difference in neonatal outcome' (Rabinovici et al 1987).

Ness did agree at this point to have an epidural sited in the interests of the second twin. She remained fearful of this and its impact to limit her ability to mobilize. Yet what subsequently took place demonstrated the art of possibility. The consultant anaesthetist that attended, having read Ness's birth plan in detail, suggested that he site the epidural but without a test dose or top up unless needed. This enabled her to continue to mobilize and her gratitude for this small freedom, was to prove significant in how she felt about the process and decisions she finally reached with regard to her management of care.

As the first day moved into the second and her uterine activity abated, Ness realized that the induction using prostaglandin gel alone, had failed to get her into labour. Although the fetal heart rates of both twins remained reactive and reassuring she was increasingly exhausted by the experience and at around 04.00 hours on the second day, she questioned what she could and should do next. In such a situation, it is easy for the midwife to seek an end to the woman's travail. The decision does not, however, rest with the midwife and by returning to what Ness had set out in her birth plan she could see the possibility of two reasonable options.

The first would be to have the epidural catheter removed, abandon the induction process and return home to await events. The second was to look at a staged approach to what could happen and to continue with the induction with artificial rupture of her membranes (ARM). Although she had wished to avoid the latter, the social circumstances in which she found herself, her tiredness and her wish to complete the process she had started, led her to make a decision to proceed to an ARM in the hope that this would succeed where other measures had failed.

Prior to the ARM, a vaginal examination showed that Ness's cervical os had changed little from the previous assessment. An ARM was carried out at 08.45 hours and in spite of the events of the previous day and the long night, Ness continued to mobilize surprised by the fact that her contractions, which had now started, were not overwhelming her as she had feared. However, as they progressed, and the pain of labour ensued, the epidural catheter that was in situ was topped up and she was provided with reasonably effective pain relief.

Although her non-interventionist approach to birth appeared to be slipping away, these small, gradual changes to her birth plan enable her to continue to discuss and make decisions, remain in control and to feel like the choices were hers. With labour well established, both twins were continuously monitored and we were able to alter the 'bed' so that Ness was in an upright, sitting position. With the change of shift, the midwife we had met on arrival at the hospital, came back on duty and once again took over Ness's care. Her gentle support and encouragement was excellent and Ness was able with our physical support, to stand as her labour advanced. Even with the epidural in place, she could adopt an upright position and a vaginal examination at 16.00 hours confirmed that she was now in the second stage of labour.

It is often the case that hospitals have protocols in place that require a large number of staff to be present during the birth of the twins. Ness had not wished this to happen and in particular, she did not want her babies taken from her unless there was a clear indication to do so. In this regard, the paediatrician who attended kept a low profile and was very sensitive to her wishes. The midwife gently encouraged Ness to use her contractions and at 17.20 hours, she gently brought her baby into the world. As a midwife myself, I was impressed with the gentleness, care and kindness that surrounded the birth of the first twin, a baby boy. Fionn, as he was to be called, had good Apgars, and looked around with wonder as he was placed in his mothers' arms.

This success, however, was not sustained as the birth was now taken over by the consultant obstetrician who intervened insisting that time was of the essence. The intense moment between mother and baby was broken, and Ness who was holding her first baby Fionn, was told that unless the second baby was born without delay, there could be serious difficulties. This was in spite of the fact that she had not wanted an imposed time limit if the second twin remained well. Such was the rush to deliver the second twin that no thought appeared to be given to whether or not Ness was contracting. As such, the issue of using Syntocinon to stimulate descent and delivery of the second twin was not even considered. The imperative was to bring the birth to a conclusion and in less than ideal circumstances Ness was told that the baby needed immediate delivery.

This was the challenge that I suspect we both knew might arise and when it did, would be difficult to deal with. The fetal heart rate of the second twin which continued to be monitored was unchanged at around 150–160 beats per minute and was reactive. He remained in a breech presentation and Ness had wanted to give him the chance to turn spontaneously or have cephalic presentation assisted by external cephalic version (ECV).

There is little robust evidence on the delivery interval between twins. Roberts et al (2003) found that in the delivery of the second twin, if the first had been born vaginally, 71% of obstetricians in Australia and New Zealand felt it was reasonable to wait up to 30 minutes before delivering the second baby, 11% would wait 30 minutes of more (range 30–130 minutes) and 18% had no time limit on the delivery of the second twin as long as the fetal condition was satisfactory.

Ness was told that unless the baby was delivered, caesarean section would be necessary. An ECV could be done to see if the baby would turn but getting him out was all important. It is true that ECV was part of Ness's birth plan, but in taking the decision to use ECV she was, with hindsight, effectively delivered into the hands of the obstetrician. The ECV was rushed, without effective pain relief and at best half hearted, with little chance of success. Quickly, the obstetrician moved to a breech extraction of the second baby, which was done with skill and efficiency but with little regard to the mother. At 17.40 hours some 20 minutes after his brother, the second twin, Callum was delivered. He was taken to the paediatrician who gently dried the baby and gave facial oxygen. His breathing was soon established, with an Apgar of 6 and 10 and sensitive to the moment,

the paediatrician quickly returned him to his mother.

Both babies were soon on the breast and feeding. The third stage, managed actively, was completed and the registrar repaired a second degree perineal laceration. Ness's labour and the boys' births was over and both mother and babies were safe and well. However, the atmosphere, because of Ness's exclusion and the obstetric takeover, was emotionally charged and we would look back at these events with mixed emotions.

The difference between the twins appearance was notable, with twin one Fionn, looking pale in comparison to his brother Callum's ruddy glow. Although there was only a slight difference in their birth weights, both the paediatrician and obstetrician raised concerns about the possibility of 'twin-to-twin' transfusion. This syndrome affects monochorionic twin pregnancies and is associated with a high risk of perinatal mortality and morbidity. However, early scans had demonstrated two placentas, two chorions and two amnions. The likelihood of twin-to-twin transfusion was remote, but careful examination of the placentas was carried out to determine chorionicity. The previous scan findings were confirmed and cord blood taken from each placenta, showed little comparative difference between either of the twins. Both placentas were sent to the laboratory for definitive confirmation of chorionicity.

STEP 5: REFLECTING ON OUTCOMES, FEELINGS AND CONSEQUENCES – THE ART OF POSTNATAL CARE

Shortly after the birth of the twins, Iain and Ness's two older children visited the hospital eager to meet the new arrivals. The social nature of this encounter was wonderful with both children helping to weigh, wash and dress their baby brothers. Ness's blood loss had been quite heavy, and a Syntocinon infusion had been established to maintain uterine tone. When this was completed and with her base line observations stable, Ness and the twins returned home.

Being able to sleep in her own bed three-hours after the birth of the twins was a great relief to Ness and helped to normalize the process and experience of her labour. One of the highlights of this was getting to examine and physically explore the bodies of their baby boys in the warmth and comfort of their own bed. Already the characters of each twin, Fionn and Callum, could be seen and this gave the other children an opportunity to welcome them home and begin their integration into the family.

Ness continued to successfully feed her babies and they thrived in their family's noisy, happy and robust household. She also made a good, if slow recovery from labour and birth, considering what she had been through. However, in the quiet hours of the morning when she woke to feed her babies, we had an opportunity for us both to reflect upon what had taken place. This reliving of the experience enabled us to debrief, give meaning and understanding to what had happened, and to place it in perspective.

Ness's birth plan had not gone as she would have liked; in retrospect, it might have been different if she had awaited the spontaneous onset of labour. Although her experience did enable her to compare what she had initially wanted to happen to that which had, nevertheless it is often a fruitless exercise to ponder what might have been. I was loathe to let anyone or anything rob Ness of her undoubted achievement in giving birth to her babies, staying as much in control as she could given the circumstances. At times we were both upset and angry about some aspects of what had taken place, but on reflection, the obstetrician had done what he thought he should do for Ness and her babies and had done it well. We also had to acknowledge and give thanks for the wonderful care and support that was given by others.

As a midwife I looked back and wondered how I might have prevented the medical take over that occurred in the birth of Callum and what was positive in what did take place. Chauhan et al (1995) in a retrospective study of 284 twin pregnancies, compared the maternal and perinatal outcomes of twins in which the nonvertex second twin was delivered by total breech extraction versus those delivered by external cephalic version. They found that total breech extraction of the nonvertex second twin was preferable to external cephalic version because it appeared to be associated with a significantly lower incidence of fetal distress and abdominal delivery with little difference in neonatal outcomes. A smaller, retro-spective study carried out by Cristalli et al (1992) also concluded that breech extraction of the second twin in their experience, was not a pernicious technique when done by trained operators within precise limits.

Ness and Iain had tried to manage their experience of the pregnancy and birth of their twins in the interests of their family and the twins themselves. In taking over control at a critical time in the labour, the obstetrician supplanted himself as the prime decision maker. It might have been the right decision, but we reflected that his actions were not based on the best available evidence or indeed the clinical situation at the time. As professionals we all need to ensure that the autonomy of women is respected; we should enable them to make decisions for themselves and to accept that responsibility and its consequences – whatever they might be.

I was privileged to be with Ness and Iain at such an important time in their lives. I learnt a lot and I trust my presence made the process for them both that much easier to understand and work with. They have generously allowed me to share their story alongside their personal and my professional reflections. Without such insights our work as midwives can become routine and unfocused and I remain indebted to the many mothers, students, midwives and doctors who, like Ness and Iain, have over the years shared their stories of pregnancy and birth with me. In the final analysis, it is often through such reflections, openly and honestly shared, that we might find answers to the uncertain world we work in and ways that will help us to improve our care and support for women and their families.

PRACTICE POINTS

- Midwives need to engage with women in an organized and reflective manner to optimize the care and advice they provide.
- Midwives need to understand the evidence on which clinical decisions are made and provide this in a manner that will enable women to make an informed choice.
- Where women make choices that are at odds with professional advice, midwives must maintain a supportive professional relationship, which facilitates the woman's autonomy and involvement in her care.

■ The midwife's duty of care lies with the woman. Within the context and involvement of the multi-professional team, the midwife while attempting to facilitate understanding with regards to the implications of choice and care, must ensure her advocacy is on behalf of the mother and not the organization.

■ There is a lack of robust evidence surrounding the management of twin pregnancies and as such, uncertainty and doubt is likely to exist in relation to many of the accepted protocols and procedures imposed upon women.

■ Multi-professional team work is an essential requirement for success as well as the safety and wellbeing of mothers and babies. Midwives and obstetricians must ensure that women are involved and central to any decision-making and that they should be the final arbitrators as to what is agreed.

References

Bastian H, Kierse M J N C, Lancaster, P A L 1998 Perinatal death associated with planned home birth in Australia: population based study. British Medical Journal 317: 384–388

Boulvain M, Stan C, Irion O 2005 Membrane sweeping for induction of labour. The Cochrane Database of Systematic Reviews: Issue 1. Wiley, Chichester, UK

Canadian Twin Birth Study. Online. Available: http://www.utoronto.ca/miru/tbs/protocol.htm accessed September 2004

Chauhan S P, Roberts W E, McLaren R A, Roach H, Morrison J C, Martin J N Jr 1995 Delivery of the nonvertex second twin: breech extraction versus external cephalic version. American Journal of Obstetrics and Gynecology October 173(4): 1015–1020

Cheung Y B, Yip P, Karlberg J 2000 Mortality of twins and singletons by gestational age: a varying-coefficient approach. American Journal of Epidemiology 152(12): 1117–1119

Cincotta R B, Flenady V, Hockey R, King J 2001 When should twins be delivered? Gestational age-specific stillbirth risk of twins vs. singletons. Perinatal Society of Australia and New Zealand, 5th Annual Congress, March 13–16; Canberra, Australia, p. 22

Crabtree S 2004 Midwives constructing 'normal birth' In: Downe S (ed.) Normal childbirth evidence and debate. Churchill Livingstone, Edinburgh, pp 85–99

Crawford J 2005 Delivering choice to women – midwifery regulation: stick, route map or suit of armour? Nursing and Midwifery Council, 3rd Annual Midwifery Conference, June 16th. SECC Glasgow, Scotland.

Cristalli B, Stella V, Heid M, Izard V, Levardon M 1992 Breech extraction of the second twin with or without version by internal manoeuvres. Journal of Gynecology, Obstetrics and Biological Reproduction (Paris) 21(6): 705–707

Crowther C A 1996 Caesarean delivery for the second twin. The Cochrane Database of Systematic Reviews, Issue 1. Art. No.: CD000047. DOI: 10.1002/14651858.CD000047.

Department of Health 1993 Changing Childbirth. Report of the Expert Maternity Group, part 1. HMSO, London

Department of Health 2004 National service framework for children, young people and maternity services. Online. Available: www.doh.gov.uk/nsf

Dodd J M, Crowther C A 2004 Elective delivery of women with a twin pregnancy from 37 weeks gestation (Cochrane Review). The Cochrane Library, Issue 3. Wiley, Chichester, UK

Downe S (ed.) 2004 Normal childbirth evidence and debate. Churchill Livingstone, Edinburgh

Downe S 2002 Preston national symposium on the evidence base for normal birth. Practising Midwife 5: 10

Evans J 1997 Can a twin birth be a positive experience? Midwifery Matters 74: 6–11. Online. Available: http://www.radmid.demon.co.uk/twins.htm (update 30 June 2000) accessed 23rd September 2004

Hodnett E D, Gates S, Hofmeyr G J, Saicala C 2003 Continuous support for women during childbirth. The Cochrane Library, Issue 4. Wiley, Chichester UK

Hogle K L, Hutton E, McBrien K A, Barrett J F, Hannah M E 2003 Caesarean delivery for twins: a systematic review and meta-analysis. American Journal of Obstetrics & Gynaecology 188(1): 220–227

Joseph K S, Marcoux S, Ohlsson A, Liu S, Allen A C, Kramer M S, Wen S W 2001 Changes in stillbirth and infant mortality associated with increases in preterm birth among twins. Pediatrics 108: 1055–1061

Keily J S 1990 The epidemiology of perinatal mortality in multiple births. Bulletin of the New York Academy of Medicine 66: 618–637

Kelly A J, Kavanagh J, Thomas J 2003 Vaginal prostaglandin (PGE2 and PGF2a) for induction of labour at term. The Cochrane Database of Systematic Reviews, Issue 4. Wiley, Chichester, UK

Luke B, Minogue J, Witter F, Keith L, Johnson T 1993 The ideal twin pregnancy: patterns of weight gain, discordancy and length of gestation. American Journal of Obstetrics and Gynecology 169: 588–597

McLaughin J 2001 EBM and risk: rhetorical resources in the articulation of professional identity. Journal of Health, Organisation and Management 15(5): 352–363

Minakami H, Sato I 1996 Re-estimating the date of delivery in multifetal pregnancies. Journal of American Medical Association 275:1432–1434

Nursing and Midwifery Council 2004 The NMC code of professional conduct: standards for conduct, performance and ethics. Online. Available: www.nmc-uk.org

Oakley A 1986 The captured womb – a history of the medical care of pregnant women. Blackwell, Oxford, p. 142

Page L A 2000 The new midwifery. Science and sensitivity in practice. Churchill Livingstone, Edinburgh

Rabinovici J, Barkai G, Reichman B, Serr D M, Mashiach S 1987 Randomised management of the second nonvertex twin: vaginal delivery or caesarean section. American Journal of Obstetrics and Gynecology 156: 52–56

Roberts C, Phipps H, Nassar N, Raynes-Grenow C 2003 The management of twin births in Australia and New Zealand. Australian & New Zealand Journal of Obstetrics and Gynaecology 43(5): 397

Smith G, Pell J B, Dobbie R 2002 Birth order, gestational age and risk of delivery related perinatal deaths in twins: a retrospective cohort study. British Medical Journal 325: 1004–1008

Suzuki S, Otsubo Y, Sawa R, Yoneyama Y, Araki T 2000 Clinical trial of induction of labour versus expectant management in twin pregnancy. Gynecological and Obstetric Investigations 49: 24–27

Walsh D, Newburn M 2002a Towards a social model of childbirth, part 1. British Journal of Midwifery 10(8): 476–481

Walsh D, Newburn M 2002b Towards a social model of childbirth, part 2. British Journal of Midwifery 10(9): 540–544

APPENDIX 1   NESS'S BIRTH PLAN

I understand fully the risks and responsibilities of having a twin birth and my rights as a mother to have control over my body and that of my babies.

I am more than willing to change my choices about the manner and process in which I give birth if the circumstances change and the evidence supports an alternative approach to that which I had originally wanted to follow.

However, I do not wish to have any form of midwifery or medical intervention performed upon myself without my informed and expressed consent. This also applies to the care and management of my twins both before and after their birth.

The following points are to inform and assist my carers, both midwives and doctors, in what I want to happen during the birth of my twin babies.

1. I wish to have my husband and my birth support partner with me and involved in my care throughout my labour. Like myself, they wish this birth to be as normal as possible and are there to help and assist in whatever way they can.

2. I have agreed to an induction because of my advancing gestation and the small but increasing risks associated with this. If my membrane sweep is unsuccessful, then I agree to a prostin induction of labour with or without an artificial rupture of membranes and will come into hospital for this.

3. I want the induction to be a step-by-step process, starting with the insertion of one milligram of prostaglandin gel. If this is unsuccessful, I want to be fully informed and understand the next stage in the process and give my consent before any further action is taken.

4. At this time, I do not wish to proceed to an artificial rupture of my membranes unless it is necessary and in the interests of my babies or myself. If the induction with prostaglandin gel is unsuccessful and I do not go into labour, providing my babies and I remain well, I would wish to revert to a conservative approach rather than have an artificial rupture of my membranes. I am happy to review this position when and if my health or social circumstances change.

5. I am more than happy for the heart rates of my babies to be monitored but I do not wish this to be continuous or unless absolutely necessary, for a fetal scalp electrode to be applied to either twin.

6. I wish to be upright and mobile for as long as I can and would want to adopt such an upright position for the birth and delivery of my babies, especially if they both remain in a cephalic presentation.

7. It is my intention to eat and drink lightly during my labour as long as I desire to do so. I am aware of the position that twin births carry a higher risk of intervention but I believe that I can birth normally and will need the energy to do so.

8. If an anaesthetic is required at any time and especially in an emergency, I would want this to be a regional block either by epidural or spinal anaesthesia. I would want to avoid a general anaesthetic unless it is absolutely indicated.

9. I do not wish to have any opiates or an epidural for pain relief. I have agreed to have an epidural line inserted towards the end of the first stage of my labour, as my obstetrician believes this is necessary in the management of the second twin. However, there is little evidence to support such an approach and I reserve my right to make a final decision on this as and when necessary.

10. I do not wish the birth to be used as an exercise in teaching and would wish the number of healthcare professionals in the room to be kept to an absolute minimum.

11. If both my babies remain in a cephalic presentation and the medical team is unable or unwilling to deliver them with myself in an upright position, I am more than happy for the births to be conducted by a midwife.

12. I do not want an episiotomy and refuse my consent for this unless in an emergency, it is to maximize manoeuvres for the effective birth of the baby and to minimize perineal trauma when such manoeuvres are being applied.

13. I want time to bond with my babies and therefore do not wish either the first or second baby to be taken from me immediately unless this is absolutely indicated. If they need resuscitation then I fully understand the need for this. However, I do not wish paediatric or midwifery staff to remove my babies for routine checks, which can wait until I have had time to hold and feed them.

14. I would like my husband to hold my first baby if it proves difficult for me to have him during the birth of my second twin.

15. If my second twin does not remain in a longitudinal lie and cephalic presentation, I want my membranes left intact and an external version to be attempted. I would like this twin to be born normally and without any unnecessary intervention if at all possible.

16. I am aware that my contractions may subside after the birth of the first twin. I wish to have the time and privacy for these to resume on their own or with the assistance of my first baby feeding at my breast.

17. If a Syntocinon infusion is required, I would wish this to be fully discussed and only be given with my full consent.

18. I am aware that it has become routine in some hospitals to minimize the birth interval between twins to no more than half an hour. However, as long as the condition of the second twin remains healthy, there is little evidence to support such an approach and I would not wish any arbitrary time limit put on the period between the birth of my first and second twin.

19. I would like both babies if they are born well, to be delivered onto my abdomen and kept close to me throughout the remainder of the labour process.

20. I recognize the potential for an increased risk of maternal haemorrhage and am happy for the third stage of my labour to be actively managed.

21. I wish to breastfeed both my babies as soon as is reasonably possible. My birth support partner is skilled in the care and management of birth and is more than happy to assist as he can and would be more than willing to help in this process if it relieves pressure on the midwifery and medical staff. He is there to support me and to work with you.

22. Providing all goes well and both my babies and I are in good condition, I would like to return home as soon as possible. I have the necessary support and know that being at home would be better in helping me establish the feeding and care of my newborn babies.

23. I fully recognise that my wishes for a normal birth may conflict with the routine approach of the hospital, medical and even midwifery systems. I do not however wish to birth in an acrimonious environment and I do not wish to be subjected to any undue pressure to change my choices unless, as I have already stated, the circumstances or the evidence dictate that this would be in the best interests of my twins or myself.

24. I would like my birth to proceed normally and to work with all members of the medical and midwifery team to achieve this.

Signed & Dated by both Parents

SECTION 2

Putting science into practice

SECTION CONTENTS

'An approach that integrates sensitivity to the individual woman and her family with scientific understanding arises from a relationship between the woman and her midwife. This relationship is both personal and professional, often being like a friendship, but a friendship with a purpose. The midwife is an expert who uses her skills, knowledge, understanding and commitment to the women in her care in order to support them around the time of the birth of their babies. The woman is also an expert, knowing her needs and understanding the changes going on in her body, with awareness of the signals her baby is giving her.'

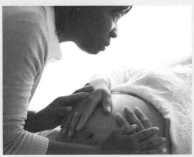

Chapter 9

Evidence-based care and twins

Belinda Ackerman and Alok Ash

INTRODUCTION

In the current climate of expectations of an open culture of medical practice, increased consumer awareness and ready access to the internet, service users are increasingly critical of the care and treatment they receive. Traditional clinical practice based on authority, anecdotes and personal beliefs has been challenged. Obstetric and maternity care are no exception. Offering evidence-based medicine and healthcare is important mainly for two reasons. Firstly, healthcare practitioners who would like to maintain a critical approach to their practice need to understand the strength of the evidence supporting any treatment or intervention they advise. Secondly, women accessing care want to evaluate for themselves the value of any suggested treatment rather than taking the advice on trust (James 2003).

But what do you do as a healthcare practitioner when working with a woman whose pregnancy would usually be considered as high risk and you find that the evidence for the management of some medical problems is either weak or non-existent, and any conventional management, which is perhaps unnecessarily interventional, is challenged by the woman and her family? In this chapter we describe our experience of being part of a team supporting Mary and her partner John through her pregnancy, labour and the birth of their twins; we discuss issues they raised with the maternity care team during Mary's pregnancy, labour and birth, and describe how clinical management was planned and informed by

addressing and dealing with the potential conflict between evidence and conventional treatment.[1]

We describe Mary's care using the five steps of evidence-based midwifery (Page 2000) and discuss the importance of good communication between the woman, obstetrician and midwife. In addition, we acknowledge the imperative to use published evidence and research to inform our practice and to share this knowledge and information with the woman and her family to reach a consensus on the way care is delivered. Where no evidence existed, we aimed to share commonly 'accepted' good practice and comply with Mary and John's requests within the boundaries of safe clinical practice.

OVERVIEW OF MARY'S PREGNANCY

Mary, a caucasian woman was 39 years old at the time of her pregnancy and birth. She had a di-chorionic di-amniotic (DCDA) twin pregnancy conceived by in-vitro fertilization (IVF) and requested a water birth in the low risk midwifery-led unit (Home from Home Birth Centre) in a teaching hospital in London, with the twins to be monitored by intermittent auscultation (IA). At the time of booking, she requested that her labour be overseen and attended by midwives with no obstetrician present, unless absolutely essential for maternal or fetal reasons. She also did not wish to have neonatologists present in the room. After the

---

1 In this chapter, we will describe the woman and her partner by their pseudonyms as Mary and John.

birth of the first twin, she requested that the midwife carry out abdominal palpation and vaginal examination to determine the presentation and position of the second twin. She wished to adopt any position she found comfortable and to avoid any medical intervention. Any intervention for the birth of the second twin would be against her wish; she wanted the second twin to be born naturally and without any time restriction imposed on the birth interval between the twins. She also declined administration of prophylactic syntometrine (Syntometrine: ergometrine 500 micrograms and oxytocin 5 units/mL) for active management of the third stage of labour.

CARE OF A TWIN PREGNANCY: BACKGROUND TO EVIDENCE AND STANDARDS CURRENTLY USED IN MIDWIFERY/OBSTETRIC PRACTICE

One of the most important resources used for pregnancy and childbirth is the Cochrane library. This has become an essential resource of high quality systematic reviews on key questions about current clinical practice in maternity care (see www.thecochranelibrary.com).

Results of Cochrane reviews are used extensively to form national clinical guidelines, for example those produced by the National Institute for Clinical Excellence (NICE). These guidelines are published to inform the healthcare professionals involved in clinical care in the NHS in England and Wales and can be accessed at www.nice.nhs.uk by the users of the service as well as the professionals.

Since 2001 NICE guidelines have been published on a range of maternity care topics including: The Use of Electronic Fetal Monitoring (NICE 2001a), Induction of Labour (NICE 2001b), Antenatal Care (NICE 2003) and Caesarean Section (NICE 2004). Guidelines covering Intrapartum Care and Care During the Post-natal Period are currently being drafted by two multi-disciplinary groups which include service users and healthcare professionals (GSTT 2005). A fundamental principal of NICE guideline development groups is that the experience, skills and knowledge of members are equally valued in terms of their contribution to developing valid and useful recommendations for clinical care.

The need to involve service users in shaping maternity care has been recognized for over a decade. For example, the Department of Health's policy document Changing Childbirth, published in 1993 acknowledged that maternity services must be woman-centred. This meant working with a woman to achieve her close involvement in planning her care, giving her 'choice, continuity and control'. Changing Childbirth sought to have a named midwife allocated to each woman throughout her pregnancy who would, in many instances, become the lead professional for care. Women who have complicated pregnancies would have their care led by obstetricians. The report emphasized the need to ensure that each woman felt respected and enabled to maintain her autonomy throughout decision-making about all aspects of her care, including place of birth. It recommended the professional team publish agreed guidelines in 'consultation with consumers' (Department of Health 1993) and be responsible for maintaining their continuing education.

More recently, the maternity module of the National Service Framework for Children, Young People and Maternity Services (Department of Health 2004), set new national standards for NHS maternity care in England. The standard addresses the requirements of women and their families during pregnancy, birth and the puerperium, emphasizing the need for women to have 'as normal a pregnancy and birth as possible, with medical interventions recommended to them only if they are of benefit to the woman or baby' (Department of Health 2004).

WORKING OUT WHETHER CARE WE OFFERED WAS EVIDENCE BASED OR NOT

One challenge for the maternity care team in providing care to Mary and her partner was in planning care for labour. We carried out a series of systematic literature searches to find reliable evidence on which to base our advice and care. Designing of the search was agreed on by the authors and one of the editors as felt relevant to this topic. Searching was performed by the authors with the results synthesized by AA. However, in many instances there was no evidence to support the practices currently used. This brought us to the realization that some aspects of 'good' practice had evolved over time and had become standardized and incorporated into the local guidelines, without a solid evidence base.

With this background, we would like to discuss the highlights of Mary's care using the five steps as a framework.

FIVE STEPS

1. Finding out what is important to the woman and her family.
2. Using information from the clinical examination.
3. Seeking and assessing evidence to inform decisions.
4. Talking it through.
5. Reflecting on outcomes, feelings and consequences.

STEP 1: FINDING OUT WHAT IS IMPORTANT TO THE WOMAN AND HER FAMILY

As this was an IVF pregnancy, Mary and her partner John had been aware of the exact date of conception. They had spent time carrying out their own research using internet sources and birth organizations before Mary's booking as well as at various stages of her pregnancy after having consulted the maternity care professionals (i.e. midwife and consultant obstetrician).

Place of birth and plan of care

The importance of a natural birth and non-intervention in labour was an overriding issue for Mary and John. They had planned for a home birth initially with an independent midwife, but when twins were confirmed on ultrasound scan, at eight weeks, they decided to use the hospital facilities with the back up of obstetric/neonatal services if required.

The hospital we are referring to here has two birth centres where women give birth: a low risk midwifery led care area, Home from Home Birth Centre (HfHBC), and a Hospital Birth Centre (HBC) where more complex pregnancies/labours are cared for by both midwifery and medical teams. Both places operate under published and referenced guidelines, with a named midwife

in-charge at each shift of the day and night. In addition, there is a designated person for overall responsibility for each area: a midwifery manager for both Birth Centres; a consultant midwife[2], clinical lead for the Home from Home Birth Centre and a consultant obstetrician, clinical lead for the Hospital Birth Centre.

At around 12 weeks gestation they had participated in a tour of the birth centres to check out what was available for their birth. From this they had understood the birthing pool would be available for use during Mary's labour and that the birth of the twins could be facilitated in the midwifery-led unit.

Mary's 'named' midwife referred them to the consultant midwife of the midwifery-led unit, in line with the unit protocol, who told them of the Home from Home Birth Centre guidelines. These excluded twin births on the grounds of inability to continuously and simultaneously monitor the fetal heart rates of the twins (NICE 2001a). Various options and suggestions were offered to facilitate Mary having an active labour; for example alternating between using the pool and having a twin cardiotocograph (CTG) carried out at regular intervals using the Hospital Birth Centre (HBC). The consultant midwife also discussed the component of the HBC guidelines which included active 'management' of the birth of the second twin (Guy's and St Thomas' Hospital NHS Trust 2004).

Following this discussion, Mary was referred to her consultant obstetrician, to discuss a formal plan of care. The consultant midwife suggested that she then meet again with them at a later date. The referral was in line with the Midwives rules and standards (Nursing and Midwifery Council 2004) that provides guidance on the midwife's sphere of practice[3].

---

2 The Consultant Midwife post was created in 1999 in England and Wales in order to create a career pathway for senior clinicians who previously moved out into management or education. This mirrors the consultant obstetrician post, the most senior doctor of the team.
3 A midwife is required to refer for medical advice following detection of abnormal conditions/deviations from the normal (Nursing and Midwifery Council 2004).

As per the hospital operational policy, the practice of Mary and John's named midwife (who is based in the community) was to offer only antenatal and postnatal care. This meant that intrapartum care was provided by the hospital midwives. It was therefore important the couple were linked to named professionals who were able to provide continuity of care and good communication between colleagues and within the hospital (Department of Health 1993). Failure in communication between health professionals is a key contribution to poor outcomes for mothers and babies and was highlighted in the most recent confidential enquiry report on maternal death in the UK: Why Mother's Die (Lewis and Drife, 2004).

It is important for midwives (and doctors) to build up a relationship with each woman and ensure they respect the woman's autonomy. This means that every woman has 'the right to decide whether to undergo any healthcare intervention – even where a refusal may result in harm or death to themselves or a fetus . . . ' (Nursing and Midwifery Council 2002).

OBSTETRIC CONSULTATION

It was essential that Mary and John had a detailed and open discussion with the obstetric consultant in order to be able to outline an agreed care plan for her labour and childbirth.

The gestational dating and chorionicity (i.e. the type of twin pregnancy – identical or non-identical) were accurately established by ultrasound (U/S) carried out at eight weeks of pregnancy. Fetal anomalies were ruled out by further U/S at 20 weeks. Right from the beginning Mary's pregnancy progressed uneventfully.

At the initial consultation with their consultant obstetrician the couple had made it clear that they wanted a non-medicalized, normal twin birth, but in a hospital setting at the Home from Home Birth Centre. The obstetrician explained to them the hospital policy and the course of a twin pregnancy with possible complications. Both Mary and John had carried out literature searches about care in labour for a twin birth. They were happy that their concerns and wishes were listened to and that the system allowed plenty of opportunity to discuss different viewpoints. However they wished to see the obstetric and midwifery con-

sultants to agree on a final care plan as well as to discuss any on-going issues through the rest of the pregnancy. Further appointments were therefore arranged at 32 weeks when Mary and John brought an updated copy of their birth plan to review with their care team, which included the following requests:

- To use the midwifery-led unit (Home from Home Birth Centre) for the labour and be attended solely by midwives.
- To be attended by partner and sister throughout the labour. No medical or midwifery students, including no obstetrician or neonatologist to be present at birth, unless complications arise.
- For the midwives in attendance to have specific experience/interest in twin births.
- No induction if possible.
- No continuous electronic fetal monitoring unless an abnormality/complication arises.
- Use of the water pool and Entonox for pain relief. No epidural or intravenous infusion as a routine.
- Active first stage using an upright position (including use of the birth ball, birth bars, mat).
- Vaginal birth for both twins – no caesarean section unless absolutely necessary.
- To allow the second twin to assume or correct its position naturally before resorting to an external cephalic version (ECV).
- No artificial rupture of membranes (ARM) or use of intravenous oxytocin infusion as a routine measure.
- Preference for a tear to an episiotomy.
- A physiological third stage of labour.
- Partner to cut the cords when they cease pulsating.
- Skin to skin contact and breastfeeding after the birth.
- No vitamin K for the babies if they are born without complications.

Non-medical aspects of care (importance of sister and partner present at the birth)

Mary had a very clear birth plan that indicated she wanted a very natural and normal twin-birth with her sister and partner present as her birthing companions. It was very important to her as she would feel most comfortable and supported by the presence of two very close family members.

Formulation of a care plan

A meeting was held between senior staff including the head of midwifery (who co-ordinated the meeting), consultant obstetrician, consultant midwifer and senior midwifery supervisors. A detailed discussion took place to reach a consensus on a care plan on the basis of the available evidence, good practice, the couple's wish and the practicality of its delivery. Effective communication was established to ensure everyone in the maternity care unit (both HfHBC and HBC) was appraised of the plan of care. Mary and John were aware of, but did not take part in, this meeting. The plan agreed at this meeting was later conveyed to them the following week by the consultant midwife and obstetrician. They happily agreed with this plan.

Hard copies of the Home from Home Birth Centre and Hospital Birth Centre guidelines together with the relevant internet and journal searches (carried out by the consultant midwife and obstetrician) were given to Mary and John for their information. Their revised birth plan including the responses agreed at the meeting were circulated by the consultant midwife to all midwifery practice leaders on the birth centres, supervisors of midwives and obstetric staff with a copy in Mary's antenatal records.

STEP 2: USING INFORMATION FROM THE CLINICAL EXAMINATION

Specific questions about twin pregnancy

A twin pregnancy is conventionally considered a high-risk pregnancy. Almost all perinatal and infant morbidity (preterm birth, low birth weight, small for gestation age, admission to neonatal intensive care unit (NICU), higher incidences of intra-partum related birth asphyxia of the second twin) occurs more frequently in twins than in singletons (Kierse & Helmerhost 1995). The New York twin study of 16 000 twin pairs born between 1978 and 1984 demonstrated rates of intra-partum stillbirth and neonatal death 3–4 times higher than in general obstetric population (Kiely 1990). A Swedish analysis of approximately one million births at term between 1988 and 1997 showed a four-fold risk of a low 5-minute Apgar score among second twins (Barrett & Ritchie 2002). A Scottish study using linked databases of pregnancy and perinatal mortality demonstrated an excess of delivery-related perinatal death among second twins born at term (Smith et al 2002).

Conventional practice is to arrange the birth of a twin pregnancy in a clinical area in which obstetricians, obstetric anaesthetist and neonatologists are readily available. In addition, easy access to epidural anaesthesia, ultrasound facilities, continuous electronic fetal monitoring, and the implementation of policies, which state optimal inter-twin delivery interval, active intervention for delivery of second twin, and active management of the third stage are usual. Mary and John however disagreed with most, if not all, of these components of care. Also, the thorough literature searches we had carried out had failed to yield any good quality evidence for recommending these aspects of conventional practice (Moll 2003).

Therefore, a mutually agreed plan of care was prepared to make a balance between the parents' choice and conventional practice for safety of the mother and the twins.

STEP 3: SEEKING AND ASSESSING EVIDENCE TO INFORM DECISIONS

In order to access all the relevant evidence in the management of labour for twins, the following areas, individuals and organizations were searched using such terms as: Multiple Pregnancy, Twins, IVF, Twin Births, Waterbirth, Home birth and Inter-twin delivery.

Electronic searches were carried out by the authors in Medline, the Cochrane library, MIDIRS (Midwives Information and Resource Service), the Royal College of Obstetricians and Gynaecologists, the Royal College of Midwives websites and overseas Colleges in order to collect evidence/good practice in international obstetric clinical practice. The consultant obstetrician also consulted the RCOG Green Top Guidelines and corresponded with the RCOG guideline committee representative. In addition, obstetric and midwifery textbooks and current hospital guidelines were reviewed. The issues were discussed with independent midwives, consultant midwives and consultant obstetricians. Multi-professional meetings took place within the hospital directorate to discuss the evidence and plans for care.

For Mary's care the main issues for which we needed to seek and assess evidence to inform decisions were:

■ **Place of birth**

Throughout the Western world the majority of twin births take place in hospital. This is despite the serious lack of sound evidence concerning the method of delivery on which to base decision about what level of care should be provided and offer advice to women about their birth choices (Hofmeyr & Drakeley 1998).

Home birth: international perspective

In the UK, two independent midwives regularly support women with twin pregnancies to have home births (Evans 1997, personal communication 2004) and individual consultant midwives in the UK have supported twin births in a birth centre (personal communication, 2004).

In the USA Ina May Gaskin supports the birth of twins on the 'Farm[4] in Tennessee (Gaskin 2003) and advises on birth techniques.

The practice of giving birth to twins at home varies between countries. Compared to other industrialized countries, the Netherlands has a high percentage (30–38%) of home births (Smeenk & ten Have 2003). Even in the highly successful Dutch system, which is regarded as a model for home birth services, there is a widely accepted list of criteria (Wiegers et al 1996) and twin pregnancy is an indication for referral to a specialist obstetrician (Eskes 1989). In Canada, a woman with a multiple pregnancy is not eligible for a home birth according to the policy set by the Home Birth Demonstration Project (HBDP) and the College of Midwives of British Columbia (CMBC) (Janssen et al 2002). The American College of Nurse-Midwives excludes multiple gestation from its criteria for home birth (American College of Nurse-Midwives 2003). Australian home birth figures show twin pregnancy as one of the two largest contributors to the perinatal death (Bastian

et al 1998). In a prospective cohort study carried out in Switzerland which compared matched pairs of hospital and home births, twin birth was not excluded from the home delivery group, although the proportion of twin births at home was much smaller (0.4%) compared with those delivered in hospital (1.9%) (Ackermann-Liebrich et al 1996).

From this it must be emphasized that although home birth for twin pregnancy is strongly discouraged, the evidence-base is limited on the safety or recommendation of twin birth in a midwifery-led unit as compared to a specialist obstetric unit. The International Federation of Gynecology and Obstetrics (FIGO) are unable to answer specific medical questions as are addressed in this article and they recommended contact with the Royal College of Obstetricians and Gynaecologists (RCOG), UK (Zamanillo: personal communication, 7 December 2004). However, neither the RCOG (Baldwin: personal communication, 15 December 2004) nor NICE (Salvidge: Personal communication, 12 January 2005) currently have any published guidelines on twin birth. It is hard to envisage that a randomized controlled trial (RCT) is likely to be carried out comparing hospital delivery with home birth for twins; this means that the evidence base for this currently relies on observational studies and consensus. For example, a consensus statement agreed by the Canadian Society of Obstetrics and Gynaecology (SOGC) suggests that twin deliveries should be planned in Level 2 (secondary care) and Level 3 (tertiary care) hospitals (Barrett & Bocking 2000). The UK Confidential Enquiry into Maternal Deaths (Lewis & Drife 2004) also recommends 'women known to be at high risk of bleeding should be delivered in centres with facilities for blood transfusion, intensive care and other interventions, and plans should be made in advance for their management'. Given the understanding that women who have twin pregnancies are at higher risk of requiring such care this means that birth at home is not usual.

Water Birth:

Water birth for twins is typically contra-indicated (Scott 2001). This is usually stated in the protocols and guidelines of the units who provide water birth, although there are reports of twin-birth in water (Ponnettee 2004).

---

4 The Farm is a 'stand-alone' birth centre in Tenessee which is run by 'lay' midwives.

Caesarean Section:

When the first twin is cephalic, no advantage for routine birth by caesarean section has been demonstrated (Dodd & Crowther 2003, Hofmeyer & Drakeley 1998, McNamara 2004, Roopnarinesingh et al 2002) and it has been shown to be more cost-effective, both physically and financially, to give birth to twins vaginally (Mauldin et al 1998).

- **Continuous electronic fetal monitoring in labour**

Although routine use of continuous electronic fetal monitoring (EFM) during singleton labour and birth has not shown any benefit in RCTs (MacDonald et al 1985), there is no evidence generated from RCTs regarding the use of EFM for twin births (Breeze & Smith 2004). However, nearly all systematic reviews of evidence, including the National Institute for Clinical Excellence (NICE 2001a), universally recommend EFM for twins.

Continuous fetal monitoring is best achieved by a combination of internal monitoring of the first twin via a scalp electrode, and external monitoring of the second twin via an abdominal transducer. The heart rates are recorded by a dual channel monitor. One observational study (Bakker et al 2004) described a significantly higher rate of signal loss from the fetal heart via an external transducer (ET) compared with via a fetal scalp electrode (FSE). During the first stage signal loss was recorded amongst 33% in ET group and 26% in FSE; in second stage 63% ET and 26% FSE. This is more than the FIGO-recommended criteria for the accepted limit of 20% signal loss (Bakker et al, 2004). Reliably recording the fetal heart for the second twin can be particularly important as some argue the delivery of the second twin can be delayed with a normal CTG (Bartnicki et al 1992).

- **Plan for birth of second twin**

Use of ultrasound to confirm position

For a number of reasons ultrasound (U/S) should not only be readily available (Barrett & Bocking 2000, Neilsen & Bajoria 2001), but be a critical and integral part of preparation for a twin delivery (Robinson & Chauhan 2004). Firstly, the presentation of the second twin strongly influences their intra-partum management and given that presen-

tation may change in up to 20% of cases after the birth of the first twin, depending on the gestation age (Houlihan & Knuppel 1996) U/S can be key in diagnosing presentation. Secondly, U/S may play an important role in locating and monitoring the heart rate of the second twin. Thirdly, if the second twin is in a non-vertex position, U/S is essential to guide obstetric manoeuvres such as external cephalic version (ECV), or internal podalic version and breech extraction.

Use of ECV

Following the birth of the first twin it is suggested that external cephalic version (ECV) should be attempted when the second twin presents by the breech. This is perceived as being less traumatic and non-invasive compared to the other intervention option for non-cephalic second twin, internal version and breech extraction. A success rate of up to 75% for ECV followed by a safe vaginal delivery has been described for the second twin weighing >1500g (Kaplan et al 1995). However the outcome may very much depend on the technique used, operator's experience and whether or not an effective epidural is in situ. Moreover, ECV may result in complications such as rupture of the membranes before it is completed and the twin is still in a transverse or oblique position. Other unintended outcomes include fetal bradycardia, failed version and non-engagement of the head, and such problems may necessitate caesarean section (Neilsen & Bajoria 2001). One study demonstrated that ECV compared poorly with internal version and breech extraction, with dramatically higher emergency caesarean section rate (38% v 3%) and fetal distress (18% v 1%) (Chauhan et al 1995). From this it would appear that if intervention is required internal version and breech extraction is safer, provided that the appropriate techniques are applied (Barrett & Ritchie 2002; Berglund & Axelsson 1989).

Artificial rupture of membranes

A consensus statement agreed by the Canadian Society of Obstetrics and Gynaecology, was conformed by well-designed cohort/case controlled studies, and suggests that it was reasonable to expedite delivery of the second twin using ECV followed by artificial rupture of membranes (ARM), and use of oxytocin, or ARM followed by

internal podalic version (Barrett & Bocking 2000).

Routine ARM following ECV assists in stabilization of the second fetus and is given as a standard clinical practice in midwifery and obstetric textbooks (Fraser et al 2003, Henderson & Macdonald 2004, MacGillivray & Campbell 1988). However, some prefer to leave the membranes intact to ensure that the cervix remains fully dilated by the fluid wedge. No RCTs have evaluated this practice in the care of the second twin and its use has evolved from clinical experience and application of evidence from studies involving singletons.

Use of Syntocinon prior to second twin

Although early routine recourse to oxytocin may accelerate descent of the second twin, this is not absolutely indicated providing labour is progressing, the presenting part descending, bleeding is minimal and the fetal heart rate (FHR) is normal (Neilsen & Bajoria 2001). In this situation there is no need for any 'rush' in uncomplicated twin births (Feng et al 1995). However oxytocin should be used to treat hypotonic uterine contractions whether this occurs before or after the birth of the first twin (Barrett & Bocking 2000).

Optimal delivery interval between the twins

What constitutes the acceptable optimal interval is debatable. Conventional practice is that the second twin should be delivered less than 15 minutes after the first, and certainly within 30 minutes (Breeze & Smith 2004). It is to be noted that these recommendations are from the era before intervention such as epidural analgesia and EFM were available. In fact these time limits have been followed in clinical practice without being subjected to rigorous evaluation. Delay beyond these time limits may be acceptable without any adverse effect on the outcome of the second twin, provided progress is being made towards a successful vaginal delivery, bleeding is minimal, and CTG is normal (Neilsen & Bajoria 2001, Midwifery Today E-News 2000). However a recent study contradicts this as it showed even with continuous EFM the risks of fetal distress and acidosis in the second twin are high when the twin-to-twin delivery interval is beyond 30 minutes (Leung et al 2002). Another study (Erdemoglu at al 2003) shows delivery interval >30 minutes is a significant predictive factor only if the second twin is in breech presentation and has a birth weight of >1900 g.

■ Use of syntometrine for third stage

There is higher incidence of uterine atony and postpartum haemorrhage (PPH) in twin births due to two placentas (dichorionic) or single placenta (monochorionic), uterine over-distension and the need for manipulation for the delivery of the second twin. The recent UK Confidential Enquiry into Maternal Deaths (Lewis & Drife 2004) reported one maternal death due to postpartum haemorrhage (PPH) associated with multiple pregnancy. Therefore an active management of third stage is recommended as there is good evidence for prophylactic oxytocin infusion to reduce the risk of PPH, compared to expectant management (Prendiville et al 2000). The report by Lewis and Drife (2004) also recommended 'women known to be at high risk of bleeding should be delivered in centres with facilities for blood transfusion, intensive care and other interventions, and plans should be made in advance for their management'.

■ No medical personnel to be present

Techniques for assisting the birth of twins and breech presentation are fundamental to a midwife's training and she should continue to maintain her skills through practice and through simulation. A range of sources to support learning and maintain skills are used by midwives and those most frequently used in the UK include Mayes (Henderson & Macdonald 2004) and Myles (Fraser et al 2003) and the Advanced Life Support in Obstetrics (ALSO) manual (American Academy of Family Physicians 2000). The advice given by these sources is to arrange for obstetric support during labour and birth. This essentially means the presence of an obstetrician competent to manage a twin birth (Barrett & Bocking 2000, Neilsen & Bajoria 2001). Some authors are very specific about the personnel to be present. For example O'Connor and Hiadzi (1996) state that two midwives, two obstetricians, one anaesthetist, one operating department assistant, one or two neonatologists should be in attendance or available immediately to support care. They do stress

the importance of mentioning this to the mother well in advance rather than causing her anxiety by their sudden arrival during delivery.

■ IVF twins

Although some authors (Moise et al 1998) found that twins conceived by IVF are at a significantly higher risk for prematurity and associated neonatal morbidity and mortality than spontaneously conceived twins, the majority of other studies do not show any evidence that twin pregnancies resulting from assisted conceptions have significantly worse perinatal outcomes compared with naturally conceived twins (Agustsson et al 1997, Bernasko et al 1997, Dhont et al 1999). More recent data also demonstrate either similar risk of neurological sequelae (Koudstaal 2000; Pinborg et al 2004a, 2004b) or even lower perinatal mortality (Helmerhorst et al 2004) in twins after assisted conception compared with natural conception, especially with DCDA twins.

THE CARE PLAN

Based on the information and evidence discussed as described under Step 1 it was agreed that there was no strong case against Mary giving birth in the Home from Home Birth Centre. Therefore a plan was drawn up to support Mary to use the birth pool during the first stage of her labour. The twins' heartbeats would be monitored simultaneously by two midwives using intermittent auscultation. She was to have an intravenous access (not a running infusion), with the actual births taking place out of the water pool. Obstetricians and neonatologists would be available, but not present in the room. Manoeuvring the second twin to achieve a longitudinal lie and cephalic presentation would be carried out only if essential. Third stage of labour would be managed physiologically with access to oxytocics, if Mary had a PPH.

As far as practicable, staffing was arranged so that two senior midwives would be available to support Mary's labour, with a senior specialist registrar and consultant obstetrician available should they be needed. Mary agreed to the admission and transfer guidelines of the unit from Home from Home Birth Centre to the Hospital Birth Centre (see Boxes 9.1 and 9.2 below).

Box 9.1 Indications for birth in the Home from Home Birth Centre

Suitable:
- All uncomplicated low risk singleton pregnancies, gestation 37–41 completed weeks, with cephalic presentation.

Not suitable:

Present pregnancy:
- Preterm labour
- Antepartum haemorrhage
- Twin pregnancy
- Pre-eclampsia
- Fetal growth restriction with or without oligohydramnios
- Pregnancy complicated by medical disorders
- Vaginal birth after caesarean section (VBAC)
- Meconium stained amniotic fluid
- Rhesus disease
- Anaemia (Hb% <9g/dL)
- BMI > 30
- Unbooked mother
- Mother requiring or requesting epidural analgesia
- Large baby (estimated fetal weight >4 Kg)

Previous pregnancy complications:
- Stillbirth/neonatal death
- Eclampsia
- Postpartum haemorrhage with or without retained placenta
- Caesarean section

THE BIRTH OF THE TWINS

Mary was admitted to the HBC at 35 weeks gestation with pre-labour premature rupture of membranes (pPROM). Later that day, established labour began. In view of the prematurity of the twins it was agreed that labour should be managed in the HBC as specified in her care plan. However, after 12 hours of labour Mary had not progressed beyond a cervical dilatation of 4 cm, despite regular contractions. At this stage ultrasound showed both twins were in a breech presentation, with the first twin in an oblique lie. Mary was offered a caesarean section in view of the

> **Box 9.2   Indications for transfer from Home from Home Birth Centre to Hospital Birth Centre**
>
> **Home Birth Centre to HBC**
> Any complication arising during or after labour that needs obstetric medical or midwifery intervention will require transfer from HfH to HBC.
>
> **Common indications:**
> - Abnormality in fetal heart rate
> - Meconium stained amniotic fluid
> - Antepartum haemorrhage
> - Need or request for epidural
> - Maternal pyrexia in labour
> - High B/P in labour
> - Failure to progress in labour
> - Abnormal presentation diagnosed during labour
> - Postpartum haemorrhage
> - Retained placenta
> - 3°/4° perineal tear
> - Inadequate staffing
> - Any other condition of concern as judged by the midwife

presentation of the twins and slow progress. She agreed and gave her written consent to this.

A spinal anaesthetic was initiated in theatre. During catheterization a vaginal examination was carried out and Mary's cervix was found to be fully dilated. This gave rise to the possibility of a vaginal breech extraction as the anaesthesia had taken effect and therefore birth by maternal effort was not an option. However, there was acute prolonged bradycardia of both twins, so following additional informed consent, an emergency caesarean section was carried out. The twins were born in good condition, the operation went well, and Mary had a smooth post-operative recovery.

STEP 4: TALKING IT THROUGH

Mary and John's reflections in the immediate postnatal period

On reflection, with the consultant obstetrician, Mary and John expressed their satisfaction with the way the whole situation was managed despite requiring an emergency caesarean section. They were very appreciative of the communication and continuity of care by the midwives and consultant obstetrician during most of the labour, and the opportunity to discuss and review each stage of the labour. However, they felt there was a lack of confidence among some junior members of staff who had looked nervous, even panicking at times. They thought that this was because they had been asked to offer care and support which was outside their normal practice. It was also evident to Mary and John that there was no midwife with *specialized* experience in twin births.

Mary's sister was upset that she was not allowed in theatre, although both Mary's partner and sister had wanted to be with her throughout her labour and childbirth. Unfortunately there was no provision in the current hospital policy for more than one family member to be with a mother in the theatre and this was a great challenge.

STEP 5: REFLECTING ON OUTCOMES, FEELINGS AND CONSEQUENCES

■ The challenge

Members of the healthcare team experienced challenges to their biases and beliefs to be involved in the care of Mary and John and their twins. Initially a negative sense prevailed that Mary and John's request could not be honoured as what was asked for was against usual practice. However, a thorough literature search failed to reveal any evidence against. In fact many aspects of their birth plan appeared reasonable and to comply with current evidence, provided their risks and benefits were appropriately discussed and documented. One has to keep in mind the fact that the autonomy of women should always be respected and that they have the legal and ethical right to refuse treatment.

■ Flexibility, forward planning and on-going communication

Keeping an open mind, willingness to respect the woman's choice, early initiation and continued discussion, flexible attitude, forward planning and effective communication were the key to achieving a way of dealing with a situation like this; so that it was possible to continue to offer effective support to Mary.

Recognition of feelings

This care was in a large institution where an effective intra- and inter-disciplinary support was readily available. Mary and John's situation is an example of how the recognition of feelings of both the couple and the professionals can be an essential part of reflection on practice! Moreover an important outcome was that Mary and John were happy on the whole with their care, and the institution learned a lot from this situation.

Lack of strong evidence

ECV confers little advantage to the fetus, and indeed may lead to more complications (Neilsen & Bajoria 2001). Instead, some recommend internal podalic version as a preferred primary procedure, as it is associated with higher success and lower complications than ECV (Chauhan et al 1995).

Flexibility and scope for an agreed care plan

Although each clinical unit will have its own guidelines and protocols covering care of women and babies with complicated needs, in some situations there should be scope for flexibility. Each case should be judged on its own merits and necessary alteration in the management plan should be made. Most importantly a woman should be able to make informed choices and design a care plan agreed by all parties.

Staffing arrangement and continuity of care

As far as possible continuity of care by the same healthcare personnel should be maintained during pregnancy, and appropriate staffing arrangements made to sustain this during labour and birth. If labour starts before the expected time, a contingency plan should be in place. Currently plans to increase midwifery group practices and personal caseloads is in hand within the maternity unit of the above maternity service, as a means to providing greater continuity of care throughout the pregnancy so that the women are familiar with individual midwives.

Staff feelings

The junior doctors and some midwives felt stressed by what they perceived as the demands of the couple outside normal practice and the fact that the twins were premature, for example, their objection to portable ultrasound to check fetal presentations, and preference for intermittent auscultation rather than continuous EFM. They were unused to these approaches to obstetric practice.

Training issues for staff

It was agreed that when providing such care in future there would be liaison with midwives with experience in care of twin births working in nearby NHS Trusts. The focus would be on training and upskilling a number of midwives to be available to offer support to colleagues for future care of twins in a midwifery-led environment. The recent hospital statistics of twins born vaginally had been shared with the couple to illustrate that our aim was to facilitate vaginal birth as far as possible (see Table 9.1. below).

Table 9.1	Twin birth statistics at Guy's and St Thomas' NHS Foundation Trust, London				
Year	Total Twin Deliveries	No. of Vaginal deliveries	Elective LSCS	Emergency LSCS	Epidurals (for vaginal delivery)
2000	84	43	16	25	30
2001	89	45	21	23	26
2002*	74	28	18	28	14
2003	97	49	15	33	24
2004	100	48	21	31	29

* Please note that during 2002 the Women's Health Unit moved site from Guy's Hospital to St Thomas' Hospital.

■ **Communication and rapport between the woman and healthcare professionals**

Effective communication all through her pregnancy between the mother (and where appropriate those who offer her social support) and members of her multi-disciplinary healthcare team is vital. The whole process should be initiated well in advance of the due date of birth with sufficient time available for both parties to reflect on information exchanged and the outcome of discussions before a decision is reached. Strategies should be implemented to ensure that staff who are not directly participant in discussions and decisions know about any changes in the woman's situation and agreed care plan. Care must be taken to ensure there is no break-up in the relationship between the woman and the healthcare professionals. Enabling continuing discussion about how the woman is experiencing care and reflection on decisions at appropriate points is key. A stepped approach with short discussions at regular intervals taking one aspect of care at a time often bears better fruit than protracted consultation to deal with all aspects at one go.

■ **Post-birth staff briefing is important for important learning issues**

Staff briefing and feedback is highly recommended as this would improve the understanding of special situations and add to learning from experience. This is also a very important issue from a risk management point of view involving the clinical risk manager, senior obstetricians and midwives and other maternity care staff. It offers an excellent opportunity for feedback and critical analysis of individual cases to improve future care from the lessons learned.

CONCLUSION

When planning pregnancy, labour and birth care with Mary and John we found that published reports do not concur with the conventional concept of higher risks of IVF (DCDA) twin pregnancy than their non-IVF matched controls. Currently there is a lack of evidence regarding the best practice of intrapartum management of twins. High quality research is needed to generate unbi-

ased and reliable results to inform clinical care. Where appropriate, randomized controlled trials should be used to evaluate alternative care options and observational methods should be used where it is considered unethical or not feasible to evaluate care using RCT methodology.

We should have an open mind in individualizing care and an agreed care plan should be made at the senior level after proper discussion. Maternal and fetal safety, however, must not be compromised while making such a plan. Risks and benefits must be explicitly documented to ensure that no false sense of security prevails for either the woman and her family or her healthcare professionals. Midwives with experience in twin births should conduct the labour, and overall, a positive attitude should be shown to earn the woman's confidence that her decision is supported and her choice respected within the limits of safety.

Mary's choices presented her healthcare team with considerable challenges and opportunities. When we presented this case to a multidisciplinary audience, most obstetricians and midwives agreed that there was insufficient evidence to deny a Home from Home Birth Centre twin birth. Mary showed how women's choices about pregnancy, labour and childbirth should be heard, listened to and respected (Department of Health 1993).

POINTERS FOR PRACTICE

- The current evidence base for best practice care of a twin birth is not robust.
- An individual care plan should be made following discussion with the woman and her birth partner (as required).
- Document the care plan clearly in the notes.
- Discuss with and circulate the care plan to the multidisciplinary team.
- Any deviation from the agreed care plan should be explained to the woman and partner and carried out with their consent.
- Evaluation/feedback from the woman and her partner should be encouraged to continuously improve practice.
- Case discussion and presentation in a multidisciplinary forum is useful as an educational tool to inform future practice.

References

Ackermann-Liebrich U, Voegeli T, Günter-Witt K, Kunz I, Züllig M, Schindler C 1996 Home vs. hospital deliveries: follow up study of matched pairs for procedures and outcome. British Medical Journal 313: 1313–1318

Agustsson T, Geirsson R T, Mires G 1997 Obstetric outcome of natural and assisted conception twin pregnancies is similar. Acta Obstetrics Gynecology Scandinavia 76(1): 45–49

American Academy of Family Physicians 2000 Advanced life support in obstetrics-provider course syllabus. 4th edn. American Academy of Family Physicians, Kansas, USA

American College of Nurse-Midwives 2003 Criteria for provision of home birth services. Clinical Bulletin #7, March. Online. Available: http://www.midwife.org/siteFiles/education/Clinical_Bulletin_7.pdf accessed 21 Dec 2005

Bakker P C, Colenbrander G J, Verstraeten A A, Van Geijn H P 2004 Quality of intrapartum cardiotocography in twin deliveries. American Journal of Obstetrics and Gynecology 191(6): 2114–2119

Barrett J F, Ritchie W K 2002 Twin delivery. Best Practice Research in Clinical Obstetrics and Gynaecology 16(1): 43–56

Barrett J, Bocking A 2000 The management of twin pregnancies (part 1) The SOGC consensus statement. Journal of the Society of Obstetricians and Gynaecologists July 91: 5–15

Bartnicki J, Meyenburg M, Saling E 1992 Time interval in twin delivery – the second twin need not always be born shortly after the first. Gynaecology Obstetric Investigations 33(1): 19–20

Bastian H, Keirse M J N C, Lancaster P A L 1998 Perinatal death associated with planned home birth in Australia: population based study. British Medical Journal 317: 384–388

Berglund L, Axelsson O 1989 Breech extraction versus cesarean section for the remaining second twin. Acta Obstetrics and Gynecology of Scandinavia 68(5): 435–438

Bernasko J, Lynch L, Lapinski R, Berkowitz RL 1997 Twin pregnancies conceived by assisted reproductive techniques: maternal and neonatal outcomes. Obstetrics and Gynecology 89(3): 368–372

Breeze A C G, Smith G C S 2004 Mode of delivery of twins. The Obstetrician and Gynaecologist 6 (4): 222–226. Online. Available: www.rcog.org.uk/togonline accessed: April 2005

Chauhan S P, Roberts W E, McLaren R A, Roach H, Morrison J C, Martin J N Jr 1995 Delivery of the nonvertex second twin: breech extraction versus external cephalic version. American Journal of Obstetrics and Gynecology 173(4): 1015–1020

Department of Health 1993 Changing childbirth part 1: report of the Expert Maternity Group. HMSO. London

Department of Health 2004 Maternity standard, national service framework for children, young people and maternity services. Department of Health, London

Dhont M, De Sutter P, Ruyssinck G, Martens G, Bekaert A 1999 Perinatal outcome of pregnancies after assisted reproduction: a case-control study. American Journal of Obstetrics and Gynecology 181(3): 688–695

Dodd J M, Crowther C A, 2003 Effective delivery of women with a twin pregnancy from 37 weeks' gestation. Cochrane Library Issue 1. Wiley, Chichester, UK

Erdemoglu E, Mungan T, Tapisiz O L, Ustunyurt E, Çaglar E 2003 Effect of inter-twin delivery time on Apgar scores of the second twin. Australia and New Zealand Journal of Obstetrics and Gynaecology 43(3): 203–206

Eskes M 1989 het Wormerveer onderzoek – Meerjare-nonderzoek maar de kwaliteit van de verloskundige zorg rond een vroedvrouwenpraktijk (dissertation). University of Amsterdam, Amsterdam. Cited by Smeenk A D J, ten Have H A M J 2003 Medicalisation and obstetric care: an analysis of developments in Dutch midwifery. Medicine, Healthcare and Philosophy 6: 153–165

Evans J 1997 Can a twin birth be a positive experience? Midwifery Matters 74: 6–8. Online. Available: www.radmid.demon.co.uk/twins.htm accessed 11 May 2004

Feng T I, Swindle R E, Huddleston J F 1995 A lack of adverse effect of prolonged delivery interval between twins. Journal of Maternal-Fetal Investigation 5(4): 222–225

Fraser D M, Cooper M A, Fletcher G 2003 Myles textbook for midwives. 14th edn. Churchill Livingstone, Edinburgh

Gaskin I M 2003 Spiritual midwifery. 4th edn. Book Publishing Co, USA

GSTT 2005 Intrapartum guidelines and Postnatal guidelines. There are numerous different guidelines under these generic headings. All available on the GSTT Intranet for all staff to use in the clinical areas.

Guy's and St Thomas' Hospital NHS Trust (GSTT) 2004 Maternity guidelines, women's health directorate. GSTT, London

Helmerhorst F M, Perquin D A M, Donker D, Keirse M J N C 2004 Perinatal outcome of singletons and twins after assisted conception: a systematic review of controlled studies. British Medical Journal 328: 261–264

Henderson C, Macdonald S 2004 Mayes' midwifery. 13th edn. Bailliere Tindall, London

Hofmeyr G J, Drakeley A J 1998 Delivery of twins. Baillieres Clinical Obstetrics & Gynaecology March 12(1): 91–108

Houlihan C, Knuppel R A 1996 Intrapartum management of multiple gestations. Clinical Perinatology 23(1): 91–116

James D 2003 Preface. In: James D, Mahomed K, Stone P, van Wijngaarden W, Hill L M (eds) Evidence-based obstetrics. Saunders, Amsterdam

Janssen P A, Lee S K, Ryan E M, Etches D J, Farquharson D F, Peacock D, Klein M C 2002 Outcomes of planned home births versus planned hospital births after regulation of midwifery in British Columbia. Canadian Medical Association Journal 166: 315–323. Online. Available: http://www.pubmedcentral.nih.gov/articlerender.fcgi?tool=pubmed&pubmedid=11868639 accessed: 14/02/2005

Kaplan B, Peled Y, Rabinerson D, Goldman G A, Nitzan Z, Neri A 1995 Successful external version of B-twin after the birth of A-twin for vertex-non-vertex twins. European Journal of Obstetrics, Gynecology and Reproductive Biology 58(2): 157–160

Keily J L 1990 The epidemiology of perinatal mortality in multiple births. Bulletin of New York Academy of Medicine 66: 616–637

Keirse M J N C, Helmerhorst F M 1995 The impact of assisted reproduction on perinatal healthcare. Sozial- und Präventiv medizin/Social and Preventive Medicine (Historical Archive) 40: 343–351

Koudstaal J, Bruinse H W, Helmerhorst F M, Vermeiden J P, Willemsen W N, Visser G H 2000 Obstetric outcome of twin pregnancies after in-vitro fertilization: a matched control study in four Dutch university hospitals. Human Reproduction 15(4): 935–940

Leung T-Y, Tam W-H, Leung T-N, Lok I H, Lau T-K 2002 Effect of twin-to-twin delivery interval on umbilical cord blood gas in the second twin. British Journal of Obstetrics and Gynaecology 109: 63–67

Lewis G, Drife J (eds) 2004 Why mothers die 2000–2002. Confidential enquiry into maternal and child health. Sixth report. of the confidential enquiries into maternal deaths in the UK. RCOG, London

MacDonald D, Grant A, Sheridan-Pereira M, Boylan P, Chalmers I 1985 The Dublin randomized controlled trial of intrapartum fetal heart rate monitoring. American Journal of Obstetrics and Gynecology 152(5): 524–539

MacGillivray I, Campbell D M 1998 Management of twin pregnancies. In: MacGillivray I, Campbell D M, Thompson B (eds) Twins and twinning. Wiley, Chichester, England, pp 111–139

Mauldin J G, Newman R B, Mauldin P D 1998 Cost effective delivery management of the vertex and nonvertex gestation. American Journal of Obstetrics and Gynecology 179(4): 864–869

McNamara D 2004 If second twin is breech, vaginal delivery still safe: study of 107 vertex-non-vertex twins. Ob/Gyn News January

Midwifery Today E-News 2000 Effect of delivery interval on twin birth outcomes. Vol 2 Issue 27, July 5

Minakami H, Sayama M, Honma Y et al 1998 Lower risks of adverse outcome in twins conceived by artificial reproductive techniques compared with spontaneously conceived twins. Human Reproduction 13(7): 2005–2008

Moise J, Laor A, Armon Y, Gur I, Gale R 1998 The outcome of twin pregnancies after IVF. Human Reproduction 13(6):1702–1705

Moll E 2003 Multiple pregnancy. In: James D, Mahomed K, Stone P, van Wijngaarden W, Hill LM (eds) Evidence-based obstetrics. 2nd edn. Saunders, London, pp 324–328

National Institute of Clinical Excellence 2001a The use of electronic fetal monitoring. NICE, London

National Institute for Clinical Excellence 2001b Induction of labour. NICE, London

National Institute for Clinical Excellence 2003 Antenatal care. NICE, London

National Institute for Clinical Excellence 2004 Caesarean section. NICE, London.

Neilson J P, Bajoria R 2001 Multiple pregnancy. In: Chamberlain G, Steer P J (eds) Turnbull's obstetrics. 3rd edn. Churchill Livingstone, Edinburgh, pp 229–246

Nursing and Midwifery Council 2002 Code of professional conduct. Nursing and Midwifery Council, London

Nursing and Midwifery Council 2004 Midwives rules and standards. Nursing and Midwifery Council, London

O'Connor R A, Hiadzi E 1996. The intra-partum management of twin pregnancies. In: Studd J (ed.) Progress in obstetrics and gynaecology. 12th edn. Churchill Livingstone, London, pp 121–134

Page L (ed.) 2000 The new midwifery: science and sensitivity in practice. Churchill Livingstone, Edinburgh

Pinborg A, Loft A, Rasmussen S, Schmidt L, Langhoff-Roos J, Greisen G, Andersen A N 2004b Neonatal outcome in a Danish national cohort of 3438 IVF/ICSI and 10,362 non-IVF/ICSI twins born between 1995 and 2000. Human Reproduction 19(2): 435–441

Pinborg A, Loft A, Schmidt L, Greisen G, Rasmussen S, Andersen A N 2004a Neurological sequelae in twins born after assisted conception: controlled national cohort study. British Medical Journal 329: 311–314

Ponnettee H 2004 An obstetrician's experience of 1600 water births including breech and twin births. Online. Available: www.birthbalance.com/resources/audiotapes.shtml (Accessed on 8 June 2004)

Prendiville W J, Elbourne D, McDonald S 2000 Active versus expectant management of the third stage of labour (Cochrane Review). In: The Cochrane Library, 2000, Issue 4. Update Software, Oxford

Robinson C, Chauhan S P 2004 Intrapartum management of twins. Clinical Obstetrics and Gynecology 47(1): 248–262

Roopnarinesingh A J, Sirjusingh A, Bassaw B, Roopnarinesingh S 2002 Vaginal breech delivery and perinatal mortality in twins. Journal of Obstetrics and Gynaecology 22(3): 291–293

Scott P 2001 Waterbirth guidelines and frequently asked questions. Online. Available: www.activebirthpools.com (Accessed on 8 June 2004)

Smeenk A D J, ten Have H A M J 2003 Medicalisation and obstetric care: an analysis of developments in Dutch midwifery. Medicine, Healthcare and Philosophy 6: 153–165

Smith G C S, Pell J B, Dobbie R 2002 Birth order, gestational age and risk of delivery related perinatal death in twins: retrospective cohort study. British Medical Journal 325: 1004–1008

Wiegers T, Keirse M, van der Zee J, Berghs G. 1996 Outcome of planned home and planned hospital births in low risk pregnancies: prospective study in midwifery practices in the Netherlands. British Medical Journal 313: 1309–1313

Chapter 10

Evidence–based midwifery: finding, appraising and applying evidence in practice

Lesley Page, Michael Corkett, Rona McCandlish

In the first edition of this book Lesley Page (Page 2000) described the experiences which began her journey of development as an evidence-based midwife saying:

> My own interest in what we now call evidence-based care started when I practised as a midwife in Canada, providing care for women and their families through the whole process of pregnancy and birth, for the first time in my experience as a midwife. As I got to know these women as individuals, I became increasingly aware of the importance of doing the right things for them as individuals. Inevitably, as we came to know each other through the course of pregnancy, the parents would start to ask why certain things were undertaken as a routine. Intuitively, I guessed that many of these routines, which were imposed in our large maternity hospital, were unfounded. It was only when I started to search for evidence, so that I could make an argument for abandoning some routines for the women in my care, that I began to realize just how senseless some of the routines were. For example, there was a very strict rule that there was to be absolutely nothing to drink or eat in labour, yet many of the women I cared for wanted the freedom to eat and drink in labour. Thus, I started to investigate the evidence on the topic. This took me many hours. I contacted others who were undertaking research in the area in question, and used the library. Now, with a number of sources of synthesized evidence, the search for evidence is easier in some areas.

As reflected in Page's words evidence-based practice requires an awareness that care affects a constellation of important outcomes, ranging from the physical and emotional, personal and family integrity, to the wider social and economic. Finding and understanding evidence to inform decisions and choices about care will mean confronting uncertainty about what is best, or better, and dealing with frustration when the usefulness of evidence may not be straightforward. Although measurements of death or serious morbidity are conventionally used as key indicators of the effectiveness and quality of care these do not encompass the reality that pregnancy, birth and family life are more than physical 'events'. Measurement of the impact of maternity care is usually more complicated than simply 'counting' outcomes.

This throws up the most challenging aspect of practising evidence-based midwifery: the need to weigh up the validity and applicability of evidence about potential benefits and risks of certain choices and decisions whilst maintaining open and honest communication with women, families and colleagues. As a consequence evidence-based practice means that midwives often find themselves questioning long-standing routines in systems that are not easy to challenge. Effective questioning demands accumulating convincing evidence about what is likely to be effective care, developing effective skills to assemble and evaluate evidence, and then using it to change practice for the better. Simply retrieving evidence is not

sufficient to practising evidence-based care; there is no point in collecting highest quality best evidence if it is not used to improve practice and outcomes of care. Therefore the approach we describe in this chapter makes responding to the needs of women and their families the starting point for asking questions.

There are two fundamental questions in evidence-based midwifery:

1. Is what I intend to do likely to do more good than harm?
2. Am I spending my time doing the right things?

Every midwife can develop key skills to ask these questions, work through the answers and apply new learning, knowledge and insights effectively in her or his practice. The skills of lifelong learning and the ability to undertake independent enquiry are therefore crucial and this has implications both for the way in which midwives learn in basic education programmes and for continuing professional education.

In this chapter we will discuss evaluating care and effective care, and briefly outline some of the influences to the development of evidence-based maternity care in the UK.

EVALUATING AND ASSESSING THE EFFECTIVENESS OF CARE

During the second half of the 20th century in the UK the drive to improve safety of birth through hospitalization and the use of technology and medical diagnosis was marked by imposition of treatments and care that were largely unevaluated. This was demonstrated for example, by routine use of perineal shaving and enemas when women were admitted to the labour ward, and more recently in the increasing proportion of women who experience induction of labour and routine use of electronic fetal monitoring. Publication of the book Effective Care in Pregnancy and Childbirth (Chalmers et al 1989) brought about a greater awareness that the effects of maternity care should be rigorously evaluated. This seminal work was an important foundation for practitioners and consumers accessing care to understand different forms of evidence, and ways of judging the strength of that evidence, in deciding the probable effects of care. In addition, it synthesized much of the relevant evidence for reference. From this, the Cochrane Collaboration and the Cochrane Library were developed (www.cochrane.org).

The ability to evaluate and understand effects of care is crucial to the practice and provision of ethical healthcare. At its most benign not knowing the effects of an inert intervention mean its continued use with consequent misuse of limited healthcare resources. At worst, lack of evidence of effectiveness means that harmful practices are applied. There are clear instances of this in pregnancy and childbirth care when there has been unquestioned adoption of innovation which has led to avoidable tragedies. For example, Silverman (1980) describes the story of the 'epidemic' of neonatal retrolental fibroplasia which took hold in the 1950s in the USA. This is a dramatic example of a well-intentioned treatment – in this case the administration of high concentrations of oxygen to premature babies – which had unknown and unsuspected adverse consequences. The oxygen regimens resulted in blindness in large numbers of the babies who had received the treatment. This unintended harm could have been minimized if practitioners who advocated the use of high-concentration oxygen had been committed to asking questions about effectiveness (Box 10.1). This would have allowed them to evaluate whether the treatment they believed would work actually caused more good than harm. Instead, extremely vulnerable babies were exposed to a regimen of oxygen therapy which caused serious life-long morbidity. For lack of rigorous evaluation this form of care was continued for a decade longer than it should have been, and the concern it caused

> ## Box 10.1
>
> Effectiveness: . . . a measure of the extent to which a specific intervention, procedure, regimen, or service, when deployed in the field in routine circumstances, does what it is intended to do for a specific population.
>
> Cochrane 1972

still acts as an impediment to carrying out research about different oxygen regimes for neonates (Silverman 1998).

One of the difficulties about the term 'effectiveness' is that it is understood differently by different people. For example, imagine a policy of routine augmentation of labour is introduced for a trial period in your local labour ward to reduce the length of time women spend in labour care and that the effectiveness of the policy was measured after six months. The results of the evaluation show a reduction in the time women spent in labour care and therefore it is proposed that the policy be adopted. However, the midwife responsible for collating unit statistics points out that compared to the 6 month period previous to the introduction of the new policy, there has been a high rate of analgesia use and a high proportion of women have said they were dissatisfied with their experience of labour. This would suggest that measuring effectiveness using length of labour alone is inadequate and that adopting the policy would be unjustified as it could be associated with more harm than good. As this example demonstrates, judgements about the effects of care during pregnancy and childbirth, as in other areas, are neither value free nor situation free. Different observers see different problems and often reach different conclusions (Susser 1984, in Chalmers et al 1989) and it is vital to take these factors into account.

EVIDENCE-BASED CARE

The movement towards 'evidence-based healthcare' (Gray 1997) has been important in helping healthcare professionals and others, including policy-makers and managers, understand that research is carried out so that the results it yields can be used. It challenges practitioners to consider whether they are simply practising in the ways they were first taught, or in response to being 'told' by someone in authority, or perhaps from decisions based on personal opinion. Evidence-based practice requires active searching for, and appraisal of, research evidence to inform decisions about tests, treatments, patterns of practice, and policy. Although personal experience is an important basis to understanding what works and

why, it is rarely wide enough to give objective answers about the effects of particular tests and treatments.

Gray (1997, p. 213) describes evidence-based clinical practice as 'the judicious use of the best evidence available so that the clinician and the patient arrive at the best decision, taking into account the needs and values of the individual patient'. Evidence should be used to inform decisions in a number of areas: policy, guidelines for practice, the appropriate organization of care, public health decisions (about the use of resources, for example), clinical decisions and information to help women's choice, health promotion and education for parenting.

Other chapters describe ways of using evidence in practice and described the sources of information used to inform decisions about care. These are:

- individual values or preferences;
- the clinical examination;
- research evidence;
- the context of care.

In that chapter, five steps for the use of evidence in practice are described:

1. finding out what is important to the woman and her family;
2. using information from the clinical examination;
3. seeking and assessing evidence to inform decisions;
4. talking it through;
5. reflecting on outcomes, feelings and consequences.

We now focus on the third step: finding and critiquing the evidence.

Although evidence-based midwifery is about using rather than doing research, in common with primary research avoiding bias is fundamental when seeking, selecting and assessing evidence.

The process of using evidence in practice includes:

- framing clear and relevant questions that will lead to an effective search;
- planning an efficient search to answer the question;
- assessing and weighing up the evidence.

FRAMING CLEAR QUESTIONS

PRINCIPLES TO GOOD QUESTIONS

A pre requisite to finding the right and best evidence is the ability to convert a precise, yet possibly vaguely expressed, need into an answerable, focused, structured question (Rosenberg & Donald 1995, Straus et al 2005). Well-structured questions have four key components:

- Population – in the case of midwifery, women.
- Intervention – cause, prognostic factor, treatment.
- Comparison – control or comparative intervention.
- Outcome – ways in which the intervention effect is measured.

These are mnemonically referred to as PICO and provide a robust framework by which to execute a search. An additional component relating to study design can also be employed, and prove particularly helpful when improving the efficiency of a search (see Planning an efficient search). The most useful types of study design that may form part of a search include:

- Systematic reviews – literature reviews focused on a single question which identify, appraise and synthesize all relevant high quality research evidence.
- Meta-analyses – systematic reviews or overviews which employ quantitative methods to summarize the results.
- Randomized controlled trials – patients are randomized into intervention and control groups, and followed up for outcomes.
- Cohort studies – identification of two groups (cohorts), one of which normally received exposure to an intervention and one which did not, and followed up for outcomes.
- Case-series – reports on a series of patients with outcomes.

When including study design in a search it is important to remain aware of potential compromises to quality. Always consider the quality of study design – the number of patients treated, or group size; the duration of the study; the objective measurement of outcomes; and, the elimination of bias.

To assist the understanding and application of PICO to the midwifery setting Table 10.1 presents a modification of the work of Sackett et al (1997) and Straus et al (2005, p. 257–259).

It is worth noting that in the maternity services the majority of women and families start off being healthy, and the aim should be to keep them that way. Because of this, the potential for doing harm is greater. One of the problems of maternity care in much of the industrialized world is the routine treatment of women as if they were a high-risk population with a high probability of adverse outcomes. In reality, the risk of an adverse outcome is lower than it has ever been. Therefore, many of the questions that midwives ask arise from the need to determine whether or not a woman is in a high-risk group; or, has the woman a higher chance than usual of an adverse outcome.

EXERCISE

Consider your own practice and think of a number of questions about the routines you undertake, then apply the PICO framework to each.

For example, you may be looking after a woman who is experiencing leg cramps. The question might be:

- In a woman with a normal pregnancy, who suffers severe leg cramps at night, is calcium supplementation likely to help; and are there any likely harmful side effects to this supplementation?

Following the PICO framework the question can be illustrated as follows:

- Population = women with a normal pregnancy, who suffer severe leg cramps at night.
- Intervention = calcium supplementation.
- Comparison = an alternative intervention, for example exercise.
- Outcome(s) = reduction of leg cramps; harmful side effects to supplementation.

Now consider the following situation:

Mrs Smith is approaching term. She has prepared a birth plan indicating that she wishes to avoid intervention in labour. At her 39 weeks visit, the fundal height is 39 cm, the fetus is active, her blood pressure is 120/85, and there is no protein

Table 10.1   Comparisons of good questions. (Adapted from Sackett et al 1997, p. 27 with kind permission)

1. Woman or problem	2. Intervention (cause, prognostic factor, treatment)	3. Comparison intervention (if necessary)	4. Outcome(s)
Tips for building			
How would I best describe a group of women similar to mine?	Which main intervention or complication or 'risk factor' am I considering?	What is the probability of adverse outcome?	What can I hope to accomplish? What else would be affected?
Examples			
In women in early pregnancy who are vomiting most of the day.	Acupressure	No Acupressure	Acupressure leads to a reduction of vomiting and the experience of nausea?
In women without other complications	Who are grand multiparous (greater than gravida 5)	When compared with women who are less than gravida 5	Is there a greater probability of excessive bleeding, a need for blood transfusion, illness or death?
In women of 26 years of age	Who have an amniocentesis for the diagnosis of Down's syndrome	Who have not had amniocentesis for diagnosis of Down's syndrome	What is the probability of miscarriage? What is the probability of Down's syndrome? What are the sensitivity and specificity of the test?
In nulliparous women without complications	Who have an elective prelabour caesarean section	Rather than allowing labour and vaginal birth	What will the effect on perinatal mortality and morbidity, and maternal mortality and morbidity be?
In pregnant women	Who are over 40 years old	Compared with women of under 40 years of age	Is there a greater probability of adverse outcomes (e.g. perinatal mortality and higher intervention rates) as a result of age alone?

in the urine. At this visit, Mrs Smith wonders whether it is enough to listen to the fetal heart regularly or whether she should think about having continuous electronic monitoring.

Using what you have learnt about the PICO framework, and the examples provided in Table 10.1, write a question to guide your search for evidence in the box opposite. (Box 10.2)

The question might read:

Box 10.2   Write your response Here

In women at term, with no problems during pregnancy, would continuous electronic fetal monitoring, rather than intermittently listening to the fetal heart, lead to lower mortality and morbidity, and how would it affect intervention rates?

OTHER TYPES OF QUESTION

The questions considered so far have been concerned with the effect of particular interventions on outcomes of care. While this represents an important part of clinical practice, a further large and important field for consideration encompasses decisions made concerning risk, or the probability of adverse outcomes.

The most effective way to answer questions in this realm is to use systematic reviews and/or meta-analyses, which combine the results of a number of studies. This approach is particularly beneficial in those areas where a considerable number of individual studies exist, and it would be beyond the available time of clinicians to read and appraise each. For example, when Olsen undertook his meta-analysis of the studies of home birth, he identified 65 separate studies that met his criteria (Olsen 1997).

Midwives are fortunate to have available to them several evidence-based medicine resources that bypass the need to read and appraise numerous individual studies. These include the National Guideline Clearing House, a repository of high-quality international clinical guidelines; clinical guidelines produced in the UK by the National Institute for Health and Clinical Excellence (NICE), in particular those concerned with women's and children's health; the Cochrane Library, an extensive collection of rigorously appraised systematic reviews; and MIDIRS, a specialist midwifery information service. Further details on these resources can be found in Table 10.2.

Table 10.2   Resources for searching for evidence

Resource	Description	Access	Availability
National Guideline Clearinghouse	Comprehensive database of evidence-based clinical practice guidelines and related documents.	www.guidelines.gov	Free of charge
National Institute for Health and Clinical Excellence (NICE)	Organization responsible for providing UK guidance on promotion of good health. Includes evidence-based guidelines on maternal health.	www.nice.org.uk	Free of charge
Cochrane Library	International organization providing regularly updated evidence-based systematic reviews. Includes systematic reviews on maternal health.	www.cochrane.org	Free of charge
National Electronic Library for Health (NeLH)	Aimed at providing UK clinicians with the best current know-how and knowledge to support healthcare-related decisions. Includes a dedicated midwifery section.	www.nelh.nhs.uk	Free of charge
MIDIRS digest	High quality research papers from journals are selected by the midwife editor and abstracted.	Hardcopy digest	Subscription

Table 10.2 *Continued*

Resource	Description	Access	Availability
MIDIRS database searches	Standard and individual searches are available that scan the content of 500 English language journals, including midwifery, obstetrics and gynaecology, paediatrics, neonatal and key general medical and consumer titles.	www.midirs.org	Subscription
Bandolier	Evidence-based healthcare journal providing concise and easy to read summaries of the latest systematic reviews and meta-analyses. Includes maternal health section.	www.ebandolier.com	Free of charge
Clinical Evidence	Summarizes current knowledge and uncertainty about the prevention and treatment of clinical conditions, based on thorough searches and appraisal of the best available evidence. Includes section on maternal health.	www.clinicalevidence.com	Free of charge
Medline	The National Library of Medicine (US) online database of approximately 15 million biomedical and pharmaceutical citations, searched via natural language and/or controlled vocabulary.		Subscription
PubMed	The National Library of Medicine service, providing access to Medline back to the 1950s. Includes links to many full text articles and related resources.	www.ncbi.nlm.nih.gov/entrez	Free of charge
Embase	A powerful database providing access to several million biomedical citations, via natural language and/or controlled vocabulary searches.		Subscription
CINAHL	Database regarded as the authoritative source of information for the professional literature of nursing, allied health, biomedicine, and healthcare.		Subscription

PLANNING AN EFFICIENT SEARCH

Having devised a structured question it is possible to begin the search for evidence. Searching for evidence has been described as an essential clinical skill that demands to be efficient (Sackett et al 1997). With the unmanageable volume of information available to health professionals well documented, the need for efficiency is crucial (Greenhalgh 1997).

When planning a search it is important to consider the kind of evidence needed, and where it is most likely to be found. Research may be published or unpublished, can be found in non-peer-reviewed or peer-reviewed journals, and vary widely in quality (see Principles of good questions). Also, it is important to know how much time can be realistically spent, not only searching for but also appraising the evidence retrieved.

Midwives may elect to use resources that bypass the need to execute searches themselves. Beyond those previously described, there are also useful journals that provide structured abstracts as a means to alert clinicians to important advances, and up-to-date books, which may prove particularly useful for understanding physiology.

Many clinicians, however, are likely to execute searches by themselves using one or more biomedical database. The best well known are Medline, Embase, and the Cumulative Index to Nursing and Allied Health Literature, commonly known as CINAHL.

It is important to appreciate that confining a search to only one database risks the exclusion of either a majority, or large minority, of the available evidence. Research has demonstrated that using only one database to identify evidence is inadequate (Suarez-Almazor et al 2000). The overlap between Medline and Embase, in terms of journals indexed, is about 40% (Smith et al 1992), and studies have demonstrated that using both databases markedly improves the coverage of literature (Biarez et al 1991, Odaka et al 1992).

A considered search strategy is important when using resources such as Medline and Embase, each consisting of several million records. While Greenhalgh (1997) says that most people can learn to carry out a basic search of either database inside an hour, it is worthwhile investing some time in preparation and design of a search strategy before the searching begins in earnest. Straus et al (2005) provide a diagram of the steps for executing a pragmatic search for evidence (Fig. 10.1).

When using databases to search for evidence problems may be experienced. A search strategy may be highly sensitive, which will result in too much evidence, or a search may prove too specific, which will considerably lessen the return of evidence.

To counter such difficulties preparation is the key. Depending upon the results of a search it may prove necessary to narrow or widen the date range being searched; limit or expand the population sub-groups; determine the quality of evidence being sought; or limit evidence to that published in English. Most important of all, understand what it is that is actually being sought. Has a focused, well-structured question been asked? Has a population, comparison, intervention, outcome, and, if necessary, study design, been identified? Are the correct resources being employed that will most likely hold the evidence sought, and best utilize the available time?

The resources listed in Table 10.2 are examples, together with descriptions, that will greatly assist the search for evidence.

BASIC MEDLINE AND EMBASE SEARCH

A basic search for evidence using Medline or Embase can be undertaken in two ways:

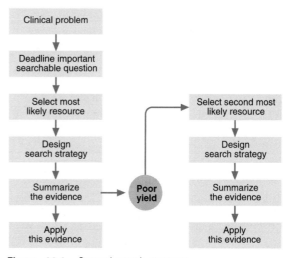

Figure. 10.1   General search strategy

- using *natural language* (text words) to seek particular authors and institutions where research is carried out, and words in the title and/or abstract;
- using *Medical Subject Headings* (MeSH), or the controlled vocabulary of the databases, that constitute powerful theasuri.

An individual's ability to search for evidence will be greatly enhanced if they acquire an understanding of the following skills, adapted from Sackett et al (1997, p.73):

- the use of *both* natural language and MeSH;
- the identification of MeSH using the thesauri;
- the ability to identify *synonyms* directly related to MeSH and incorporate them into a search;
- the appropriate use of *search field tags* (e.g. abstract = .ab; author = .au; paper title word = .ti; textword = .tw);
- the ability to use search field tags as *limiters* (e.g. publication type = .pt; publication year = .py);
- the appropriate *truncation* of natural language and use of *wildcards* to replace characters within words;
- the ability to employ *adjacency commands* so linking words or phrases to each other;
- combining natural language, including search field tags, and MeSH by using *Booleon operators* (AND, OR, NOT) to expand and limit a search.

Medical librarians and information specialists have historically been regarded as experts in the field of searching for evidence; however, today there are many opportunities, via dedicated training courses and/or self-tuition, for health professionals to learn how to conduct effective and efficient searches.

ASSESSING AND INTERPRETING THE EVIDENCE

Once you consider that you have found the appropriate information to answer your question, it is necessary to assess the quality of the information to ensure that it is right for your purposes and that it provides valid evidence to answer your question. There are several accessible books that detail structured approaches to assessing research

reports (see especially Greenhalgh 1997, Gray 1997, Sackett et al 1997, Straus et al 2005).

An essential first step in assessing the evidence is to discard poor-quality or irrelevant reports. Greenhalgh (1997) emphasizes the need to 'trash' papers and suggests that 'some purists would say 99% of published articles belong in the bin' (p. 34). She makes a strong argument that the quality of a paper is best assessed through the methods section and that the article should be 'trashed' on methods alone before looking at the results. She suggests three preliminary and basic questions as a way of getting an orientation to the paper are:

1. Why was the study done, what were the hypotheses, and what were the authors testing?
2. What type of study was carried out?
3. Was this research appropriate to the broad field of research studied?

Sackett et al (1997) propose the following questions to assess evidence:

- Is it true (valid)?
- Are the valid results important?
- Does it apply to the woman/women in my care?

VALIDITY (BOX 10.3)

When reviewing evidence from a study both internal and external validity (Box 10.3) of the results need to be considered. Internal validity is concerned with whether selection of groups and the way comparisons were carried out between the study's groups were sufficiently robust so that any reported difference is likely to be attributable to the effect being measured. External validity is concerned with the extent to which research findings can be generalized to people who are

---

Box 10.3

Validity: The degree to which the inference drawn from a study, especially generalizations extending beyond the study sample, are warranted when account is taken of the study methods, the representativeness of the study sample, and the nature of the population from which it is drawn.

Last 1995

similar to the participants but who did not take part in the study. A fundamental point when assessing evidence, and the validity of a study, is to question whether the methodology used is appropriate to the question posed (Box 10.4).

IMPORTANCE

Assessment of importance is related to the

- size and potential benefits of the effects measured in a study;
- probability of outcomes occurring over time;

Box 10.4   Broad topics of research

Most research studies are concerned with one or more of the following:

- Therapy – testing the efficacy of drug treatments, surgical procedures, alternative methods of service delivery, or other interventions. Preferred study design is randomized controlled trial.
- Diagnosis – demonstrating whether a new diagnostic test is valid (can we trust it?) and reliable (would we get the same results every time?). Preferred study design is cross sectional survey . . . in which both the new test and the gold standard test are performed
- Screening – demonstrating the value of tests that can be applied to large populations and that pick up disease at a presymptomatic stage. Preferred study design is cross sectional survey.
- Prognosis–determining what is likely to happen to someone whose disease is picked up at an early stage. Preferred study design is longitudinal cohort study.
- Causation–determining whether a putative harmful agent, such as environmental pollution, is related to the development of illness. Preferred study design is cohort or case-control study, depending on how rare the disease is . . . but case reports . . . may also provide crucial information.

Reproduced from Greenhalgh T 1997 How to read a paper. With kind permission from BMJ Books, BMJ Publishing Group.

- strength of association between the outcomes (either harmful or good) and interventions;
- increased probability of particular outcomes in different groups;
- precision of the estimates of effect.

Established methods are applied to numerical data reported in a study which are used to assess the importance of the results. For example, Straus et al (2005) describe the method to calculate how many people need to be treated to avoid an adverse outcome (number needed to treat; NNT) or to harm one person (number needed to harm; NNH). Measures of importance, strength of association and precision include relative risks, absolute risk reduction, Number needed to treat (NNT), and number needed to harm (NNH), odds, odds ratios and confidence intervals. The explanations of the terms by Straus et al (1998, pp. 141–145, 2005 pp.281–284) are outlined below:

- Odds – a ratio of non-events to events. If the event rate for a disease is 0.1 (10%), its non-event rate is 0.9 and therefore its odds are 9:1. Note this is not the same as the inverse of event rate.
- Odds ratio (OR) – is the odds of having the target disorder in the experimental group relative to the odds in favour of having the target disorder in the control group or the odds of being exposed in subjects with the target disorder divided by the odds in favour of being exposed in control subjects (without the target disorder).
- Risk ratio (RR) – is the ratio of risk in the treated group (EER) to the risk in the control group (CER) RR = ERR/CER.
- Relative risk reduction (RRR) – the proportional reduction in rates of bad outcomes between experimental and control groups.
- Absolute risk reduction (ARR) – the absolute arithmetic difference in rates of bad outcomes between experimental and control groups.
- Number needed to treat (NNT) – the number of patients who need to be treated to achieve one additional favourable outcome, calculated as 1/ARR and accompanied by a 95% confidence interval. If the ARR is 25% 1/25% = 4.
- Number Needed to Harm – the number of patients who need to be treated to achieve one additional unfavourable outcome, calculated as

1/ARR and accompanied by a 95% confidence interval. If the ARR is 25% 1/25% = 4.

- Confidence interval (CI) – expresses the range within which we would expect the true value of a statistical measure to fall. Few studies can be carried out amongst all of the people who would be eligible to experience the care or therapy being assessed. Therefore for a particular research study a sample is selected comprising people who it is hoped will be representative of the relevant population. This means that the results of that study should be considered as an estimate of measured effect(s), and need to be placed in the context of the likely upper and lower value of the effect should the same study be repeated with different representative samples. CIs are usually accompanied by a percentage value, which shows the level of confidence that we have that true value lies within this range. For example, for an NNT of 10 with a 95% CI of 5–15, we would have 95% confidence that the true value of NNT values was between 5–15.

APPLICATION TO WOMEN AND FAMILIES IN YOUR CARE

Questions of application are concerned with the similarity between the women and families in your care and those in reported research and should take into account their individual preferences and values.

APPRAISING EVIDENCE FOR VALIDITY AND IMPORTANCE

The assessment of the validity of particular studies will depend on the type of evidence used. Sackett et al (1997) propose the following categories:

- diagnosis
- prognosis
- harm
- therapy
- systematic reviews
- decision analysis
- qualitative research.

The following is based on the work of Straus et al (1998, 2005), using their categories for structured steps for appraisal. We have summarized many of the suggestions from three sources: Sackett et al (1997), Straus et al (1998, 2005) and the handbook from the 1998 Oxford workshop on teaching evidence-based medicine (University of Oxford 1998).

DIAGNOSIS

One of the most rapidly changing fields of maternity care lies in diagnosis and screening, particularly during the antenatal period. Midwives should be able to appraise current evidence and convey the accuracy of results to the women and families in their care. This area is perhaps one of the most complex of practice (see Chapter 11), and an understanding of key terms, such as sensitivity and specificity (see Box 10.5), is crucial not only to interpreting evidence, but also to interpreting test results and understanding their predictive value in practice.

> **Box 10.5   Diagnostic tests: key terms (reproduced from Sackett et al 1997, with permission)**
>
> Sensitivity: the proportion of people with the target disorder who have a positive test. It is used to assist in assessing and selecting a diagnostic test/sign/symptom.
>
> SnNout: when a sign/test/symptom has a high sensitivity, a negative result rules out the diagnosis.
>
> Specificity: the proportion of people without the target disorder who have a negative test. It is used to assist in assessing and selecting a diagnostic test/sign/symptom.
>
> SpPin: when a sign/symptom has a high specificity, a positive result rules in the diagnosis.
>
> Positive predictive value: the proportion of people with a positive test who have the target disorder.
>
> Negative predictive value: the proportion of people with a negative test who are free of the target disorder.

Results There were a positive, highly significant association between increasing maternal age and obstetric intervention prelabour ($P < 0.001$) and emergency ($P < 0.001$) caesarean section, instrumental vaginal delivery (spontaneous labour $P < 0.001$; induced labour $P = 0.001$), induction of labour ($P < 0.001$). Epidural usage in induced labour and the incidence of small for gestational age newborns did not increase with increasing maternal age ($P = 0.68$ and $P = 0.50$, respectively).

Conclusions This study demonstrates that increasing age is associated with an incremental increase in obstetric intervention. Previous studies have demonstrated a significant effect in women older than 35 years of age, but these data show changes on a continuum from teenage years. This finding may reflect a progressive, age-related deterioration in myometrial function.

(Reproduced with kind permission from Blackwell Science Ltd.)

We can look at this paper against the framework of two of Sackett et al's (1997) questions:

Was a defined, representative sample of patients assembled at a common (usually early) point in the course of their disease?

This was a retrospective review of what is described as 'prospectively' gathered data which had been routinely collected. Information that might help to explain and define some of the measures (for example, the definition and diagnosis of fetal distress) was missing from the data collection. There are important gaps in the reported data, for example about the early pregnancy of women who participated in the study and about diagnosis of fetal distress. There are a number of indications in the report that the population studied may be different from the normal population of women giving birth. For example, the intervention rate in the hospital in which the study took place was described as higher than average and the women who were part of the study were described as having a higher than average age, and a larger proportion of 'career women'. This limits the confidence with which we might generalize the findings as the women in this study may not be representative of women in other populations. Length of follow-up was appropriate in a study that was concerned only with intervention rates.

Were objective criteria applied in a blind fashion?

Some of the criteria, for example operative delivery, are objective; others, such as failure to progress and fetal distress, are more subjective measures. There is no clear definition of criteria for the diagnosis of fetal distress and failure to progress (both of these being prone to bias in clinical interpretation). There is no mention of blinding for interpretation or for analysis. There was also no adjustment for prognostic factors. It is also possible that higher anxiety experienced by health professionals attending older women may be a factor in increasing the rate of interventions in older women, and as this study has not tested this important hypothesis. In studies examining the effect of maternal age on outcome that are adequately controlled for factors which may confound the outcomes, no significant differences are found (Harker & Thorpe 1992). There is no control or reanalysis for confounding factors, such as raised blood pressure, in this study.

The higher incidence of epidural analgesia in spontaneous labour may well have been an independent factor in increasing the intervention rate. Moreover, there is no mention of the fetal monitoring rate, which is likely to have been higher in this group of women, and which is in itself associated with a higher rate of intervention and a falsely high rate of diagnosis of fetal distress. A number of factors, including mobility and position in labour, may have affected the outcome; but none of these are described in the report. In addition, the lack of clear definition of failure to progress and fetal distress, which may be highly subjective assessments, is a fundamental flaw in this study. Attendant anxiety may well have affected the judgements made, in itself leading to a higher rate of intervention.

In assessing this study it is important to be aware of the idea that labelling particular women as being at increasing risk of intervention in labour becomes a self-fulfilling prophecy. It is quite likely that attendant anxiety or perception is likely to affect the outcome of labour (and this has not been refuted by this study). There is a danger of the outcomes of such studies being confounded, that is, being affected by other factors than the one under study, in this case increasing age. Examples of potential confounders in this group of women would be the pre-existence of medical problems in subgroups of older women, or the tendency of health professionals to treat older women as being at higher risk, leading to a higher rate of continuous electronic fetal monitoring, which in itself produces a higher intervention rate. Unfortunately, the authors of this study did not heed the warnings of one of the papers they referenced (Harker & Thorpe 1992) and did not control for such confounding factors.

Is this evidence about prognosis important?

In relation to importance, two questions are relevant:

1. How probable are the outcomes over time?
2. How precise are the prognostic estimates?

Given the flaws of the study, its validity is in doubt and therefore it would not be appropriate to determine the importance.

Two further questions then follow.

Were the study patients similar to your own, and will this evidence make a clinically important impact on your conclusions about what to offer or tell your patients?

In this case, the flaws which have been identified in response to the questions above lead to the conclusion that the results are not valid. Therefore it would not be appropriate to change practice on the basis of the evidence from this study. Perhaps the only change in practice that should be considered would be to be more aware that bias caused by regarding older women as inherently at risk of adverse outcomes can itself increase the intervention rate.

HARM

Is this evidence about harm valid?

Straus et al (2005, p. 179) propose the following questions to assess the validity of studies to evaluate the possibility of harm:

1. Were there clearly defined groups of patients, similar in all-important ways other than exposure to the treatment or other cause?

2. Were treatment exposures and clinical outcomes measured the same ways in both groups (e.g. was the assessment of outcomes either objective (for example, death) or blinded to exposure)?
3. Was the follow up of study patients complete and long enough?
4. Do the results satisfy some 'diagnostic tests for causation'?
   - Is it clear that the exposure preceded the onset of the outcome?
   - Is there a dose response gradient?
   - Is there positive evidence from a challenge–rechallenge study?
   - Is the association consistent from study to study?
   - Does the association make biological sense?

This is a question of whether or not a treatment *caused* the harmful outcome experienced and thus, as Sackett et al (1997) tell us, 'benefits from what has been learned from classical epidemiology'. There are four possible designs for a study of the harmful effects of treatments. These are the randomized controlled trial, the cohort study, the case control study, or reports of one or two patients who have suffered from something that is unique and rare. Table 10.3 is a summary of the advantages and disadvantages of these approaches, as described by Sackett et al 1997.

Using evidence to inform practice

Let us look at the above questions with regard to a study to examine the effect of neonatal exposure to vitamin K on the risk of childhood cancer (Klebanoff et al 1993). The relationship between vitamin K and cancer was examined in a nested case control study that used data from the Collaborative Perinatal Project, a multicentre, prospective study of pregnancy, delivery and childhood that took place in the USA. Among 54,795 children born between 1959 and 1966, 48 cases of cancer were diagnosed after the first day of life and before the eighth birthday. Each case child was matched with randomly selected controls whose last study visit occurred at or after the age when the case child's cancer was diagnosed.

Table 10.3 Advantages and disadvantages of different kinds of harm study. (From Sackett et al 1997, with kind permission)

Type of study	Advantages	Disadvantages
Randomized controlled trial	Randomization would make groups similar for all other features that would cause harm	For rare events, very large trials would be needed (one per thousand would need 3000 patients in order to be 95% certain of seeing at least one adverse reaction)
Cohort study	Next most powerful design	The groups of patients (cohorts) may not be identical in every respect. Other things apart from the treatment being evaluated such as severity of illness may affect outcome. Same problem of size applies
Case control studies	For rare or late complications of treatment, need to rely on studies in which those who already have the disease are assembled and compared with a group who do not have the disease	The problem of confounding (of prognosis with exposure) is worse with case control studies because it may be impossible to measure confounders in a case even if they are known
Case reports and case series	Reports of one or two patients who developed a complication while under treatment (e.g. phocomelia in children born to women who took thalidomide)	May be enough but usually point to the need for further studies

Were there clearly defined groups of patients, similar in all-important ways other than exposure to the treatment or other cause?
The rarity of the disease in this case makes a randomized controlled trial impractical for answering the question of harm and makes the case control study the only practical design. Attempts were made to adjust for factors that might be associated with the development of childhood cancer (for example, race, sex, birth weight, maternal age, exposure to X-rays during pregnancy, and breastfeeding). Nevertheless, we cannot be confident that the groups were similar in every respect.

Were treatment exposures and clinical outcomes measured in the same ways in both groups (e.g. was the assessment of outcomes either objective, for example death, or blinded to exposure)?
The report states that 'two investigators who were

blinded to the child's vitamin K status examined all records of children with cancer. Definite cases of cancer were required to have a histologically proved diagnosis of cancer, a clinical course including treatment consistent with the diagnosis or both' (Klebanoff et al 1993, p. 905).

Was the follow-up study of patients complete and long enough? There is no account of loss to follow-up, but the authors state that, afterwards, loss to follow-up was accounted for by life table methods. The study followed children up to 8 years of age.

Do the results satisfy some diagnostic tests for causation?
- *Is it clear that the exposure preceded the onset of the outcome?* It is as clear as can be that the exposure preceded the outcome. There was

reclassification for children with cancer before their first birthday, and therefore with the possibility that the cancer started in pregnancy.

■ *Is there a dose–response gradient?* No dose–response gradient was available, but babies whose mothers were given vitamin K in the intrapartum period were excluded. All babies received the intramuscular vitamin K. In addition, there was an analysis of effect according to the brand of vitamin K used. There was then reanalysis to exclude the children in whom the administration of vitamin K was uncertain.

Because this was part of a larger study not aimed primarily at the evaluation of the effect of vitamin K, it is particularly important to be sure that vitamin K was actually administered when it was recorded and that all vitamin K was recorded when given. Recording in this situation was probably more careful because this was part of a research study with special documentation that was checked for completeness. In addition, there was recording by an observer in the delivery room of any drugs administered.

■ *Is there positive evidence from a challenge–rechallenge study?* The challenge–rechallenge question (seeing what happens if a drug is withdrawn or re-administered) is not appropriate to this drug.
■ *Is the result consistent from study to study?* The answer to this is no. The authors comment on two earlier studies including an evaluation of the effect of the administration of oral vitamin K that found twice the expected risk of cancer

during childhood with the administration of vitamin K.
■ *Does the association make biological sense?* There is no biological link made explicit in this study, but the fact that the incidence of childhood cancer has not increased with the frequent administration of vitamin K at birth increases confidence in the findings of the study.

Are the valid results from this harm study important?

Importance is evaluated against an estimation of the strength of the association between receiving the treatment and suffering the adverse effect. Strength here means the risk or odds of the adverse effect, with, as opposed to without, exposure to the treatment; the higher the risk or odds, the greater the strength and the more one should be impressed with it. Different tactics are used for estimating the strength of the association for different research methods. This is illustated in Table 10.4.

Using the data presented in the paper on vitamin K (Klebanoff et al 1993), this calculation is as shown in Table 10.5 and shows that, in this case, there is no association between Vitamin K and cancer.

Can the study results be extrapolated to your patient?

Given the situation in the USA, with such different demographic characteristics, direct extrapolation is not appropriate. One factor that is pointed out by the authors as being different is that the vehicle

Table 10.4 Calculating the strength of an association between a treatment and subsequent adverse outcomes. (Reproduced from Sackett et al 1997, with kind permission)

		Adverse outcome		Totals
		Present (Case)	Absent (Control)	
Exposed to the treatment	Yes (Cohort)	a	b	a+b
	No (Cohort)	c	d	c+d
	Totals	a+c	b+d	a+b+c+d

In a randomized trial or cohort study: relative risk = RR = [a/(a+b)]/[c/(c+d)] In a case-control study: relative odds = RO = ad/bc

Table 10.5 Calculating the strength of an association between vitamin K and cancer

		Adverse Outcome	
		Present (Case)	Absent (Control)
Exposed to the treatment	Yes vitamin K	33 a	171 b
	No vitamin K Controls	c 15	d 69
		$\dfrac{33.69}{15.171}$	$\dfrac{2277}{2565} = 0.89$

of administration of the vitamin K differs between the USA and the UK.

THERAPY

If one wants to find out whether a treatment is likely to be of benefit, the most appropriate methodology to answer the question is a randomized controlled trial. There are so many factors that might influence the outcome of treatment that the only good way to control for possible sources of bias is to allocate people randomly to different treatment conditions.

In this section, we will look at assessing the evidence from a single study. If several studies are available, the investigator should first look for a systematic review and use that as a starting point.

Before going on to assess the results of a study, one must first ask the following questions.

Are the results of this single study valid?

The key questions to answer, following Straus et al (2005, p. 117) are:

1. Was the assignment of patients to treatments randomized?
2. And was the randomization list concealed?
3. Were patients and clinicians kept blind to which treatment was being received?
4. Aside from the experimental treatment, were the groups treated equally?
5. Were the groups similar at the start of the trial?

Studies of treatment (or therapy) compare outcomes in groups receiving the treatment with outcomes in groups either not receiving treatment or receiving an alternative treatment. It is essential that, at the outset, the groups being compared are as alike as possible. The only way to avoid bias when assigning people to groups is to make the assignments random. This does not guarantee that the groups will be identical, but it does ensure that any differences are more likely to be caused by chance alone.

For example, imagine that you are looking for a treatment for pregnancy-induced nausea and have heard that acupuncture worked. You decide to test this out by carrying out a randomized controlled trial to compare women who have been allocated acupuncture with those who have not. If you are testing the effectiveness of acupuncture compared to another form of care you would want to make sure that your groups consisted of a mixture of women with different severities of the condition, different lifestyles and a different tolerance of the symptoms: Uneven distribution of these factors between groups may confound your results by providing an alternative explanation for any result that you see, for example by exaggerating, counteracting or even cancelling out the effects of the therapy. If the random allocation is concealed from clinicians, they will be unaware of the treatment that the patient is receiving and will not be able to distort the effect, either consciously or unconsciously.

It would be important to set up a system so that you can ensure that you can account for all the women who were randomized, right through to the end of follow-up. This means that you would make every effort to account for women who were randomized but who dropped out from follow-up It is possible to analyse and report the results of a trial even when there has been 'loss' to follow-up by assigning those participants the 'worst' value of the outcome of interest. In the example of acupuncture for nausea in pregnancy, all the participants who did not contribute information to follow-up might be considered to have experienced no improvement in nausea. However, as a rule of thumb, this approach is not useful if more than 20% of participants are lost to follow-up.

The correct method for a randomized controlled trial is to analyse results by 'intention-to-treat'. This means that the data are analysed according to the groups to which the participants were assigned when they were first randomized in the trial, and not according to their experience of care after assignment. For example, in a randomized controlled trial of home birth to assess the effect of home birth on intervention rates a number of women are likely to be transferred to hospital to give birth because of failure to progress or some other problem. If intention-to-treat analysis was not used to analyse the results, and outcomes are evaluated according to the location of birth, there would be a falsely low intervention rate in the home birth group. An intention to treat analysis provides an estimate of the effects of interventions in practice, by taking into account the reality that care and therapies do not always happen exactly as defined or prescribed.

In real practice it is often impossible to conceal (blind) the nature of allocated treatment/care for participants and clinicians. However it may be possible to have the outcomes being evaluated assessed by people who are unaware of what the original allocation was.

Are the results of this single preventive or therapeutic trial important?

Straus et al (2005, pp 126–130) propose calculating the number needed to treat (NNT), as a way of concealing how relevant and important the results of a study would be to the people you are working with. If a valid study found, for example, that you needed to treat four people to have one respond to the treatment, this gives a clear indication of how many people you would need to treat and the chance of a response in the population of people you are caring for. The view of these numbers differs for the midwife and the childbearing woman. A midwife may want to know that for every four women she treats, one will respond to treatment. For the childbearing woman, the most useful presentation of these figures is that she has a 1 in 4 chance of responding to therapy.

SYSTEMATIC REVIEW AND META-ANALYSIS

Although it is important to critically appraise the results of individual research studies, there are instances when it is possible to identify topics for which major work has already been achieved to synthesize and review evidence from several studies. In maternity care the Cochrane Library (www.cochrane org) is probably the most well-known important resource of reliable reviews of evidence. Increasingly other agencies are publishing the results of commissioned reviews to inform care (for example NICE May 2005, HTA 2005). Differences between systematic review and meta-analysis are outlined below.

A systematic review is a review that includes explicit and detailed description of why and how it was conducted so that it should be possible to replicate it (Jahad 1998). In should clearly state a research question and methods used to assemble data, explicitly taking into account issues such as bias, confounding and chance in interpretation of findings. Ideally its authors should seek to bring together research from all relevant evidence sources. It should clearly present the results of individual studies but should not combine results unless it is appropriate statistically to do so and issues such as bias and heterogeneity between studies have been satisfactorily dealt with.

Meta-analysis is a method of combining statistically the results of independent research studies, which are sufficiently similar, to generate a single estimate of effect for a particular treatment or therapy. The benefit to using this method is that it can increase the precision of the estimate of effect, thereby reducing uncertainty about what the range of the estimate is likely to be.

Straus et al (2005, p. 148) propose the following questions to test the validity of a systematic review:

1. Is it an overview of RCTs of the treatment you are interested in?
2. Does it include a methods section that describes:
   a. Finding and including all the relevant trials?

b. Assessing their individual validity?

3. Were the results consistent from study to study?

The first question asks whether you are sure that the treatment is the same as the one you are interested in and the others whether all the studies were carried out at the same, most powerful level of evidence.

For example, if a randomized controlled trial of vitamin K prophylaxis were available and you wanted to know whether oral vitamin K were effective, you would want to ask whether it was oral or IM vitamin K that had been tested.

Some overviews combine randomized and non-randomized studies. It is wrong to combine results from these different research methods and we would advise that you should not use results from such reviews to change practice.

DOES IT INCLUDE A METHODS SECTION THAT DESCRIBES (A) FINDING AND INCLUDING ALL THE RELEVANT TRIALS, AND (B) ASSESSING THEIR INDIVIDUAL VALIDITY?

The most important point to remember is that carrying out a systematic review is just like carrying out research. In other words, it uses the same approach as research to avoid bias and should be reported like research. As in the assessment of research, look carefully at the methods section. This should include a description of how the studies were identified which were included and excluded, and why. Straus et al (2005, p. 149) describe the importance of having sought unpublished results and of hand-searching for reports. The methods section should also say how the validity of the study was judged.

Were the results consistent from study to study?

Although we should not expect all trials to show exactly the same degree of effectiveness, it is reassuring if the results are not widely different.

Are the results of this systematic review important?

Deciding whether or not a treatment is important depends on the size and potential benefits of the effects of the treatment you are interested in.

Do these results apply to your patient?

- Is your patient so different from those in the overview that its results can't help you?
- How great would the potential benefit of therapy actually be for your individual patient (e.g. what is the NNT/NNH)?
- Do your patients and you have a clear assessment of their values and preferences?
- Are they met by this regimen and its consequences?

It is crucial to remember that systematic reviews and meta-analyses are no better than the studies they combine therefore applying critical appraisal methods to both is necessary.

ASSESSING QUALITATIVE RESEARCH

Qualitative research is important to all professionals working in the maternity services, but it is perhaps most important to midwives. Midwives hold the potential for strong and intimate relationships with childbearing women and their families as well as the potential for changing the experience of care and of pregnancy and birth.

Greenhalgh (1997, p. 151) describes clearly the limitations of quantitative research and the importance of qualitative research in 'seeking a deeper truth'. She quotes the aim of qualitative research as being 'to study things in their natural setting, attempting to make sense of, or interpret, phenomena in terms of the meanings that people bring to them', and that researchers use a 'holistic perspective which preserves the complexity of human behaviour (Denzin & Lincoln 1994)'. The contribution of social science and anthropology in researching maternity care is immense and provides a mine of information regarding the perspectives of childbearing women using the maternity services and their experiences, to inform midwives who want to understand better and improve care.

Greenhalgh (1997, see pp 155–61) suggests the following questions for assessing qualitative research. She is clear about the limits of such a checklist, and it should be used with caution. Qualitative research is by its very nature non-standard; and this list of questions is taken from

Greenhalgh to provide a structure. However, it is advisable to read Greenhalgh's chapter in full and to refer to the list of further reading at the end of that chapter.

DID THE PAPER DESCRIBE AN IMPORTANT CLINICAL PROBLEM EXAMINED THROUGH A CLEARLY FORMULATED QUESTION?

As with quantitative research, the topic area needs to be clearly defined. The process is iterative so the question may emerge more clearly at the end of the project, although it should still be clearly stated.

WAS A QUALITATIVE APPROACH APPROPRIATE?

It is most appropriate when the objective is to explore, interpret or obtain a deeper understanding of a particular issue.

HOW WERE THE SETTING AND SUBJECTS SELECTED?

The study should go beyond a convenience sample to a theoretical sample. Instead of taking an average view, the aim is to achieve an in-depth understanding of particular individuals, for example, a group of Somali women receiving maternity care in west London.

WHAT WAS THE RESEARCHER'S VIEW, AND HAS THIS BEEN TAKEN INTO ACCOUNT?

It is important to recognize that there is no way of controlling for observer bias in qualitative research. It is thus important that the investigator's personal perspective is fully explained.

WHAT METHODS DID THE RESEARCHER USE FOR COLLECTING DATA, AND ARE THESE DESCRIBED IN ENOUGH DETAIL?

The methods section is likely to be lengthy and discursive. You should ask the question. 'Have I been given enough information on methods?' There are no hard and fast rules.

WHAT METHODS DID THE RESEARCHER USE TO ANALYSE THE DATA, AND WHAT QUALITY CONTROL MEASURES WERE IMPLEMENTED?

The researcher must have found a systematic way of analysing the data. A number of methods are available, which include content analysis. A good paper will describe a method of quality control; in other words, it will not depend on just the interpretation of one person.

ARE THE RESULTS CREDIBLE?

The results should be independently and objectively verifiable. Are they sensible and believable, and do they matter in practice?

WHAT CONCLUSIONS WERE DRAWN, AND WERE THEY JUSTIFIED BY THE RESULTS?

Greenhalgh suggests using these three questions:

- How well does this analysis explain why people behave in the way they do?
- How comprehensive would this explanation be to a thoughtful participant in the setting?
- How well does the explanation cohere with what we already know? (Mays & Pope 1996).

CONCLUSION

It is easy to feel overwhelmed by the never-ending deluge of information about developments and changes in practice and care. The world-wide web has given everyone with access the possibility of finding almost infinite sources of information and sources of evidence that healthcare practitioners use are increasingly available to the women and families using maternity services. This should lead to invigorating information-sharing and into exciting and innovative realms of practice. However it must not mean abdication of responsibility by midwives for retrieving and appraising evidence, and thinking through its implications to midwifery practice and to the wellbeing and health of women and families. In this chapter we outlined structured and systematic approaches to use to find, assess and evaluate evidence. Just as you would apply a structure when undertaking a clinical examination, this framework will help you to make sure that you have covered key issues and think through whether there is anything important that has been missed out.

It is important not to be intimidated by the mystique and sense of élitism that sometimes surrounds research in midwifery. Do not be afraid to make judgements about whether or not research findings make sense on a basic level. Your everyday experience and the knowledge you gain from practice give you an important basis for judging whether or not things simply make sense. Although you should be aware of the limitations of personal knowledge in making generalizations, your general sense about whether or not a piece of research is 'somehow just not right' can be an invaluable tool to cut through the information 'jungle'.

We believe that asking questions that arise from practice and being able to find, evaluate, and implement the findings of research are crucial to ensuring that midwifery care is likely to be beneficial and to avoid harm. However, we often find that there is no strong evidence to help answer questions arising from practice. In that case, the challenge is to be honest about the sources we use for answering questions and dealing with uncertainty. For us, and we think for midwifery practice generally, the guiding principals of effective evidence-based midwifery are to make use of the best evidence possible to underpin ethical maternity care for all women and their families. And always to be prepared to challenge ourselves – as much as others!

POINTERS FOR PRACTICE

- Above all, evidence-based practice demands that practitioners constantly question whether or not they are doing good or harm.
- Clear and well-constructed questions are fundamental for evidence-based care.
- Systematic and planned approaches are necessary to find and assess evidence.
- The outcomes of maternity care that are of concern to midwives and women and families are broader than just measures of mortality and physical morbidity and encompass such issues as psychosocial wellbeing, personal and family safety, economic outcomes.
- There are a number of specialist resources for midwives (for example MIDIRS), and these should be available and used whenever possible.

References

Biarez O, Sarrut B, Doreau C G, Etienne J 1991 Comparison and evaluation of nine bibliographic databases concerning adverse drug reactions. Drug Intelligence and Clinical Pharmacy 25: 1062–1065

Chalmers I, Enkin M E, Kierse M J N C 1989 Effective care in pregnancy and childbirth. Oxford University Press, Oxford

Cochrane A 1972 Effectiveness and efficiency; random reflections on health services. The Nuffield Provincial Hospitals Trust, London

Denzin N K, Lincoln Y S 1994 Handbook of qualitative research. Sage, London

Gray J A Muir 1997 Evidence-based healthcare: how to make health policy and management decisions. Churchill Livingstone, Edinburgh

Greenhalgh T 1997 How to read a paper: the basics of evidence-based medicine. BMJ Publishing Group, London

Harker L H, Thorpe K 1992 'The last egg in the basket'? Elderly primiparity – a review of findings. Birth 19(1): 23–28

HTA Online. Available: http://www.hta.nhsweb.nhs.uk/projectdata/3_project_record_published.asp?PjtId=1011 (accessed 8th August 2005)

Jahad J 1998 Randomised controlled trials. BMJ, London

Klebanoff M A, Read J S, Mills J L, Shiono P H 1993 The risk of childhood cancer after neonatal exposure to vitamin K. New England Journal of Medicine 329(13): 905–908

Last J M 1995 A dictionary of epidemiology. 3rd edn. Oxford University Press, Oxford

Mays N, Pope C 1996 Qualitative research in healthcare. BMJ Publishing Group, London

NICE May 2005 Breastfeeding for longer – what works. Systematic review summary. Online.

Available: http://www.publichealth.nice.org.uk/
page.aspx?o=511618 accessed October 19th 2005

Odaka T, Nakayana A, Akazawa K, Sakamoto M,
Kinukawa N, Kamakura T et al 1992 The effect of a
multiple literature database search. A numerical
evaluation in the domain of Japanese life science.
Journal of Medical Systems 16(4): 177–181

Olsen O 1997 Meta analysis of the safety of home
birth. Birth 24: 4–13

Page L 2000 Using evidence to inform practice. In:
Page L (ed.) The new midwifery. Science and
sensitivity in practice. Churchill Livingstone,
London, p. 45

Rosenberg W, Donald A 1995 Evidence-based
medicine: an approach to clinical problem-solving.
British Medical Journal 310: 1122–1125

Rosenthal A, Paterson-Brown S 1998 Is there an
incremental risk of obstetric intervention with
increasing maternal age? British Journal of
Obstetrics and Gynaecology 105: 1064–1069

Sackett D L, Richardson W S, Rosenberg W, Haynes B
R 1997 Evidence-based medicine: how to practise
and teach EBM. Churchill Livingstone, Edinburgh

Silverman W A 1980 Retrolental fibroplasia: a modern
parable. Academic Press, London.

Silverman WA 1998 Where's the evidence. Debates in
modern medicine. OUP, Oxford

Smith B, Darzins P, Quinn M, Heller R F 1992 Modern
methods of searching the medical literature.
Medical Journal of Australia 157: 603–611

Straus E S, Badenoch D, Scott Richardson W,
Rosenberge W, Sackett D L 1998 Practising
evidence-based medicine. Tutor's manual. 3rd edn.
Radcliffe Medical, Oxford

Straus E S, Scott Richardson W, Glasziou P,
Haynes R B 2005 Evidence based medicine: how to
teach and practice EBM. 3rd edn. Elsevier,
Edinburgh

Suarez-Almazor M E, Belseck E, Homik J, Dorgan M,
Ramos-Remus C 2000 Identifying clinical trials in
the medical literature with electronic databases:
Medline alone is not enough. Controlled Clinical
Trials 21: 476–487

University of Oxford 1998 Manual of Oxford
workshop on teaching evidence-based medicine.
University of Oxford, Oxford

USEFUL ADDRESSES

National Institute for Health and Clinical Excellence
Mid City Place
71 High Holborn
London
WC1V 6NA
www.nice.org.uk

MIDIRS
9 Elmdale Road
Clifton
Bristol
BS8 1SL
www.midirs.org

Chapter 11

Risk: theoretical or actual?

Sally Tracy

This chapter is intended to help midwives think about their practice in light of society's prevailing preoccupation with risk. Some midwives will be familiar with the concepts that are discussed here, but for others, the chapter will identify concepts that are operating at an almost subliminal level as our profession continues to become subsumed into techno-rational science and away from our 'with women' focus. Childbirth in resource rich nations enjoys on the one hand an unprecedented level of safety and on the other an unprecedented obsession with the concept of risk. Ironically, there is a cyclical aspect to the exercise of risk assessment. Through the identification of risk, we introduce intervention which itself poses new risks. In fact, we could argue that risk assessment does not really predict problems; rather it has become an important way of controlling women's choices and is indeed a form of social control. The preoccupation with risk is changing women's sense of themselves. Social control is further strengthened by forms of technological surveillance and the gaze of biomedicine and genetic screening. Medical technologies such as ultrasonography and fetal monitoring render pregnancy increasingly 'transparent' to both doctors and the public at large. Most important, this newfound transparency bestows enhanced personhood as well as patient status on the fetus.

The notion that health is first and foremost a medical product excludes our assessment and evaluation of other social and economic factors that influence health in such a profound way. Identification of risk factors for the fetus as distinct from the mother heralds the emergence of the fetus as 'patient' and contributes to the perception of maternal–fetal conflict. Such a perception may have a far reaching and potentially damaging effect on the symbiotic and biologically crucial relationship between mother and baby.

The nature of risk in pregnancy and childbirth has many changing facets. Preoccupation with risk and the complexity of its nature, shape every interaction and procedure between women and their midwives as they negotiate a safe and fulfilling path through pregnancy and childbirth. Some will be discussed here in depth; others will be mentioned in passing.

RISK: AND 'REDUCTIO AD ABSURDUM'

In a public lecture in 1989 Ann Oakley described the way risk was central to the obstetric definition of birth as a medical event because it helped doctors identify in advance those things that might 'go wrong', and that the general failure of this exercise has led to the 'reductio ad absurdum' of the risk approach! That is, 'every women and foetus is at risk until proved otherwise' (Oakley 1993, p. 135). The labelling of women as 'high-risk' or 'low-risk' is an integral part of the language of childbirth and is one with which many pregnant women and most midwives are all too familiar.

Studies exploring the way women feel, however, show quite conclusively that women feel differently, from midwives and from health professionals, about these concepts. The women in Oakley's study did not believe birth to be a medical event. Oakley found that the emphasis on normality exists in mother's accounts of childbirth and that women believe that birth is a normal process describing it as a 'continuous part of a woman's life' (Oakley 1993, p. 134).

Notwithstanding these women's views and those of birth activists and consumers in many resource rich nations (Goer 2004), we are still faced with the questions: 'Why has such a strong technical focus become acceptable? Why don't more women have normal births? Where is the evidence that this technology-intensive model of care does more good than harm?' (Albers 2005). The birth activists claim that although an astonishing amount has been accomplished by voluntary groups of women with limited resources, the grassroots movement has had little overall impact on the difficulties for women resulting from the 'hegemony of conventional obstetric management' worldwide (Goer 2004).

QUANTIFYING RISK: THE PURPOSE AND EFFICACY OF RISK-SCORING SYSTEMS

Opinions on the validity of scoring systems for determining risk in labour and birth vary widely and their efficacy has yet to be determined (Enkin et al 2000). The lack of precision in risk identification tools means there is no factual 'scientific' basis for denying women choice regarding their care or for insisting that all women give birth in an institutional setting. Medicine has had the power to define what is normal in childbirth, so that any deviation from this standard is viewed as 'abnormal' and justifies the further surveillance of pregnant women (Arney 1982, Lupton 1999). The range of normal has shifted drastically throughout the 20th century as new tests, procedures and technology redefine it. Rothman (1982) observed that conditions of pregnancy and childbirth that would have been considered normal or marginal in the past are now being labelled high risk. In contrast, that which is presently considered 'high risk' may, at a later date, turn out to be within the 'normal' range (Overall 1989).

Clinicians have long identified risk markers in pregnancy, but formalized risk-scoring systems did not become common until the 1960s, when computerized databanks became available to collate and analyse information about large numbers of observations from pregnant women and fetuses. Dozens of scoring systems were developed, some are still widely in use and others having been abandoned (Enkin et al 2000). The primary *purpose* of a risk-scoring system is to 'permit classification of individual women into different categories, for which actions can then be planned, advised and implemented' (Enkin et al 2000, p. 49). The *goal* of risk assessment from a public health perspective is to understand the rate of occurrence of a condition in a given population and calculate the risk that other population groups have of developing the same condition (Handwerker 1994). There are questions of whether risk-scoring systems can be generalized from one population to another, if . . . many of the values we measure are probably only surrogates for the true etiologic variable' (Spasoff & McDowell, quoted in Hayes 1992, p. 406). According to Murphy (1994, p. 67) '. . . most risk factors, even if they are strongly associated with outcomes in populations, do not predict adverse outcomes very well for individuals'.

In essence risk-scoring is a screening test and should meet the criteria of any screening test in helping a woman and her midwife discriminate clearly between those who are and those who are not at risk of developing a certain problem. Risk-scoring involves allocating a number to each adverse factor and totalling them to achieve an overall score. These cumulative scores are then assigned a category of risk from low to high, although they often display unequal weighting of risk factors and fail to address how to account for compounding risk factors (Lazarus 1990, Lilford & Chard 1983). For example, in a risk-scoring system developed by Hobel (1978), a maternal age of 35 years or more has the same weight as acute pyelonephritis, habitual abortion, rhesus sensitization and excessive drug use. Furthermore, there is little consensus on what the appropriate risk factors are, much less on how to weigh them (Alexander & Keirse 1989). Hall (1994) observes that 'there is no evidence that a woman with a risk factor of 9 is three times more likely to have a problem than a woman whose score is 3'.

It would appear that a formal risk-scoring tool should be more accurate than the rather subjective process of clinical impressions. However, risk factors are only statistically *associated* with the outcome being scored for and are not the *cause* of the adverse outcome. Since certainty is rare, risk can only be defined in terms of the *probability* that the risk factor will lead to a poor outcome (Murphy 1994). Therefore, removing or correcting the risk factor does not eliminate the possibility of an adverse outcome. Lilford & Chard (1983) have argued that risk-scoring systems do not make a precise prediction of the chances of an adverse outcome and therefore cannot be used in formal decision analysis. In order for risk assessments to be effective, the 'poor outcomes' for which a woman is at risk must be clearly specified, otherwise 'the outcome measures are so prone to bias that the scoring system can easily become no more than a self-fulfilling prophecy' (Alexander & Keirse 1989, p. 347).

To the expectant woman, the label of 'high risk' is only beneficial when something can be done to decrease or eliminate the risk factor. It is not useful to predict a poor outcome if it is too late in the pregnancy to positively influence the outcome predicted (Enkin 1994). While some antepartum problems can be prevented and corrected, Hall (1994, p. 1241) asserts that, when this occurs '. . . the risk score should be reduced, but typically risk scores are never deflated'. Unfortunately, risk assessment tools only take the woman and her baby up the ladder of risk, rarely down, even if the factors that caused her to be labelled as high risk have disappeared (Handwerker 1994, Perkins 1994). Also, as pregnancy risk is dynamic and complex in nature, a screening test applied even at serial points during pregnancy can never effectively assess the dynamic character of pregnancy (Wall 1988).

HOW WELL DO FORMAL 'RISK-SCORING' SYSTEMS WORK?

Alexander & Keirse (1989, p. 350) noted that, with formal risk-scoring '. . . women may be assigned to the high-risk group because of rigid definitions of the risk markers, whereas a capable clinician could have assessed the situation more sensitively

thanks to implicit clinical judgment'. Risk scoring systems have never been evaluated with well designed randomized controlled trials and seem to have lost favour in the past five to ten years. They have been superseded in part by the risk assessment guidelines which will be discussed more fully later in the chapter.

According to Perkins (1994, p. 24), more than 20 risk assessment instruments have been developed in the USA, while in Canada, there are currently at least 12 risk-scoring systems reported in use, with varying degrees of compliance and success (Hall 1994). Although it has been well established that low socio-economic status is associated with increased perinatal risk (see, for example, Handwerker 1994, Lazarus 1990, Osofsky & Kendall 1973), only 2 out of the 12 scoring systems make provision for any social factors. In addition, seven do not include either smoking or alcohol use as predictors of risk (Hall 1994).

The consequences of false negative results (high-risk women being classified as low-risk) may result in increased mortality or morbidity for the mother or baby. Conversely, the consequences of a false positive result (low-risk women being classified as high risk) may subject women to unnecessary and potentially harmful interventions (Murphy 1994). According to Wall (1988, p. 155), 'seventy percent or more of adverse perinatal outcomes appear to be unpredictable by existing assessment methods'. Very small improvements have been made in terms of the sensitivity of risk assessment systems since those devised by Hobel et al (1973) which predicted poor outcomes in only one-third of women thought to be high risk.

Even the presence of many risk factors is no guarantee that a bad outcome will occur. The validity of a screening test is defined as the ability of a test to distinguish between those who have the outcome of interest and those who do not. The sensitivity of the test is defined as the ability of the test to identify correctly those who *have* the outcome of interest; whereas the sensitivity of the test is defined as the ability of the test to identify correctly those who do *not have* the outcome of interest (Gordis 1996) (see Box 11.1). The combination of poor specificity (a test with many false positives) and the low prevalence of most adverse outcomes creates a low predictive value for positive test results. The appearance of benefit,

Box 11.1 Diagnostic tests: key terms (reproduced from Sackett et al 1997, with permission)

Sensitivity: the proportion of people with the target disorder who have a positive test. It is used to assist in assessing and selecting a diagnostic test/sign/symptom.

SnNout: when a sign/test/symptom has a high sensitivity, a negative result rules out the diagnosis.

Specificity: the proportion of people without the target disorder who have a negative test. It is used to assist in assessing and selecting a diagnostic test/sign/symptom.

SpPin: when a sign/symptom has a high specificity, a positive result rules in the diagnosis.

Positive predictive value: the proportion of people with a positive test who have the target disorder.

Negative predictive value: the proportion of people with a negative test who are free of the target disorder.

Likelihood ratio: the likelihood that a given test result would be expected in a patient with the target disorder compared with the likelihood that the same result would be expected in a patient without the target disorder.

however, reinforces the perceived value of risk screening and timely intervention and makes it difficult to question whether assessment and intervention programmes are beneficial (Murphy 1994).

Many attempts have been made to design risk scoring systems, though most continue to be fraught with poor positive predictive value and a lack of sensitivity (Koong et al 1997; Low et al 1995).

There is a burgeoning industry around inventing decision aids to 'help' women through the maze of deciding which risks to take and how to weigh them up. This area promises strong growth in the future as women navigate their way though the screening, surveillance and intervention procedures that continue to evolve around pregnancy and childbirth. For example,

■ the Paling Perspective Scale is a graphic tool with a logarithmic graph ranging from 'one in

a million' to 'one in one' that sits above a visual numerical scale representing the relative likelihood of the risk of a particular outcome (Stallings & Paling 2001);

■ an evidence-based decision-aid for pregnant women who have experienced previous caesarean section and who are considering options for birth in a subsequent pregnancy is currently undergoing a randomized trial for the evaluation of its effectiveness (Shorten et al 2004);

■ one of the latest medical 'risk scoring' enterprises aims at giving women their personal 'score' to predict their achievement of vaginal birth after a previous caesarean section. Gonen et al (2004) recently published a set of variables associated with vaginal birth after caesarean section (VBAC) and set out to define and to develop a scoring system for the prediction of successful VBAC. Combined with the ever increasing primary caesarean section rate, this will prove fertile ground for those who engage in developing scores for managing childbirth.

DEALING WITH RISK 'HOLISTICALLY'

Objecting to the risk management approach to childbirth is difficult, because the idea of risk management is a product of the culture we live in. It is so basic to maternity care today that it is difficult to imagine any other model of care.

Enkin 1994, p. 133

As early as 1950, numerous studies demonstrated that psychological and/or social factors play a role in pregnancy outcome and that interventions in these areas can decrease the incidence of problems (Chalmers 1982, Crandon 1979, Gorsuch & Key 1974, Kapp et al 1963, Katchner 1950, Laukaran & van den Berg 1980, McDonald 1968, Nuckolls et al 1972, Oakley 1992). In 1983, Grimes et al developed a holistic, phenomenological approach to risk-screening to test for accuracy against a more traditional medical approach. As well as her medical and obstetric history, consideration was given to a woman's nutritional status, life and relationship stress, behavioural patterns, coping styles, beliefs and attitudes about childbirth, and energy levels in relation to strength.

The authors concluded, 'this alternative method of risk assessment is more successful than traditional medical methodology' (Grimes et al 1983, p. 27).

Smilkstein et al (1984) developed and applied a 'biopsychosocial' model of risk-screening to 93 pregnant women and compared the results with those of a control group screened using only biomedical risk factors. They found that while biomedical risk factors alone were not substantially related to complications, psychosocial risk was related to both delivery and postpartum complications. Family function and biomedical risk also reliably predicted complications. The authors suggest that an interaction of biomedical and psychosocial risk screening 'will offer significant improvement in identifying women who may experience pregnancy complications' (Smilkstein et al 1984, p. 315).

The use of selection criteria to decide where to book to give birth is a rational attempt to predict a safe outcome. But being labelled 'high risk' is only meaningful when there is evidence to show that booking at a different place will alter the nature and magnitude of that risk. A review published in the British Journal of Obstetrics and Gynaecology by Rona Campbell in 1999 described and assessed selection criteria used for advising women where to book in to give birth. The cross sectional survey was carried out in the South and West region of England and sampled the booking criteria from 27 NHS trusts who provided maternity care. The study looked at selection criteria used when booking pregnant women for different places of birth; length of time the criteria had been in use and whether the criteria was applied individually or as part of a risk score. Campbell (1999) also looked at how the criteria had been developed. Eighty one percent of the units surveyed responded. The study found that not one of the 128 individual risk criteria identified was common to all 21 obstetric unit policies, including previous stillbirth and previous caesarean section. None of the trusts who responded used the criteria in order to calculate a risk score. All except one of the policies were for selection of women to give birth outside the tertiary consultant-led maternity unit. Only two trusts used sets of criteria which identified, to any extent, outcomes for which women could be at risk and strategies that should be implemented to reduce that risk. Over half the

trusts were able to identify a rationale for the particular set of criteria which they used but in only two cases was any reference made to an evidence base. Although effective selection criteria should be able to demonstrate a clear association between adverse outcome and place of birth there was no evidence that this was how they were being used. The author concluded that given the 'diversity of the criteria used and the absence of any clear evidence of their effectiveness, . . . the application of these criteria amounts to constraint on a woman's choice' (Campbell 1999, p. 554).

THE GROWING SPIRAL OF CONTROL AND ANXIETY

For several decades now, sociologists and academics have contended that to be 'at risk' is to be threatened by uncertainty and hazards both within and around us (Beck 1992, Giddens 1990, 1991).

Being at risk is also increasingly defined in terms of individual or personal responsibility rather than in terms of social constraints and collective responsibilities (Hallowell & Lawton 2002). Similarly the advice offered to solve such uncertainty engendered by being 'at risk' is to take individual responsibility and to modify behaviour and lifestyles (Fitzpatrick 2000). Paradoxically this is seen as the solution despite the effects of poverty, environment and health systems over which women very often have little control. In resource rich countries however, health risk management is not only endemic, it has become a moral exercise, and those who fail to modify their lifestyle and continue to indulge their desires are seen as morally wanton (Fitzpatrick 2000, Lupton 1993, 1995, Peterson & Lupton 1996).

Managing a risky body takes a certain amount of self sacrifice and restraint. It may involve modification of diet and exercise and avoiding dangerous desires. According to some critics '. . . epidemiologists have affected our way of eating and drinking, our physical activity, our relationship with sunshine, our working environment and our sexual behaviour, without balancing this with an ethical debate on the societal effects of increasing a population of worried well' (Forde 1998, p. 1155).

Theoretically then, for modern women 'being-at-risk' constitutes a new social identity (Scott et al 2005). Women who become pregnant are identified within a risk grouping of 'low' or 'high risk' which may ultimately determine where she gives birth and with whom. The inevitability of risk causes increasing numbers of women to surrender control at the beginning of the birth process, turning to a doctor to confirm pregnancy, and an ultrasound to predict the date of birth. From that moment onwards they are on a conveyor belt which it is very difficult to step off. They no longer weigh up the risks and choose their own path (Greer 1999). 'Risk' has become one of the defining cultural characteristics of modern Western society (Douglas 1994), and the creation and accentuation of 'risk' is itself a means of establishing a professional power base (de Vries 1996, Lupton 1995, Mander 2001).

Is contemporary social life improved by such sustained attention to medical information and medically informed solutions? Does this emphasis on screening for the unknown and suspected risk not only increase uncertainty but also further increase an individual's perception of being at risk? A public health scientist examining the social and ethical implications of biotechnology and the relationship between prevailing discourses on risk and emerging diagnostic/screening technologies asserts that there is such a relationship between the perception of being at risk, the diagnostic and screening mechanisms that provide an answer to such questions and the reproduction of more uncertainty so that each feeds on the other and reproduces in an ever expanding spiral (Robertson 2001).

Could the fascination and preoccupation with risk be a greater danger to the public and society than the material risks themselves? The dream of security is confounded by the insecurity of contemporary social conditions and, ironically, by insecurity generated by efforts for protection. The contradiction at the heart of medical culture is that the continuing expansion of knowledge about threats to health, the prolific communication and insatiable consumption of that knowledge and the professional and lay mandate to protect and improve health, together aggravate the very insecurities they are designed to quell. The preoccupation with safety engenders alarm, a heightened sensitivity to danger and a sense of personal vulnerability. Anxiety about health, though over-determined, is aggravated by a medical culture compelled to identify dangers in order to control them' (Crawford 2004, p. 506).

Without a doubt the preoccupation of modern medicine with managing risk status rather than recognizing and dealing with signs and symptoms of actual bodily pathology has had considerable implications for women and midwives and for health provision in general. The focus on the *potential* presence of a problem is part of a much wider movement which some commentators have highlighted as a new stage of development in the relationships between healers and patients in the modern world (Scott et al 2005). The new stage is referred to as that of 'biomedicalization' in contrast with its predecessor, referred to as 'medicalization'. Biomedicalization includes a focus on health and risk (rather than illness and disease), it transforms the way biomedical knowledge is distributed, and transforms bodies and personal identities in line with the increasingly 'techno scientific' nature of biomedical practices (Clarke et al 2003). In particular, the development of genetic testing and screening technologies has enabled clinicians to make visible an individual's risk of disease well before it manifests. Screening technologies provide a new biological reductionism that assigns future disease states to corporeal risks, partially displacing previous emphasis on germs enzymes and biochemical compounds with (sub) molecular levels of proteins, individual genes and genomes.

The 'embodied' or 'corporeal risks' made visible by genetic screening occupy a unique position within the healthcare system, and this is especially so in the world of clinical genetics. In that world, the direct interpersonal contact and focus on the patient's body is re-drafted in a number of ways. The 'gaze' of the clinical practitioner shifts from body and cell to DNA, from individual patient to family group, from bedside to laboratory, and to family counselling sessions (Scott et al 2005). For example, when a woman has an abnormal cervical smear test she is confronted with knowing that there are cells in her body that may predispose her to the risk of getting cancer. This embodied or corporeal risk imposes a threat from within the body (Kavanagh & Broom 1998).

It defines who a person *is* rather than what they *do* (lifestyle risk) or what is *done to* them (environmental risk). In pregnancy the manifestations of environment, lifestyle and corporeal risks very often overlap. For example, in gestational diabetes the implication that there may be genes that confer insulin resistance and impaired insulin secretion are likely to add to the relative risk that affects women's predisposition to gestational diabetes mellitus (Allan et al 1997), along with her age, weight and country of origin. To be labelled 'at risk' genetically for example makes being 'at risk' a reality – possibly for the first time. It may provoke an increased sense of vulnerability, or unsettle a previous understanding of oneself as perfect and somehow immune (Kavanagh & Broom 1998). So that, for such individuals, to be 'at risk' is to feel well, to be asymptomatic, yet always to be aware of the potential for becoming otherwise. Such 'beings-at-risk' must consequently confront the possibility of their future self as suffering from a bodily pathology that is probable rather than actual (Scott et al 2005).

Although those with genetic mutations are not held personally responsible for being at genetic risk, the discourse of the 'genetic clinic' constructs them as responsible for managing these risks and where they fail to do so by refusing genetic screening or surveillance they may be regarded as morally questionable (Hallowell & Lawton 2002).

However, while the rhetoric of the new genetics constructs genetic information as providing individuals with new 'choices' for health risk management, it has been observed that, in reality, those who are in a position to use genetic information perceive their choices as constrained in a variety of ways (Hallowell 1999). It is argued that genetic information is constructed as empowering, it supposedly holds the promise of the ability to control future health and to end uncertainty (Petersen 1998, Wilkinson 2001). But do genetic discourses actually foster a myth of control for the person whose genetic makeup has been assessed? The estimation of genetic risk makes what is essentially an uncertain future appear more certain; it renders the unpredictable more predictable. Thus, probabilistic information about inherited health risks (to self and others) is constructed as a resource, which can be used to inform individuals' risk management choices and thus, potentially

allay their anxiety about their future health (Hallowell et al 2004).

Contrary to this opinion the drive to achieve security through acquisition of medical knowledge and adoption of individual, self-protective practices motivates more finely tuned awareness of possibilities and unforeseen events, and still more elaborate efforts in pursuit of an elusive state of health. In short, our efforts to control risk are almost invariably accompanied by an ever increasing array of possibilities that are just out of our reach in a bid for further control (Crawford 2004). This in turn gives rise to 'an escalating spiral of control and anxiety' (Crawford 2004, Wilkinson 2001).

RISK SURVEILLANCE AND SOCIAL CONTROL

> This new medical intrusion in the lives of women may be diffuse, but it is certainly insidious, legitimating its interventions and its discourse not only in the name of science, as it has up to now, but in the name of the foetus itself.
>
> Queniart 1992, p. 163

Oakley (1992) asserts that risk-scoring systems are used to control women, ostensibly in the interests of their own health and that of their babies, while Sapolsky (1990) infers that people's fears about risks can be used to maintain control by the institutions that have the power to define and categorize these risks. In childbirth the imposition of a risk category on all women acts in a regulatory role, requiring women to acquiesce (in their best interests) to medical intervention (Lane 1995).

What women *wanted* was viewed in the 1920s and 1930s as an important force shaping maternity care. After the 1950s, women's wishes came to be seen as a 'luxury' and incompatible with the medical determination of risk (Oakley 1984). Obstetricians began to dominate higher levels of policy-making, control the introduction of new procedures and define who was at risk. Riessman & Nathanson (1986) argue that the development of the concept of risk was essential to the maintenance of birth as a medical problem and that obstetrics extended its boundary over clearly pathological birth by expanding the concept of risk to include births that were *potentially* pathological (Ehrenreich & English 1973). In 1985, the 17th edition of Williams' Obstetrics added to 'high-risk' and 'low-risk' the new category of 'growing risk', broadening the definition of what constitutes risk (Queniart 1992). Arney (1982, p. 26) states that 'The concepts of "normal" and "abnormal" took on a new relationship to one another. No longer was there a clear demarcation between the two; a grey area had been created that was capable of taking on added dimensionality'.

In Discipline and Punish, Foucault (1979) describes a panopticon, a structure of power that has the capacity for constant and total surveillance, which effects a new form of control based on behaviour that is self-regulated through the fear of observation. Arney (1982) relates the panopticon to obstetrics, in which women are subjected to constant and total visibility, and in which technologies and monitoring allow obstetrics to extend into every aspect of women's pregnancies. Power and control are magnified by making risk factors more 'known' through multiple monitoring schemes; 'risk-scores thus became a vehicle for expanding the scope of surveillance to all aspects of a woman's life' (Foucault 1979, p. 143). Foucault observed that tests are instruments of control. They provide the means to compare, differentiate, homogenize and exclude. The power to define the normal can impose standards of conformity, while the ability to measure individual deviations can justify classification and hierarchy (Foucault 1975, 1979).

Douglas & Wildavsky (1982) contend that the selection of risk is a social process: the risks selected may be concerned with issues of little or no danger, but they are culturally identified as important. For women in resource rich countries childbirth has never been safer, and Arney (1982, p. 137), believes that obstetricians have now become fetal advocates, drastically altering the orientation of obstetrics. The fetus is becoming increasingly more autonomous and is gradually being perceived as the primary patient (Maier 1992). Duden (1993) discusses how 'seeing' the fetus with ultrasound and the publication of Nilsson's (1965) photographs of the fetus in utero have changed the public's perception of pregnancy and allowed physicians, friends, family members, judges and strangers the freedom to judge and condemn women for their 'risky' behaviour. Society has now shifted its gaze to the fetus, and the resulting social control over pregnant women is legitimated in the name of fetal protection (Rodgers 1989). As prenatal testing and other medical interventions become more routinized and therefore accepted as a 'normal' part of care, expectations about women's behaviour will expand. It becomes very difficult for women to refuse testing and interventions when they are presented as being 'for the good of the baby' (Gregg 1993).

In recent years, some physicians have asserted their control over the definition of risk by using the judicial system to apprehend the baby in utero if the mother is not complying with medical advice. A woman's right to refuse medical treatment and surgery has been overruled by the courts in North America (Rodgers 1989). Recent legal developments threaten pregnant women's privacy and autonomy by using control measures in court 'whenever [a woman's] behaviour is seen to be detrimental to the fetus she carries' (Rodgers 1989, p. 174). The identification of the fetus as having a risk distinct from that of the mother has enormous implications for the future of risk assessment in pregnancy and childbirth. Such a perception may have a far reaching and potentially damaging effect on the symbiotic and biologically crucial relationship between mother and baby. However, Nelkin (1989) argues that these definitions of risk tend to apportion blame upon stigmatized minorities. This is supported by the findings of Kolder et al (1987), who reported an alarming increase in attempts to prosecute what essentially constitute poor pregnant women, primarily from ethnic minorities, for failing to follow medical advice. It is noteworthy that Maier (1992) found, in cases of court-ordered caesarean sections sought to protect the baby from the mother's non-compliance, that women who *did not* undergo surgery delivered safely with no adverse outcome.

Medicine and society are now defining what constitutes *risky behaviour* (Gregg 1993). When risk is believed to be internally imposed because of a lack of self-control or willpower, blame is placed on the 'lifestyle choices' made by the individual. Yet there has never been a clear demarcation between socially produced risks (poverty, illiteracy, abuse issues, drug addiction and lack of housing) and biologically produced risks (genetic traits, age and blood type). When socially produced risks are identified, pregnancy surveillance is increased and women are cautioned to avoid harming the baby. Interventions in the root causes of the risk are rarely carried out; they include more money, educational programme, better and safe housing, addiction treatment and counselling (Oakley 1992). A new trend that views pregnant women and their unborn babies in an antagonistic relationship raises serious questions about 'pregnant women's right to privacy and autonomy . . . through direct pressures and explicit social sanctions regarding their choices' (Gregg 1993, p. 67). This alarming violation of women's reproductive freedom and the assessment of the fetus as having a risk distinct from the mother's health has enormous implications for the future of risk assessment in obstetrics.

THE EFFECT OF BIOMEDICALIZATION AND GENETIC SCREENING ON SURVEILLANCE

With the advent of biomedicalization and genetic screening for risk there is a consequent extension and strengthening of the risk focus into 'surveillance medicine' (Armstrong 1995). Risk and surveillance mutually construct one another: risks are calculated and assessed in order to rationalize surveillance, and through surveillance risks are conceptualized and standardized into ever more precise calculations and algorithms (Howson 1998; Lupton 1995, 1999).

Risk and surveillance are aspects of biomedicalization and the medical gaze that are in a quintessential Foucauldian sense, no longer contained in the hospital, clinic, or even within the doctor–patient relationship (Armstrong 1995). Rather, they implicate each of us and whole populations through constructions of risk factors (Clarke et al 2003).

There has been a transformation of antenatal care of the mother by the addition of the technical surveillance of the fetus. Ultrasound imaging is now firmly embedded although whether it should be used routinely or used selectively has not as yet been firmly established (Enkin et al 2000). Currently the number of routine scans differs according to national health system context and public versus private funding. In Germany, Austria and Canada pregnant women are offered two routine

ultrasound scans during pregnancy. In UK the National Institute for Clinical Excellence (NICE) commisioned an evidence-based clinical guideline for the NHS in England and Wales in 2003 which recommended that two scans should be offered to healthy pregnant women: one at 10–13 weeks gestation to determine gestational age and another at 18–20 weeks gestation to assess structural abnormalities (Royal College of Obstetricians and Gynaecologists 2003). In Iceland and Norway women are offered one scan and in Greece women may have a scan at every visit (Harris et al 2004). In the United States, despite a statement from the American College of Obstetricians and Gynecologists (ACOG) recommending against routine ultrasound, ACOG itself has estimated that between 60 and 70 percent of pregnant women have a 'routine' scan (American College of Obstetricians and Gynecologists 1997).

Ann Oakley in her essay on ultrasound in obstetrics reasons that 'technology brings about a profound shift in the knowledge base of medicine . . . it substitutes so-called "objective" data for the earlier patient-generated kind . . . both X-rays and ultrasound are stages in a long history of clinicians attempts to secure a better knowledge of what is happening inside the womb than mothers themselves have . . . (Oakley 1993, p. 190–191). Oakley argues that claims to safety are based on the mistaken logic that because serious bioeffects have not been demonstrated, ultrasound is safe (Oakley 1993). It is further assumed that the level of 'certainty' about safety increases directly with the length of time the technology has been in use, rather than through scrutiny to which it has been subjected. The dangers of such assumptions are highlighted by the parallels between the use of X-rays and ultrasound in obstetrics. Both proceeded before being subjected to controlled trials and both were claimed safe on the basis of the personal conviction of advocates (Oakley 1993).

HOW DO WOMEN THEMSELVES INTERPRET SURVEILLANCE?

In a qualitative study undertaken by Harris and colleagues (2004) pregnant women's conceptions and interpretations of the significance of ultrasound were sought through multiple interviews with 34 study participants. Informants were purposively selected to include women of English-speaking background, primiparous delivery, and low-risk (Harris et al 2004). All women in the study underwent a 18–20-week scan, while 27 (79%) also had scans at other stages of the pregnancy. The researchers drew heavily on Foucauldian concepts to examine the discursive constructs underpinning women's involvement with obstetric scans.

Among the women in the study, most were unaware of any possible screening outcomes in relation to the 18–20-week test. The scan was perceived as 'normal' and 'routine' and a responsible thing to do. 'So I had the routine two blood tests and the routine two ultrasounds.' . . . 'I think that's why you, it's more important to look after it while it's there, it's your responsibility' (Angela) (Harris et al 2004, p. 31) The ultrasound was embraced by women themselves for a variety of reasons, including the pleasures of seeing the baby while still in utero, and the sense that ultrasound scans are part of the responsible management of pregnancy that enhance the chances of a positive outcome.

The authors stated that the 'normalization' of ultrasound in antenatal care, by both women and practitioners, has the potential to obfuscate many issues including ethical issues around abortion and disability rights, and the right to decline tests (Harris et al 2004, p. 32). The concept of 'normalcy' was also linked to reassurance following scan results. Women spoke of 'normal' and 'average' babies: 'It was really good, the baby was average size' (Iona) (Harris et al 2004, p. 32).

The researchers found that the production of risk discourse particularly about pregnancy increased the anxiety levels and concerns experienced by pregnant women and only two women stated they did not experience any anxiety in relation to scanning. 'Like I think I'm young, I'm healthy, I'm fit, everything's just got to be fine, but at the same time, you know, it's just in the back of your mind' (Natalie) (Harris et al 2004, p. 31).

Generally, women experienced the greatest anxiety in relation to their first scan and the combined anxiety and relief posed by the results of the nuchal translucency (NT) test: 'It was just a horrible thing to actually deal with, that the relief afterwards was quite remarkable . . . I said to my husband, I wasn't aware of how tense I was up until then and he was a little bit the same as well, because there was all this unspoken stuff that you avoided. What if? What if it's not right?' (Leah) (Harris et al 2004, p. 33).

The study found that even amongst women who perceived the scan to be risky, the potential harm to mother or baby did not outweigh the risk of rejecting the scan and thus foregoing a (perceived) chance to help the baby, or the chance to terminate the pregnancy. These reasons are linked to the importance of having control over the pregnancy (and if necessary, foreknowledge of an adverse outcome). The pregnant woman is exhorted to be a responsible agent acting in the interests of the fetus, while also subject to the rationality of expert medical knowledge. Those women who chose to minimize screening because they would not terminate the pregnancy considered control more in terms of their embodied experiences: controlling their anxiety levels and enjoying their pregnancies (Harris et al 2004).

The researchers concluded as others have that scanning in pregnancy both reinforces and relieves pre-existing anxieties, and that the pre-existing anxieties relate, in part, to ways in which antenatal technologies enforce the notion of the hazards of pregnancy, situating all pregnancies as 'at risk' and making the 'no-risk' pregnancy obsolete (Lupton 1999, p. 68).

Harris et al (2004) report that surveillance technologies are where epidemiologically based notions of risk become individualized and are described as such. For example, in relation to nuchal translucency scanning, comments such as Leah's were common: 'So combining the results of the blood test and the scan, my age, they then count the odds of genetic disorders and Down syndrome. And those odds were quite long, so I was quite pleased with that' (Harris et al 2004, p. 36).

Lupton, in a study of first-time motherhood describes another example of the way women's concepts of risk differ considerably from those of the expert. Lupton found that where the expert relies on statistical concepts of probability, 'women draw not only from expert knowledges but from their own experiences, their knowledge of other's experiences and lay concepts of risk which circulate in their cultural context' (Lupton 1999, p. 76). Other researchers have described ambiguities of risk which stem from its translation from epidemiological findings into clinical knowledge and practice and thus to lay experiences of health and illness as a clear dilemma. Similarly these researchers describe 'What mattered was their position in relation to the boundaries of normalcy' (Adelsward & Sachs 1996, p. 1186).

The introduction of new screening and surveillance measures continues at such a pace that it is beyond the scope of a conventionally published text to inform readers of the very latest techniques. For example, at the time of writing, one of the more promising areas of screening currently being researched is analysis of fetal cells and fetal DNA and RNA from the maternal circulation. If this is effective it holds considerable possibilities for changing the way that prenatal diagnosis is carried out. It is speculated that new technologies involving sampling maternal plasma with cell-free fetal DNA may play a bigger role in non-invasive prenatal genetic diagnosis of aneuploidy by helping to identify pregnancies at sufficient risk for trisomy 21 or 18 without women having to undergo an invasive diagnostic procedure for definitive diagnosis such as amniocentesis or chorionic villous sampling (CVS). Circulating fetal DNA has also been targeted as a marker for assessing feto-maternal wellbeing. Increased fetal DNA concentrations have been reported for several pregnancy-related complications including pre-eclampsia. So far, various forms of circulating DNA in plasma have been observed: shed cells, apoptotic bodies, nucleosomes, other nucleoproteins, and free DNA (Bischoff et al 2005). This fast-moving area will continue to change and challenge the way that midwives offer care and support for women and their families.

INVISIBLE FORMS OF SOCIAL CONTROL AND SURVEILLANCE – 'IMPERCEPTIBLE SURVEILLANCE CREEP'

In shifting the gaze from 'body' to invisible 'gene' and away from the direct supervisory techniques such as ultrasound described above, and famously analysed by Foucault (1975), are the technologies of sensing and recording. These have enabled a massive growth in the *invisible monitoring* of individuals and groups without the need for constant direct observation (Graham & Wood 2003). The new era in surveillance manifests itself in the data bases constructed from personal data taken from individuals and in, for example, the networked remote fetal monitoring that occurs in large hospital labour suites. The move from paper based to digital or automatic technology facilitates a steep change in the power, intensity and scope of surveillance. Electronic records that monitor, sort and track information on events as they happen (in real time) allows a much more sophisticated level of observation. Computers are commonplace in homes and hospitals. Although public health medicine and epidemiology have a long history of surveillant practices, mainly in notification and monitoring infectious disease (Mooney 1999), the advent of electronic patient records and genetic data bases has moved this surveillance to a new level (Kitzinger & Reilly 1997, Nelkin & Andrews 1999). Although in principal we should have no real cause to be suspicious of the large databases of personal and other facts accumulated within patient records, Mooney (1999) relates the possibility of 'for the public good' winning out against the privacy of the personal rights of an individual. Nelkin and Andrews (1999) observe a dichotomous stance on the merits of data bases. On the one hand they have been referred to as 'almost imperceptible surveillance creep, marked by subtle invisible involuntary forms of social control' (Nelkin & Andrews 1999, p. 690). On the other hand they are proclaimed as essential and inevitable in complex societies that require formalized systems of data gathering, and that they are not in themselves a problem. The issue is how can they be regulated to avoid abuse (Nelkin & Andrews 1999, p. 670). Some commentators describe the potential threat of electronic and digitalized surveillance in terms of a danger to privacy and freedom, as 'Big Brother' style observation (Orwell 1949). Graham and Wood (2003) also highlight cause for concern in the increasing influence of the private sector in health care provision. The relationship between public database holders and the private sector is a key issue, one that is again complicated by digitization. Modern medical research, and in particular genetics, depends increasingly on high-powered computing. Only through the eyes of computers could we hope to map and sequence the human genome in a practical period of time' (Graham & Wood 2003).

This sentiment is echoed in the work of Nelkin who states 'Science is now more about money than scholarly endeavour. It is "the promise of profits" that motivates many scientists' (Nelkin 1998, p. 893). Nelkin has for a long time warned of the impact and social implications of the advances in genetics and neurosciences. She warns that the impact of the new faith in the apparent exactness of biological determinism in our daily lives will eventually determine an individual's fitness for life itself (Nelkin & Tancredi 1994). The power of commerce is revealed by Nelkin who claims that it took a *fatality* in a clinical trial for a gene therapy product to provoke critical press coverage about both the commercialization of genetic research and its medical risks (Nelkin 2001).

In assessing the concerns that public health professionals hold towards identification of genetic risk, Halliday et al (2004) contend that at a time when there are moves to address inequalities in socioeconomic and political factors affecting health, the emphasis on identifying genetic risk might move us back towards the 'single cause for single disease' paradigm (analogous to the 'germ theory' of the 19th and 20th centuries (Worboys 2000). 'A reductionist approach can be useful for identifying genetic associations with disease and elucidating aetiological pathways in a research setting, but does not reflect the way genes operate in complex biological systems. Genetic information may motivate people to improve their health behaviour, or, at the other extreme, it may lead to a fatalistic view of genetic risk with people shunning preventive behaviours or treatments' (Halliday et al 2004). They maintain that 'the main objective for using genetic information in public health today is not to enhance, change, or remove one's genes, but to promote their optimal expression' (Halliday et al 2004, p. 895). They concede, however, that 'the possibility of a new eugenics era cannot be ruled out, and neither can changes in social values and economic influences. Therefore concern about eugenic activities should be taken seriously and the scientific community is responsible for engaging the public in informed debate around this issue' (Halliday et al 2004, p. 895).

The information revealed by genetic testing/pedigree analysis is constructed or described in terms of providing individuals with 'foresight'. For a test that identifies a single gene defect resulting in severe disease or early death, the nature of the choice and the consequences of a pregnancy with a fetus carrying such a defect are clear. The estimation of genetic risk makes what is essentially an uncertain future appear more certain; it renders the unpredictable more predictable. Thus, probabilistic information about inherited health risks (to self and others) is constructed as a resource, which can be used to inform individuals' risk management choices and thus, potentially allay their anxiety about their future health (Clarke et al 2003).

BIG BUSINESS AND THE CONSTRUCTION OF RISK

The impact of patents on gene sequences and of pharmacogenetics is clearly outside the scope of this chapter, but as Halliday et al (2004) assert, they potentially have much greater public health implications. The alarming alliance between industry and medicine is brought to our attention in an essay by Moynihan et al (2002) who point out that a lot of money can be made from telling healthy people they are sick. They claim that big business in the form of pharmaceutical companies may now be better described as disease mongers. They are 'widening the boundaries of treatable illness in order to expand markets for those who sell and deliver treatments. Pharmaceutical companies are actively involved in sponsoring the definition of diseases and promoting them to both prescribers and consumers. The social construction of illness is being replaced by the corporate construction of disease' (Moynihan et al 2002, p. 886). Pathologizing normal physiology is not unknown in midwifery and it is wise to keep a healthy index of suspicion when research studies funded by industry claim to have found 'new' risks to pregnant women or 'new solutions' to improve childbirth and a 'new' prevalence in some condition that in fact has remained quite stable in the population.

The corporatization of medicine in many parts of the developed world and the advent of private sector control in health have contributed to some of the startling activities around the 'sell off' of genetic information (Graham & Wood 2003). For example, the government of Iceland has licensed its entire national genetic database to the American genetics company deCODE for research and commercial purposes and Estonia is also planning a genetic database of its citizens. Although as Graham and Wood (2003) concede, the Icelandic public knew of this venture, they claim, however, that a leaked health Green Paper by the UK Labour government shows that the American company group proposed making the results of DNA sampling in NHS hospitals available to pharmaceutical companies (Graham & Wood 2003). Nelkin and Tancredi (1994) ask, 'who is responsible for the drive to biologically categorize the individual?' They agree with Graham and Wood (2003) that the wellbeing of the population may indeed drive the health imperative of genetic research, but there are ominous signs. That which is useful to doctors and patients for health, and which is based on a personal, individualistic and humanistic approach, is used by insurers and corporations in an impersonal, statistical way to increase profits by exclusion (Nelkin & Tancredi 1994). Being refused insurance cover has serious implications for personal wellbeing when individuals are increasingly forced to find private health care and rely less upon decreasing state provision. Those whose genetic records make them too financially risky for insurance companies could find themselves bypassed by neo-liberal health policies (Graham & Wood 2003).

COMMUNICATING RISK

What are the ethics of assessing all women to identify hypothetical risk factors (that may or may not predict disease with accuracy) in order to prescribe interventions (which may be of dubious value and possible harm) in the hopes of preventing an outcome (that will never happen to most of those subjected to this process)?

Murphy 1994, p. 68

In order to facilitate informed decision-making, women require their midwives to provide information that is objective, evidence based and unswayed by emotion and ideologies. They must

also be fully informed of the risks *as we know them to be* without slanting or biasing the information. Clearly women learn to make decisions long before they first meet a midwife. These decisions take place in a range of contexts – of feeling and of prior experience and learning. They learn to make decisions that 'feel right' to them (Bursztajn et al 1990). Women do not define risk solely as the number of deaths or injuries likely to happen as a result of their exposure to something, but as how well they can control their exposure and whether they have assumed the risk voluntarily (Radford 1997). The label of high risk can create stress and anxiety in a pregnant woman, which can cause a diminished sense of competence and a loss of confidence in her ability to give birth safely (Chalmers 1982). However, there is virtually no human activity that can be completely free from risk, and it is up to the individual to decide what constitutes an acceptable risk. Despite the anxiety that risk-taking can induce, successful risk-taking can induce a feeling of euphoria, with a sense of power to reinvent everyday life.

In their study of the factors influencing pregnant women's perception of risk, Heanen and colleagues (2004) found that women do not necessarily use known statistical odds in making their risk assessments, but rather use their own personal data or 'rules of thumb'. The process of risk assessment was multidimensional and influenced by more than statistical ratios. Consistent with the findings of other studies of midwives and women in Canada (Saxell & Midwifery Group 1999), Heamen et al (2004) found that women determined their risk by considering both factors that intensified risk and factors that ameliorated risk. Women constructed their risk as potential based on past and present conditions. Past reproductive experiences and present health states played a major role in risk determination (Heamen et al 2004, p. 115).

For medicine, risk is a statistical artefact, while for the woman, risk is a subjective experience. All risk calculations involve the juggling of personal understanding about not just the danger, but also experience (Gabe 1995). Risk can take on a different content and meaning depending on whether the language being used to describe it is epidemiological, clinical or lay. While the epidemiologist may quote the number of deaths per 1000 babies that occur with a given complication, the clinical risk can be expressed in comments such as 'I have seen 10 babies die . . . '. Women who know someone who has had a stillbirth are much more aware of that hazard than those who do not. For professionals, those who have dealt with a serious complication are subsequently more likely to see the risk of that complication as being higher than it actually is. Kaufert and O'Neil (1993) found, when talking with health professionals, that their fear of childbirth was related to concerns about competence and being able to cope in an emergency. The burden of responsibility is enormous, and the experience of the last case can inordinately affect judgement. In labour, care decisions can be influenced by fear of litigation, the common response often being over use of investigation or of treatment, subjecting labouring women to treatment regimens based on hospital policies rather than an individualized care plan.

Even in situations where the diagnosis is certain, the appropriate treatment may be far from certain (Harvey 1996). However, when women express a desire to deviate from the recommended standard of care, for example by seeking to give birth at home rather than in a hospital, risk discourse often moves into the emotional realm. This involves the clinician conjuring up images of past obstetric disasters.

The individualization of risk has legitimated the routine use of invasive techniques such as the augmentation of uterine activity and drug administration in pregnancy and childbirth, all potentially hazardous. When labour is not progressing 'normally', an assumption is made that women and their babies are at risk because of the pending failure of their bodies. A large number of interventions are begun for 'failure to progress in labour,' which incorporates the lack of progressive dilatation of the cervix and maternal exhaustion. Lane argues that this term merely describes an existing state: 'They are not reasons, but states of being. These states of being may seem legitimate reasons for medical intervention, but they do not provide a causal explanation' Lane (1995, p. 63).

Contextual factors, including positive and negative social exchanges and emotional responses to physical surroundings, are rarely examined or considered in the causal framework. However, these contextual factors may be the primary determinants of risk precipitating medical intervention.

Lupton (1993) observed that the discourse of risk is weighted toward disaster and anxiety rather than peace of mind. Oakley (1993) writes about the connection between peace of mind and a competent cervix, and emotional confidence and a coordinated uterus.

QUANTIFYING THE RISKS OF 'INFORMED COMPLIANCE'

During 2002, three very important studies, a survey, a cluster randomized controlled trial and an adjunct qualitative study were published by a group of midwives and others based in Sheffield, England (Kirkham 2004). The themes that emerged are sobering signposts pointing to some of the contemporary risks that women currently face in the maternity services. The researchers set out to determine the extent to which women using maternity services perceive that they have exercised informed choice. In addition the researchers investigated the use of evidence-based leaflets on informed choice and the effect of leaflets on promoting informed choice for women (O'Cathain et al 2002a, 2002b, Stapleton et al 2002). The results from all three studies illustrate clearly the overwhelming 'risks' that women face today in the maternity services in terms of 'compliance' and 'coercion'.

O'Cathain et al (2002a) carried out a survey about the perceived involvement of women in making informed decisions, that when women said they had made an informed choice at any of the decision points during their care this was strongly associated with the perception of having made informed choices about all the things that happened during their maternity care. Over half of the women 54% (905) felt that they had made informed choices about all the things that happened during their maternity care in both the antenatal and the postnatal samples. The perception of informed choice was lower for fetal heart monitoring at 31% (513) and higher for the screening test for Down's syndrome and spina bifida in the baby 73% (996) and feeding the baby 70% (1184) (O'Cathain et al 2002a).

Overall informed choice was defined as 'having enough information and discussion with midwives or doctors to make choices together about all the things that happened during maternity care'. In this first study responses were analysed to evaluate the level of informed choice operating at each of the following decision points: support in labour, listening to the baby's heartbeat during labour, deciding whether to have an ultrasound scan, having a choice of positions in labour and at birth, having an epidural for pain relief in labour, feeding baby with breast or bottle, screening for Down's syndrome and spina bifida in pregnancy and where to have the baby – in hospital or at home? In the researchers own words 'findings from this study imply that women's perceptions may overestimate the extent to which informed choice actually occurs and may measure the extent to which 'informed compliance' occurs' (O'Cathain et al 2002a).

The clustered randomized trial was carried out in 13 maternity units in Wales which were allocated to 10 paired clusters. This meant that the units were divided into five pairs and then each pair was randomly allocated to the 'intervention' care, in which evidence-based leaflets were introduced to antenatal care, or to 'control' care, which meant usual care was offered to women. The main aim was to assess the effect of evidence-based leaflets on promoting informed choice in women using maternity services. Four separate samples of women in the participating units responded to a study questionnaire about information in maternity care. Before leaflets were introduced in the intervention clusters, 1386 pregnant women (707 intervention, 679 control) and 1741 postnatal women (922 intervention, 819 control) responded to the questionnaire. After the introduction of the leaflets in the interventions clusters, 1678 pregnant women (935 intervention, 843 control) and 1547 postnatal women (886 intervention, 661 control) responded to the same questions. The study demonstrated that use of the leaflets did not change the proportion of women who reported exercising informed choice, or components or consequences of informed choice, in maternity care (O'Cathain et al 2002b). There was no change in the proportion of women who reported that they exercised informed choice in the 'intervention' units compared with the 'control' units for either antenatal or postnatal women. There was a small increase in satisfaction with information in the intervention units compared with the control units (odds ratio 1.40, 95% confidence interval 1.05 to 1.88). Only three quarters of women in the intervention units reported being given at least one of the leaflets, indicating problems with the implementation of the intervention. This led the researchers to conclude that in everyday practice, evidence-based leaflets were not effective in promoting informed choice in women using maternity services (O'Cathain et al 2002b).

A qualitative study was undertaken alongside this randomized controlled trial and it provides a rich insight into what was happening with the information leaflets. It found that the way in which the leaflets were disseminated affected the way informed choice was promoted (Stapleton et al 2002). The culture into which the leaflets were introduced supported existing normative patterns of care and this ensured informed compliance rather than informed choice (Stapleton et al 2002).

As with all sound research, many questions remain at the end of the project. The researchers identified that we need further research to answer questions relating to the *perceived* involvement in decision making, and whether this is more important to consumers of healthcare than *actual* involvement. Further research is needed to determine why women have different preferences for the extent to which they want to be involved in making decisions and why were women who preferred a non-participatory style more likely to perceive that they exercised informed choice? According to the researchers these women were more likely to be multiparous, with lower educational status and from manual social occupations (O'Cathain et al 2002a). The authors concluded that if women's views developed from a position of power and understanding, then their views should be respected and followed. However, if they are developed from a position of resignation or ignorance then we may wish to tackle this from an educational perspective (O'Cathain et al 2002a).

The results of the randomized trial assessing the use of information leaflets as a decision aid in everyday clinical practice leave several questions unanswered which must concern all midwives engaged in evidence-based practice. At the conclusion of their study the researchers ask:

- Regardless of the fact that decision aids are considered effective under certain circumstances, are they in fact effective in the real world?
- Under what circumstances should we believe women have truly been involved in the decision making around giving birth to their babies?

The results from the qualitative study (Stapleton et al 2002) found that doctors and midwives were positive about the leaflets and their potential to assist women in making informed choices, but they were usually too busy, and women perceived they were too busy to answer many questions. This undermined their effective use. Some midwives also made assumptions about the ability and willingness of women to participate in decision making. These assumptions were sometimes incorrect (Stapleton et al 2002). Some technological interventions, such as ultrasound scanning and monitoring in labour, have become so routine in maternity care that health professionals no longer perceive them as optional. Women sometimes made choices on the basis of their previous experiences of childbirth but were often met with resistance if their preferences contradicted established clinical norms. Staff sometimes expressed a strong dislike for an option covered by the leaflets to the extent that distribution of some leaflets was terminated on some sites (Stapleton et al 2002, p. 641). Researchers observed health professionals driving decision making towards technological intervention by conveying information which either minimized the risk of the intervention or emphasized the potential for harm without the intervention. This seemed to make it difficult for women to hear alternative messages, even from obstetricians. Both fear of litigation and bullying were involved in promoting notions of 'right' choices with which clinicians felt clinically secure.

QUANTIFYING THE RISKS FOR INTERVENTION

Alongside this lack of informed decision making in pregnancy and childbirth is the risk imposed by rising levels of obstetric intervention in birth. In her essay 'The medical model of the body as a site of risk' Karen Lane points to amongst other things, the risks women face in the iatrogenic risk of interventions (Lane 1995, p. 56).

The disabling power of intervention in birth is described in the following account of a woman who had a caesarean section for the birth of her first baby. 'In my delivery I was an adjunct; I had almost no role. There was nothing I could do to contribute to the birthing process if I wanted to, which I badly did before epidural essentially neutered my faculties and will. From what we had been told about the (CTG) monitors reading, my husband and I understood that the baby's life was at stake. No parent would risk the health of his or her child by questioning the procedures the medical establishment had decreed were necessary. I did not dare risk doing anything other than what the doctors and nurses told us I must do. I lay down passively on the birthing bed, letting them tie and tether me down and anaesthetize me' (Wolf 2001, p. 117).

In all industrialized countries the levels of obstetric intervention during childbirth, including caesarean section, have risen dramatically since the 1960s without a concomitant dramatic fall in rates of maternal and neonatal morbidity (Thacker et al 2004, Wagner 2001). In developed countries, obstetric management and medical intervention have become routine without evidence of effectiveness (Hofmeyr 2004). The effect of business management principles and production and marketing models of maternity care in Australia and the US have promoted routine use of excessive interventions during childbirth. The prevailing business imperatives underlying medical care define, determine, and distort that care (Perkins 2004).

THE RISKS OF CASCADE OF INTERVENTION

In 2000, 2002 and 2005 a multidisciplinary group of researchers undertook several population based studies on the effect of obstetric intervention and the risk of the 'cascade effect' of interventions in labour and birth (Roberts et al 2000, 2002, Tracy et al 2006). The studies showed the association between interventions introduced in labour with the resulting intervention at the time of birth amongst women who were considered to be of low obstetric risk for any intervention in labour. The study populations were also classified according to whether they employed a private obstetrician or gave birth in a private hospital. The first study was designed to identify the 'risks' associated with private obstetric care in comparison to public hospital care. It included 171,000 births in New South Wales between 1996 and 1997 and found that amongst low-risk first time mothers, labour was induced or augmented with oxytocin for one in three women who gave birth in a public hospital and half the women who gave birth in a private hospital with a private obstetrician. A quarter of all public women and a half of the privately insured women used epidural anaesthesia. Forceps procedures or vacuum extraction were used to deliver one in every five babies born in a public hospital and one in every three born in a private hospital. One in three public women and half of all private women received an episiotomy. Overall, less than one in four first time mothers in a public hospital and less than one in every two first time mothers in private hospitals give birth without obstetric intervention of any sort (Roberts et al 2000). The study concluded that the risk of intervention in labour and birth was more highly associated with having private obstetric care than with identified risk markers in pregnancy (Roberts et al 2000).

A study was undertaken the following year aimed at estimating the economic impact of these interventions on the public health system and to identify the potential savings from lowering intervention rates (Tracy & Tracy 2003). When a cost formula was applied to these levels of intervention, the relative cost of birth increased by up to 50% for low-risk primiparous women and up to 36% for low-risk multiparous women as labour interventions accumulated. An epidural was associated with a sharp increase in cost of up to 32% for some primiparous low-risk women, and up to 36% for some multiparous low-risk women. Private obstetric care increased the overall relative cost by 9% for primiparous low-risk women and 4% for multiparous low-risk women (Tracy & Tracy 2003). (see Fig. 11.1).

To ascertain the trends in intervention, another study into the trends in labour and birth interventions in NSW was undertaken (Roberts et al 2002). For a population of 336,189 women categorised as low risk of a poor pregnancy outcome over an eight year period (1990–1997), fewer than 40% of 'low-risk' first time mothers had a vaginal birth following an epidural (Roberts et al 2002). Women who had no identified pregnancy risk markers and were having a first baby were five times more likely to have an instrumental birth following an epidural. For multiparous women without identified risk markers the risk was ten times higher after an epidural (Roberts et al 2002).

In the most recent study undertaken in Australia by Tracy et al (2006) the cascade of interventions that begin in pregnancy and build up through labour and birth is again demonstrated. This population based study of all women (1,017,958) who gave birth in Australia between 1999–2002 shows the 'cascade' where women with uncomplicated pregnancies (medically low-risk women) were more likely to have an instrumental birth (vacuum or forceps) or a caesarean section than a vaginal birth following an epidural (Tracy et al 2005). The following illustration demonstrates what happens following the introduction of interventions into labour in a pre specified cascade effect by grouping them in a chronological sequence – those interventions that occur during labour but before birth (epidural and induction of labour) followed by those that occur at the time of birth (episiotomy and type of delivery) (Fig. 11.2).

When women are offered interventions in labour such as induction and epidurals, they may not be informed of the cascade of interventions in labour and birth that almost inevitably follow. Unnecessary intervention allocates scarce resources to a group of women who do not need them. However, appropriate and meaningful information on the outcomes associated with the various interventions may ultimately influence their choices. The rising rates of obstetric intervention in labour are concerning for both women and those who oversee maternity service policy and funding. Although some interventions in obstetrics are appropriate and have led to improved perinatal outcome, no intervention is absolutely free of risk of unintended harm. Wagner goes

Low risk Primiparous women

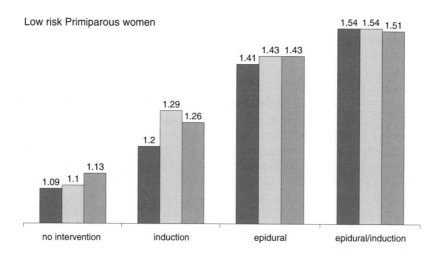

Low risk Multiparous women

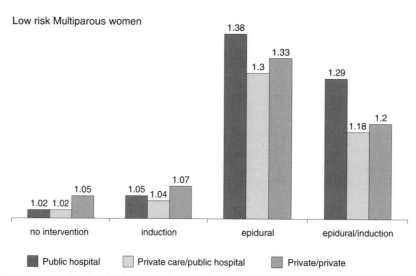

■ Public hospital   ▢ Private care/public hospital   ▢ Private/private

Figure 11.1   Costing the cascade: the rise in cost units associated with the introduction of increased levels of intervention for low-risk women in different systems of care. There is an incremental rise in cost (measured in cost units) as interventions such as induction and epidurals are used in labour and birth (Tracy & Tracy 2003)

even further to note 'Western, medicalized, high tech maternity care under obstetric control usually dehumanizes, often leads to unnecessary, costly, dangerous, invasive obstetric interventions and should never be exported to developing countries' (Wagner 2001, p. S26).

SOLUTIONS: WOMEN AND MIDWIVES MAKING DECISIONS TOGETHER

There are ways to effect a change in this all encompassing and apparently all consuming context of risk in pregnancy and childbirth. One of the most

promising is the method of 'walking' through care in pregnancy and childbirth prompted by a series of 'decision points' which remind midwives and women to discuss together the need for addressing certain issues as they arise. In New Zealand women and midwives have a special booklet to help them navigate their way through the risks that present themselves during pregnancy and labour. The New Zealand Midwives Handbook for Practice (New Zealand College of Midwives 2004) is a comprehensive guide for establishing information sharing and 'partnership' (Guilliland & Pairman 1995) between women

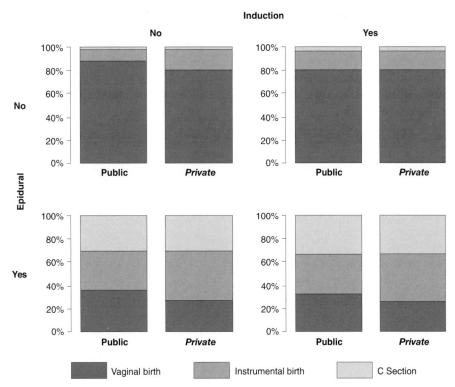

Induction

No   Yes

Figure 11.2   The cascade of labour and birth interventions for first time mothers who were medically low risk in Australia, 1999–2002 by location of labour and birth: public hospitals (public) and women who were attended by private obstetricians in private hospitals (*private*). As the interventions are introduced in a chronological sequence the association with further intervention demonstrates the 'cascade of interventions'

and their caregivers. It is a widely available practical guide written for midwives, women and the general public and aims to set in place a system for the profession and the public to measure both individual midwife practices and midwifery services. Rather than prescribing a course of action including medical 'visits' at monthly and fortnightly intervals as most antenatal guidelines do, the handbook is set out using a format of 'decision points' for the woman and midwife to negotiate through the entire pregnancy, birth and postpartum spectrum. This offers a unique opportunity for women to plan with their midwife, the strategies and actions needed to make their pregnancy and birth both safe and fulfilling. It reinforces the notion that women are paramount in the decision making around childbirth, as well as providing comprehensive information on public health interventions that are attainable during pregnancy and childbirth. It prompts health behaviours such as

choices for self-care and lifestyle including education about smoking, diet, exercise, breastfeeding and childhood vaccination, information about community agencies, social services, and consumer agencies. It raises public issues with women such as the need to educate the medical and midwifery workforce for the future, and invites women to consider participating. It also spells out the rights women have, to make a complaint about their care, and how to access resolution processes when problems arise. The handbook is a practical reminder of the fact that although women are confronted almost daily with the notion of pregnancy and labour as a risky undertaking, it helps women to map out good reasons for requiring anything that would interfere with the normal process, and weigh up the evidence to show that any intervention about to be undertaken will have been well considered from an informed perspective. The prompt for women and midwives to discuss and evaluate together each decision in the context of appropriate and adequate information helps to avoid many unnecessary interventions.

CONCLUSION

Strategies for the future include a vision of care for all childbearing women in which care is continuous, personalized and non-authoritarian, responding to a woman's physical, social, emotional and cultural needs (Page 2000). Care is thus built on a model of cooperation between women and their healthcare providers, women being encouraged to participate and make choices regarding their care (Donley 1986, Guililland 1990). Midwifery, in partnership with women, must develop and clearly define its own model or framework for risk assessment, based on principles that are holistic in scope and incorporate what midwives refer to as a *midwifery philosophy* of care.

POINTERS FOR PRACTICE

- The label of 'high risk' is intended to direct attention and provide specialized care for particular women or groups of women. It may, however, be used by institutions to control women, and may make women feel inadequate.
- Clinical judgement should be used in determining treatment for individual women, along with evidence-based guidelines for consultation and referral.
- Pregnant women depend on care-givers' advice. Their decision-making will be influenced by how the information is presented.
- It is up to the individual woman to decide what constitutes an acceptable risk to her.
- Risk assessment tools and strategies lack precision and are of poor predictive value.
- Do risk factors exist? Women may have risk *markers* that alert her midwife to the need for careful observation or consultation. Markers other than medical factors are often ignored.

References

Adelsward V, Sachs L 1996 The meaning of 6.8: numeracy and normality in health information talks. Sociology Science Medicine 43(8): 1179–1187

Albers L L 2005 Overtreatment of normal childbirth in U.S. hospitals. Birth 32: 67

Alexander S, Keirse M J N C 1989 Formal risk scoring during pregnancy. In: Chalmers I, Enkin M, Keirse M J N C (eds) Effective care in pregnancy and childbirth, vol. 1. Oxford University Press, Oxford

Allan C J, Argyropoulos G, Bowker M et al 1997 Gestational diabetes mellitus and gene mutations which affect insulin secretion. Diabetes Research and Clinical Practice 36(3): 135–141

American College of Obstetrics and Gynecologists 1997 Routine ultrasound in low-risk pregnancy, ACOG practice patterns: evidence-based guidelines for clinical issues. International Journal of Gynecology and Obstetrics 59(3): 273–278

Armstrong D 1995 The rise of surveillance medicine. Sociology of Health and Illness 17(3): 394–404

Arney W R 1982 Power and the profession of obstetrics. University of Chicago Press, Chicago

Beck U 1992 Risk society: towards a new modernity. Sage, London

Bischoff F Z, Lewis D E, Simpson J L 2005 Cell-free fetal DNA in maternal blood: kinetics, source and structure. Human Reproduction Update 11(1): 59–67

Bursztajn H J, Feinbloom R I, Hamm R M, Brodsky A 1990 Medical choices, medical chances: how patients, families, and physicians can cope with uncertainty. 2nd edn. Routledge/Chapman & Hall, New York

Campbell R 1999 Review and assessment of selection criteria used when booking pregnant women at different places of birth. British Journal of Obstetrics and Gynaecology 106: 550–556

Chalmers B 1982 Psychological aspects of pregnancy: some thoughts for the eighties. Social Science and Medicine 6: 323–331

Clarke A, Shim J K, Mamo L, Forsket J R, Fishman J R 2003 Biomedicalization: technoscientific transformations of health, illness, and US biomedicine. American Sociological Review 66: 161–194

Crandon A J 1979 Maternal anxiety and obstetric complications. Journal of Psychosomatic Research 23: 109–111

Crawford R 2004 Risk ritual and the management of control and anxiety in medical culture. Health 8(4): 505–528

de Vries R 1996 The midwife's place: an international comparison of the status of midwives. In: Murray S F (ed.) Midwives and safer motherhood. Mosby, London, pp 159–174

Donley J 1986 Save the midwife. New Women's Press, Auckland, New Zealand

Douglas M 1994 Risk and blame. Essays in cultural theory. Routledge, London

Douglas M, Wildavsky A 1982 Risk and culture. Basil Blackwell, Oxford

Duden B 1993 Disembodying women: perspectives on pregnancy and the unborn. Harvard University Press, Cambridge

Edwards A, Elwyn G, Smith C et al 2001 Consumers' views of quality in the consultation and their relevance to 'shared decision-making' approaches. Health Expectations 4: 151–161

Edwards NP 2000 Women planning homebirths: their own views on their relationships with midwives. In: Kirkham M (ed.) The midwife–mother relationship. Macmillan, London

Ehrenreich B, English D 1973 Witches, midwives and nurses: a history of women healers. Feminist Press, New York

Enkin M 1994 Risk in pregnancy: the reality, the perception, and the concept. Birth 21(3): 131–134

Enkin M, Keirse M J N C, Neilson J, Crowther C, Duley L, Hodnett E, Hofmeyer J 2000 A guide to effective care in pregnancy and childbirth. Oxford University Press, Oxford

Fitzpatrick M 2000 The tyranny of health: doctors and the regulation of lifestyle. Routledge, London

Forde O H 1998 Is imposing risk awareness cultural imperialism? Social Science Medicine 47(9): 1155–1159

Foucault M 1975 The birth of the clinic: an archeology of medical perception. Vintage Books, New York

Foucault M 1979 Discipline and punish: the birth of the prison. Random House/Vintage Books, New York

Gabe J (ed.) 1995 Medicine, health and risk: sociological approaches. Blackwell, Oxford

Giddens A 1990 The consequences of modernity. Polity Press, Cambridge

Giddens A 1991 Modernity and self-identity: self and society in the late modern age. Polity Press, Cambridge

Goer H 2004 Humanizing birth: a global grassroots movement. Birth 31(4): 308–314

Gonen R, Tamir A, Degani S, Ohel G 2004 Variables associated with successful vaginal birth after one cesarean section: a proposed vaginal birth after cesarean section score. American Journal of Perinatology 21(8): 447–453

Gordis L 1996 Epidemiology. WB Saunders, Pennsylvania

Gorsuch R L, Key M K 1974 Abnormalities of pregnancy as a function of anxiety and life stress. Psychosomatic Medicine 36: 352–362

Graham S, Wood D 2003 Digitizing surveillance: categorization, space, inequality. Critical Social Policy 23(2): 227–248

Greer G 1999 Keynote address: homebirth Australia conference. September 11th, Byron Bay, Australia

Gregg R 1993 'Choice' as a double-edged sword: information, guilt and mother-blaming in a high-tech age. Women and Health 20(3): 53–73

Grimes L, Mehl L, McRae J, Peterson G 1983 Phenomenological risk screening for childbirth: successful prospective differentiation of risk for medically low-risk mothers. Journal of Nurse Midwifery 28: 27–30

Guililland K 1990 Women and midwives: a partnership in progress. Proceedings of the International Confederation of Midwives 21st International Congress of Midwives, Kobe, Japan

Guililand K, Pairman S 1995 The midwifery partnership: a model for practice. Department of Nursing and Midwifery Monograph Series 95/1. Victoria University of Wellington, New Zealand

Hall P F 1994 Editorial: rethinking risk. Canadian Family Physician 40: 1239–1244

Halliday J L, Collins V R, Aitken M A et al 2004 Genetics and public health–evolution, or revolution? Journal Epidemiology and Community Health 58: 894–899

Hallowell N 1999 Advising on the management of genetic risk: offering choice or prescribing action? Health, Risk and Society 1: 267–281

Hallowell N, Foster C, Eeles R et al 2004 Accommodating risk: responses to BRCA1/2 genetic testing of women who have had cancer. Social Science and Medicine 59: 553–565

Hallowell N, Lawton J 2002 Negotiating present and future selves: managing the risk of hereditary ovarian cancer by prophylactic surgery. Health 6(4): 423–443

Handwerker L 1994 Medical risk: implicating poor pregnant women. Social Science and Medicine 38(5): 66–75

Harris G, Connor L, Bisits A, Higginbotham N 2004 'Seeing the Baby': pleasures and dilemmas of ultrasound technologies for primiparous Australian women. Medical Anthropology Quarterly 18(1): 23–48

Harvey J 1996 Achieving the indeterminate: accomplishing degrees of certainty in life and death situations. Editorial Board of Sociological Review. Blackwell, Oxford

Hayes M V 1992 On the epistemology of risk: language, logic and social science. Social Science and Medicine 35(4): 401–407

Heamen M, Gupton A, Gregory D 2004 Factors influencing women's perception of risk during pregnancy. MCN 29(2): 111–116

Hobel C J 1978 Risk assessment in perinatal medicine. Clinical Obstetrics and Gynecology 21(2): 287–295

Hobel C J, Hyvarinen M A, Okada D M, Oh W 1973 Prenatal and intrapartum high-risk screening: prediction of the high-risk neonate. American Journal of Obstetrics and Gynecology 117: 1–9

Hodnett E D 2004 Continuity of caregivers for care during pregnancy and childbirth (Cochrane Review). The Cochrane Library, Issue 3, 2004. Wiley, Chichester, UK

Hofmeyr G J 2004 Evidence-based intrapartum care Best Practice & Research Clinical Obstetrics and Gynaecology 20(30): 1–13

Howson 1998 Surveillance, knowledge, and risk: the embodied experience of cervical screening. Health 2: 195–215

Kapp F T, Hornstein S, Graham V T 1963 Some psychological factors in prolonged labor due to inefficient uterine action. Comparative Psychiatry 4: 9–13

Katchner F D 1950 A study of the emotional reactions during labor. American Journal of Obstetrics and Gynecology 60: 19–29

Kaufert P A, O'Neil J 1993 Analysis of a dialogue on risks in childbirth: clinicians, epidemiologists, and Inuit women. In: Lindenbaum S, Lock M (eds) Knowledge, power and practice: the anthropology of medicine and everyday life. University of California Press, Los Angeles

Kavanagh A M, Broom D H 1998 Embodied risk: my body, myself? Social Science and Medicine 46: 437–444

Kirkham M 2004 Informed choice in maternity care. Palgrave Macmillan. Hampshire, UK

Kitzinger J, Reilly J 1997 The rise and fall of risk reporting. Media coverage of human genetics research, 'false memory syndrome' and 'mad cow disease'. European Journal of Communication 12: 31950

Kolder V, Gallagher J, Parsons M 1987 Court-ordered obstetrical interventions. New England Journal of Medicine 316(19): 1192–1196

Koong D, Evans S, Mayes C, McDonald S, Newnham J 1997 A scoring system for the prediction of successful delivery in low-risk birthing units. Obstetrics and Gynecology 89(5): 654–659

Lane K 1995 The medical model of the body as a site of risk: a case study of childbirth. In: Gabe J (ed.) Medicine, health and risk: sociological approaches. Blackwell, Oxford

Laukaran V H, van den Berg B J 1980 The relationship of maternal attitude to pregnancy outcomes and obstetric complications. American Journal of Obstetrics and Gynecology 136: 374–379

Lazarus E S 1990 Falling through the cracks: contradictions and barriers to care in a prenatal clinic. Medical Anthropology Quarterly 12: 269–287

Lilford R J, Chard T 1983 Problems and pitfalls of risk assessment in antenatal care. British Journal of Obstetrics and Gynaecology 90: 507–510

Low J A, Simpson L L, Toni G, Chamberlain S et al 1995 Limitations in the clinical prediction of intrapartum fetal asphyxia. American Journal Obstetrics and Gynecology 72: 801–804

Lupton D 1993 Risk as moral danger: the social and political functions of risk discourse in public health. International Health Surveys 23(3): 425–435

Lupton D 1995 The imperative of health: public health and the regulated body. Sage, Thousand Oaks, CA

Lupton D 1999 Risk. Routledge, New York

Maier K E 1992 Forced cesarean section as reproductive control and violence: a feminist social work perspective on the 'Baby R' case. Unpublished Master's thesis, Women's Studies, Simon Fraser University, Canada

Mander R 2001 Response to male appropriation and medicalization of childbirth: an historical analysis. Journal of Advanced Nursing 35(3): 390–391

McDonald R L 1968 The role of emotional factors in obstetric complications: a review. Psychosomatic Medicine 30(2): 222–237

Mooney G 1999 Public health versus private practice: the contested development of compulsory disease notification in late nineteenth century Britain. Bulletin of the History of Medicine 73(2): 238–267

Moynihan R, Heath I, Henry D 2002 Selling sickness: the pharmaceutical industry and disease mongering. British Medical Journal 324: 886–891

Murphy P A 1994 Editorial: Risk, risk assessment and risk labels. Journal of Nurse Midwifery 39(2): 67–69

Nelkin D 1989 Communicating technological risk: social construction of risk perception. Annual Review of Public Health 10: 95–113

Nelkin D 1998 letters The Lancet 352(9131): 893

Nelkin D 2001 Beyond risk. Reporting about genetics in the post-Asilomar press. Biology and Medicine 44: 199–207

Nelkin D, Andrews L 1999 DNA identification and surveillance creep. Sociology of Health and Illness 21(5): 689–706

Nelkin D, Tancredi L 1994 Dangerous diagnostics: the social power of biological information 2nd edn. University of Chicago Press, Chicago

New Zealand College of Midwives 2004 Handbook for practice. NZCOM, Christchurch, NZ

Nilsson L 1965 A child is born – the drama of life before birth. Dell, New York

Nuckolls K, Cassel J, Kaplan B 1972 Psychosocial assets, life crisis and the prognosis of pregnancy. American Journal of Epidemiology 95(5): 431–41

O'Cathain A, Thomas K, Walters S J, Nicholl J, Kirkham M 2002a Women's perceptions of informed choice in maternity care. Midwifery 18: 136–144

O'Cathain A, Walters S J, Nicholl J P, Thomas K J, Kirkham M 2002b Use of evidence based leaflets to promote informed choice in maternity care: randomised controlled trial in everyday practice. British Medical Journal 324: 643–646

Oakley A 1984 The captured womb: a history of the medical care of pregnant women. Blackwell, Oxford

Oakley A 1992 Social support and motherhood: the natural history of a research project. Blackwell, Oxford

Oakley A 1993 Essays on women, medicine and health. Edinburgh University Press, Edinburgh

Orwell G 1949 Nineteen eighty-four. New American Library, New York

Osofsky H J, Kendall N 1973 Poverty as a criterion of risk. Clinical Obstetrics and Gynecology 18: 103–109

Overall C (ed.) 1989 The future of human reproduction. Women's Press, Toronto

Page L A (ed.) 2000 The new midwifery:science and sensitivity in practice. Churchill Livingstone, Edinburgh

Perkins B B 1994 Intensity, stratification, and risk in perinatal care: redefining problems and restructuring levels. Women and Health 21(1): 17–31

Perkins B B 2004 The medical delivery business: health reform, childbirth, and the economic order. Rutgers University Press, New Brunswick, New Jersey

Petersen A 1998 The new genetics and the politics of public health. Critical Public Health 8: 59–72

Petersen A, Lupton D 1996 The new public health: health and self in the screening decisions: age of risk. Sage, London

Queniart A 1992 Risky business: medical definitions of pregnancy. In: Currie D H, Raoul V (eds) Anatomy of gender: women's struggle for the body. Carleton University Press, Ontario

Radford T 1997 Juggling life's comical odds. Guardian, 5 December, p. 21

RCOG 2003 Antenatal care: routine care for the health pregnant woman. Royal College of Obstetricians and Gynaecologists, London

Riessman C K, Nathanson C A 1986 The management of reproduction: social construction of risk and responsibility. In: Aiken L H, Mechanic D (eds) Applications of social science: to clinical medicine and health policy. Rutgers University Press, New Jersey

Roberts C L, Algert C, Peat B, Tracy S, Douglas I 2002 Trends in labour and birth interventions among low-risk women in an Australian population. Australia and New Zealand Journal Obstetrics and Gynaecology 42(2): 176–181

Roberts C, Tracy S, Peat B 2000 Rates for obstetric intervention rates among private and public patients in Australia: population based descriptive study. British Medical Journal 321(7254): 137–141

Robertson A 2001 Biotechnology, political rationality and discourses on health risk. Health 5(3): 293–309

Rodgers S 1989 Pregnancy as justification for loss of juridical autonomy In: Overall C (ed.) The future of human reproduction. Women's Press, Toronto

Rothman B 1982 In labor: women and power in the birthplace. WW Norton, New York

Sapolsky R A 1990 The politics of risk. Daedalus 119: 83–96

Saxell L, The Midwifery Group 1999 Nulliparous women's perception of the risk of pregnancy after age 35. Health and Canadian Society 4: 367–388

Scott S, Prior F, Wood L, Gray J 2005 Repositioning the patient: the implications of being 'at risk'. Social Science and Medicine 60(8): 1869–1879

Shorten A, Chamberlain M, Shorten B, Karaminia A 2004 Making choices for childbirth: development and testing of a decision-aid for women who have experienced previous caesarean. Patient Education and Counseling 52: 307–313

Smilkstein G, Helsper-Lucas A, Ashworth C, Montano D, Pagel M 1984 Predictions of pregnancy complications: an application of the biopsychosocial model. Social Science and Medicine 18(4): 315–321

Stallings S P, Paling J 2001 New tool for presenting risk. Obstetrics and Gynecology 98: 345–349

Stapleton H, Kirkham M, Thomas G 2002 Qualitative study of evidence based leaflets in maternity care. British Medical Journal 324: 639–643

Thacker S B, Stroup D, Chang M 2004 Continuous electronic heart rate monitoring for fetal assessment during labor (Cochrane Review). In The Cochrane Library, Issue 1. Wiley, Chichester

Tracy S, Tracy M 2006 Revisiting the cascade of interventions in birth. Unpublished manuscript.

Tracy S, Tracy M 2003 Costing the cascade: estimating the cost of increased obstetric intervention in childbirth using population data. British Journal Obstetric and Gynaecology 110: 717–724

Wagner M 2001 Fish can't see water: the need to humanize birth. International Journal of Gynecology and Obstetrics 75: S25–S37

Wajcman J 1994 Delivered into men's hands? The social construction of reproductive technology. In: Sen G, Snow R C (eds) Power and decision: the social control of reproduction. Harvard University Press, Boston, pp 153–175

Wall E M 1988 Assessing obstetric risk: a review of obstetric risk-scoring systems. Journal of Family Practice 27(2): 43–45

Wilkinson I 2001 Anxiety in a risk society. Routledge, London

Wolf N 2001 Misconceptions: truth, lies and the unexpected on the journey to motherhood. Chatto and Windus, London

Worboys M 2000 Spreading germs: disease theories and medical practice in Britain, 1865–1900. Cambridge University Press, Cambridge, UK

Chapter 12

Why do research?

Jane Sandall and Rona McCandlish

All that we do as health professionals is based on a mixture of formal knowledge, experience and judgement. Every day midwives combine these knowledge and information sources to work with women and their families, advising and supporting them in their decisions to provide the 'best' quality care. Evidence generated by research is an ingredient in the mix, and in the UK and many parts of the world is an increasingly significant influence on practice. For example, clinical guidelines such as those developed by the National Institute for Health and Clinical Excellence (NICE) (see www.nice.org.uk) and service delivery guidelines such as the National Service Framework for Children, Young People and Maternity Services (Department of Health 2004) are based on 'best' evidence. What is considered to be best evidence, how is it produced, and most importantly how midwives and women can judge the strengths and limitations of such evidence is discussed in Chapter 10. Although much evidence is based on research, some midwives find it hard to see the relevance of research to their own everyday practice, and find it even harder to engage with it directly. We feel this is because 'doing' research, just as attending birth, cannot be learnt solely from books, but is learnt by 'doing', which means building on formal knowledge, accumulated experience and reflection. We also consider that research for midwifery is too important to be 'someone else's business' and so we want all midwives to be part of it, to take ownership, and make sure that midwifery research works for women, families and midwives.

With this in mind we decided that this would not be a chapter about 'how to do' research, although it will give pointers about where to find information about different research methods and how to apply them. Instead it aims to convince readers that research is important and to give examples of how midwifery research has made a difference to the care of women and their families. We hope it will give some insight into the political and social context of midwifery research and demonstrate why engaging with research is vital to ensuring that midwifery practice remains relevant and responsive to the needs of women and families.

WE WANT TO:

1. ask and answer the question 'Why do research'?;
2. reflect on how research for midwifery has become reality during our working lives;
3. think about the political and social context of research;
4. demonstrate the importance of setting relevant and answerable research questions;
5. consider what methods are used and how research evidence is generated.

Our journeys in midwifery began as students in the UK in the 1980s at a time when asking questions about care was not greatly encouraged. The following quotation, from the foreword to the well-known and widely used midwifery textbook by Margaret Myles was first published in 1953 and republished with each edition of that book until

1985; and it captures attitudes to learning, enquiry and unquestioned acceptance of expert opinion that were then prevalent in midwifery:

> No bibliographical references have been given because of the vast number of sources which have been tapped in compiling the text and because pupil midwives become confused when they study from more than one or two text-books. Few . . . pupils would find time to read widely; for . . . pupils who desire to broaden their field of study the midwife teacher will recommend suitable books.
>
> Myles 1953, p. vii

In the twenty-five years since the last appearance of these words in Myles, an information revolution has swept through healthcare which has challenged conventional deference to expert opinion. It has also had the potential to empower women and families by providing them with access to the information that healthcare professionals draw on. As a result anyone who now claims the knowledge and professional expertise to be a midwife needs to be prepared to question whether the care they offer is based on evidence that it is likely to cause more good than harm for women and families, and to acknowledge when there is a lack of evidence and talk through that uncertainty in partnership with women. Evidence and information generated by robust research is therefore fundamental to practising contemporary midwifery and the foreword to the most recent edition of Myles Textbook for Midwives vividly illustrates this. In it Gillian Fletcher (2003), then President of the National Childbirth Trust (the UK's largest 'lay' organization which aims to provide wide-ranging support to new parents (http://www.nctpregnancyandbabycare.com/) said

> The editors of this new edition . . . have done an excellent job of weaving both the art and the science of midwifery throughout . . . [the text is] . . . brimming with up-to-date research.
>
> Fletcher 2003, p. xi

Many midwives who have moved into research did so with a desire to challenge inhumane and ineffective practice that did more harm than good.

The aim was to generate new knowledge by asking different questions that would improve the care that women and families receive. This desire underpinned the development of MIDIRS Midwifery Information Service (http://www.midirs.org/), to make such knowledge accessible to a wider audience. During the 1980s, student midwives were not trained within a university system and midwives and service users did not have automatic rights of access to medical libraries to assess the quality of the evidence that such policies were based upon. Since these early, rather naïve, days where it was felt that the production of high quality evidence was all that was needed for practice to change, there has been the development of the evidence based health movement, which seeks to address the complexities and politics of how practice changes come about. Maternity care has always been a political arena for debate where women and professionals draw on evidence to support their case. For example, in the UK in the 1980s, there were many public and professional arguments about the use of new technologies in pregnancy and childbirth such as active management of labour, and about whether home birth is safe (Bourgeault et al 2001). Such debates continue today, for example, about new technologies such as one stop prenatal screening (Williams et al 2005) and midwife led units (Walsh & Downe 2004).

Being a midwife is truly a journey of life-long learning. We believe that active understanding of, and involvement in research about midwifery is fundamental to effective, relevant, responsive midwifery. The exhilaration of being a 21st century midwife is being able to work with women and families during the most significant experiences of life, and use the best knowledge and evidence we have, combined with the skill and art of midwifery, to support them.

WHY DO RESEARCH?

Very little UK based work has formally reviewed the development of midwifery research and the impact on policy and practice to answer the question 'why do research?'. Rafferty and Traynor (2002) and Renfrew and Smith (2000) have discussed the place of nursing and midwifery research in the UK research and development strategy. Reasons for the difficulties that midwife researchers encounter in getting their findings valued and implemented by the midwifery profession have been discussed by Hicks (1995). However we have set out the following possible six responses to the question (you'll notice that we have stated the replies as questions – we don't think that any one is the 'right' answer!).

1. TO DEVELOP NEW MIDWIFERY KNOWLEDGE?

There is a view that its professional status is legitimized by the movement of midwifery training into higher education and by an involvement in research. It has also been suggested that midwifery needs to develop a body of knowledge to underpin practice (Bryar 1995).

2. TO IMPROVE THE EXPERIENCE OF CHILDBIRTH FOR WOMEN AND TO GIVE WOMEN A VOICE?

Some research has been inspired by a commitment towards giving women a voice and using their perspectives and experiences to inform a feminist political agenda. Much of this work has been carried out not by midwives but by social scientists (for example, Cartwright 1979, Green et al 1990, Macintyre 1977). It has highlighted the competing views of women and doctors (Graham & Oakley 1981), and placed women's experiences of reproduction into a wider theoretical framework examining the impact of patriarchy on women in society (Oakley 1980). Other researchers have focused on the needs of women from various ethnic groups (Baxter 1996). Clark (2000) summarizes this saying that

> It could be argued that this early social science research laid the foundation for the broad research base that now characterizes the research undertaken by midwives today. Right from the start, the views and experiences of women have been regarded as centrally important, thereby challenging the medical model of maternity care with its emphasis on cause and effect relationships and the effectiveness of forms of care, often at the expense of listening to

women themselves and knowledge of their experiences.

Clark 2000, p. 37

3. TO CHANGE PRACTICE AND MAKE SURE THAT CARE IS EFFECTIVE?

Individual midwives have often embarked on research because of their unhappiness with current practice. They have been motivated by a desire to demonstrate that a different way of doing things has a better outcome. Such research uses scientific principles to challenge the supremacy of clinical experience and opinion. Initiated by medical epidemiologists (Chalmers & Richards 1977) and using the controlled trial to evaluate effectiveness, iatrogenic consequences arising from obstetric technologies have been uncovered (Chalmers et al 1989). Midwives have been involved in this movement from an early stage, and midwives collaborating with epidemiologists have examined the effectiveness of common midwifery practices such as perineal care, and nipple preparation for breastfeeding (Alexander 1996, Kettle et al 2002, Sleep 1991). The Cochrane Library (http://www.cochrane.org/reviews/clibintro. htm) is the key information source for reviews of (mainly) trials in healthcare.

4. TO EXAMINE THE ROLE OF HEALTH PROFESSIONALS AND THE ORGANIZATION OF CARE?

In general, research in this area has focused on place of midwifery care in a health system, or the organization and delivery of care. It has generally been conducted by social scientists using methods such as surveys, interviews and observation. For example, cross cultural perspectives have been explored by Davis-Floyd and Sargent (1997) and de Vries et al (2001), and Benoit (2005) looked at the role of midwifery in Northern Europe and North America. Such work aims to understand the political and social context of maternity care, and the role of midwives within it, and how this impacts on the services that women and their families receive.

Robinson et al (1983) investigated the limited scope of midwifery practice and their findings highlighted medical domination of maternity care and the constrained role of the midwife, particularly in specialist units. Subsequent research has focused on the provision of less medicalized, woman-centred midwifery care (Green et al 1986) and the impact of midwifery policies on practice (Garcia & Garforth 1991). A second strand of research into occupational roles has examined the organization of care and the implementation of new developments (Davies & Evans 1991). Research into the organization of care proliferated following the government report Changing Childbirth (Department of Health 1993a). Studies have looked at team and caseload midwifery (Allen et al 1997, McCourt et al 1998, Wraight et al 1993), but most not all (Declerq 1998) of this work has been descriptive and has had a strong evaluative component, which has resulted in the under theorization of broader issues. Some research has explored in a reflective sense the experiences of midwives as workers, and the impact of emotion work in midwifery has been examined by Hunter and Deery (2005). The support needs for midwives have begun to be examined (e.g. Deery 2003) and workforce issues, for example recruitment and retention (Curtis et al 2003), the social shaping of Changing Childbirth Policy (Sandall 1996), and its impact on the midwifery workforce have been explored (Sandall 1998).

5. TO EXAMINE THE PROCESS OF MIDWIFERY CARE?

This stream of midwifery research has been concerned with the components of 'sensitive midwifery' and has usually been conducted by midwives, tending to focus on the primacy of the midwife–woman relationship. Examples include communication (Kirkham 1987), informed choice (Kirkham 2003), and continuity of care and carer (Flint et al 1989, McCourt et al 1998). The examination of the effectiveness of the psychosocial aspects of care has mainly been undertaken by social scientists drawing on a broader theoretical framework of similar work in other areas of healthcare, for example Oakley et al's (1996) work looking at the effect of social support in pregnancy and work on the impact of control in childbirth (Green & Baston 2003).

6. AS HISTORICAL RESEARCH?

There has been a stream of historical study into midwifery, usually undertaken by historians and sociologists. A wide range of research has examined the historical aspects of midwifery in Britain and abroad (e.g. Donnison 1988, Marland & Rafferty 1997). Other work has viewed midwifery history from a critical perspective: Heagerty (1997) and Hannam (1996), for example, have examined the role of the Midwives Institute (RCM), while Witz (1992), Leap & Hunter (1993) and Sandall (1996) have looked at the development of midwifery as a profession and the relationship between gender and social class. Yet other research (Oakley 1984, Williams 1997) has looked more broadly at women's experiences of motherhood and maternity care during the 20th century.

7. AS PART OF A COURSE REQUIREMENT OR JOB?

Many midwives are now being required to undertake small-scale projects as part of their job. As in any other area of midwifery practice, midwives should be trained and competent to do the work. Thus, midwives who are asked to do research should make sure that they have training and adequate supervision for the project. Other midwives have to carry out research as a requirement for a higher degree. It is important to remember that the reason for this involvement is that it is considered to be part of the educational and personal development of that particular midwife. Such midwives are often tempted into taking on large and complex research projects, which should really be the remit of midwives who have professional research training and experience.

WHERE DO OUR QUESTIONS COME FROM?

PERSONAL DRIVERS

Research should be driven by curiosity, and the questions that arise daily in midwifery work. However, although enthusiasm for asking questions is fundamental in developing research, it is essential to ask whether what is to be investigated or explored is an important and relevant issue, and is amenable to research. It helps to think through how would midwifery policy and practice, and women's experiences of care be changed if the research question(s) were answered?

For many midwives the drive to carry out research comes from their own uncertainty about whether care that they and other midwives are offering really does have the best results for women and families. The impact of this kind of research can be substantial. For example, the results of Sleep's work questioning whether using routine episiotomy is beneficial (Sleep 1991) have undoubtedly influenced practice, knowledge and information. However, not even such important work can answer all the questions about episiotomy. For example, the long-term effect of policies for routine and restricted use of episiotomy on women's long-term pelvic floor health remains under-evaluated.

At an individual level, questions come from a wide range of sources including listening to women, observing and reflecting on practice, personal experiences, reading newspapers, watching television, reading professional journals and learning about results of previous research, and talking to colleagues. At an institutional level, questions come from examining audit data and statistics, and making comparisons with other sites. At a national level, a more systematic way has developed of developing topics for research. Research is often determined by policy initiatives. For example, Standard 11 of the National Service Framework for Children's, Young People and Maternity Services (Department of Health 2004) set out the national standards about the content and delivery of care and outcomes.

POLITICAL DRIVERS

Deciding what and how topics get researched can be subject to political influences. Clearly the people who set the research agenda hold a powerful position in determining what research questions are asked and what are not. The danger is that what gets researched is driven by the interests of powerful professional groups and a government's policy agenda. In these circumstances issues that are more important to users and to the improvement of health in a broader sense can get neglected. At worst this could lead to reluctance on the part of government to fund research that might yield uncomfortable evidence questioning or challenging policy (Pollit et al 1990). An attempt to address these concerns in the UK has been the promotion of the involvement of users in research (Oliver et al 2004, and see INVOLVE web site http://www.involve.org.uk/).

In the 1990s policy initiatives were informed by the Centrally Commissioned Research Programme of the Department of Health, the purpose of which was to provide a knowledge base for health and social policies directed at the health of the population as a whole. The NHS Research and Development (R & D) strategy, in its goal of producing knowledge-based health care, created a national and regional infrastructure for identifying and prioritizing NHS research requirements. This resulted in a major research and development programme on NHS and nursing (Department of Health 1993b) priority topics. Details of the completed projects can be accessed on the Mother and Child Health pages of the Department of Health's website (http://www.dh.gov.uk). Other agencies in the NHS such as the NHS Service Delivery and Organisation (SDO) R & D Programme, which was established in 2000 to consolidate and develop the evidence base on the organization, management and delivery of healthcare services, and the Health Technology Programme (http://www.ncchta.org/) who aim to provide high-quality information on the costs, effectiveness and broader impact of healthcare treatments and tests support research into aspects of midwifery care. In addition clinical guidelines produced by the National Institute for Health and Clinical Excellence (NICE) now identify research priorities. Policy initiatives specific to maternity care; for example, Changing Childbirth (Department of Health 1993a) outlined 10 indicators of success to be met by the year 2000 and funded projects to develop and evaluate this initiative along with research funded from other sources. New policies such as the National Service Framework for Children's, Young People and Maternity Services (Department of Health 2004) was informed by reviews of evidence and feed into new research commissioned by the Department of Health.

Questions also arise from theoretical considerations, and here, clinicians and social scientists may take quite different approaches to questions relating to health. For example, and very simply, the medical approach defines the problem as beginning with a disease or a stage of healthcare. Psychological approaches are concerned with people's responses to health and illness, while sociologists would look at the implications of the provision of care both for women and society in general. Table 12.1 highlights the types of question that arise from differing perspectives, using pre-natal screening as an example.

WHAT METHOD IS BEST AT ANSWERING A QUESTION?

It may seem obvious but different research methods or designs are appropriate for answering different research questions. Normally you do not start by deciding what method you are going to use, the research design is largely determined by the research questions and by what is already known about particular aspects of a research topic. Although more than one research design may be used in any one particular study because, for example, even well-designed controlled trials can answer questions about effectiveness but cannot address process questions, which are best answered by qualitative research. A systematic review about continuous support in labour published in the Cochrane Library illustrates this (Hodnett et al 2003). It tells us that continuous support in labour improves maternal and child health outcomes and those outcomes are best when someone who is not a member of staff offers the support. However, important questions remain such as the impact of male birth partners or male staff compared to support from a female, and how and why support during childbirth leads to a better outcome. Only qualitative work may provide answers, while further trials can answer the question of who is most effective at providing support during childbirth. In summary, the types of questions we ask demand different methods to answer them. Table 12.2 gives specific examples of how different questions about the induction of labour could most appropriately be answered.

THE RESEARCH CONTINUUM

Within the broader and often-used terms of 'qualitative' and 'quantitative' research, there are categories or groups of research design. One way of describing these is by drawing a research continuum: (Box 12.1).

However, it must be emphasized that 'travel' along the research continuum may be in either direction and depends on the level of understanding and knowledge about an issue (See Further Reading at the end of the chapter for suggested sources for details of these approaches). At one end of the research continuum, if little is known about a particular aspect of a topic, *exploratory* research may be undertaken, in which the researcher is essentially asking individuals about their experiences in an open-ended, narrative way.

Imagine that we want to research place of birth. Using the research continuum, and acknowledging that there are many important questions that

Table 12.1	Different perspectives on prenatal screening
Epidemiology	What is the uptake, specificity, sensitivity, effectiveness, efficacy of a particular programme?
Health economist	What is the cost / effectiveness of a prenatal screening programme? What should the outcome measure be?
Psychologist	What are the effects of antenatal serum screening on pregnant women?
Sociologist	How do perceptions of risk differ between the lay public and experts?
	What is the relationship between prenatal screening and the eugenics movement?
Midwife	How can midwives support women in making an informed choice about screening?
Anthropologist	How is the way we think about pregnancy being changed by prenatal screening?
Ethics	What are the ethical issues of genetic screening?

Table 12.2 Answering questions

What is the effect of induction on clinical outcomes?	Randomized controlled trial Case control study
What is the effect of induction on psychosocial outcomes?	Randomized controlled trial or survey
What do women feel about induction?	In depth interviews with women and observation
How are decisions to induce made? Who makes them?	Observation and interviews with clinical staff

How many women are induced in the UK?
  – In this hospital?
  – Does it vary by class, ethnicity, parity, consultant, and hospital?
What are the variations in practice?
	Survey or secondary analysis

What is the history of inductions?	Documentary analysis
How did induction become implemented as an innovation?	Interviews with 'experts' and key informant

---

Box 12.1

Exploratory → Descriptive → Correlational →
Quasi Experimental → Experimental

---

can be asked, we could start by conducting an exploratory study whose purpose was:

> To understand the meaning of birth experiences of women who gave birth in 2005 attended by NHS maternity care health professionals at home or in a midwifery-led alongside unit, or a midwifery-led free-standing unit or an obstetric-led unit.

As more information becomes available we 'travel' on the research continuum and could choose a *correlational* design to investigate relationships between two or more variables. For example to ask the question:

> Is there a relationship between a woman's gratification with her place of birth and her emotional well being at six weeks after the birth?

At the other end of the research continuum, building on the knowledge and evidence generated by the other research methods, a *quasi-experimental* or

true experimental study may be appropriate. This allows midwives to evaluate specific protocols or treatments and test hypotheses.

For example the following hypothesis could be tested:

> Women who are at low risk of complications during labour and birth and the immediate postnatal period who give birth in a midwife-led free-standing birth centre have significantly higher levels of emotional wellbeing at six weeks after the birth compared to women who give birth in standard obstetric-led units.

Within each of these broad categories, a number of different research approaches or designs would be appropriate and the choice of these is dependent on the question that is being asked. The next section of the chapter provides a brief overview of these approaches.

EXPLORATORY RESEARCH

Exploratory research largely seeks to observe, describe or explore aspects of a situation. Such studies are conducted in areas where little knowledge exists, largely seeking to describe and explore a person's understanding or experience of given situations (Parse 1996). Within the broad category of exploratory research, a number of approaches may be used, for example phenomenological, grounded theory, ethnographic or historical (Cresswell 1998). One major focus of qualitative research is to generate hypotheses and develop theories (Smith & Hunt 1997).

DESCRIPTIVE AND CORRELATIONAL RESEARCH

Descriptive research is used to obtain more information about a particular area or topic. Descriptive–correlational research moves a step further in that it investigates relationships between variables or groups, correlational research seeking to establish a relationship between variables. Within the broad categories of descriptive and correlational research, a number of approaches may be used. Epidemiologists often use quantitative descriptive designs, which may be either retrospective or prospective. While correlational designs cannot always establish causal relationships they nevertheless form a critical part of health evaluation. They are rich in realism and can be used for the many problems not appropriate for experimental designs (Britten et al 1998).

Good correlational studies with a careful design and tightly worded hypotheses may be used in prediction (Burns & Grove 1993). For example, in the case of thalidomide, a retrospective approach was used to look at infants born with birth defects who were then identified as having been exposed to thalidomide during pregnancy (Chalmers 1989). However, because in such situations no control is possible over the presumed causative factor, the relationship is correlational rather than causal. Correlational studies are also commonly used in workforce research (Sandall 1998) and patient satisfaction and the methodological issues addressed (Crow et al 2002, McColl et al 2001).

It is important to remember that identifying a correlation does not imply causation. When a significant correlation exists between two variables, it is not always possible to specify the direction of causation. For example, a correlation between a higher level of birth interventions and lower levels of emotional wellbeing could mean a) that a high level of birth interventions leads to lower emotional wellbeing or b) that women with a low emotional wellbeing end up having a higher level of birth interventions. One way to unpick this is to measure emotional wellbeing at two points in time, which is what prospective studies aim to do.

EXPERIMENTAL DESIGNS

Experimental research usually begins with an explanation, predicts what should be found on observation and then tests these predictions. The purpose of most experimental research is to predict a causal relationship between an independent and a dependent variable. That is a change in one factor will be related to a change in another factor. Within the broad category of experimental research, a number of research designs or approaches are available, for example the randomized trial. Again, these are described in detail in many resources (for example Burns & Grove 1993, Polit & Hungler 1991, Procter & Renfrew 2000). The two most common kinds of experimental designs are true experimental and quasi-experimental.

True experimental designs. A true experimental design must have the following features:

- *Random assignment.* Random assignment means each participant in the study has an equal chance of being in either the intervention group or the control group. Neither the person assigning a participant's group nor the participant herself can choose the allocated group.
- *Control group*: treatment and care for participants in the control group should not be changed from that which would be offered normally. Their outcomes and experiences are the standard against which those of the intervention group are compared.
- *Experimental group*: The participants in this group are allocated to receive care or treatment that differs in a key aspect from the control group. An independent variable is changed for this group to test its relationship to a dependent variable. For example, in a trial to compare routine episiotomy with restricted episiotomy on the rate of perineal trauma involving anal sphincter and rectal injury, the independent

variable is episiotomy use and the dependent variable is perineal trauma.

A well-conducted randomized controlled trial (RCT) is the most powerful method for evaluating cause-and-effect relationships – for asking 'What works?' The aim of an RCT is to reduce the likelihood that findings can be explained by bias or confounding variables (Jadad 1998). The main disadvantage of true experimental designs is that a large number of human characteristics cannot be controlled. Ethically, it is often not possible to assign people randomly into comparison groups. Imagine the outcry if women were randomly assigned to give birth at home or hospital regardless of their own wishes. In addition, the results demonstrated in a trial may not translate so impressively to real life or clinical situations in which the people accessing care are likely to be more mixed than those who took part in a study. Nevertheless, trials are increasingly being used in research on social and policy interventions and in health (MRC 2000). These studies present considerable challenges and are much more complex than conventional clinical trials to carry out and to interpret (Oakley et al 2005). In these circumstances particular methodological issues associated with the complexity of the interventions and factors being evaluated must be addressed (Ukoumunne et al 1999).

Quasi-experimental designs. Quasi-experimental research usually lacks one or more of the characteristics of control, manipulation of an independent variable and random assignment. While it is often not possible randomly to assign individuals into groups, it is still possible in many instances to have a control group. Naturally occurring groups may, however, be non-equivalent. In other words (using the home birth example), women who have a home birth may be inherently different from those who give birth in hospital. There are advantages to quasi-experimental studies in that they are practical, feasible and can be more realistic. However, because of a decreased control over competing causes between the independent and dependent variables, there may be alternative explanations for the research findings. It is, therefore, more difficult to establish a causal relationship between the independent and dependent variables and to make inferences and predictions from the results of such studies.

WHAT ARE THE STRENGTHS AND WEAKNESSES OF EACH PARTICULAR DESIGN AND METHOD?

There has been much debate regarding the choice of research methods. We would like to suggest that the study method is chosen as a result of the research question. To illustrate this, Table 12.3 has deliberately created a typology of the extreme differences between quantitative and qualitative research. The aim is to demonstrate the strengths and weaknesses of each method rather than to create a hierarchy of evidence as is often presented, with randomized controlled trials given as the 'gold standard'. This is only the case when the question to be answered is one of effectiveness. As we have seen above, there are many other equally valid questions so what we need to reflect on is why the 'effect' questions are so often given priority in research funding.

SIMILARITIES BETWEEN QUANTITATIVE AND QUALITATIVE RESEARCH

All data are analysed qualitatively irrespective of the method used to collect them insofar as the act of analysis is an interpretation. Qualitative judgements are made each time one moves further away from the point of data collection. For example, in a questionnaire, the researcher has to consider issues such as whether the question was understood by the respondent in the way that was intended, whether this class of response is equivalent to another, and whether it is correct to aggregate responses to different questions. Some procedures, such as factor analysis, depend on an intuitive understanding of the data to identify underlying factors; some quantitative research is descriptive and does not always test hypotheses, and some qualitative work tests hypotheses.

MULTIPLE METHODS

From what we have discussed, it would appear that using different methods is a good idea, and the term 'triangulation' has been used to describe such a process. The term was originally derived

Table 12.3   Strengths and weaknesses of quantitative and qualitative approaches

Aspect	'NUMBER CRUNCHERS' Quantitative	'NAVAL GAZERS' Qualitative
Type of research	Randomized Controlled Trial (RCT) Case control study Survey Questionnaire	In depth interview Participant observation Ethnography Conversation analysis
Research questions	How much, how many, how often, what is the effect of	What is the experience, feeling regarding, opinions of
Type of question	Precise, requiring numeric answer	Broad, requiring verbal answer
Use of hypothesis	Present at the start and tested on data	May emerge as a result of the study
Treatment of data	Isolates and defines variables	Starts with general concepts that may change during research
Sample size	Large	Small
Sampling	Random or representative – to infer from sample to population	Theoretical – to minimize and maximize differences
Issues /items described	Through eyes of researcher	Through eyes of respondents
Data collection	Extensive Pre-designed instrument	Intensive Uses self as instrument
Logic of generalization	Hypothesis testing against data to see how many cases it explains. Statistical generalizability	By examining data to determine axiom that fits all cases. Theoretical generalizability of concepts and categories
Analytical approach	Deductive	Inductive
Strengths	Causal inferences Analysis explicit	Explores lived experience of respondents
Sources of bias	Poor allocation in randomized controlled trial Poor case control Biased sample	Selecting data to fit a preconceived idea Selecting the exotic at the expense of the mundane Sample selection
Weaknesses	RCT – lower external validity i.e. does it work in the real world	Lower internal validity/difficulty establishing cause and effect Analysis less explicit (before computers)

from land surveying, in which two landmarks rather than one is used to establish more 'truly' where a location point is (Denzin 1970). Thus, if different kinds of data produced from different methods come to the same conclusion, our confidence in the results should be increased. It may be possible to combine different types of data or different researchers, or test competing theories. Increasingly the term multiple methods is used in recognition that there may not be an objective truth, but simply different viewpoints. Although the idea of using multiple methods seems attractive, there are pitfalls (Bryman 1988). Such research is more expensive in researchers' time and the amount of data needed, and it may not necessarily provide a clearer picture. Brannen (1995) describes the following ways in which qualitative and quantitative data can be combined:

- Qualitative work can assist quantitative work by:
  - the development and piloting of research instruments, questionnaires and scales;
  - the interpretation and clarification of quantitative data;
  - providing exemplars of qualitative data;
  - exploration of subgroups where the quantitative method is inappropriate.
- Quantitative work can assist qualitative work by:
  - providing a survey sample that can be used to identify individuals for qualitative study;
  - correcting the 'elite bias' of field methods that overemphasize the articulate and those with high status;
  - providing a background context for qualitative data often derived from official statistics or the secondary analysis of official data.
- Qualitative and quantitative approaches are given equal weight:
  - which may result in two separate but linked studies that are distinct from each other at all stages of the research process; alternatively, they may be integrated into one study, the linkage occurring in the fieldwork, the analysis or the writing up.

ETHICAL CONSIDERATIONS IN THE RESEARCH PROCESS

Research poses ethical dilemmas relating to the interests of individual participants versus the pursuit of knowledge with potential benefit to the population in general. These dilemmas are inherent in *all* aspects of the research process, even at the end, with issues relating to publication and the final storage of data; it is wise to clarify them and resolve potential conflicts prior to starting any study. There are, however, no simple guidelines. Although the need for ethical consideration is universal, different types of research and each research situation present unique dilemmas that require specific resolution. For a detailed consideration of the issues, readers are advised to consult reputable texts appropriate to the specific research designs (Bowling 2002) and to examine guidelines from governing bodies, for example,

Department of Health Research Governance Definition. September 2002. www.dh.gov.uk

PRACTITIONER–RESEARCHERS

Many midwives are now undertaking some forms of research and, in exploring midwifery, such 'insider' perspectives can provide valuable insights. However, as Field's (1991) notable quote 'if you want to study water don't ask a goldfish' suggests, these perspectives cannot be exclusive and may prove problematic. The advantages that practitioner-researchers may gain in terms of negotiating access and maintaining an unobtrusive field role have to be considered against the more problematic areas: the danger of imposing a personal 'world view' and the unrecognized hidden assumptions that may bias the data collected. In ethical terms, there is a need to avoid the potential exploitation of colleagues, clients or students. Practitioner-researchers may also need to resolve conflicting responsibilities that arise from an adherence to a variety of codes of ethical conduct, towards their professional community (colleagues), the research community, the professional bodies (e.g. the NMC Code of Professional Conduct), the research participants and, not least, but often forgotten, themselves, as well as from legal restrictions such as observing the Data Protection Act (1989). In addition, there are ethical issues in the design of studies that require consideration (Edwards et al 1998).

All research involves the use of limited resources, particularly time (the participants' and the researcher's) and funding, so it is important to ensure that these are not used inappropriately. Thus, when undertaking some form of research it may be helpful to consider:

- *Area:* Not all areas are suitable for research. Particular groups, or women attending units with large research communities, need to be protected against being 'over-researched', a situation that can be annoying for the client and can influence the quality of the data collected.
- *Experience:* Matching the researcher to the research is important as research undertaken by people with inappropriate experience can be damaging to women and is unethical. Complex

research designs, such as large-scale randomized controlled trials, require more than basic research skills, while working in sensitive areas, for example exploring reactions following a termination for fetal abnormalities, or working with vulnerable groups, such as abused women, requires particular communication skills.

CONSENT

The idea of gaining 'informed consent' from participants is generally accepted as a principle of research, although it is not universal: midwives may be familiar with laboratory research being conducted on placentae on the basis that, as the tissue is being thrown away, consent is superfluous. Informed consent usually involves the following:

- Informed:
  - that all pertinent aspects of what is to occur and what might occur are disclosed to the participant;
  - that the participant should be able to comprehend this information.
- Consent:
  - that the participant is competent to make a rational and mature judgement;
  - that the agreement to participate should be voluntary, free from coercion and undue influence.

However, these principles may prove more problematic in practice, as the following discussion shows.

Whose consent?

Although desirable, it may in some situations be considered impossible or inappropriate to gain everyone's consent. For example, in observational research, the consent of authority figures may be gained, but what about the consent of those observed? In institutional and crowd behaviour studies in particular, how do you contact everyone who might be included? It is frequently the less powerful who are ignored: for example, consent for observation in a clinical area may be gained from the doctors, midwives and clients involved but not the cleaners, who are equally essential.

In the maternity services a dilemma may arise if the mother actively wants to participate but her partner disagrees; an example may be the use of the placenta for laboratory research purposes. Whose wishes are paramount? There is also the problem of reactivity. People may feel inhibited and self-conscious as a consequence of being researched so may not behave in the 'normal' manner that the researcher needs to observe.

For what?

Not all research has clearly defined outcomes. Some studies involve a dynamic process and may develop and alter radically, as in, for example, exploratory studies or action research, where the risks and benefits are not necessarily obvious. When the full implications of a study are unknown even by the researcher, at what stage can truly informed consent be sought? In addressing this problem, Munhall (1991) describes a proposal for process consent, which involves a more negotiated, flexible agreement that reflects the reality of the situation and the mutual involvement of the participant and researcher. Another area to consider involves secondary analysis, in which other researchers may use the data gathered for one study at a later time for a different purpose. Ethically, this may be viewed positively as an appropriate use of a valuable resource, but does anonymity negate the requirement for the participants' consent? In recognition of this reality, funding organizations that store such data (e.g. the Economic and Social Research Council) have developed a consent form for qualitative data that contains different levels of consent. Here, the participant agrees to assist with the primary study, either anonymously or named, and then again for the data to be stored for secondary analysis. This difficulty relates to the final ownership of data gathered, a point that it may be advantageous to clarify prior to starting the research. This has particular relevance when undertaking government-sponsored research as the results could be modified, delayed or even suppressed if considered unacceptable, the publication of the Black Report (Townsend & Davidson 1982) being a notorious example of this.

When?

Identifying the appropriate timing for consent can be difficult. Many midwives will be familiar with the highly undesirable situation of mothers in labour being asked to participate in research. Much potential distress could be avoided by women being informed of possible research participation requests at 'booking' and by a notice board of ongoing research being made available within the hospital or GP practice. Thus, when approached, couples might be more informed and confident in their response. This idea has been promoted within the AIMS/NCT Charter for Ethical Research in Maternity Care (1997). In addition, people need to understand what they are consenting to, and difficulties have been highlighted regarding clinical trials (Robinson et al 2005).

How?

Consent may be obtained in different ways. Written consent is usually required, especially for intervention studies involving specific clinical procedures. Survey studies may assume consent by the participant completing and returning the questionnaire, and in personal contact situations such as interviews, written consent is increasingly considered necessary. However, in obtaining any form of informed consent, meeting the language and level of information needs of individual participants is hard to achieve. Can we be sure that translations provided by family and friends ensure an informed consent by the woman? The alternative of providing translated information leaflets does not address the different educational levels of a multicultural clientele – and how much information is it appropriate to give? Some participants may be particularly interested in the research and demand high levels of information, while others readily agree before a full explanation has been provided. In acknowledging a 'right to know', do participants have a 'right not to know'?

By whom?

The dilemma surrounding who is best placed to gain consent from women – the known midwife versus the strange researcher – relates to the timing and place in which the consent is sought. The researcher is better placed to provide information about the study and reassurance that refusal will have no detrimental effect on care.

Nevertheless, it is frequently the midwife who is asked to recruit participants, generally for pragmatic reasons but also on the assumption that women prefer not to see many strangers. This itself would provide an interesting area for research. Again, such research needs explicitly to address the ethics of those in a position of power conducting research within their own institution. The difficulties of shedding the professional perspective when carrying out ethnographic research in this area have been raised by Hunt & Symons (1995).

CONFIDENTIALITY

The assurance of confidentiality through anonymity is another central principle of ethical research in the belief that:

- participants will respond more openly and honestly if they cannot be identified from the data;
- participants should not be harmed in any way by the research, for example by an individual's views becoming public knowledge.

In much research, identification of the individual is not required. Demographic data about age, sex and so on are sufficient, and confidentiality is achieved through the use of codes and the avoidance of names and addresses. However, in case studies, ethnographies and action research, the situation is more complex. With the current imperative to publish both the evaluations of midwifery service developments and research undertaken by midwives within their own clinical area, these issues are of particular relevance, as total anonymity cannot be assured.

Simple strategies such as processing raw data off-site, for example in transcription of tapes, and storing primary data away from the research area, with clearly defined and limited access, may be advisable when undertaking research focusing on professionals in specific units. Nevertheless, this only ensures partial anonymity; studies undertaken in specific areas may be impossible to disguise. For example, publications resulting from the ethnographic study of a high-profile development such as One-to-One midwifery practice require extremely sensitive writing to avoid individuals being compromised.

Discussing these difficulties in her study of ward sisters, Lathlean (1996) notes how her adherence to the principle of anonymity in a nationally recognized innovative development resulted in a very 'bland' presentation and that the 'essence of the experience' had been lost. In research that involves feedback and enables participants to reflect on and react to the findings, Lathlean questions how appropriate it is to guarantee confidentiality, suggesting that it may be more useful to negotiate other arrangements.

A consideration of these ideas is integral to the concepts of greater consumer involvement in research, an approach that has recently been promoted with the development of the Standing Advisory Group on Consumer Involvement in the NHS R & D programme; they are particularly appropriate when considering midwifery research. Not only are the users and providers of maternity care asked to participate in research, but also their values and views are central to the questions that are posed and explored, and the way in which the results are presented in subsequent publications; they become active participants rather than subjects. This loss of control may appear a risky concept to researchers, but it offers exciting new dimensions for research within the maternity services.

In the context of a health service which recognizes that research is vital to the development of improved healthcare and its delivery, the welfare of people taking part in research is paramount (Central Office for Research Ethics Committees www.corec.org.uk) major research funding bodies, such as the Medical Research Council (MRC) and the Economic and Social Research Council (ESTRC) have set out clearly their position on research ethics (ESRC 2005, MRC 2005). The resources they publish are entirely congruent and are based on the belief that the research process should be transparent and open to scrutiny.

In the NHS, standards of research governance to which all Trusts must adhere (Department of Health 2005) mean that before it begins research involving patients and staff should be subject to ethical review by a Local Research Ethics Committee (LREC), or if it is being conducted across several sites, a Multi Centre Research Committee (MREC). The role of a Trust in research governance includes ensuring that ethical approval and

informed consent processes have been approved and that legal requirements, for example systems to ensure that the requirements of the Data Protection Act are met (Department of Health 2005). The processes for obtaining ethical approval to conduct research are subject to change and development and therefore it is essential to access the most up-to-date information about these matters via web sites, such as the Department of Health in England (www.dh.gov.uk). It is important to recognize that ethical and research governance issues are not only the concern of LRECs/MRECs or NHS Trust managers. Once approval has been granted for a study it is the midwives and other healthcare professionals working with women and families who must be alert to whether implementation of the research methods is conducted ethically.

CONCLUSION

Knowledge about research is a component of effective midwifery practice. Different levels of knowledge are needed depending on where midwives are working. For example, all midwives will need to be critical users of research findings, as women seek information and discussion about various options for pregnancy and childbirth and as new technologies are introduced. Some midwives are involved in audit and local practice development projects and will need a more in-depth knowledge of the research process. A few may wish to pursue a full-time research career, necessitating formal research training.

For those who are undertaking research, it is important to see the activity of research as a craft, a technical skill, that improves with practise, just as learning to be an experienced midwife takes time. As with learning to 'do' midwifery, research cannot be picked up from a textbook: it is important to learn from and work with experienced researchers. It is also important to know that research never happens in the way in which it is written up for publication. Research is messy: deadlines overlap, budgets get miscalculated, questionnaires get lost, respondents refuse to cooperate, access to sites is refused and ethics committees refuse to give approval. These 'housekeeping' issues of research are rarely written about, which is why it is so important for novice researchers to pair up with more experienced researchers. Similarly, ethical issues are also rarely acknowledged in published research, often being consigned to working papers and methodology chapters in reports and theses.

Being research minded and basing practice on best evidence means asking questions, challenging oneself and others, and being prepared to commit time and effort to get meaningful answers. Asking and answering questions is most rewarding when it can be done in partnership, with women and families, and with colleagues. Many issues that require answers arise from listening to women and observing practice, being open to alternative explanations and experiences. Sensitization to issues, however, often needs an awareness of the broader literature and the political and social context within which women give birth and within which their healthcare is provided.

Research has the potential to be a powerful lever for change. It can provide answers that help midwives and women to challenge existing practice, to make things better. To do this, one needs to understand the strengths and limitations of all the methods used in research to establish what works and what does not, and to find out why and how women receive the care they do. However, we also need to recognize that knowledge by itself will not change practice or the organization of care. Awareness of and the ability to negotiate political dimensions and structural constraints of power relations in organizations are necessary when trying to initiate change.

Finally, drawing on other disciplines such as anthropology, sociology and social history allows us to place maternity care and childbirth in a wider context and step outside a narrow professional viewpoint to enrich the possibilities for research for midwifery.

POINTERS FOR PRACTICE

- Ideas for research come from many sources, for example, wider society, national policy and research strategies, scientific advances and women's and midwives' experiences of care.
- Different research questions require different methods to answer them, each method having strengths and weaknesses.
- To conduct high quality research requires high-quality training, varied experience and supportive mentorship, just as being a good midwife does.
- All research should be considered for the ethical impact that it may have on women and their families, students and health professionals, and all research findings need to be disseminated to participants and the wider community.

References

AIMS/NCT 1997 Ethical research in maternity care. Association for Improvements in Maternity Care, London

Alexander J 1996 The Southampton randomised controlled trial of breast shells and Hoffman's exercises for inverted and non-protractile nipples. In: Robinson S, Thomson A (eds) Midwives, research and childbirth, Vol. 4. Chapman & Hall, London

Allen I, Bourke Dowling S, Williams S 1997 A leading role for midwives? Evaluation of Midwifery Group Practice Development Projects. Policy Studies Institute, London

Baxter C 1996 Working from a multi-racial perspective. In: Kroll D (ed.) Midwifery care for the future, meeting the challenge. Baillière Tindall, London

Benoit C, Wrede S, Bourgeault I, Sandall J, de Vries R, van Teijlingen E R 2005 Understanding the social organisation of maternity care systems: midwifery as a touchstone. Sociology of Health and Illness 27: 6

Bourgeault I, Declerq E, Sandall J 2001 Changing birth: interest groups and maternity care policy. In: DeVries R, Benoit C, van Teijlingen E, Wrede S (eds) Birth by design: pregnancy, maternity care and midwifery in North America and Europe. Routledge, New York, pp 51–69

Bowling A 2002 Research methods in health. 2nd edn. Open University Press, Maidenhead

Brannen J (ed.) 1995 Mixing methods: qualitative and quantitative research. Avebury, Aldershot

Britton A, McKee M, Black N, McPherson K, Sanderson C, Bain C 1998 Choosing between randomised and non-randomised studies: a systematic review. Health Technology Assessment 2(13)

Bryar R 1995 Theory for midwifery practice. Macmillan, London

Bryman A 1988 Quantity and quality in social research. Unwin Hyman, Aldershot

Burns N, Grove S K 1993 The practice of nursing research: conduct, critique and utilization. WB Saunders, Philadelphia

Cartwright A 1979 Dignity of labour. Tavistock, London

Chalmers I 1989. Evaluating the effects of care during pregnancy and childbirth. In: Chalmers I, Enkin M, Kierse M J (eds) Effective care in pregnancy and childbirth, Vol 1. OUP, Oxford, pp 4–8

Chalmers I, Enkin M, Keirse M J N C 1989 Effective care in pregnancy and childbirth. Oxford University Press, Oxford

Chalmers I, Richards M 1977 Intervention and causal inference in obstetric practice. In: Chard T, Richards M (eds) Benefits and hazards of the new obstetrics. Spastics International Medical Publications, London

Clark E 2000 Historical context of research in midwifery In: Proctor S, Renfrew M (eds) Linking research and practice in midwifery. Baillière Tindall, London

Cresswell D 1998 Qualitative inquiry and research design: choosing among five traditions. Sage, Thousand Oaks, California

Crow R, Gage H, Hampson S, Hart J, Kimber A, Storey L et al 2002 The measurement of satisfaction with healthcare: implications for practice from a systematic review of the literature. Health Technology Assessment 6(32)

Curtis P, Ball L, Kirkham M 2003 Why do midwives leave? Talking to managers. Royal College of Midwives, London

Davies J, Evans F 1991 The Newcastle community midwifery care project. In: Robinson S, Thomson A (eds) Midwives, research and childbirth, vol. 2. Chapman & Hall, London

Davis-Floyd R, Sargent E C 1997 Childbirth and authoritative knowledge: cross cultural perspectives. University of California Press, Los Angeles

de Vries R, Benoit C et al 2001 Birth by design: pregnancy, maternity care and midwifery in North America and Northern Europe. Routledge, New York

Declerq E 1998 Changing childbirth in the United Kingdom: lessons for US Health policy. Journal of Health Politics, Policy and Law 23: 833–859

Deery R 2003 Engaging with clinical supervision in a community midwifery setting: an action research study. Unpublished PhD Thesis, University of Sheffield, UK

Denzin N K 1970 The research act in sociology. Butterworths, London

Department of Health 1993a Changing childbirth, Part 1. Report of the Expert Maternity Group. HMSO, London

Department of Health 1993b Report of the Taskforce on the Strategy for Research in Nursing, Midwifery and Health Visiting. Department of Health, London

Department of Health 2004 Maternity standard, national service framework for children, young people and maternity services. Department of Health, London

Department of Health 2005 The research governance framework for health and social care. 2nd edn. April 2005. Online. Available: http://www.dh.gov.uk

Donnison J 1988 Midwives and medical men: a history of the struggle for control of childbirth. 2nd edn. Historical Publications, New Barnet

Edwards S J L, Lilford R J, Braunholtz D A, Jackson J C, Hewison J, Thornton J. 1998 Ethical issues in the design and conduct of controlled trials. Health Technology Assessment 2(15)

ESRC 2005 Research ethics framework. July. ESRC, London. Online: Available: www.esrc.ac.uk

Field P A 1991 Doing fieldwork in your own culture. In: Morse J M (ed.) Qualitative nursing research: a contemporary dialogue. Sage, Newbury Park, CA

Fletcher G 2003 Foreword. In: Fraser D, Cooper M (eds) Myles Textbook for midwives 14th edn. Churchill Livingstone, Edinburgh, p. xi

Flint C, Poulengeris P, Grant A 1989 The 'Know your Midwife' scheme – a controlled trial of continuity of care by a team of midwives. Midwifery 5: 11–16

Garcia J, Garforth S 1991 Midwifery policies and policymaking. In: Robinson S, Thomson A (eds) Midwives research and childbirth, vol. 2. Chapman & Hall, London

Graham H, Oakley A 1981 Competing ideologies of reproduction: In Roberts H (ed.) Women, health and reproduction. Routledge, London

Green J M, Baston H A 2003 Feeling in control during labor: concepts, correlates, and consequences. Birth 30(4): 235–247

Green J M, Coupland V A, Kitzinger J V 1990 Expectations, experiences and psychological outcomes of childbirth: a prospective study of 825 women. Birth 17(1): 15–24

Green V A, Kitzinger J V, Coupland J M 1986 The division of labour: implications for staffing structure for doctors and midwives on the labour ward. Child Care and Development Group, University of Cambridge, Cambridge

Hannam J 1996 Some aspects of the history of the Royal College of Midwives. In: Robinson S, Thomson A M (eds) Midwives, research and childbirth, vol. 4. Chapman & Hall, London

Heagerty B V 1997 Willing handmaidens of science? The struggle over the new midwife in early twentieth-century England. In: Kirkham M J, Perkins E R (eds) Reflections on midwifery. Baillière Tindall, London

Hicks C 1995 Good researcher, poor midwife: an investigation into the impact of central trait assumptions of professional competencies. Midwifery 11: 81–87

Hodnett E D, Gates S, Hofmeyr G J, Sakala C 2003 Continuous support for women during childbirth. The Cochrane Database of Systematic Reviews 2003, Issue 3. Art. No.: CD003766.

Hunt S, Symons A 1995 The social meaning of midwifery. Macmillan, Basingstoke

Hunter B, Deery R 2005 Building our knowledge about emotion work in midwifery: combining and comparing findings from two different research studies. RCM Evidence Based Midwifery 3(1): 10–15

Jadad A 1998 Controlled trials. BMJ Publishing, London

Kettle C, Hill R K, Jones P et al 2002 Continuous versus interrupted perineal repair with standard or rapidly absorbed sutures after spontaneous birth: a randomized controlled trial. Lancet 359: 2217–2223

Kirkham M 1987 Basic supportive care in labour: interaction with and around labouring women. Unpublished PhD thesis, Faculty of Medicine, Manchester University

Kirkham M 2003 (ed.) Informed choice in maternity care. Palgrave Macmillan, Hampshire

Lathlean J 1996 Ethical issues for nursing research: a methodological focus. Nursing Times Research 1(3): 175–183

Leap N, Hunter B 1993 The midwives tale: an oral history from handywoman to professional midwife. Scarlet Press, London

Macintyre S 1977 The management of childbirth: a review of the sociological research issues. Social Science and Medicine 11: 477–484

Marland H, Rafferty A M (eds) 1997 Midwives, society and childbirth: debates and controversies in the modern period. Routledge, London

McColl E, Jacoby A, Thomas L, Soutter J, Bamford C, Steen N et al 2001 Design and use of questionnaires: a review of best practice applicable to surveys of health staff and patients. Health Technology Assessment 5(31)

McCourt C, Page L, Hewison J, Vail A 1998 Evaluation of One-to-One midwifery: women's responses to care. Birth 25(2): 73–80

MRC 2005 Position statement on research regulation and ethics. January. MRC, London. Online. Available: www.mrc.ac.uk

MRC 2000 A framework for development and evaluation of RCTs for complex interventions to improve health. April 2000 MRC London and www.mrc.ac.uk

Munhall P L 1991 Institutional review of qualitative research proposals. In: Morse J M (ed.) Qualitative nursing research: a contemporary dialogue, revd edn. Sage, Newbury Park, CA

Myles M 1953 Preface to the first edition. A textbook for midwives. Churchill Livingstone, Edinburgh, p. vii

Nuffield Council on Bioethics 1993 Genetic screening: ethical issues. Nuffield Council on Bioethics, London

Oakley A 1980 Women confined: towards a sociology of childbirth. Martin Robertson, Oxford

Oakley A 1984 The captured womb: a history of the medical care of pregnant women. Basil Blackwell, Oxford

Oakley A, Gough D, Oliver S, Thomas J 2005 The politics of evidence and methodology: lessons from the EPPI-Centre. Evidence & Policy 1(1): 5–31

Oakley A, Hickey D, Rajan L 1996 Social support in pregnancy: does it have long term effects? Journal of Reproductive and Infant Psychology 14: 7–22

Oliver S, Clarke-Jones L, Rees R, Milne R, Buchanan P, Gabbay J et al 2004 Involving consumers in research and development agenda setting for the NHS: developing an evidence-based approach. Health Technology Assessment 8(15)

Parse R R 1996 Building knowledge through: a road much less travelled. Nursing Science Quarterly 9(1): 10–16

Polit D, Hungler B 1991 Nursing research: principles and methods. 4th edn. Lippincott, Philadelphia

Pollit C, Harrison S, Hunter D, Marnoch G 1990 No hiding place: on the discomforts of researching the contemporary policy process. Journal of Social Policy 19(2): 169–190

Pope C, Mays N 1995 Reaching the parts other methods cannot reach: an introduction to qualitative methods in health and health services research. British Medical Journal 311: 42–45

Proctor S, Renfrew M (eds) 2000 Linking research and practice in midwifery. Baillière Tindall, London

Rafferty A M, Traynor M 2002 Exemplary research for nursing and midwifery. Routledge, London

Renfrew M, Smith M 2000 Research and development in the NHS. In. Proctor S, Renfrew M (eds) Linking research and practice in midwifery. Baillière Tindall, London

Robinson E J, Kerr C E P, Stevens A J, Lilford R J, Braunholtz D A, Edwards S J et al 2005 Lay public's understanding of equipoise and ation in controlled trials. Health Technology Assessment 9(8)

Robinson S, Golden J, Bradley S 1983 A study of the role and responsibilities of the midwife. NERU Report No. 1. Kings College, University of London, London

Sandall J 1996 Continuity of midwifery care in England: a new professional project? Gender, Work and Organization 3(4): 215–226

Sandall J 1998 Occupational burnout in midwives: new ways of working and the relationship between organisational factors and psychological health and wellbeing, Risk, Decision & Policy 3(3): 213–232

Sleep J 1991 Perineal care: a series of five controlled trials. In Robinson S, Thomson A (eds) Midwives research and childbirth, vol. 2. Chapman & Hall, London

Smith P, Hunt J M (eds) 1997 Research mindedness for practice. Churchill Livingstone, London

Townsend P, Davidson N 1982 Inequalities in health: the Black report. Penguin, Harmondsworth

Ukoumunne O C, Gulliford M C, Chinn S, Sterne J A C, Burney P G J 1999 Methods for evaluating area-wide and organisation-based interventions in health and health care: a systematic review. Health Technology Assessment 3(5)

Walsh D, Downe S 2004 Outcomes of free-standing, midwifery-led birth centres: a structured review. Birth 31(3): 222–229

Williams C, Sandall J, Lewando Hundt G, Grellier R, Heyman B, Spencer K 2005 Women as 'moral pioneers'?: experiences of first trimester nuchal translucency screening. Social Science and Medicine 61: 1983–1992

Williams S A 1997 Women and childbirth in the twentieth century. Sutton, Stroud

Witz A 1992 Professions and patriarchy. Routledge, London

Wraight A, Ball J, Seccombe I, Stock J 1993 Mapping team midwifery, a report to the Department of Health. IMS Report series 242. Institute Manpower Studies, Brighton

Further reading

Bowling A 2002 Research methods in health. 2nd edn. Open University Press, Maidenhead

Experimental research methods

Black N, Brazier J, Fitzpatrick R, Reeves B (eds) 1998 Health services research methods: a guide to best practice. BMJ Books, London, Chapters 6 & 7

Cook D C, Campbell D T 1979 Quasi-experimentation: Design and analysis issues for field settings. Houghton Mifflin, Boston, Chapters 2& 3

Jadad A 1998 (ed.) Controlled trials. BMJ, London

Pocock S 2000 Clinical trials: a practical approach. Wiley, London

Qualitative research methods

Cresswell D 1998 Qualitative inquiry and research design: choosing among five traditions. Sage, California.

Denzin N, Lincoln Y S 2005 Sage handbook qualitative research. 3rd edn. Sage, London

Green J, Thorogood N 2004 Qualitative methods for health research. Sage, London.

Mays N, Pope C 1995 Reaching the parts other methods cannot reach: an introduction to qualitative methods in health and health services research. British Medical Journal 311: 42–45

Murphy E, Dingwall R, Greatbatch D, Parker S, Watson P 1998 Qualitative research methods in health technology assessment: a review of the literature. Health Technology Assessment 2(16)

Sampling for qualitative research

Coyne I 1997 Sampling in qualitative research. Purposeful and theoretical sampling: merging or clear boundaries? Journal of Advanced Nursing 26: 623–630

Faugier J, Sargeant M 1997 Sampling hard to reach populations. Journal of Advanced Nursing 26: 790–796

Morse J 1995 The significance of saturation. Qualitative Health Research 5(2): 147–149

Sandelowski J 1995 Sample size in qualitative research. Research in Nursing and Health 18: 179–183

Analysing qualitative data

Burnard P 1991 A method of analysing interview transcripts in qualitative research. Nurse Education Today 11: 461–466

Morrison M, Moir J 1998 The role of computer software in the analysis of qualitative data:

efficient clerk, research assistant or Trojan horse? Journal of Advanced Nursing 28 (1): 106–116

Morse J 1995 The significance of saturation. Qualitative Health Research 5(2): 147–149

Pope C, Ziebland S, Mays N 2000 Qualitative research: Analysing qualitative data. British Medical Journal 320: 114–116

Ritchie J, Spencer L 1994 Qualitative data analysis for applied policy research. In: Bryman A, Burgess R(eds) Analysing qualitative data. Routledge, London

Assessing quality of qualitative research

Bloor M 1998 Techniques of validation in qualitative research: a critical commentary. In: Miller G, Dingwall R (eds) Context and method in qualitative research. Sage, London

Mays N, Pope C 2000 Qualitative research: assessing quality in qualitative research. British Medical Journal 320(7226): 50–52

Survey research

De Vaus 2002 Surveys in social research. 5th edn. Routledge, London

Fink A 1995 The survey kit. Sage, Thousand Oaks, California, Vols 5–9

Pallant J 2001 SPSS survival manual. Open University Press, Buckingham

Questionnaire design

McColl E, Jacoby A, Thomas L, Soutter J, Bamford C, Steen N et al 2001 Design and use of questionnaires: a review of best practice applicable to surveys of health service staff and patients. Health Technology Assessment 5 (31)

Focus groups

Barbour R S, Kitzinger J 1999 Developing focus group research. Sage, London

Bloor M, Frankland J, Thomas M, Robson K 2001 Focus groups in social research. Sage, London

Coughlan D, Brannick T 2002 Doing action research in your own organisation. Sage, London

Fulop N, Allen P, Clarke A, Black N 2001 Studying the organisation and delivery of health services. Research methods. Routledge, London

Kitzinger J 1995 Introducing focus groups. British Medical Journal 311: 299–302

Krueger A, Morgan D L 1998 The focus group kit. Sage, London

Meyer J 2000 Using qualitative methods in health related action research. British Medical Journal 320: 178–181

Research in organisations

Winter R, Munn-Giddings C 2001 A handbook for action research for health and social care. Routledge, London

Evaluation

Atkinson P, Coffey A, Delamont S et al 2001 Sage handbook of ethnography. Sage, London

Mays N, Pope C 1995 Qualitative research: observational methods in health care settings. British Medical Journal 311: 182–184

Observation/Ethnography

Pawson R, Tilley N 1998 Realistic evaluation. Sage, London

Rossi P, Freeman H E 1993 Evaluation. A systematic approach. 5th edn. Sage, Newbury Park, CA

Combining methods

Brannen J (ed.) 1992 Mixing methods: qualitative and quantitative research. Ashgate, Brookfield, VT

Campbell M, Fitzpatrick R, Haines A et al (2000) Framework for design and evaluation of complex interventions to improve health. British Medical Journal 321: 694–696

Cresswell J W 1994 Qualitative and quantitative approaches. Sage, London

Herman J L 1988 Program evaluation kit. Sage, London

MRC 2000 A framework for development and evaluation of RCTs for complex interventions to improve health. April. MRC, London. Online. Available: www.mrc.ac.uk

Wolff N (ed.) 2001 Trials of socially complex interventions: promise or peril? Journal of Health Services Research and Policy 6: 123–126

Research design

For further information about developing a protocol and doing a research study the web site of the National Network of Research and Development Support Units is an invaluable resource http://www.rdinfo.org.uk

Ethics

Department of Health 2005 The research governance framework for health and social care. 2nd edn. DOH, London. Online. Available: www.dh.gov.uk

ESRC 2005 Research ethics framework. July. ESRC, London. Online. Available: www.esrc.ac.uk

MRC 2005 Position statement on research regulation and ethics. January MRC, London. Online. Available: www.mrc.ac.uk

Chapter 13

Jenna's care story: post-term pregnancy

Sara Wickham

Jenna was expecting her first baby and, at the time this story begins, she was 41 weeks and 5 days pregnant, which meant that, as her midwife, I had become increasingly aware of the issue of post-term pregnancy and the possible risks that this is thought to carry. At this time, I was working independently and, although I was Jenna's primary midwife, I worked with other midwives in a small group where we would support each other at births, and in talking through issues when one of us needed another perspective. This chapter explores the story of the interactions between Jenna and myself, between myself and my midwife friends, and between the different kinds of knowledge that we explored in making the decisions surrounding the issues involved when Jenna's pregnancy continued beyond 42 weeks.

I have used Lesley Page's (2000) Five Steps of Evidence-based Midwifery (Box 13.1) as a basic framework for this discussion of how Jenna and I worked through the issues. Inevitably, using any kind of framework simplifies what is, in reality, a complex process, and I have tried, throughout this chapter, to simultaneously show how our decisions and experiences happened approximately within this framework, while also giving a sense of the complexity of the journey we took together. When I contacted Jenna recently to ask her permission to use her story for this chapter, and to ask her a couple of questions about things I was not sure I remembered accurately, we found ourselves remembering the process as a winding journey. Jenna commented that:

> Box 13.1 The five steps of evidence-based midwifery (Page 2000)
>
> 1. Finding out what is important to the woman and her family.
> 2. Using information from the clinical examination.
> 3. Seeking and assessing evidence to inform decisions.
> 4. Talking it through.
> 5. Reflecting on outcomes, feelings and consequences.

I remember our journey side-tracking a lot, you know, like winding off onto other paths . . . and some were interesting but not really helpful, and some were useful . . . some were just dead-ends! And I do remember one evening, when it seemed like I was going round in circles and then Dev said something like, you know, it seems like you just have to choose one route and then go with it, because by not choosing you're actually choosing to wait, even if you're just waiting another few minutes while you think and talk some more, so if it's in your heart to wait then why not just choose that road for as long as it feels good and then you can relax and enjoy it?' That was the realization point for me.

FINDING OUT WHAT IS IMPORTANT TO THE WOMAN AND HER FAMILY

Jenna and her partner, Dev, had planned a home birth for two main reasons. Firstly, as Pagans, they both held very strong beliefs about non-interference and allowing things to take a natural course. Secondly, as a sociology graduate, Jenna was (in her own words), 'well-versed in the culture and power-politics of Western medicine'. She felt that, once women entered maternity care systems, they were at risk of losing their personal power and control over their bodies.

Although Jenna was always happy to have her blood pressure and urine checked, and for me to do an abdominal examination and listen to her baby's heartbeat with a fetoscope, she had chosen not to have any other antenatal screening, apart from a blood test at the beginning of her pregnancy to determine her blood group and rhesus type. We had also discussed the use of Doppler in labour and had agreed that, where possible, I would use a fetoscope and only use a Doppler if the fetal heart was impossible to hear with a fetoscope, or if I was genuinely worried. Jenna and Dev were very committed to each other and to their beliefs and, while it would probably be inaccurate to say that Dev felt just as strongly about some of the issues as Jenna did, he was devoted to her and totally supportive of her beliefs and wishes.

We had talked at length during Jenna's pregnancy about what would happen if some aspect of her pregnancy or birth did cause us to think that things might no longer be within what is considered 'normal', as I felt it very important to know both how she would feel and what my situation would be if this occurred. Ultimately, Jenna was not opposed to pharmaceutical drugs, medical treatment or hospital admission if it were truly essential for the wellbeing of her or her baby, but she had wanted to have a midwife who was very comfortable with physiological birth, with the use of holistic remedies and therapies before resorting to drugs and with the choices she had made around screening. The choices she had made were well within the limits of my own 'comfort zone' and we were both happy that our philosophy and approach to birth and health was similar.

Of course, one of the key tasks of the midwife is to determine, in conjunction with women, when an aspect of pregnancy and birth is 'normal', or when something indicates that a deviation from the normal has occurred, and this was what I needed to do, along with Jenna. This is a complex process which, for me, involves making constant comparisons between what the woman I am with is feeling and experiencing (and what I am experiencing when I feel her abdomen, or take her blood pressure) with the 'norms' that exist for me as a midwife. My own norms come from a number of sources; I learned some as a student, I generate others from reading books or research articles, from attending conferences, from my experience of working with lots of other pregnant and birthing women and, especially where I haven't encountered something before, I often talk to other midwives about their experiences and norms. These norms aren't static; they often change as we learn or think new things, and they are also affected by other things, such as beliefs. I believe they are also influenced by the kinds of knowledge that are very difficult to pin down, such as intuition, or gut feelings. Somehow, this all melts down in an interaction between the woman and her midwife, and results in decisions about whether everything is well, or whether some kind of action needs to be taken.

USING INFORMATION FROM THE CLINICAL EXAMINATION

I had actually seen Jenna for an antenatal visit in her home a few days earlier, when she was 41 weeks pregnant, and she and her baby were both doing well. It was during this visit that I suggested we met again later that week to talk further about what we would do if she did not go into labour by 42 weeks. I knew that she would not want her labour to be medically induced unless it was warranted, for reasons explained above, and I wanted to give her as long as possible to go into labour naturally before we discussed options which would include going into the hospital. Another part of my rationale included that I could spend more time with Jenna considering and discussing this particular issue, having talked through her other questions at the earlier visit.

Jenna's expected date of birth (EDB) had been calculated from menstrual dates and from her menstrual chart, as she and Dev had used natural family planning in the past and she had continued to chart her temperature and periods so that she would know when they conceived. This meant that we were able to pinpoint conception to within two or three days, and calculated the EDB from the date of conception rather than the first day of her last period.

The following questions (in Box 13.2) covered both general and specific areas relevant to Jenna's

decision. Generally, there was a need to determine whether both Jenna and her baby were well and if there was any reason to be particularly concerned at this time. Specifically, we needed to consider a number of issues relating to this area, including the accuracy of her EDB, the condition of the baby in relation to the length of pregnancy and whether a longer-than-normal pregnancy was normal or unusual in Jenna's case.

I already knew the answers to many of these questions because I had attended Jenna

---

Box 13.2 Using information from the clinical examination – Based on Page (2000)

General Questions:

History:
- Is the woman generally healthy and well-nourished?
- Is the woman emotionally healthy?
  - Does she feel happy and well supported?
  - Does she feel good about pregnancy and birth?
  - Does she have any unresolved fears or concerns?
  - Does she feel that everything is OK with herself and her baby?
- Are there any factors in her history that may indicate a possible risk or problem?
  - Drug use (pharmaceutical or recreational), smoking, heavy alcohol consumption.
  - Illnesses or medical problems (past or current).
  - Obstetric problems (past or current).
  - Relevant family history.

Clinical:
- Are the results of any antenatal screening tests that consider the woman's wellbeing within normal limits, or are any problems indicated?
  - General examination (e.g. heart, lungs, kidneys, skin, eyes).
  - Blood pressure, pulse.
  - Urinalysis.
  - Other antenatal tests which check the woman's wellbeing, such as blood values.
- Are the results of any antenatal screening tests that consider the baby's wellbeing within normal limits, or are any problems indicated?

- Abdominal palpation (size, growth, lie, presentation, position, amount of amniotic fluid).
- Fetal heartbeat (within normal range, variable, reactive to stimulation).
- Other antenatal tests which check the baby's wellbeing, such as ultrasound.
- Are there any other signs of disease or abnormality that might indicate a problem for either the mother or baby? (e.g. any vaginal bleeding, unusual physical signs or symptoms)

Case-Specific Questions:
- Is the pregnancy truly post-term? / Is the EDB accurate?
  - How was the EDB calculated? Has it been revised? If so, why?
  - Does the woman have particularly long menstrual cycles, which could make a normally-calculated EBD a few days too early?
  - Does the woman have any other factors in her personal history or this pregnancy which might alter the EDB?
  - Is there a family history of pregnancies which last longer than average?
- Apart from the general concerns about post-term pregnancy, is there any reason to be especially concerned about this particular baby remaining in the womb for another few days?
  - Is the baby excessively large?
  - Is the woman worried about the baby?
  - How does the woman feel about induction of labour?

throughout her pregnancy. Her own health was excellent and she was well-nourished, although she did experience significant nausea during the first three months of her pregnancy. Nothing in her history was of concern; her full blood count at the beginning of pregnancy was normal, her blood pressure had been within normal limits throughout her pregnancy and the only 'blip' on her urinalysis chart was a single episode of proteinurea at around 20 weeks which coincided with a minor urinary infection. Jenna had treated this by taking herbs, drinking lots of water and avoiding sugar, and it had not recurred.

Jenna's baby had grown steadily, but was not over-large. He had always been active and playful when I examined her abdomen, and I had no concerns. As above, Jenna had declined ultrasound but it was easy to determine that the baby had an adequate amount of amniotic fluid from abdominal examination. She felt very comfortable with the idea of still being pregnant at this point, and felt confident that both she and the baby were doing well.

SEEKING AND ASSESSING EVIDENCE TO INFORM DECISIONS (PART 1)

It is only in reflecting on this experience for this chapter that I realized something fairly key to this part of Jenna's story, and probably to the practice of many midwives. Before we started to search for and analyse literature which we hoped would provide answers to some of our questions, we spent time talking not only about what we already knew (for instance, Jenna was well aware of the aspects of induction which she wanted to avoid if possible), but also in figuring out the questions that Jenna was *not* looking for answers to.

Although there is a growing body of literature considering the accuracy of the due date (e.g. Baskett & Nagele 2000, Bergsjo et al 1990, Olsen & Clausen 1997, Rosser 2000), this did not seem an especially important question in this situation because Jenna was so sure about the date on which she conceived. A few studies have considered individual factors when calculating the due date (Purrett 2004), but the only factor relevant in Jenna's case was that this was her first baby, which Mittendorf et al (1990) suggested means an average

gestation of 288 days rather than the 280 days generally used to calculate due date.

It was also very clear to me that, as far as Jenna was concerned, the only 'good' reason for induction was if there was clear evidence showing that continuing with pregnancy beyond 42 weeks was going to be potentially hazardous for her baby. She was not particularly concerned about whether there was a difference in the risks to herself, mainly because she remained convinced in her own mind that it was far better to avoid medical intervention if possible. Therefore, while some of the studies cited below did look at outcomes such as differences in the caesarean section rate, this was not something which, by her own admission, would have changed Jenna's mind, and so it is not considered here.

We were then left with two questions which seemed the most important in Jenna's case:

1. Once pregnancy becomes 'post-term', is it safer for the baby for labour to be induced rather than to remain pregnant?
2. If post-term pregnancy carries greater risk to the baby than continuing with the pregnancy, yet (as in Jenna's case) the woman wants to avoid medical care if possible, are there effective and safe non-medical ways of inducing labour?

A literature review showed that there were a fair number of relevant studies which offered data relevant to the first of our questions. Details of the studies identified are summarized in Table 13.1. Although a number of (mostly older) studies evaluated the use of induction before or at 41 weeks (Breart et al 1982, Cole et al 1975, Egarter et al 1989, Martin et al 1978, Sande et al 1983, Tylleskar et al 1979), these were omitted as irrelevant in this case because Jenna was already past 41 weeks of pregnancy. It may be useful to note, however, that not one of these studies showed any benefit to induction at 41 weeks as far as perinatal mortality or any other factor was concerned.

Fetal and/or neonatal deaths occurred in one or both groups in over half of the trials. In no case, however, did this prove to be a statistically significant indicator of a difference between induction and 'watchful waiting'. The remaining trials had no perinatal deaths in either group, therefore showing no difference in relation to perinatal

Table 13.1   Studies comparing watchful waiting with induction of labour at 41–42 weeks

Author	Participants	Objective	Methods	Outcome measures	Results/ conclusions
Augensen et al 1987	409 women who were 'around the 42nd week of pregnancy': 214 in the induction group and 195 assigned to a week of conservative management (after which labour was induced).	Comparison of early versus late induction of labour in post-term pregnancy.	RCT	Measurement of labour duration and outcome and neonatal outcomes.	No significant differences in neonatal outcomes except for a higher chance of babies in the induced group needing phototherapy for hyperbilirubin-aemia.
Bergsjo et al 1989	188 pregnant women; 94 in each of the induction and expectant management groups.	To determine the proper management of pregnancy in uncomplicated cases going beyond 42 weeks.	RCT	Mode of delivery, maternal and perinatal mortality and morbidity (APGAR; neonatal problems such as hyperbilirubinaemia and respiratory distress).	No statistically significant outcomes.
Cardozo et al 1986	402 women: 207 allocated to conservative management and 195 to induction.	To compare the effects of conservative management of prolonged pregnancy with routine induction of labour at 42 weeks	RCT	Maternal and labour outcomes; neonatal outcomes including perinatal mortality and morbidity (APGAR, meconium, admission to SCBU).	No significant differences in neonatal outcome, although babies in the induction group were more likely to need intubation and were more likely to have a lower cord venous pH.
Dyson et al 1987	302 'low-risk' women at 41 weeks of pregnancy or more: 152 in induction group; 150 in the antepartum fetal test group.	Comparison of induction with antepartum fetal testing.	RCT	Perinatal outcomes included mortality, APGAR, meconium, macrosomia and length of infant hospital stay.	One minute APGARs higher in induction group (5 minute APGARs similar), more meconium and fetal distress in expectant management group.

Continues

Table 13.1 *Continued*

Author	Participants	Objective	Methods	Outcome measures	Results/ conclusions
Hannah et al 1992	3407 women; 1701 in the induction group and 1706 in the monitoring group.	Comparison of induction with serial antenatal monitoring	RCT	Perinatal mortality, neonatal morbidity, fetal distress, presence of meconium, APGAR, caesarean section rate.	Babies in the monitoring group had slightly more fetal distress and meconium; no other statistically significant neonatal differences. Caesarean section lower in the induction group.
Heden et al 1991	238 women with a gestational age of 42 weeks (dating by scan). Women randomized to immediate induction (109) or expectant management (129).	To compare induction of labour with conservative management in prolonged pregnancy.	RCT	Fetal heart monitoring, APGAR, admission to NICU.	Maternal and fetal outcomes good in both groups. 'Uterine inertia' more common in expectant group.
Herabuyta et al 1992	108 women who were at least 42 weeks pregnant; 57 were induced, 51 continued without intervention.	To compare induction with conservative management in relation to perinatal mortality/ morbidity and other measures.	RCT	Labour outcomes, APGAR.	No differences in meconium staining, fetal distress, APGAR. More babies in the non-induced group needed intubation.
Katz et al 1983	156 women who had reached 42 weeks; 78 in each of the study (conservative management) and control (induction) groups.	To test a non-aggressive management of post-date pregnancies.	RCT	Maternal and birth outcomes; neonatal assessment by PMR, APGAR and examination by a neonatologist to identify any morbidity.	One neonatal death in each group. No significant differences in fetal or neonatal pathology or in meconium staining.

Table 13.1 *Continued*

Author	Participants	Objective	Methods	Outcome measures	Results/ conclusions
Martin et al 1989	22 women: ten who experienced conservative management and twelve whose labours were induced.	1) To compare induction/ antepartum surveillance after 41 weeks. 2) To determine which appears to be associated with better perinatal outcome.	RCT	APGAR, neonatal course, meconium.	No significant differences.
Matijeviae 1998	124 women at 42 weeks of pregnancy matched with 124 women at term. Women matched by age and parity.	Assessment of perinatal mortality and feto–maternal morbidity relating to post–term pregnancy.	Case-control study.	Perinatal mortality (SB / NND), morbidity (APGAR <7 at 1 minute, cord abnormalities, abnormal blood pH / base excess, admission to NICU, presence of meconium).	No statistically significant differences in perinatal mortality. Higher maternal and neonatal abnormal CTG morbidity, in the post–term group but the researchers felt these risks were biased by more monitoring leading to increased intervention rates.
NICH 1994	440 women at 41 weeks randomized to immediate induction of labour (265) or expectant management (175).	Comparison of induction of labour and expectant management in postterm pregnancy.	RCT	Perinatal death or adverse outcome (seizures, intercranial haemorrhage, need for ventilation, nerve injury).	No significant differences.
Suikkari et al 1983	119 women 10 days or more post-dates; 66 in the induced group and 53 in the expectant management group.	Comparison of induction or observation.	Prospective case series	Several indicators of maternal wellbeing, plus APGAR, birth weight, perinatal mortality rate and paediatric evaluation of neonates.	Neither of the methods influenced the fetal wellbeing perinatally.

Continues

Table 13.1 *Continued*

Author	Participants	Objective	Methods	Outcome measures	Results/ conclusions
Witter and Weitz 1987	200 women at 41 weeks or more: 97 randomised to expectant management, 103 to induction.	Comparison of induction versus expectant management in postdates pregnancy.	RCT	Maternal and birth outcomes and a range of neonatal outcomes including APGAR, BPD, fetal distress, anomalies and meconium aspiration.	Induction group had statistically higher 5 minute APGARs though this was not clinically significant: induction group had fewer babies deemed small for gestational age.

RCT = Randomized controlled trial

mortality. A few of the studies found one or two areas where there was a statistically significant difference in relation to perinatal morbidity, but there was no consistency between which method (induction or watchful waiting) was preferable. It is possible that this could be due to chance findings because there were too few women and babies in some of the studies to answer questions about benefit or harm, or from 'observer bias', which happens when clinicians are more likely to pick up problems in babies who have experienced what they perceive to be the poorer approach. The results of some studies show induction is slightly preferable while others show that watchful waiting is slightly preferable and therefore to use this information in practice an overall view becomes essential, which is explored further below.

There is also a need to look at the absolute numbers and rates of morbidity in the studies as well as the size of differences reported between the two groups. Another important issue is whether statistically significant differences have any clinical importance. For instance, in Witter and Weitz's (1987) study, babies in the induction group had slightly higher APGARs than babies in the watchful waiting group, but this was not clinically significant. APGAR scoring is carried out in whole numbers, and no baby receives an APGAR of, say, 8.76. However, when APGAR scores are averaged, the calculation is very likely to result in a figure which includes numbers after a decimal

point. In this study, the figures after the decimal point revealed that the average APGAR was slightly higher in the induction group, but the average APGAR scores in the two groups both rounded up to 9, which is why they were said to not be clinically significant.

Of the studies which compared watchful waiting with induction after 42 weeks, those carried out by Bergsjo et al (1989), Herabuyta et al (1992) and Heden et al (1991) were linked trials, where women either had their labours induced at 42 weeks, or underwent fetal monitoring until 43 weeks, with induction only offered when specifically indicated. The studies found no difference in perinatal mortality, which might in theory offer reassurance that continuing with pregnancy is no less hazardous than induction up to 43 weeks of pregnancy, yet even when the data is pooled the studies which evaluate outcomes after this stage of pregnancy include smaller numbers of women than would be needed to establish whether or not there is a difference in the number of babies who died.

It became very evident when reading these studies that several of the authors already had a clear preference for either induction or watchful waiting, and were relatively honest in the introduction to their paper (whether intentionally or otherwise) about the kind of management they felt was preferable; that is, whether it was induction or watchful waiting that needed to prove its worth. When compiling these tables, I noticed a general correlation between the attitude of the research team towards the different approaches to 'management' and the conclusions they drew from their results. Even in a randomized controlled trial a strong belief one way or the other can lead to observer bias, as mentioned above, for instance in the unintentional over or under ascertainment of 'soft' outcome measures. These include aspects of care or outcomes that are measured subjectively and on the basis of clinical opinion, such as APGAR, or the decision that a procedure such as intubation is required. While women may be randomized very effectively, clinicians in the delivery room can hardly be 'blinded' to the clinical details which are necessary to inform their care of women.

Midwives should be well aware of this potential for bias in medical research. For instance, three of the studies in Table 13.1 had similar results, all showing that there was no significant differences between induction of labour and watchful waiting (Martin et al 1989, NICH 1994, Suikkari et al 1983). However, they all drew different conclusions from these similar results: Martin et al (1989) concluded that there did not seem to be any reason to not offer watchful waiting, NICH (1994) concluded that either option was acceptable, and Suikkari et al (1983) concluded that women may as well be induced, especially because watchful waiting was perceived by the doctors to be laborious.

The point of the assessment was to determine whether there was a significant advantage to Jenna's baby in her labour being induced, and, overall, this did not appear to be the case. From these studies, we did not see any overall advantage (in terms of the risk of perinatal morbidity or mortality) in inducing labour at or before 42 weeks of pregnancy compared with 'watchful waiting'. Of course, it could equally be said, as some of the authors have done above, that there is no advantage to waiting. My overall view from this, then, is that it comes down to the question of what the individual woman would prefer. Having said that, I also have a sense, as a midwife, that it is generally better not to interfere with nature and the natural course of pregnancy and labour unless there is good reason to do so.

TALKING IT THROUGH (PART 1)

As is often the case, the 'talking it through' process was not a simple interaction between myself and Jenna. It involved a spiralling series of conversations between myself and Jenna, which also included Dev when he could be around, and also between myself and other midwives, for instance when I needed to find out something that I did not know or could not find in the literature, or, on one occasion, when I felt I needed to talk through my own feelings in order to be able to better help Jenna.

Initially, Jenna and I talked through the findings of the above studies, and it very quickly became apparent that Jenna and I both felt the same way: while there was no option which offered guarantees (as is the case with both birth and life in general), the data did not provide us with any evidence that medical induction at or before 42 weeks was safer than watchful waiting. While this led to our decision not to pursue the second question we had discussed (concerning non-medical methods of induction), we found we had generated two more areas we needed to consider:

1. What is the best kind of 'watchful waiting'?
2. How long should we 'watchfully wait' before reassessing the issues?

SEEKING AND ASSESSING EVIDENCE TO INFORM DECISIONS (PART 2)

I was able to talk to Jenna about ' watchful waiting' that same day, having anticipated this question. The studies which had compared this with induction had used a variety of methods of 'watchful waiting' (or, as they sometimes term it, 'conservative management', a term which has not been used here because of its somewhat patriarchal overtones). The assessment methods used in each of the studies are summarized in Table 13.2, along with the criteria for inducing women in the 'watchful waiting' group; that is the signs that were seen as problematic and therefore reasons to induce labour.

It seemed to me that these could be summarized relatively simply – generally, three things were being measured:

Table 13.2   Methods of 'watchful waiting'

Study	Method of 'Watchful Waiting'/ 'Conservative Management'		Criteria for Decision to Induce
	Up to the end of 42 weeks	After 42 weeks	
Augensen et al 1987	Not relevant	'CTG non-stress test on day of referral and day 3 or 4 if still undelivered. If birth had not occurred by day 7 labour was induced.'	Not stated.
Bergsjo et al 1989	Not relevant	'No special intervention for one week {after 42 weeks} unless complications arose.' After 43 weeks, all women stayed at the hospital 'due to poor transportation facilities' and had 'close daily clinical surveillance' (685) including daily fetal movement test, atropine test, ultrasound and urinary estriol excretion tests.	'Complications'.
Cardozo et al 1986	Ultrasound (sometime between 40+12 and 40+16 weeks gestation) to determine ratio of head circumference to abdominal circumference. Daily kick count charts; CTG on alternate days.	Ultrasound (sometime between 40+12 and 40+16 weeks gestation) to determine ratio of head circumference to abdominal circumference. Daily kick count charts; CTG on alternate days.	'Asymmetric intrauterine growth retardation together with an abnormal cardiotocogram, premature rupture of membranes or the onset of hypertension.'
Dyson et al 1987	Twice weekly non-stress test (CTG). Weekly pelvic examination and determination of amniotic fluid volume (method not stated).	Twice weekly non-stress test (CTG). Twice weekly pelvic examination and determination of amniotic fluid volume (method not stated).	Nonreactive non-stress test; variable decelerations on non-stress test; oligohydramnios; cervical score became equal to or more than 6 (scoring system not outlined).
Hannah et al 1992	Fetal kick counts; twice weekly NST and amniotic fluid volume.	Not relevant	Evidence of fetal or maternal compromise.
Heden et al 1991	Not relevant	Clinical examination (not defined further) and assessment of cervical score and non-stress test. If non-stress test was unreactive, an oxytocin stress-test was performed. Weekly ultrasound.	Ominous non-stress test/ ominous stress test/ oligohydramnios.

Table 13.2 *Continued*

Study	Method of 'Watchful Waiting'/ 'Conservative Management'		Criteria for Decision to Induce
	Up to the end of 42 weeks	After 42 weeks	
Herabuyta et al 1992	Once-weekly non-stress test until 43 weeks: twice weekly non-stress test after 43 weeks.	Once-weekly non-stress test until 43 weeks: twice weekly non-stress test after 43 weeks.	'(1) abnormalities on antepartum fetal testing such as a nonreactive non-stress test, or variable decelerations on non-stress testing (2) Bishop score becomes more than 6, (3) on reaching 44 completed weeks of gestation.' (255)
Katz et al 1983	Not relevant	Twice-daily fetal movement counts carried out by the women in their own homes. Women were asked to attend the hospital for vaginal examination, amnioscopy and an oxytocin challenge test (OCT or stress test) should they note a drop in home fetal movement count. Otherwise, these tests were carried out every three days.	Induction only carried out if cervical score was above 4 (method not stated) or in the presence of one of the three critical parameters: inadequate fetal movement, presence of meconium on amnioscopy or unsatisfactory response to OCT.
Martin et al 1989	Weekly antepartum monitoring: amniotic fluid volume estimation by ultrasound, non-stress test/contraction test, cervical examination.	Weekly antepartum monitoring: amniotic fluid volume estimation by ultrasound, non-stress test/contraction test, cervical examination.	Oligohydramnios/evidence of fetal distress on non-stress or stress testing.
NICH 1994	Weekly cervical examination. Twice-weekly non-stress test and ultrasonic examination of amniotic fluid volume.	Weekly cervical examination. Twice-weekly non-stress test and ultrasonic examination of amniotic fluid volume.	Bishop score greater than 6/estimated fetal weight greater than 4.5 kg/medical or obstetric indication/ oligohydramnios/ abnormal non-stress test.
Suikkari et al 1983	Checks every 3 days, including 'obstetric examination' (details not given), non-stress test, s–HPL and s–estriol tests and amniotic fluid determination by ultrasonography.	Checks every 3 days, including 'obstetric examination' (details not given), non-stress test, s–HPL and s–estriol tests and amniotic fluid determination by ultrasonography.	Not stated.

Continues

Table 13.2   *Continued*

Study	Method of 'Watchful Waiting'/ 'Conservative Management'		Criteria for Decision to Induce
	Up to the end of 42 weeks	After 42 weeks	
Witter and Weitz 1987	All women had a 24-hour urinary estriol creatinine ratio determined between 41 and 42 weeks. N.B. Although fetal wellbeing was assessed at this time, the study evaluated induction at 42 weeks.	Fetal movement charts three times a day. Decreased fetal motion assessed by an oxytocin challenge test.	Failed oxytocin challenge test.

NST = non-stress test

- Fetal wellbeing (kick charts to measure fetal movements, CTG/non-stress test and sometimes OCT/stress test to measure fetal heart).
- Level of amniotic fluid (usually by ultrasound, method sometimes not stated).
- Cervical 'score'.

TALKING IT THROUGH (PART 2)

This aspect of the research evidence was useful, in that it enabled us to see how the researchers had defined 'watchful waiting'/'conservative management'. Were we not able to analyse this aspect of the research studies, there would be little point in applying the results to Jenna's situation. However, much as it is important in theory to be able to follow a particular set of guidelines in aiming for the best care and decisions possible, it does not necessarily follow that the guidelines used in the studies are the only, or the best, options for care. In practice, Jenna and I used this information as a yardstick rather than a set of fixed rules, not least because we could find no evidence which appropriately evaluated these forms of assessment and measured their effectiveness as markers of fetal wellbeing against other possible markers.

Jenna felt that she was already measuring her baby's wellbeing on an ongoing basis and that her connection with her baby and awareness of his movements was already providing the information sought by the 'kick chart' approach. She had a strong preference not to have any ultrasound examinations unless one or both of us felt this was truly necessary and was very nervous about the idea of involving an obstetrician, because she felt that there was a danger that her choices might not be respected and that attempts would be made to cajole her into the hospital. She said she was happy for me to examine her at home to assess the state of her cervix as often as I felt it necessary, but in this case it was me who did not see how this would benefit the situation at this point. I was concerned about the slight risk of introducing infection, and could not see a reason to justify this at that point. I suspected, from reading the research studies, that vaginal examinations weren't actually done to assess wellbeing, but because the clinicians wanted to induce labour as soon as this was deemed possible by the cervical score; this was certainly explicitly stated in a number of the studies.

I was already aware that it was possible to introduce a 'midwifery version' of several of the other markers used in the studies, although I did not have much personal experience of these, and so I had drawn on the experience of other midwives. With the help of my colleagues, it was relatively easy to devise a set of low-tech 'watchful waiting' guidelines, using both the research and midwifery experience as a basis, whereby I would see Jenna every three days and assess abdominal fluid volume by palpation and listen to the fetal heart every two minutes in a 20-minute period to assess rate, variability and response to movement. Combined with Jenna's assessment of her baby's wellbeing, which included taking note of whether her clothes became tighter or looser and how she felt the baby's position was changing, we felt this would provide as much information as possible within Jenna's comfort zone.

As far as the question of when we should next evaluate the situation was concerned, we were able to draw upon the results of some of the studies in Table 13.1, because a few of them had 'allowed' women in the conservative management groups to continue until 43 or 44 weeks before they induced labour (unless, of course, there was reason to suspect a problem). However, these studies were among those with the smallest numbers, and further than this there was no good evidence either way. I let Jenna know I wanted to discuss this issue with other midwives; to draw on their experience and thoughts as well as reflecting on the issue myself. Jenna and I agreed to meet again in three days time, when she would be 42 weeks pregnant, and decided that, as a general rule, we would keep in fairly close contact with each other and be very honest with each other about our thoughts and feelings. We agreed that Jenna would assess her baby's wellbeing and call me if she was concerned – I secretly rather hoped that, having had her mind put at ease by the results of the studies, she might be calling me soon to tell me she was in labour!

SEEKING AND ASSESSING EVIDENCE TO INFORM DECISIONS (PART 3)

Having just about exhausted the quantitative research evidence in this area, I turned again to another form of knowledge which has been well used for centuries, though is sadly less respected than quantitative research. I spent several hours talking to other midwives, some of whom had many years of out-of-hospital experience, and reflecting on the situation and the best way forward.

As far as the question of what happens after 42 weeks was concerned, some of the midwives I

talked to had either personal or indirect experience of women whose pregnancies had lasted up to 44 weeks. In most of these cases, the baby was fine, although one midwife had cared for a woman who went into labour at 43 weeks, but gave birth to a stillborn baby after transfer to a hospital when the fetal heart could not be heard. In this case, there was no ultimate conclusion on the cause of death. Another midwife knew of a woman whose baby had died in utero at 42 and a half weeks. Clearly, this kind of information is one of the things which can lead to an over-cautious approach, yet one-off experiences, while very real for the women and midwives who live through them, need to be considered in context.

One of the problems when looking at this area is that, sadly, some babies die during every week of gestation, and there is a need to separate out whether the babies who die after 42 weeks would have died anyway, or whether the cause of death is specifically linked to post-term pregnancy. Unfortunately, these data were simply not available. I could tell Jenna only two things with certainty:

1. Obstetric received wisdom suggests that induction is preferable to continuing pregnancy beyond 42 weeks, but in the case of perinatal mortality and morbidity this is not backed up by sound research evidence.
2. A number of midwives have known women whose pregnancies have lasted as long as 44 weeks of pregnancy with no ill-effects to them or their babies. Some of these midwives also know women whose babies have died, but without being able to say whether the baby's death was related to gestation or would have happened anyway.

TALKING IT THROUGH (PART 3)

When I talked to Jenna at 42 weeks, she was quite distressed, as her family had started to involve themselves in this decision and were pressuring her to go to hospital for induction. Her mother had both of her labours induced for prolonged pregnancy and did not understand why Jenna was afraid of hospitals and doctors. (As an aside, the fact that Jenna's mother experienced long pregnancies actually reassured me somewhat; I thought it may mean that Jenna had a genetic predisposition to longer pregnancies, and that this might therefore be 'normal for her'.) While Jenna's instinct was still to remain at home, she felt that she had picked up some of her family's fear and was now unsure whether she was doing the right thing by waiting and trusting her body and her baby.

I drove over to Jenna's house and we went out to a park together, where we talked for a couple of hours about the different options, about her feelings and about what she wanted to do. I had to leave before she had come to a conclusion, and, at Jenna's request, left her one of my fetoscopes, so that she and Dev could listen to the baby if they were worried. I left them to talk their decision through further, and, at Jenna's request, went off to research one of my original questions: to find out whether, if Jenna decided she wanted her labour induced, there was a safe and effective method of 'natural induction' which could be used to get Jenna into labour at home. With Jenna's permission, I also spoke to an obstetrician who was sympathetic to home birth, to arrange friendly back-up in the case of transfer to hospital at any stage.

SEEKING AND ASSESSING EVIDENCE TO INFORM DECISIONS (PART 4)

As far as the question of non-medical (that is, non-pharmacological and non-mechanical) methods of induction is concerned, the Cochrane team have released a small number of reviews on alternative methods of induction over the past few years, including acupuncture (Smith & Crowther 2004), breast stimulation (Kavanagh et al 2004a), castor oil, bath and/or enema (Kelly et al 2004), homeopathy (Smith 2004), membrane sweeping (Boulvain et al 2004) and sexual intercourse (Kavanagh et al 2004b). Each of these reviews concludes that there is either not enough data to assess the safety of these methods or not enough evidence of efficacy. This, then, meant that, again, the only way to gather any kind of information on this subject was to talk to other midwives. However, there is wide variation of opinion in this area; some midwives feel that it is best to avoid any kind of interference, some see no problem with suggesting the use of castor oil, acupuncture or homeopathy and others realize that some of the 'natural' methods of induction

include things that women may do anyway (e.g. making love, eating spicy foods). I realized that the only thing I could do for her was to offer Jenna the range of opinions in this area and help her work through what was right for her.

TALKING IT THROUGH (PART 4)

Jenna had called me the evening after we went to the park, sounding much happier. Dev had been able to help her talk through her feelings further and, with more knowledge of her relationship with her family than I had, was able to put the situation into context. It was at this point that Dev apparently made the comment in Jenna's quote at the beginning of this chapter, and she decided that, although she knew there might be additional risks in waiting, there were also risks in going to the hospital and she would rather remain at home and wait for as long as that felt comfortable to her. She and Dev made arrangements that would prevent Jenna from being further exposed to the views of her family until the baby was born (that is, they unplugged the phone and gave me the phone number of a friendly neighbour). Jenna decided she would like me to examine her cervix when we next met, and do a 'stretch and sweep' if possible. After that she would take it 'day by day', see how she felt, and continue seeing me every three days for fetal heart and amniotic fluid volume assessment.

THE OUTCOME OF THE STORY

Jenna and I met three more times before she went into labour; each time the fetal heart was variable and reactive, I was happy that there was still plenty of amniotic fluid around the baby and Jenna was happy. Jenna had a VE at 42 and a half weeks; her cervix was partly effaced, mostly closed and admitted a finger, I attempted a stretch and sweep but what I actually managed might be better termed 'cervical jiggling'! Jenna then (unsurprisingly) had a 'show' later that evening, but no contractions. Jenna did use some of the low-tech 'old midwives' tricks to encourage her body to go into labour, such as fresh pineapple, spicy food, long walks and making love. I am not sure whether these worked, or whether the fact that she spent those extra few days working through some of her fears and simply 'being' (with the phone unplugged) had something to do with it. There are so many aspects of women's lives and bodies that we know so little about, and that we will never find out about through prospective trials.

Jenna called me late one evening when she had been pregnant for 43 weeks and 1 day. I already knew that she had been having mild, irregular contractions for the past 24 hours, and she said that she and Dev had spent a really lovely evening together, eating curry and making love. She had then got into a bath and found the contractions increased in strength and frequency. I went over to their house and Jenna laboured for another few hours before giving birth to a baby boy as the sun rose. He weighed eight and a half pounds, and had very little vernix but was – and remains – very healthy.

REFLECTING ON OUTCOMES, FEELINGS AND CONSEQUENCES

I am very conscious that a good proportion of midwives who will read this chapter will not be working, as I was, in independent practice, but will, to a greater or lesser extent, have aspects of their practice directed by policies and guidelines. It is a source of endless fascination to me that there is so often a conflict between what midwives perceive the evidence to show and what happens in practice, especially where that practice is guided by reviews of the evidence carried out from a risk management or medical model perspective. While I have a strong belief that we need to use multiple forms of knowledge and evidence in practice, I also believe that, even if one simply looks at the quantitative research evidence, it so often supports a hands-off, midwifery approach rather than the medicalized practice which so many women encounter. Yet our assessment of any kind of evidence depends almost entirely on our own philosophy and on the questions we ask.

This chapter has looked at the studies which were available at the time Jenna and Dev had their baby; since then, two key responses to the research in this area have occurred which highlight this issue. Firstly, meta-analysis of the prospective studies (including many of those cited here) concluded that, if you pool the study results and analyse the results together, it is possible to argue that induction of labour is preferable to watchful waiting. This has led to a number of documents stating that induction is preferable to watchful waiting (NICE 2001, RCOG 2001) and, in some cases, has created significant changes in policies which in turn have a huge impact on women.

The second debate has arisen following the publication of a paper written by Menticoglou and Hall (2002). Their response to the meta-analysis was ground-breaking: they realized that, while pooling of the research results in the meta-analysis might show different perinatal mortality rates in the groups of women who were induced or not, this was not the only question of importance. They showed that it was also important to look at the babies who had died in the watchful waiting group and to ask whether induction of labour would have prevented their deaths. The answer was that, in most cases, it would not. Furthermore, when they removed from the analysis the babies whose deaths could not have been prevented by earlier induction of labour, there was, again, no difference between induction and watchful waiting in terms of perinatal mortality or morbidity.

One conclusion which can be drawn from an exploration of the conflict between a midwifery appraisal of the evidence and the evidence-based guidelines developed by medical model proponents is that research appraisal is no more objective than any other human activity; our biases and philosophy guide the way we look at evidence. For instance some people will be seeking proof that they can trust what they perceive to be a risk-laden process, while others will be seeking proof that it is effective to intervene in what they see as a natural and normal event. I feel it is crucial that we consider this and understand that, in practice, objectivity is an incredibly difficult place to reach.

The question of whether, when, why, where and how labour should be induced is a huge one, with no easy answers. It is not simply a case of looking at one kind of evidence and applying it to all women; there are a multitude of individual factors to be taken into account. I was very grateful that Jenna had been using natural family planning and knew her conception date; I have also worked with other women where the issues have been even more complex, principally because many women cannot be this certain around the date of conception or their last period. With some women, it matters less to them that there is little evidence of the efficacy of non-medical ways of inducing labour than that they feel they are 'doing something'. For others, acupuncture, homeopathy or other ways of encouraging their body to go into labour might not be their first choice, but they turn to these therapies in order to attempt to avoid the medical induction which they feel is otherwise inevitable.

Jenna's story also highlights the hugely important yet massively under-researched issue of the impact that our beliefs, experiences and psyche can have on what our bodies are doing. At one point in Jenna's pregnancy, I had a very strong sense (based on no evidence except my own intuition) that the opinions that some members of her family were sharing with her were serving to inhibit her ability to relax and allow her body to go into labour. I was relieved when she and Dev were able to work through these issues and especially when they made the decision to unplug the phone; as soon as they had done this, in tandem with arranging other ways for me to get in touch with them should the need arise, Jenna visibly relaxed.

I believe midwives have always known that life and birth are uncertain events; it is really only in the past few decades that we have been seduced away from this belief towards the idea that we can 'manage' pregnancy and birth. I do believe that the majority of women will go into labour at the time that is right for them and their babies; I don't know whether I believe that some women develop some kind of pathology which means they will not go into labour at the right time – this is just one of literally hundreds of questions in this area

for which we do not have a good answer. However, my experience as Jenna's midwife led me to realize that there is no good evidence to support the practice of routinely forcing an artificial end to pregnancy.

PRACTICE POINTERS

- Questions surrounding induction of labour for post-dates are complex and intertwined and care is needed to determine whether, for any given woman, the primary question(s) relate to dating, appropriateness of induction, the comparative safety and/or effectiveness of methods of induction or other issues.
- The factors that can affect a woman's experience and the decisions she makes are also complex and, as here, include issues such as family dynamics which are not always easy to uncover where time is pressured.
- Although there is no difference in perinatal mortality between induction and 'watchful waiting' until 42 weeks of pregnancy, the research evidence concerning the comparative difference in perinatal mortality after this point of pregnancy is less clear because of a lack of large, well-conducted studies.
- There is little agreement about what is meant by 'watchful waiting' and guidance in this area appears to be based on clinician opinion and philosophy rather than research evidence.
- Ultimately, because there is no good evidence to support artificially forcing an end to pregnancy before 42 weeks and little evidence either way after this point, decisions around this area need to be made only after women are fully aware of both the consequences of intervention/non-intervention and the knowledge that no course of action can offer any kind of guarantee.

References

Augensen K, Bergsjo P, Eikeland T, Ashvik K, Carlsen J 1987 Randomized comparison of early versus late induction of labour in post-term pregnancy. British Medical Journal 294: 1192–1195

Baskett T, Nagele F 2000 Naegele's rule: a reappraisal. British Journal of Obstetrics and Gynaecology 107: 1433–1435

Bergsjo P, Daniel W, Denman III D W et al 1990 Duration of human singleton pregnancy; a population-based study. Acta Obstetrica Gynecologica Scandinavica 69: 197–207

Bergsjo P, Gui-dan H, Su-qin Y, Zhi-zeng G, Bakketeig L S 1989 Comparison of induced vs. non-induced labor in post-term pregnancy. Acta Obstetricia Gynecologica Scandinavica 68: 683–687

Boulvain M, Stan C, Irion O 2004 Membrane sweeping for induction of labour (Cochrane Review). In: The Cochrane Library, Issue 3, 2004. Wiley, Chichester

Breart G, Goujard J, Maillard F et al 1982 Comparison of two obstetrical policies with regard to artificial induction of labour at term. A randomised trial. Journal d'Obstetrique, de la Gynocologie et de la Reproducion (Paris) 11: 107–112

Cardozo L, Fysh J, Pearce J M 1986 Prolonged pregnancy: the management debate. British Medical Journal 293: 1059–1063

Cole R A, Howie P W, MacNaughton M C 1975 Elective induction of labour. A randomised prospective trial. Lancet 1: 767–770

Duff C, Sinclair M 2000 Exploring the risks associated with induction of labour: a retrospective study using the NIMATS database. Journal of Advanced Nursing 31(2): 410–417

Dyson D, Miller P D, Armstrong M A 1987 Management of prolonged pregnancy: induction of labour versus antepartum testing. American Journal of Obstetrics and Gynecology 156: 928–934

Egarter C H, Kofler E, Fitz R, Husselein P 1989 Is induction of labour indicated in prolonged pregnancy? Results of a prospective randomised trial. Gynecological and Obstetric Investigations 27: 6–9

Hannah M E, Hannah W J, Hellman J ey al 1992 Canadian Multicenter Post-Term Pregnancy Trial Group. Induction of labour as compared with serial antenatal monitoring in post-term pregnancy. A randomized controlled trial. New England Journal of Medicine 326: 1587–1592

Heden L, Ingemarsson I, Ahlstrom H, Solum T 1991 Induction of labor vs. conservative management in prolonged pregnancy: controlled study. International Journal of Feto-maternal Medicine 4(4): 148–152

Herabutya Y, Prasertsawat P O, Tongyai T, Isarangura Na Ayudthya N 1992 Prolonged pregnancy: the management dilemma. International Journal of Gynecology and Obstetrics 37: 253–258

Katz Z, Yemini M, Lancet M, Mogilner B M, Ben-Hur H, Caspi B 1983 Non-aggressive management of post-date pregnancies. European Journal of Obstetrics Gynecology & Reproductive Biology 15: 71–79

Kavanagh J, Kelly A J, Thomas J 2004a Breast stimulation for cervical ripening and induction of labour (Cochrane Review). In: The Cochrane Library, Issue 3, 2004. Wiley, Chichester

Kavanagh J, Kelly A J, Thomas J 2004b Sexual intercourse for cervical ripening and induction of labour (Cochrane Review). In: The Cochrane Library, Issue 3, 2004. Wiley, Chichester

Kelly A J, Kavanagh J, Thomas J 2004 Castor oil, bath and/or enema for cervical priming and induction of labour (Cochrane Review). In: The Cochrane Library, Issue 3, 2004. Wilet, Chichester

Martin D H, Thompson W, Pinkerton J H M 1978 A randomised controlled trial of selective planned delivery. British Journal of Obstetrics and Gynaecology 85: 109–113

Martin J N, Sessums J K, Howard P, Martin R W, Morrison J C 1989 Alternative approaches to the management of gravidas with prolonged post-term postdate pregnancies. Journal of the Missouri State Medical Association 30: 105–111

Matijeviae R 1998 Outcome of post-term pregnancy; a matched pair case-control study. Croatian Medical Journal 39(4): 11–14

Menticoglou S M, Hall P F 2002 Routine induction of labour at 41 weeks gestation: nonsensus consensus. BJOG: An International Journal of Obstetrics and Gynaecology 109(5): 485–491

Mittendorf R, Williams M A, Berkey C S et al 1990 The length of uncomplicated human gestation. Obstetrics and Gynecology 75: 929–932

NICE (National Institute for Clinical Excellence) 2001 Induction of labour: inherited clinical guideline D. National Institute for Clinical Excellence, London

NIC (National Institute of Child Health and Human Development Network of Maternal-Fetal Medicine Units 1994 A clinical trial of induction of labor versus expectant management in postterm pregnancy. American Journal of Obstetrics and Gynecology 170: 716–723

Olsen O, Clausen J A 1997 Routine ultrasound dating has not been shown to be more accurate than the calendar method. British Journal of Obstetrics and Gynecology 104: 1221–1222

Page L (ed.) 2000. The new midwifery: science and sensitivity in practice. Churchill Livingstone, Oxford

Purrett G 2004 Individualised due dates. In Wickham S 2004 Midwifery best practice, Volume 2. Books for Midwives, Oxford, pp 17–20

RCOG (Royal College of Obstetricians and Gynaecologists) 2001 Induction of labour. Evidence-based clinical guideline, Number 9. RCOG, London

Rosser J 2000 Calculating the EDD; which is more accurate, scan or LMP? The Practising Midwife 3(3): 28–29

Sande H A, Tuveng J, Fonstelien T 1983 A prospective randomised study of induction of labor.

International Journal of Gynaecology and Obstetrics 21: 333–336

Smith C A 2004 Homeopathy for induction of labour (Cochrane Review). In: The Cochrane Library, Issue 3, 2004. Wiley, Chichester

Smith C A, Crowther C A 2004 Acupuncture for induction of labour (Cochrane Review). In: The Cochrane Library, Issue 3, 2004. Wiley, Chichester

Suikkari A M, Jalkanen M, Heiskala H, Koskela O 1983 Prolonged pregnancy: induction or observation. Acta Obstetrica Gynecoogical Scandinavica Supplement 116: 58

Tylleskar J, Finnstrom O, Leijon I, Hedenskog S, Ryden G 1979 Spontaneous labor and elective induction – a prospective randomized study. Effects on mother and fetus. Acta Obstetrica Gynecoogical Scandinavica 58: 513–518

Witter F R, Weitz C M 1987 A randomised trial of induction at 42 weeks of gestation vs. expectant management for postdates pregnancies. American Journal of Perinatology 4: 206–211

SECTION 3

Promoting healthy birth, using midwifery skills and the organization of practice

'I see what I do now as a complete job not part of it or bits of it or half of it, because what you and the woman decide antenatally impacts on what happens postnatally . . . it's given me freedom in that I am my own boss and I will make decisions with the woman about what happens.'

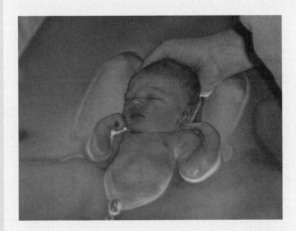

Chapter **14**

A public health view of the maternity services

Jean Chapple

This chapter looks at the common aims of personal and public health services, how health needs of pregnant women are assessed for a community and how an evidence-based policy of care provided by midwives acting as public health practitioners can help to improve the health of mothers, babies and families.

ACHIEVING BETTER OUTCOMES OF MATERNITY SERVICES: THE ROLE OF PUBLIC HEALTH

WHAT IS PUBLIC HEALTH?

Public health is the science and art of preventing disease, prolonging life and promoting health through the organized efforts of society (Acheson 1988). Public health specialists differ from the nurses, midwives and doctors involved in clinical medicine in that their 'patients' are whole communities rather than the individuals who make up that community. This creates a potential tension between those making health policy decisions that affect society as a whole and those who have day-to-day contact with individuals and who need resources to deliver that clinical care.

In general, what is good for the individual is also good for society, but this is not inevitably the case. Every parent contemplating immunization for their child would like every other parent to get their child immunized in order to provide herd immunity. This would mean that their own child would not come into contact with the disease and would be protected without encountering any of the extremely small but individually important risks of immunization. This argument is not sustainable for the country as a whole: living in a democratic community means compromise. We have to follow rules and forego some individual choices to live in harmony with others. Imagine the chaos if we did not follow laws to drive on a given side of the road or to dispose of rubbish in an hygienic manner. Similar rules must apply if we are to have a publicly funded health service. We cannot all have every diagnostic test or treatment that we might desire or the health service bank will run dry at an even faster rate than it already does; diagnosing and treating one person might mean that no resources are left to diagnose and treat another. We often face similar decisions in our home budgets – having to choose between a new suite of furniture or a holiday, or to compromise by opting for having both but selecting the cheaper options available. These are opportunity costs, the opportunity for one clinician to treat one person being affected by the decisions made by another. Dr Paul may be robbing Dr Peter of his chance to treat the patient sitting in front of him (Mooney 1992).

SETTING PRIORITIES THROUGH HEALTH NEEDS ASSESSMENT

As health service resources are finite, tough decisions are needed on what services should be provided and for which members of the community. Care in publicly funded healthcare systems is rarely rationed (given as a fixed allowance to restrict supply) but is prioritized or ranked in order of preference. Public health specialists help in this process through needs assessment to ensure that resources are targeted to those who need them most. Some specific groups, such as people who are mentally ill, the elderly and those with learning disabilities, will lose out in a system in which the person or service that shouts loudest gets most. In an ideal world, public health would cover more than just health services – it would also cover the health impact of plans formulated by other parts of government, for example those dealing with education, housing, social policy on benefits and environmental issues such as new roads and air pollution. This is finally being recognized by the UK Government in national policy (Department of Health 2004).

Health needs assessment is not an exact science but studies:

- how common any given condition is and its impact on the health of the affected individual and the population;
- changes in disease patterns, for example, the re-emergence of old diseases such as tuberculosis and syphilis and the development of new ones such as HIV and AIDS;
- the development of new healthcare interventions, new drugs and new techniques in terms of *effectiveness* (does it change the natural history of the disease?) (Cochrane 1972) and *efficiency* (is it used in a way which produces the best results for the total population?) as judged by scientifically rigorous studies – *evidence-based medicine*;
- the effects of national initiatives to improve quality of care, such as Changing Childbirth (Department of Health 1993) and the National Service Framework for Children – Maternity (Department of Health 2004);
- what the public expects from the healthcare services for which it pays through taxes.

The chief tool of public health and needs assessment is *epidemiology*.

WHAT IS EPIDEMIOLOGY AND WHAT DOES IT HAVE TO OFFER MIDWIVES?

Epidemiology is the study of the distribution and determinants of disease: who gets what disease, where they live, and when and why they get it. There is a need to put an individual patient in the context of the community of which he or she is a member. For example, we know through population-based studies that a woman with insulin-dependent diabetes has five times the risk of losing her baby than does her neighbour without this disease (Casson et al 1997, Hawthorne et al 1997). We therefore focus attention on this individual before and during pregnancy – even if she appears well and has no social or other disadvantages – because, in general, women like her have a higher risk of having a baby with a congenital malformation and macrosomia. Midwives can use epidemiology to tell them which members of their local community are at higher risk of a complication of pregnancy and thus need more monitoring and support.

POPULATIONS WITH PROBLEMS: WHAT IS RISK?

We never say that there is a risk we may win the lottery but that we think we have a chance of winning (Silman 1997). This implies that the term 'risk' adds a negative emotive element to the *probability* or *likelihood* of an event happening. This element is also subjective: the risk of any event may be viewed and expressed in a very different light by different people (Calman & Royston 1997). Contraceptive pill scares in the media produce the common phenomenon of a woman rushing to her doctor and appearing surprised that the doctor is far more concerned about the risk of thrombosis from her smoking habit – which she refuses to contemplate giving up – than about changing her pill.

There is also a conflict here between a population and a personal health approach. Epidemiological studies can supply accurate figures on the probability or chance of having a baby with an abnormality on which to base informed consent, but if you are one of the small percentage of high-risk patients in a total population of a thousand, that is 100% of you. It is the value judgements linked to this probability by clinicians and their patients that may cause conflict and concern.

IDENTIFYING PEOPLE WITH PROBLEMS IN THE POPULATION

METHODS

There are three methods of identifying high risk populations:

1. needs assessment to identify high risk groups with features that predispose them to problems within a population;
2. case finding to identify high risk individuals within a population attending for healthcare;
3. screening to identify high risk individuals within a population invited for screening.

Needs assessment can identify the characteristics of the local population and alert both those commissioning care and those providing it to specific services that are needed. Anonymous HIV testing in neonates (which acts as a proxy for maternal HIV infection) identified that, in London, there are populations in whom the prevalence (the proportion of people in the population with HIV at any given time) is 1 in 150 pregnant women. Services to encourage all women to be screened for HIV, to look after mothers and to minimize the transmission to their babies are needed in these districts. In other parts of the UK, prevalence assessed through neonatal screening was so low that screening for HIV was targeted at women with a known high-risk lifestyle, such as those injecting drugs (Nicoll et al 1998). However, current prevalence is higher in all parts of the UK, so that HIV screening is now offered to all women (National Institute for Clinical Excellence 2003).

Case-finding involves clinicians looking for illness or its predictors whenever a patient presents to them for another reason, seen, for example, in checking blood pressure when a woman comes to a clinic for a cervical smear. Case-finding is usually carried out at the same place where definitive diagnosis and therapy are offered (for example, in a primary care setting), so there are few problems

linking those identified as high risk to a source of care (Sackett et al 1991).

Antenatal care usually involves case-finding as midwives check for a range of social and clinical complications, ranging from evidence of domestic violence (Mezey & Bewley 1997) to signs of pregnancy hypertension, at each visit. Formal counselling or permission to case-find is not usually sought as most women and their carers accept that this is a normal part of pregnancy care, although midwives take care to explain what they are doing and why. Ultrasound scanning is a very nonspecific type of case-finding; a woman may be informed that the scan is to confirm her dates, but the ultrasonographer may then measure the nuchal skinfold thickness as a 'routine' part of the scanning process to assess the risk of Down's syndrome without formal or informed consent.

Screening involves inviting the public to undergo screening tests to separate them into groups with higher and lower probabilities of disease. Those with a high probability of disease will be offered a diagnostic test. Specific screening programmes are set within pregnancy care, for example offering testing for Down's syndrome through serum screening, or screening for rhesus status. These screening programmes usually involve some form of pretest counselling and are formalized, with protocols and literature for women to take away and discuss with their partners.

NEEDS ASSESSMENT AND CASE-fiNDING: WHICH GROUPS OF WOMEN DEVELOP WHICH PREGNANCY COMPLICATIONS AND WHEN?

Risks before and during conception and early pregnancy

Some women are at risk even before they conceive as they are aware that they carry genes for severe disease and seek advice before pregnancy. Good family history taking may also unearth potentially heritable problems.

Random errors in the division of the egg can lead to fetal chromosomal abnormalities or multiple pregnancy, both of which are more common in older mothers. Some trisomies, such as trisomy 18 (Edwards' syndrome) and trisomy 13 (Patau's syndrome), are rapidly lethal, often in the middle or third trimester, but others, for example trisomy

21 (Down's syndrome), may produce a viable fetus if there is no major structural abnormality such as a congenital heart defect.

Multiple births are exposed to many hazards and are becoming more common with the increasing use of infertility treatment. Multiple placentation and increased nutritional demands made by two or more fetuses can result in fetal growth retardation. In monozygous twins, cords can become entangled in a single amniotic sac, competition for placental tissues may occur, or one twin may transfuse blood into the other, resulting in a marked size difference between them or the death of one twin. The rate of premature delivery is also very high, especially in higher-order births.

Some maternal infections, such as rubella, cytomegalovirus and toxoplasmosis, may be transmitted vertically from mother to child and cause severe malformation without causing symptoms in the mother. The birth prevalence in developed countries of severe malformation and death caused by these infections is very low, but it remains to be seen whether public health programmes to prevent the spread of toxoplasmosis through personal and food hygiene (Royal College of Obstetricians and Gynaecologists 1992) and to prevent neural tube defects by a periconceptional increase in maternal folic acid intake (Czeizel & Dudas 1992, Czeizel 1993, MRC Vitamin Study Research Group 1991) will result in the primary prevention of malformation. It is likely that congenital rubella will recur in the UK because of the low uptake by some parents of measles mumps and rubella vaccine for their children. The ease of intercontinental travel to countries where rubella is common and immigration of women from countries where rubella vaccine is not offered will also increase the risk of congenital rubella (Mehta & Thomas 2002). Other organisms, such as *Listeria*, *Salmonella* and Parvovirus (fifth disease) can cause death through miscarriage or prematurity with or without intrauterine or neonatal infection.

ENVIRONMENTAL FACTORS ACTING IN PREGNANCY

External environment

Exposure to occupational or environmental hazards such as radiation or lead can contribute to perinatal mortality, but the literature is unclear on the risk, mainly because the numbers of births considered are generally too small to achieve sufficient statistical power to assess risk (Rosenberg et al 1987, Savitz et al 1989). A retrospective case control study of over 1000 perinatal deaths in Leicester between 1976 and 1982 showed that leather-workers were at increased risk of perinatal death, particularly from congenital malformation and macerated stillbirth, compared with other manual workers in the same class (Clarke & Mason 1985).

The effect of occupational hazards on perinatal mortality may also be mediated through an increased risk of prematurity or low birth weight, both of which have a major influence on the risk of a baby dying. In a large study in Scotland between 1981 and 1984 (Sanjose et al 1991), the risk of preterm delivery and low birth weight was shown to be over 50% higher in the children of women who worked with electrical, metal or leather goods than in other female manual workers and was more frequent in the children of mothers and fathers employed in manual rather than non-manual jobs. Women in jobs for which high physical exertion is needed have a higher rate of preterm and low birth weight delivery (Homer et al 1990).

In utero environment

The effects on the fetus of maternal smoking have been intensively studied since the 1950s. The actual contribution made by maternal smoking to the risk of perinatal death is not direct but appears to depend on the presence of other adverse factors as smoking reduces fetal growth rate and therefore adds to other detrimental influences. However, its importance is shown by the estimate that, in England and Wales in 1984, 18% of instances of low birth weight were attributable to maternal smoking (Simpson & Armand Smith 1986). Women who stop smoking by the third trimester are not at increased risk of a low birth weight baby compared with non-smokers, but women who begin smoking during the second or third trimester have a risk of a low birth weight baby similar to that of women who have smoked throughout their pregnancy. The risk in the third trimester is also dose related: the more cigarettes smoked, the higher the risk of a small baby (Liberman et al 1994).

The role of undernutrition and specific dietary constituents is still uncertain (Naismith 1981) but will also vary with the underlying health of the mother. A study carried out in London showed that mothers of low birth weight babies are not randomly distributed among mothers at all nutritional levels but are concentrated among mothers of poor nutritional status (Wynn et al 1991). This study also found that vitamin and mineral supplementation in the last two trimesters of pregnancy had no significant effect on birth dimensions; thus diet may have its maximum effect during ovulatory maturation and early embryonic development (Doyle et al 1990).

Maternal nutrition may have an even more longlasting effect. There is currently much debate about the Barker programming hypothesis – that it is earlier rather than later adverse circumstances that have the major impact on diseases seen later in life. The hypothesis is that a programming stimulus or insult (such as a drug or hormone) during certain critical periods of development have a lasting or lifelong effect on the structure or function of organs, tissues and body functions. Work initially done on the midwifery records of a cohort of males born in Hertfordshire from 1911 onwards who were followed up many years later suggests that cardiovascular and chronic lung disease in adult life may have important causes in fetal and early life, such as poor maternal nutrition (Barker 1992).

SOCIAL FACTORS CAUSING PROBLEMS

Most social factors act through causing prematurity and/or growth retardation.

Hellier (1977) showed that almost a quarter of the reduction in perinatal mortality rate that occurred in England and Wales between 1953 and 1978 was explained by the demographic changes in maternal age, parity and social class that had occurred. These included:

- more women bearing children at a safer age;
- improvements in the standard of living, with relative poverty (being poor in a rich society) becoming more of a problem than absolute poverty (being poor in a poor country) (Kawachi & Kennedy 1997);

- a decrease in the number of mothers of very large families;
- a general rise in the standard of nutrition and stature of women;
- more widespread use of contraception;
- the legalization of abortion following the 1967 Act.

'Elderly' primiparae and women with more than four previous births are often seen as high-risk patients. The data on which this perception is based are collected through national record systems that produce cross-sectional data at one point in time. Such studies of pregnancy loss show a U-shaped curve for the distribution of perinatal mortality rate and parity, the death rate being high for first births, dipping to a lower level for first births and women under 20 years of age, and rising for fourth and subsequent births and for women aged over 35. Analysis in this way gives an erroneous view of the risks, as reproductive compensation may apply to women who have previously lost babies. Women who lose babies usually go on to have further pregnancies in order to achieve the size of family they want. They are at high risk because of the previous poor outcome and are therefore of higher parity and, of necessity, older. Longitudinal studies follow the same women over a period of time by linking each episode of healthcare. They show that fetal mortality for each pregnancy goes down as the mother's parity increases (Bakketeig & Hoffman 1979, 1981, Billewicz 1973, Roman et al 1978). For babies of the same mother, the risk of each baby dying seems to fall steadily with each pregnancy, but children from families that end up large are all at higher risk of perinatal death regardless of their birth order compared with children from small families. Higher age and parity in subsequent pregnancies may be the result of poor pregnancy outcome rather than its cause.

Longitudinal studies can also examine the effects of birth interval: a close spacing of pregnancy may contribute to an increased risk of perinatal death, and there is also a tendency for repeated perinatal death with the same mothers.

There is still great disparity between perinatal mortality rates in different social classes in Britain, although the increasing proportion of babies born to unmarried women – now over one-third – has meant that illegitimate babies are now less disadvantaged at birth than they once were.

Women from minority ethnic groups appear to have a higher risk of perinatal death than do indigenous mothers. A minor part of this may be the result of a difference in birth weight distribution, but the incidence of malformation may be very different. The increased incidence of lethal congenital malformations in British Pakistanis made a large contribution to a perinatal mortality rate of 18 per 1000 in 1984 for this group compared with 12 per 1000 in other ethnic groups – a 50% excess (Balarajan & Botting 1989, Chitty & Winter 1989). The access to and use of maternity services may also affect outcome (Clarke et al 1988).

Table 14.1 shows some of the relationships between external factors and the health and wellbeing of women and babies.

MIDWIVES AS PUBLIC HEALTH PRACTITIONERS

While public health specialists can help to identify at risk groups and develop evidence-based strategies for improving health, there is a point at which policies for whole communities have to be taken to and 'sold' to the individuals who make up the community. There is much debate about the balance between the 'nanny state' – for example, banning smoking in public places – against the rights of the individual. 'The Public Health White Paper Choosing Health: Making Healthier Choices Easier' (Department of Health 2004) makes the case for promoting and protecting health through changes in lifestyle and to encourage investment in health promotion as well as disease diagnosis and treatment.

Table 14.1 Relationship between external factors and health and wellbeing of women and babies

KEY DETERMINANTS OF HEALTH OUTCOME	IMPACT ONTO HEALTH & WELLBEING OF MOTHER AND BABY
SOCIAL CLASS Women in social classes IV and V are more likely to experience:	Low birth weight (associated with increased risk of death in first year and increased risk of disability and special educational need Preterm birth Stillbirth and infant mortality Maternal death Smoking Lower rates of successful breastfeeding
DEPRIVATION[1]	Stillbirth and infant mortality Perinatal deaths due to congenital abnormalities Smoking Lower rates of successful breastfeeding
TEENAGE PARENTING	Postnatal depression Smoking Domestic violence Inadequate diet Establishing successful breastfeeding
ETHNIC ORIGIN[2]	Low birth weight (associated with increased risk of death in first year and increased risk of disability and special education need Maternal death Establishing successful breastfeeding (inverse relationship)
FIRST LANGUAGE NOT ENGLISH	Higher caesarean section rate?
SMOKING	Low birthweight Fetal and neonatal death Sudden infant death syndrome Childhood development

Continued

Table 14.1 *Continued*

KEY DETERMINANTS OF HEALTH OUTCOME	IMPACT ONTO HEALTH & WELLBEING OF MOTHER AND BABY
INADEQUATE DIET	Low birthweight Coronary heart disease Diabetes
DRUG AND ALCOHOL MISUSE	Miscarriage Developmental abnormalities Fetal alcohol syndrome Sudden infant death syndrome (SIDS)
DOMESTIC VIOLENCE (associated with younger couples, separation, financial pressures, drug/alcohol abuse, Asian populations, refugees)	Premature death Low birthweight Placental abruption Fetal injury
LACK OF SOCIAL SUPPORT HOMELESSNESS	Postnatal depression Low birthweight Miscarriage Stillbirth Infant mortality Childhood accidents
ASYLUM SEEKERS	Rape Poor maternal health Depression Poor nutrition
DISABILITY	Accessing services Communication

[1] Measured by receipt of welfare benefits, unemployment, younger parents, low educational attainment poor and over-crowded housing

[2] Existing data relates only to women born outside the UK

Midwives, with their links to local communities and standing with pregnant women, play a vital role as public health practitioners in individualizing public policy and helping women and their families to lead healthier lives. The poor and disadvantaged in society often find it difficult to become empowered enough to make healthy choices. All midwives are aware of the need to target marginalized groups through interventions such as Sure Start. This is a government programme to deliver the best start in life for every child by bringing together early education, childcare, health and family support. It has had much positive support from parents (Department for Education and Skills 2005).

Midwives need to reach every pregnant woman. Some are 'hidden' in society – asylum seekers who may be moved round the country, the 4500 women in UK prisons (two thirds of whom are mothers), homeless and travelling women, disabled women and the 21 000 girls under 18 who become mothers each year, of whom 3400 are under 16. Women who abuse alcohol or drugs may be afraid to approach midwives if they fear that social services may become involved with their other children. Women with disabilities may not be able to access care physically. It is also important not to forget that wealth does not protect against postnatal depression, isolation or anxiety.

Minimizing the effects of inequalities is an integral part of maternity care. Research shows that all women, regardless of colour, culture, religion, background, circumstances and age, want and value the same aspects of care – respect, good communication, information, choice and control. The evidence on interventions to promote healthy lifestyles suggests that for all aspects, an individualized approach tailored to each woman's needs is more effective than a blunderbuss approach that tries to target all things to all women. Care needs to be individual, flexible and personal for each woman with consideration of her circumstances. It is unhelpful to identify groups of women who are 'unequal' as this view does not respect women as individuals but instead encourages stereotyping and categorization of women. Many women may be in more than one disadvantaged group.

Maternity services can respond to the challenge of addressing health inequalities by adopting three key principles:

- Identifying women who are likely to experience inequalities of access or outcome
- Planning, commissioning and delivering care that is individual and personal for each woman.
- Recognizing that care of a pregnant woman and her family is not exclusive to the Health Service.

Those planning and delivering maternity services to reduce inequalities need to understand their local community, deliver flexible patterns of service, collaborate with local agencies such as social services and involve service users.

SPECIFIC PUBLIC HEALTH INTERVENTIONS

Smoking

Antenatal care gives an opportunity to encourage and help women give up smoking for the benefit of their own health as well as their children's (Health Education Authority 1994). The government target is to reduce the percentage of pregnant women who smoke from 23% to 15% by 2010. Nonetheless, interventions designed to motivate or assist women give up smoking have fairly low rates of success.

Over a quarter of pregnant women who smoke will continue in pregnancy, but pregnancy itself seems to be a prime motivator to stop. The majority of women who quit smoking during pregnancy do so spontaneously. Of 100 women still smoking at the time of their first antenatal visit, about 10 will stop with normal care and a further 6 or 7 with a special programme (Coleman 2004, Lumley et al 2003). Acceptance of group sessions for smoking cessation is very poor. Local specialist cessation services are a central component of any local anti-smoking strategy to provide on going individually tailored support including home visits. Tailoring interventions and addressing barriers to behavioural change and the concerns of pregnant women lead to greater acceptance of interventions (Health Development Agency 2004).

Individualizing smoking cessation support means taking account of women's feelings about smoking, such as their fears that giving up will lead to a big baby and a difficult birth, guilt about smoking, and their capacity to cope with adverse circumstances. Disadvantaged women use smoking to cope with the difficulties of their lives. Working class mothers report that cigarettes are their only luxury, their only leisure activity, their only item of personal expenditure, and are a quick and easy way of coping with stress. Smoking relieves boredom and is a social activity, which also demarcates adult time away from the children (Dorsett & Marsh 1998, Graham 1987, 1993).

A systematic review of randomized controlled trials found that, in general, behavioural self-help approaches to smoking cessation were more effective than advice and feedback in reducing smoking in pregnancy (Arblaster et al 1998). However, a cluster randomized trial of self help smoking cessation using standardized booklets with outcomes validated by urinary cotinine levels showed that although self help intervention was acceptable it was ineffective when implemented during routine antenatal care. It also showed that validated smoking cessation rates among pregnant women are substantially lower than self reported rates (19% validated smoking cessation with the intervention compared to 26% self reported, 21% validated cessation for at least 7 days in the normal care group compared to 29% self reported) (Moore et al 2002). Computer-generated, individually tailored materials are generally more effective than standardized booklets (Lancaster & Staed 2003). Antenatal counselling of at least 10 minutes person to person contact, combined with written materials tailored to pregnancy, can double cessation rates (NHS Centre 1998).

It is important to assess a pregnant smoker's 'stage of change' at the start of antenatal care in order to offer appropriate advice, because pregnant smokers are much less likely to agree with a list of statements about the dangers of maternal smoking than non-smokers, and a woman's stage of change is related both to the number of health risks she agrees with and her level of conviction (Haslam & Draper, 2000). Since women whose partners give up smoking during the pregnancy are themselves much more likely to give up, partners also need access to smoking cessation services through the antenatal clinics (Holmes 2001).

As nicotine may cause harm through placental vasoconstriction, health professionals are anxious about the use of nicotine replacement therapy during pregnancy, and the pharmaceuticals are not licensed for use in pregnancy. (Bupropion (Zyban) is specifically contraindicated in pregnancy). Nicotine replacement therapy should be used during pregnancy if the benefits of using it (increased likelihood of cessation) outweigh the risks (from extra nicotine if women use the therapy and continue to smoke). Midwives should be able to prescribe nicotine replacement therapy after full explanation of the pros and cons.

Mental health

There is little evidence to support the effectiveness of universal screening for depression either antenatally or postnatally. Continuity of care is highly valued by individuals experiencing mental illness (Bindman et al 2000) and this applies equally to maternity care, where midwives are available to discuss women's feelings of depression and also to identify mood changes over time (Mauthner 1997).

Baby massage may improve the mental health of mothers with postnatal depression (Onozawa et al 2000), possibly by promoting mother-infant bonding or by providing social contact with other mothers through baby massage classes (Hart et al 2003).

Breastfeeding

There are two challenges in promoting breastfeeding: to increase the number of women who start breastfeeding (initiation), and to increase the length of time for which they breastfeed (duration). Some consider breastfeeding a 'learned art' and specific help, support and encouragement may be needed, especially by mothers from a peer group where bottle-feeding is the norm. For women on a low income, the decision to initiate breastfeeding has been found to be influenced more by embodied knowledge gained from seeing breastfeeding than from theoretical knowledge about its benefits (Hoddinott & Pill, 1999). Many women who start breastfeeding give up before they have even left hospital, so teaching basic technique and practicalities is important.

Support to mothers during pregnancy, labour and after birth increases both initiation and duration of breastfeeding, and can be effective among women on low incomes and from ethnic minority groups. Three different types of interventions can help with initiation: informal, small group health education delivered during the antenatal period, one-to-one support and peer support programmes delivered postnatally. Effective packages include a peer support programme and/or media campaign combined with structural changes to the health sector and/or health education activities (Fairbank et al 2000).

Extra professional support of any kind appears to increase initiation of breastfeeding and lay support is effective in reducing the cessation of exclusive breastfeeding (Sikorski et al 2002).

Diet

Knowledge alone does not change behaviour - a study of the impact of specially designed written nutrition education materials on pregnant women found that although the intervention significantly increased participants' nutritional knowledge, it did not affect their dietary intake or attitudes to food (Anderson et al 1995). A randomized controlled trial of brief counselling by nurses in the general (non-pregnant) UK population, which compared straightforward nutritional counselling with individual behavioural counselling based on the stage of change model, found that both types of counselling were effective in increasing fruit and vegetable consumption but behavioural counselling produced twice as great an increase in the numbers of portions consumed by people with a low income (Steptoe et al 2003).

Pregnant women living in poverty have a fairly high awareness of the main constituents of a healthy diet, but the main reason women receiving income support cite for not eating more 'healthy' foods is the cost. One third of those who receive advice on diet in pregnancy find the advice unhelpful because it does not take account of their tight budgets and lack of local shops selling healthy food. A promising approach is to promote healthy food in the community, with input from local councils, community groups and the food industry and to provide help in learning to prepare and cook raw foods rather than rely on more expensive and less healthy processed meals.

SOCIAL SUPPORT

Generally the effect of social support during pregnancy (targeted at women believed to be at risk) on birthweight and preterm births appears to be quite weak (Hodnett 2002a, 2002b, 2002c, Hodnett & Fredericks 2003). However, individual trials have found success with particular vulnerable groups. A small study of one-to-one visits and regular telephone contact for African-American women lacking support from a partner or mother achieved a substantial reduction in low birthweight (Norbeck et al 1996). Another trial of weekly telephone calls from a registered nurse found a significant reduction in preterm births among African-American women aged 19 or over (but not for White women or women under 19) (Moore et al 1998). One participant in a small American study of weekly 'listening' telephone calls for disadvantaged pregnant women commented: 'The telephone is best because if it would be face-to-face it would have taken time to house clean and it would have been formal . . . A visit would have added more stress' (Bullock et al 2002). Midwives might like to consider how new technology can help – phone calls, text messages or even e-mails to women who have access to computers may all help to keep in touch.

Research shows that women receiving social support are less likely to feel unhappy, nervous and worried during pregnancy, are more likely to feel 'in control', to attend antenatal classes and to have a companion with them during labour. Postnatally, they are more likely to be breastfeeding on discharge from hospital and at six weeks are also less likely than controls to be feeling physically unwell. Their babies are less likely to have worrying health problems following hospital discharge (Elbourne et al 1989). One follow-up study found that improvements in physical and emotional health in the babies of disadvantaged mothers who had received support from midwives in the form of 'listening' home visits and 24-hour telephone availability were still present seven years later (Oakley et al 1996).

The evidence suggests that effective support for parents needs to act at a number of levels: relief of poverty and social isolation, community-based interventions, as well as individual and group-based support.

WOMEN FROM ETHNIC MINORITIES AND WOMEN WHO DO NOT SPEAK ENGLISH

There are a number of inconsistencies and confusion about the role, function and definition of interpreters, translators, link workers and advocates.

The role of the *interpreter/translator* is to facilitate communication between two people or groups of people by providing a literal translation of one language into another.
The role of the *link worker* is to interpret and offer advice about cultural and religious issues, acting as a link between staff and patients. Link workers are generally employed by NHS trusts.
The role of *bilingual advocate* is to act as an interpreter, and to empower users by ensuring that they have access to information and services.

Women want a good interpreting service but link workers recruited by the health authorities to work with health professionals may have a clear structural allegiance to the health service. The most successful link worker schemes are those in which the worker has a clear base and accountability to the community.

An evaluation of a health advocacy programme for non-English speaking women in east London found significant differences in three outcomes: reduced antenatal admissions and antenatal length of stay, reduced inductions and mode of delivery (Parsons & Day 1992) with a fall in the caesarean section rate. The authors conclude that although these changes cannot be directly attributed to health advocacy, it was reasonable to deduce that improved communication could have influenced clinical practice.

A project in Newcastle provided enhanced midwifery care specifically to Bangladeshi women, 70% of whom expressed difficulty with English, and who had a high incidence of postnatal complications. Two midwives with a bilingual health worker provided a high level of continuity on a 'domino' model with as many home visits as necessary and were available to women 24 hours a day by pager. They also held specific parentcraft classes which included the mothers-in-law, and produced written and tailored health education material in Bengali script, and videos in Bengali. The project saw statistically significant improvements (compared with controls) in attendance at parentcraft, breastfeeding rates, and incidence of poor weight gain in the babies, and also reduced defaulting on appointments (Sen & Holmes 1996).

Other interventions have aimed to improve physical access to antenatal clinics. The 'Maternity Bus Stop' in Bradford was started in response to a high number of women from one area, who were mostly Asian, defaulting booking appointments at the health centre. A coach was fitted out as a mobile clinic and parked near the school where women dropped off their older children and opposite the supermarket where they shopped, resulting in a dramatic increase in uptake of services (Wilkinson 1995).

The national service framework for maternity services (Department of Health 2004) requires the NHS to make provision for translation, interpreting and advocacy services based on an assessment of the needs of the local population. Provision includes a mixed economy of interpreting and advocacy services – for home visiting, out-of-hours services, ante-natal classes. It also requires Primary Care Trusts and maternity service providers design, review and improve maternity services through a programme of consultation with women who use the services, their link-workers and advocates, and their families, building on the work of existing local groups including Maternity Service Liaison Committees. The programme includes individual feedback and review of complaints, surveys, focus groups, audit and reviewgroups, peer/user group input and community groups.

FINDING PROBLEMS BY SCREENING

Needs assessment and case finding target interventions on specific groups in communities. However, there are some problems in pregnancy which can affect any group. These are found by screening programmes. The National Screening Committee (NSC) was set up in 1998 to oversee the implementation and management of these public health services at large population levels to monitor quality effectively. The NSC defines screening as 'a public health service in which members of a defined population, who do not necessarily perceive they are at risk of, or are already affected by a disease or its complications, are asked a question or offered a test, to identify those individuals who are more likely to be helped than harmed by further tests or treatment to reduce the risk of a disease or its complications' (National Screening Committee 1998). Public health specialists evaluate how well screening tests perform in picking up individuals who will develop disease.

Screening can be carried out by specific questions or by tests using blood samples or ultrasound. For example, the questions 'How old are you?' and 'What ethnic group do you belong to?' are both screening tests to determine a subgroup who are at higher risk of having a baby with a problem than the general population: trisomy 21 in the case of maternal age, and sickle cell anaemia, thalassaemia or Tay–Sachs disease in the case of ethnic group. We treat questions as part of case-finding and as of little importance. We certainly do not counsel people before we ask their age, and may not warn that we are measuring nuchal skin-fold when we perform a dating scan, and a woman needs to make a definite move to opt out of this type of screening. However, we should reflect on why the offer of a blood test to estimate the risk of Down's syndrome triggers long sessions explaining the condition and the screening process, and relies on the woman opting in and giving verbal informed consent. It is important that counselling or questioning is non-directive – enabling rather than prescriptive – and does not involve carers in putting their own views forward, although with the best will in the world, body language and intonation of voice can betray one's own thoughts (Hollingsworth & Daly-Jones 2003).

A screening test is not usually in itself diagnostic; it detects a subgroup of those tested who are at higher risk of having the disease or disorder than the original population screened. This subgroup needs further investigation with a diagnostic test that is usually more time-consuming, invasive and expensive than the screening test.

SCREENING PROGRAMMES

Prenatal screening is a two-edged sword that can do good and harm, often at the same time to the same person (Abramsky 2003). To maximize benefit and minimize detriment, screening should not be introduced because a screening test has just been devised, but should be part of a planned and evaluated programme that is:

- cost-effective, with the costs of screening weighed against the benefits gained from the programme and the opportunity of using the money for other projects that are foregone;
- planned, with an agreed policy on who to screen;
- preceded by a campaign of education of both professionals and those who are being offered screening;
- offering good, sympathetic, non-directive counselling;
- monitored to see that it is, and continues to be, effective;
- continuous rather than one-off;
- providing treatment services for those who are missed by screening or do not take up the offer of screening, prenatal diagnosis or therapeutic abortion for whatever reason.

Any screening programme must be preceded by good diagnostic and treatment facilities. It is no good offering a neonatal hearing screening service

if there is a 6-month wait for an audiology appointment to diagnose the child and to fit hearing aids.

Some sort of cost–benefit evaluation is needed for all screening programmes, together with surveys on what those who are most affected by the results – the parents – think of what is offered to them.

WHAT INFRASTRUCTURE IS NEEDED FOR A SCREENING PROGRAMME?

Without a functioning infrastructure in place, any genetic screening programme is likely to cause more problems than it alleviates and run into disrepute. Any screening programme needs (Modell 1990):

- a programme of information and education for health professionals and the target population;
- a system for collecting samples from a cohort of the population and delivering them to the laboratory where the tests will be conducted, or a system for imaging, such as ultrasound;
- a network of diagnostic laboratories and ultrasound departments with a quality control system;
- an information storage and retrieval system;
- a system for notifying results to those tested and their medical advisors and for storing the results in their medical records;
- an information and counselling service for the target population;
- an adequate number of expert centres for counselling couples at risk and providing prenatal diagnosis;
- a system of monitoring the service.

WHAT IS AN IDEAL DISEASE TO SCREEN FOR?

There are many sets of criteria by which to judge whether a screening programme is likely to bring benefits to those screened (Cochrane & Holland 1971, Cuckle & Wald 1984, McKeown 1968, Thorner & Remein 1961, Wilson & Jungner 1968).

In summary, screening programmes work well if the disease they are intended to pick up is:

- well defined;
- of known natural history;

- an important health problem for the individual and for the community as it is severe, common or both;
- of known incidence and prevalence;
- preventable by acceptable methods.

CASE STUDY: ROUTINE SCREENING FOR GROUP B STREPTOCOCCUS

The main cause of serious neonatal infection in the UK is Group B streptococcus (GBS). About 28% of women in the UK carry GBS in their intestines or vagina The majority have no symptoms and they and their carers are unaware that they are carriers (Hasting et al 1986). All babies born to mothers colonized with GBS are theoretically at risk of being infected and could develop sepsis, pneumonia and meningitis but transmission occurs in only 1 to 2%. Of these, between 3 to 12% develop bacteraemia, and 5 to 10% of babies developing disease in the first week of life die. The parent group Group B Strep Support calls for routine screening of all pregnant women by taking vaginal swabs. Giving intravenous prophylactic antibiotics during labour to women who are found to be carriers could prevent transmission of infection to babies.

Mortality from GBS varies with gestational age at birth. In the UK, 17% of early onset GBS disease occurs in preterm babies but 68% of the deaths are in this preterm group (Moses et al 1998). A 2001 surveillance study in the UK found a prevalence of early onset GBS infection of 0.5 per 1000 births – 376 cases with 39 deaths (Health Protection Agency 2002). This compares to 2519 neonatal deaths from all causes. Policy makers therefore need to look at the pros and cons of screening all pregnant women (about 600 000 a year in England and Wales) and finding the 180 000 or so who may be carriers who need to be treated to prevent a relatively low number of infections and deaths. The debate on universal screening ranges through the acceptability to all women of having vaginal and rectal swabs taken (women can take swabs themselves), the ability of swabs to identify only four out of five colonized women correctly, the medicalization of labour for large numbers of women by the need to give intravenous antibiotics in labour, the risk to the mother's health from unexpected anaphylactic shock from IV antibiot-

ics and a lack of evidence that giving intrapartum antibiotics prevents neonatal deaths (Smaill 1999). It is estimated that fewer than 1.4 cases of early onset GBS disease will be prevented for every 1000 women treated with intrapartum antibiotics.

Cost–benefit analyses do not support universal screening for GBS at current prevalence levels (National Institute for Clinical Excellence 2003). This is disappointing for well informed and highly motivated pressure groups of families who have discovered that their child has been killed by a potentially detectable and treatable disease. The cost per case prevented, however beneficial to the individual family concerned, is simply too high. However, the case for screening all normal healthy pregnancies could change if the prevalence of GBS disease changes. It is also essential that women who are found to be at risk during pregnancy are treated. At risk groups include pregnant women who have already had a baby who developed a GBS infection, or who develop preterm rupture of membranes, prolonged rupture of membranes (more than 18 hours before delivery) or a raised temperature over 37.8°C.

CASE STUDY: 'NORMALITY' – WHAT MESSAGES DO WE GIVE BY SCREENING?

There are now numerous ways of screening for Down's syndrome: asking for maternal age, fetal nuchal translucency measurement with ultrasonography and the use of a variety of biochemical markers from maternal blood in combination with maternal age. None of these programmes picks up all cases of trisomy 21, and all produce false positive results that cause untold worry and may lead to the loss of a pregnancy after an invasive diagnostic test. Counselling about these tests takes considerable time and effort.

Smoking overall produces more ill-health in women and babies than any genetic disorder; however, we do not routinely offer clinical screening for smoking but instead rely on self-reporting. Why do clinicians and the general public pay so much attention to the Down's screening programme but pay less attention to, and use fewer resources on, other more important health messages?

What messages are we giving to women by these programmes? Do women think that people with trisomy 21 have such a poor quality of life that clinicians are determined on a 'search and destroy policy' by inventing more and more tests? As the birth prevalence of the disorder decreases with increased testing, fewer lay people and professional staff will come into contact with families who have a member with trisomy 21. There is a high risk that continued emphasis on screening for the most common chromosomal disorder in liveborn babies will present a skewed public view of its effects and a stigmatization of families and people with the syndrome.

Amniocentesis will pick up chromosomal variations other than trisomy 21, but parents are often not forewarned that this may happen. Some (trisomy 13 and trisomy 18) are lethal, but many, such as a sex chromosome trisomy, an apparently balanced structural rearrangement or a mosaicism, are not. These are often reported as chromosomal abnormalities rather than variations. What messages does this give to parents and clinicians?

It is difficult to give a prognosis with respect to the physical or intellectual effect of many of these variations. Many perceptions are based on data that are collected in a way which is biased. Males with XXY chromosomes (Klinefelter's syndrome) are found in approximately 1 in 1000 male births. Not long ago, the traditional textbook description of a Klinefelter's syndrome was of a mentally retarded male, lacking in male secondary characteristics and with breast enlargement – an alarming prospect for future parents. This picture resulted from a bias in selection, since originally only those boys with the most severe physical manifestations had their chromosomes analysed. Long-term prospective and population studies suggest that many people with Klinefelter's syndrome look and act 'normally' and may not be found to have the syndrome until karyotyping is carried out as part of investigations for infertility (Abramsky & Chapple 1997, Robinson et al 1992).

WHAT ARE THE CHARACTERISTICS OF AN IDEAL SCREENING TEST?

The screening test must:

- be simple, safe and acceptable;
- be valid, that is, both sensitive and specific, with a high predictive value;

- be repeatable;
- be relatively inexpensive;
- have a distribution of test values in affected and unaffected individuals that is known, a sufficiently small extent of overlap and a suitable, defined, cut-off level.

As screening tests are applied to people who are regarded as being fit and well in an attempt to stop future ill-health, it is vital that the tests are acceptable and do not cause iatrogenic disease. Acceptability varies according to culture and perceived seriousness of the disorder. It is accepted in Western countries that women should not mind having a vaginal examination with a speculum in order for a cervical smear to be taken because it is perceived that the screening procedure will have a significant effect on mortality from cervical cancer.

In any screening programme, it is inevitable that certain individuals will be subjected to what is later proved to be unnecessary worry and that some will be falsely reassured, thus being even more devastated by the birth of a child with a congenital malformation. The evaluation of screening programmes is therefore essential if individuals in society are to have access to appropriate technology that, overall, does more good than harm.

MEASURING BETTER OUTCOMES OF MATERNITY SERVICES

The aim of needs assessment, case finding and screening programmes is to target resources at women who will benefit most from them. This is done with the aim of improving the outcome of pregnancy for the woman, her child and her family. How can we measure whether we are achieving this aim?

Modern technology gives us countless methods of investigating and treating health and disease. However, many of the procedures carried out by health professionals are ineffective and do not produce a better state of health for those individuals who have sought clinical help (Enkin et al 1989). In a tax-funded healthcare system such as the NHS, it is inevitable that interest focuses on funding good results, or outcomes, of healthcare rather than on emphasizing the processes (such as the number of operations or other procedures).

Health is not merely the absence of disease and infirmity but a state of complete physical, mental and social well-being (World Health Organization 1992), and should be a universal human right (Saracci 1997). Better health outcomes will therefore also include social aspects of pregnancy and childbirth, but these may be difficult to measure. For example, a good outcome is for every woman to be satisfied with the support she has received during pregnancy, delivery and the postpartum period, and to feel that she and her baby have been at the centre of care. Some tools to measure this are available (Audit Commission 1997, Lamping & Rowe 1996, Mason 1989). In small surveys, a response rate of about 70% can be expected with postal questionnaires, but there will be a bias in those who respond: women with visual problems or learning disabilities, or who do not speak English, will find it difficult to give their views. It is also difficult to look at changes in behaviour as a result of care; a good outcome would be for smokers to reduce or give up smoking during pregnancy and afterwards, but monitoring this is difficult if it relies on self-assessment (Moore et al 2002, Walsh et al 1996) and intrusive if it requires urinary testing for cotinine, a byproduct of nicotine. Some physical problems after childbirth, such as urinary or faecal incontinence, are also important but are often hidden by women. Many of these outcome measures are not included in routinely collected data systems but would need special surveys to monitor them. It is therefore unsurprising to see that the chief measure of outcome used in the past has been death, an event that has to be registered in the UK by law, as does birth, so figures are readily available.

LOOKING AT DEATH AS AN OUTCOME

Staff working in maternity services have a long history of investigating deaths through confidential enquiries, a form of external clinical audit. In such studies, each death is reviewed individually by a group of clinicians from different disciplines concerned in maternity care, and 'avoidable', 'adverse' or 'notable' factors that may have contributed to the death are ascertained. The identification of less than optimal resources and practice can be

fed back anonymously to all clinicians to make them rethink how they provide maternity care.

From 1928 onwards, the main concern of obstetricians was maternal rather than perinatal death, as the maternal mortality rate was 4.4 deaths per 1000 total births, or 3000 mothers dying each year in England and Wales. In 1952, this led to a national confidential enquiry into maternal deaths. The persisting difference in the rates of death of babies between countries and between regions in England and Wales in the 1970s led to interest in applying the methodology of confidential enquiries to perinatal deaths, although as there were then 10 perinatal deaths for each maternal death, the task was much greater (Chalmers 1979, Chalmers & McIlwaine 1980). A full national Confidential Enquiry into Stillbirths and Deaths in Infancy (CESDI) was instituted in England, Wales and Northern Ireland from 1 January 1993. Slightly contrary to its name, CESDI covered all deaths from the 20th week of pregnancy to the end of the first year of life. The maternal and CESDI enquiries were put under one roof in April 2003, when the Confidential Enquiry into Maternal and Child Health (CEMACH) was formed. By this time, there were 106 direct and 261 indirect maternal deaths over the three year period 2000–2002 (13.1 deaths per 100 000 maternities) and 4886 perinatal deaths (7.9 per 1000 births) of babies in 2002 (Confidential Enquiry into Maternal and Child Health 2004).

ARE PERINATAL MORTALITY RATES A GOOD OUTCOME MEASURE OF MATERNITY AND NEONATAL CARE?

There are several factors that make the continued use of perinatal mortality rates as a measure of the effectiveness of maternity and neonatal care increasingly unsafe.

Perinatal rates include only deaths in the first week of life. Many babies who would previously have died within this period are now, thanks to improved paediatric care, surviving beyond the first week but still die before they are a month old. There is a strong case for including late neonatal deaths in analyses of deaths occurring round the time of delivery to prevent the postponement of death artificially lowering perinatal rates.

Low and very low birth weight are such strong determinants of perinatal survival that any maternity hospital with a neonatal unit, especially one that takes tertiary referrals, will have a high crude perinatal rate simply because of the types of cases for which it cares. Evaluating its services on this basis is akin to castigating a geriatric hospital because of its high number of deaths – units looking after high-risk patients have high death rates. Some effort should be made to adjust perinatal rates for case mix and referral patterns to produce a meaningful result (Clarke et al 1993). Calculating birth weight-specific perinatal rates may help, although the number at individual hospitals will again be very small.

While all perinatal deaths are tragic and should not be dismissed lightly, there is concern that death may be preferable to severe long-term impairment and anxiety about the quality of life for some very small babies who would have become part of the perinatal mortality statistics had modern technology not been used to save them. It is important that, in the future, as much attention is paid to morbidity arising in the antenatal and perinatal period as has been paid to perinatal mortality in the past. This will require better information systems to collect data on each pregnancy as a routine part of care. It is also important that data from child health information systems can be linked to details of the pregnancy that produced that child to provide long-term follow-up. Midwives have a vital part to play in collecting reliable and clinically relevant information to link the health of the mother to the outcome for the baby.

POINTERS FOR PRACTICE

- Public health specialists have as their patients whole communities.
- Epidemiology (the study of the distribution and determinants of disease) is the chief tool of public health.
- A number of environmental factors, both external and acting in utero, may affect pregnancy, especially size at birth and the risk of exposure to environmental hazards is associated with socio-economic status.
- Midwives acting as public health practitioners play a vital role in empowering all pregnant women to live healthier lives – but need to seek out the 'hidden' women in their communities.
- Public health programmes must be targeted to individuals and their unique circumstances to be effective.
- Screening detects the predisposition towards a particular disease at its early treatable stages in people who are generally considered to be disease free when the screen is carried out; a screening test is not usually in itself diagnostic.
- In any screening programme, certain individuals will be subject to unnecessary worry and some falsely reassured. An evaluation of the screening programme is essential to ensure that it does more good than harm.
- Death rates are not in themselves a good outcome measure of maternity and neonatal care.

References

Abramsky L 2003 In: Abramsky L, Chapple J (eds) Prenatal diagnosis – the human side. 2nd edn. Nelson Thornes, Cheltenham

Abramsky L, Chapple J 1997 47,XXY (Klinefelter syndrome) and 47,XYY: estimated rates and indication for postnatal diagnosis with implications for prenatal counselling. Prenatal Diagnosis 14(4): 363–368

Acheson D 1988 Public health in England – the report of the committee of enquiry into the future development of the public health function. London HO Cm 289. HMSO, London

Anderson A S, Campbell D M, Shepherd R 1995 The influence of dietary advice on nutrient intake during pregnancy. British Journal of Nutrition 73(2): 163–177

Arblaster L, Entwhistle V, Fullerton D et al 1998 A review of the effectiveness of health promotion interventions aimed at reducing inequalities in health. NHS Centre for Reviews and Dissemination, York

Audit Commission 1997 First class delivery: improving maternity services in England and Wales. Audit Commission, London

Bakketeig L S, Hoffman H J 1979 Perinatal mortality by birth order within cohorts based on sibship size. British Medical Journal 2: 693–696

Bakketeig L S, Hoffman H J 1981 Epidemiology of preterm birth. In: Elder M G, Hendricks C H (eds) Results from a longitudinal study of births in Norway in preterm labour. Butterworths International Medical Reviews. Butterworth, London

Balarajan R, Botting B 1989 Perinatal mortality in England and Wales: variations by mother's country of birth (1982–1985). Health Trends 21: 79–84

Barker D J P 1992 Fetal and infant origins of adult disease. BMJ, London

Billewicz W Z 1973 Some implications of self selection for pregnancy. British Journal of Preventive and Social Medicine 27: 49–52

Bindman J, Johnson S, Szmucker G et al 2000 Continuity of care and clinical outcome: a prospective cohort study. Social Psychiatry and Psychiatric Epidemiology 35: 242–247

Bullock LFC, Browning C, Geden E 2002 Telephone social support for low-income pregnant women. Journal of Obstetric Gynecologic and Neonatal Nursing 31: 659–664

Calman K C, Royston G H D 1997 Risk language and dialects. British Medical Journal 315: 939–942

Casson I F, Clarke C A, Howard C V et al 1997 Outcomes of pregnancy in insulin dependent diabetic women: results of a five year population cohort study. British Medical Journal 315: 275–278

Chalmers I 1979 Desirability and feasibility of a 4th National Perinatal Survey: report submitted to the Children's and Reproductive Research Liaison Group's Research Division of the DHSS. National Perinatal Epidemiology Unit, Oxford

Chalmers I, McIlwaine G (eds) 1980 Perinatal audit and surveillance. Proceedings of the 8th study group. Royal College of Obstetricians, London

Chitty L S, Winter R M 1989 Perinatal mortality in different ethnic groups. Archives of Disease in Childhood 64: 1036–1041

Clarke M, Clayton D G, Mason E S, MacVicar J 1988 Asian mothers' risk factors for perinatal death – the same or different? A ten year review of Leicestershire perinatal deaths. British Medical Journal 297: 384–387

Clarke M, Mason E S 1985 Leatherwork: a possible hazard to reproduction. British Medical Journal 290: 1235–1237

Clarke M, Mason E S, MacVicar J, Clayton D G 1993 Evaluating perinatal mortality rates: effects of referral and case mix. British Medical Journal 306: 824–827

Cochrane A L 1972 Effectiveness and efficiency – random reflections on health services. Nuffield Provincial Hospitals Trust, London

Cochrane A L, Holland W W 1971 Validation of screening procedures. British Medical Bulletin 27: 3

Coleman T 2004 ABC of smoking cessation: Special groups of smokers. British Medical Journal 328: 575–577

Confidential Enquiry into Maternal and Child Health 2004 Online. Available: http://www.cemach.org. uk/publications.htm accessed 16th December 2005

Cuckle H S, Wald N J 1984 Principles of screening. In: Wald N J (ed.) Antenatal and neonatal screening. Oxford University Press, Oxford

Czeizel A E 1993 Prevention of congenital abnormalities by periconceptional multivitamin supplementation. British Medical Journal 306: 1645–1648

Czeizel A E, Dudas I 1992 Prevention of the first occurrence of neural tube defects by periconceptional vitamin supplementation. New England Journal of Medicine 327: 1832–1835

Department for Education and Skills 2005 Implementing Sure Start local programmes: an in-depth study. Ref NESS/FR/2005/007 Department for Education and Skills, Nottingham

Department of Health 1993 Changing childbirth. Report of the Expert Maternity Group (Cumberlege report). HMSO, London

Department of Health 2004 Maternity – national service framework for children. young people and maternity services 2004 reference 40498 Department of Health, London

Department of Health Public Health White Paper 2004 Choosing health: making healthier choices easier. Department of Health, London

Dorsett R, Marsh A 1998 The health trap: poverty, smoking and lone parenthood. Policy Studies Institute, London

Doyle W, Crawford M, Wynn A, Wynn S 1990 The association between maternal diet and birth dimensions. Journal of Nutritional Medicine 1: 9–17

Elbourne D, Oakley A, Chalmers I 1989 Social and psychological support during pregnancy. In: Chalmers I, Enkin M, Keirse M, (eds) Effective care in pregnancy and childbirth, vol. 1. Oxford University Press, Oxford

Enkin M, Keirse J N C, Chalmers I 1989 A guide to effective care in pregnancy and childbirth. Oxford University Press, Oxford

Fairbank L et al 2000 A systematic review to evaluate the effectiveness of interventions to promote the initiation of breastfeeding. Health Technology Assessment 4: 25

Graham H 1987 Women's smoking and family health. Social Science and Medicine 25; 1: 47–56

Graham H 1993 When life's a drag: women, smoking and disadvantage. HMSO, London

Hart J, Davidson A, Clarke C, Gibb C 2003 Health visitor run baby massage classes: investigating the effects. Community Practitioner 76(4): 138–142

Haslam C, Draper E 2000 Stage of change is associated with assessment of the health risks of maternal smoking among pregnant women. Social Science and Medicine 51(8): 1189–1196

Hawthorne G, Robson S, Ryall E A, Sen D, Roberts S H, Ward Platt M P 1997 Prospective population based survey of outcome of pregnancy in diabetic women: results of the Northern Diabetic Pregnancy Audit. British Medical Journal 315: 279–281

Health Development Agency 2004 Smoking and public health: a review of reviews of interventions to increase smoking cessation, reduce smoking initiation and prevent further uptake of smoking. Health Development Agency, London

Health Education Authority 1994 Smoking in pregnancy: guide for purchasers and providers. Health Education Authority, London

Health Protection Agency 2002 Incidence of Group B Streptococcal disease in infants aged less than 90 days old. CDR Weekly 12(16): 3

Hellier J 1977 Perinatal mortality 1950 and 1973. Population Trends 10: 13–15

Hoddinott P, Pill R 1999 Qualitative study of decisions about infant feeding among women in the east end of London. British Medical Journal 318: 30–34

Hodnett E D 2002a Continuity of caregivers for care during pregnancy and childbirth (Cochrane Review). In: The Cochrane Library, Issue 4, Update Software, Oxford

Hodnett E D 2002b Caregiver support for women during childbirth (Cochrane Review). In: The Cochrane Library, Issue 4, Update Software, Oxford

Hodnett E D 2002c Support during pregnancy for women at increased risk of low birthweight babies (Cochrane Review). In: The Cochrane Library, Issue 4, 2002. Update Software, Oxford

Hodnett E D, Fredericks S 2003 Support during pregnancy for women at increased risk of low birthweight babies (Cochrane Review). In: The Cochrane Library, Issue 3 Update Software, Oxford

Hollingsworth J, Daly-Jones E 2003 The sonographer's dilemma. In: Abramsky L, Chapple J (eds) Prenatal diagnosis – the human side. 2nd edn. Nelson Thornes, Cheltenham

Holmes C 2001 Partner involvement in smoking cessation. British Journal of Midwifery 9; 6: 357–361

Homer C J, Beresford S A, James S A, Siegel E, Wilcox S 1990 Work-related physical exertion and risk of preterm low birth weight delivery. Paediatric and Perinatal Epidemiology 4(2): 161–174

Kawachi I, Kennedy B P 1997 Health and social cohesion: why care about income inequality? British Medical Journal 314: 1037–1040

Lamping D L, Rowe P 1996 Survey of women's experience of maternity services (short form): user's manual for purchasers and providers. Health Services Research Unit, London School of Hygiene and Tropical Medicine, London

Lancaster T, Staed L F 2003 Self-help interventions for smoking cessation (Cochrane Review). In: The Cochrane Library, Issue 1. Update Software, Oxford

Liberman E, Gremy I, Lang J M, Cohen A P 1994 Low birthweight at term and the timing of fetal exposure to maternal smoking. American Journal of Public Health 84(7): 1127–1131

Lumley J, Oliver S, Waters E 2003 Interventions for promoting smoking cessation during pregnancy. In: The Cochrane Library, Issue 1. Update Software, Oxford

Mason V 1989 Women's experience of maternity care – a survey manual. HMSO, London

Mauthner S 1997 Postnatal depression: how can midwives help? Midwifery 13(4): 163–171

McKeown T 1968 Validation of screening procedures. In: Screening in medical care. Reviewing the evidence. Nuffield Provincial Hospital Trust/ Oxford University Press, Oxford

Mehta N M, Thomas R 2002 Antenatal screening for rubella–infection or immunity? British Medical Journal 2002(325): 90–91

Mezey G C, Bewley S 1997 Domestic violence and pregnancy. British Journal of Obstetrics and Gynaecology 104: 528–531

Modell B 1990 Cystic fibrosis screening and community genetics. Journal of Medical Genetics 27: 475–479

Mooney G 1992 Economics, medicine and healthcare. 2nd edn. Harvester Wheatsheaf, England

Moore L, Campbell R, Whelan A, Mills N, Lupton P, Misselbrook E, Frohlich J. 2002 Self help smoking cessation in pregnancy: cluster randomised controlled trial. British Medical Journal 325: 1383–1386

Moore M L, Meis P J, Ernest J M, Wells H B, Zaccaro D J 1998 A randomised trial of nurse intervention to reduce preterm and low birthweight births. Obstetrics and Gynecology 91(5pt1): 656–661

Moses LM, Heath PT, Wilkinson AR, Jeffery HE, Isaacs 1998 Early onset group B streptococcal neonatal infection in Oxford 1985-96. Archives of Disease I Childhood Fetal and Neonatal Edition 79: F148-F149

MRC Vitamin Study Research Group 1991 Prevention of neural tube defects: results of the Medical Research Council Vitamin Study. Lancet 338: 131–137

Naismith D J 1981 Diet during pregnancy – a rationale for prescription. In: Dobbing J (ed.) Maternal nutrition in pregnancy. Eating for two? Academic Press, London

National Institute for Clinical Excellence 2003 Antenatal care: routine care for the healthy pregnant woman. RCOG Press, London

National Screening Committee 1998 Online. Available: http://libraries.nelh.nhs.uk/screening/ accessed 16th December 2005

NHS Centre 1998 Smoking cessation: What the Health Service can do. NHS centre for Reviews and Dissemination, The University of York 3, Issue 1.

Nicoll A, McGarrigle C, Brady A R et al 1998 Epidemiology and detection of HIV-1 among pregnant women in the United Kingdom: results from a national surveillance 1988–96. British Medical Journal 316: 253–258

Norbeck J S, DeJoseph J F, Smith R T 1996 A randomised trial of an empirically derived social support intervention to prevent low birthweight among African-American women. Social Science and Medicine 43(6): 947–954

Oakley A, Hickey O, Rajan L, Hickey A 1996 Social support in pregnancy: does it have long term effects? Journal of Reproductive and Infant Psychology 14: 7–22

Onozawa K, Glover V, Kumer C, Potts J, Adams D, Dore C 2000 Infant massage improves mother-infant interaction for mothers with postnatal depression. Journal of Affective Disorders 63: 201–207

Parsons L, Day S 1992 Improving obstetric outcomes in ethnic minorities: an evaluation of health advocacy in Hackney. Journal of Public Health Medicine 14(2): 183–191

Robinson A, Bender B G, Linden M G 1992 Prognosis of prenatally diagnosed children with sex chromosome aneuploidy. American Journal of Medical Genetics 44: 365–368

Roman E, Doyle P, Beral V, Alberman E, Pharoah P 1978 Fetal loss, gravidity and pregnancy order. Early Human Development 2: 131–138

Rosenberg M J, Feldblum P J, Marshall E G 1987 Occupational influences on reproduction: a review of the recent literature. Journal of Occupational Medicine 29: 584–591

Royal College of Obstetricians and Gynaecologists, Multidisciplinary Working Group 1992 Prenatal screening for toxoplasmosis in the United Kingdom. Royal College of Obstetricians and Gynaecologists, London

Sackett D L, Haynes R B, Guyatt G H, Tugwell P 1991 Clinical epidemiology – a basic science for clinical medicine. 2nd edn. Little, Brown, Boston

Sanjose S, Roman E, Beral V 1991 Low birthweight and preterm delivery, Scotland, 1981–1984: effect of parents' occupation. Lancet 338: 428–431

Saracci R 1997 The World Health Organisation needs to reconsider its definition of health. British Medical Journal 314: 1409–1410

Savitz D A, Whelan E A, Kleckner R C 1989 Effect of parents' occupational exposures on risk of stillbirths, preterm delivery, and small for gestational age infants. American Journal of Epidemiology 129: 1201–1218

Sen D M, Holmes C 1996 Newcastle Bangladeshi midwifery project. MIDIRS Midwifery Digest 6(2): 225–229

Sikorski J, Renfrew M J, Pindoria S, Wade A 2002 Support for breastfeeding mothers Cochrane Database of Systematic Reviews; (1): CD001141

Silman R 1997 The social and ethical issues of risk assessment. In: Grudzinskas J G, Ward R H T (eds) Screening for Down syndrome in the first trimester. RCOG, London

Simpson R J, Armand Smith N G 1986 Maternal smoking and low birthweight: implications for antenatal care. Journal of Epidemiology and Community Helath 40: 223–227

Smaill F 1999 Intrapartum antibiotics for group B streptococcal colonisation. Cochrane Database of Systematic Reviews (3): 1–5

Steptoe A, Perkins-Porras L, McKay C, Rink E, Hilton H, Cappuccio F 2003 Behavioural counselling to increase consumption of fruit and vegetables in low income adults: randomised trial. British Medical Journal 326: 855–858

Thorner R M, Remein Q R 1961 Principles and procedures in the evaluation of screening for disease. Public Health Monograph No. 67. US Department of Health Education and Welfare. Public Health Service Publication No. 846. US Department of Health and Human Services, Public

Health Service, National Institutes of Health, Besthesda

Walsh R A, Redman S, Adamson L 1996 The accuracy of self report of smoking status in pregnant women. Addictive Behaviours 21: 675–679

Wilkinson A 1995 All Aboard in Bradford. MIDIRS Midwifery Digest 5(3): 302–303

Wilson J M C, Jungner G 1968 Principles and practice of screening for disease. Public Health Papers No. 34. WHO, Geneva

World Health Organization 1992 Basic document, 39th edn. WHO, Geneva

Wynn A, Crawford M, Doyle W, Wynn S 1991 Nutrition of women in anticipation of pregnancy. Nutrition and Health 7: 69–88

Chatper **15**

Reducing inequalities in childbirth: the midwife's role in public health

Jacqueline Dunkley-Bent

Inequalities in health and healthcare provision continue to exist across the world in both developed and developing countries. Health and life expectancy are still linked to social circumstances and childhood poverty. Poorer health and reduced quality of life experienced from before birth and through childhood may subsequently contribute to poor health during pregnancy. And compromise in maternal health can have effects for fetal development, growth and have life-long consequences (Barker et al 1993).

Evidence suggests a strong correlation between deprivation and maternal death. Women living in the most deprived areas of England have been shown to have a 45% higher death rate than those who live in more affluent areas (Department of Health 2004a). Action to reduce health inequality continues at political and social theory level and also involves communities taking an active role. Midwives have an important role in enhancing the health of the woman and her family throughout the childbirth continuum. The impact of the midwives' work has the potential to influence the inter-generational cycle of poor health and the wider social determinants of ill health that perpetuate family life cycles. Addressing these complex socio-political issues requires commitment at national and local level to achieve health improvement, education and social care policy.

My experience of work in health promotion and public health issues for women and their families has been carried out in the United Kingdom and stems from my role as a consultant midwife. My clinical work is predominantly focused within the community where I hold weekly clinics. Women are referred to my clinics by midwives, obstetricians, GPs, health visitors, the refugee council and legal centre. Reasons why women are referred includes, previous traumatic life experience, this may include previous traumatic childbirth and/or rape and sexual assault, request for caesarean section for none medical reasons, women who have had a previous caesarean section and wish to discuss mode of delivery for the current pregnancy, and fear of childbirth. I also support the lead midwife during the labour of women who are pregnant as a result of rape. Home visits are a frequent requirement, particularly for those women who miss clinic appointments. My ability to carry out this work is supported by my study of health promotion issues, experience of working in partnership with community and primary care colleagues and my experience as a rape and sexual assault counsellor.

In this chapter I will explore the realities of inequalities in health and health service provision within the context of midwifery care in the UK and focus on key practice issues. These include well-known issues such as smoking tobacco, diet, nutrition and breastfeeding, teenage pregnancy and the following less common but crucial challenges for some women who access maternity care: women seeking asylum, refugees, female genital mutilation, and the traumatic experiences of women who are pregnant as a result of rape. Throughout the chapter I have used clinical examples to illustrate the points made and help midwives think about ways they may tackle practice issues of this nature.

GOVERNMENT ACTION TO REDUCE HEALTH INEQUALITIES – THE LAST TWENTY FIVE YEARS

The major determinants of health were described in an important government report about public health written almost 25 years ago (Black et al 1982). The main factors associated with health concerned social class, economic conditions, geographical location and gender. The recommendations focus on reducing the socio economic and health disadvantage of the poorer social groups and include, the need for a programme of health education sponsored by the government, increases in the level of child benefit, increase in the maternity grant to £100, an infant care allowance should be introduced over a 5 year period beginning with all babies born in a year following a date to be chosen by the government and stronger measures should be adopted to reduce cigarette smoking. Unfortunately the recommendations were not endorsed but this report was successful in keeping health inequalities at the forefront of the public health agenda. In 1998 the government commissioned an independent enquiry into health inequalities chaired by Sir Donald Acheson to contribute to the development of strategy for health and action on inequalities in the longer term.

Thirty nine recommendations were made and included:

- increasing social benefits to reduce the level of poverty;
- development of policies which improve the nutritional health of women of childbearing age and their families;
- development of policies that increase the accessibility and affordility of foodstuff;
- development of policies that will promote the social and emotional support for expectant parents;
- education including effective programmes that will enable pregnant women to give up smoking;
- development of policies that will increase the prevalence of breastfeeding;

- strategies that would enable families who wish to combine working with parenting to do so, by removing social barriers to participation and the provison of affordable and accessible childcare (Acheson 1998).

The report largely contributed to the health strategy Saving Lives: Our Healthier Nation (Department of Health 1999). This proposed a contract for better health which meant that everyone from those in government, people working at a national level, healthcare providers, support agencies, and communities would be required to contribute to improvement. This included recognition of the responsibility of families and individuals for their own health.

Reducing Health Inequalities: An Action Report (Secretary of State for Health 2004) was published at the same time and set out what action was being taken across government to tackle the underlying causes of ill health, including socio-economic factors, building on the recommendations of the Acheson report (Acheson 1998). Subsequently the NHS Plan (Department of Health 2000) clearly identified the importance of health and health inequality. The NHS Plan detailed the commitment by government to ensure that local targets for reducing health inequalities are reinforced by the creation of national health targets concerned with reducing inequality.

Subsequently the Programme for Action (PaG) (Secretary of State for Health 2004) was developed as a result of a cross cutting review on health inequalities. This report set out plans to tackle health inequalities over the three years following its publication. It established the foundations for achieving the national target of reducing the gap in infant mortality across social groups and raising life expectancy in the most disadvantaged groups by 2010. The PaG is intended to improve the health of the poorest fastest. By 2010 one of the declared targets is to reduce inequalities in health outcome by 10% as measured by infant mortality and life expectancy.

Specific interventions likely to have an impact on disadvantaged groups include:

- Improving the quality and accessibility of antenatal care and early years support in disadvantaged areas.

- Reducing smoking and improving nutrition in pregnancy and early years.
- Preventing teenage pregnancy and supporting teenage parents.
- Improving housing conditions for children in disadvantaged areas (Secretary of State for Health 2004).

The plethora of reports, strategies, targets and commitment from government over the last two decades has ensured that inequality in health remains high on the political agenda. But unless those who are at the front line of health promotion and public health work are appropriately resourced then improvements in health and healthcare provision will not progress.

In the NHS maternity services are provided within the primary, secondary and tertiary healthcare sectors and make a direct and indirect contribution to health gain. A key theme of the National Service Framework for Children's, Young People's and Maternity Services for England and for Wales is to reduce inequalities in health and improve access to services (Department of Health 2004b, Welsh National Service Framework 2004). In some areas across the UK maternity services have implemented new developments in this area, focusing care delivery toward the areas of greatest need. Examples of service development in this context include working with pregnant teenagers, homeless women, and women who are seeking asylum (Department of Health 2003). Other areas where midwives have made positive contributions toward health improvement programmes are evident within Sure Start projects (Department for Education and Employment 2000).

SURE START

Sure Start developed from the concept that tackling inequalities which affect children and families in terms of health, education and social inclusion demanded complex inter-agency approaches. This government funded programme in England, Wales and Scotland is designed to deliver the best start in life for every child by bringing together services and support for early education, childcare, health and family support (Department for Education and Employment

2000). The first Sure Start project was set up in 1999. The plan was to have up to 500 projects serving families with children aged 0–4 in defined areas of need across England by 2004, but this target has been surpassed and current figures estimate that Sure Start is well on track to help 400 000 children over the next two years (Cooper 2004). In Scotland, Sure Start funding has been allocated to all local authorities in recognition of there being need across Scotland (Sure Start Scotland 2005). Funding for Sure Start programmes in Wales will grow to 51 million in 2005–2006. This includes funding provision for the establishment of children's centres (Sure Start Wales 2005).

An effective multidisciplinary, multi-agency approach to health and social care has the potential to support a woman and her family above and beyond the care the midwife is able to provide. Sure Start aims bring relevant agencies together to pool resources and to reduce the potential for a disjointed approach to health and social care provision.

Each local Sure Start programme is charged with addressing specified national targets to improve health and reduce inequalities. This is achieved by involvement from local communities in decisions about what services will be offered and how they will be delivered. The overall focus of the Sure Start health strategy is on prevention and early identification of needs. Midwives in England have been actively involved in Sure Start programmes that aim to support families to ensure the best possible start in life and break the intergenerational cycle of poor health. This provides midwives with the opportunity to be practitioners of public health.

The following example of midwifery involvement in Sure Start programmes in London demonstrates the scope of midwifery practice in this complex area of healthcare provision. In these programmes six midwives have been responsible for driving forward a specific focus of healthcare provision. Their roles include a focus on mental health, support for asylum seekers and refugees, physical and psychological adaptation to parenthood and a group of midwives who deliver personal caseload midwifery to women living in the area served by a Sure Start programme. This way of working provides exciting opportunities for maternity services to create vital collaborative links in a multi-agency environment to take forward the public health agenda with childbearing women and their families.

Because funding of Sure Start was never intended to be permanent there are natural concerns about mainstreaming services. However good planning will ensure that valuable, efficient services are embraced and funded by mainstream care providers so that they can be sustained. The Government's plans to mainstream Sure Start programmes is complex and includes housing those services that have been shown to be effective within Children's Centres. Children's Centres will offer education, childcare, health and family support services to 650 000 children in England and Wales by 2006 (Sure Start 2005). This is an exciting opportunity for maternity services to have vital collaborative links in this multi-agency environment, taking forward the public health agenda among childbearing women and their families. In order for public health work to be effective it is important that midwives have an understanding of what the public health role of the midwife is and how best to fulfil this role.

WHAT IS PUBLIC HEALTH AND ARE MIDWIVES PUBLIC HEALTH PRACTITIONERS?

Public health is defined as

> The use of theory, experience and evidence derived from the population sciences aimed at improving the health of the population in a way that best meets the implicit and explicit needs of the community.
>
> Heller et al 2003

The Royal College of Midwives (RCM) describes midwives as public health practitioners and details clearly the midwives role within the public health arena (Royal College of Midwives 2000). Public health is developed by policy makers, driven by government and stakeholders and delivered by public health practitioners.

The role of midwives as practitioners of public health is not always fully understood and it is important that midwives themselves recognize the substantial contribution they already make to public health by promoting the long-term well being of the woman and her family (Royal College

of Midwives 2001). The health promotion activity of the midwife which involves interventions aimed at enabling people to enhance their health, is frequently undervalued and underestimated and as such is not readily identified as public health work. For example, a study that sought to identify the public health workforce did not recognize midwives as public health practitioners (Walters et al 2002). The researchers developed a tool to identify the public health workforce, including those people whose work contributes to the wider public health function. Those identified as public health practitioners included health visitors, school nurses and dentists. Perhaps midwives were not recognized because in the UK they deliver public health at the individual level rather than adopting the population approach used by public health specialists who work largely with whole communities.

ANTENATAL CARE: A WINDOW OF OPPORTUNITY OR A CLOSED DOOR?

Working with a woman during her pregnancy provides a midwife with a unique opportunity to offer holistic, focused, individual and flexible care and support. For example, the privileged relationship between a woman and her midwife has the potential to influence healthy lifestyle choices and opportunities for a woman to be empowered to enhance her wellbeing. The woman may share information about the social, spiritual, sexual, emotional and psychological aspects of her life. She may disclose information to a midwife that she has never shared with others, including sexual abuse and domestic violence. Such sensitive, personal information is shared because the woman perceives her relationship with her midwife to be one of trust and mutual respect. However this opportunity may be lost if interactions are not confidential and unrushed. Busy schedules often dictate the duration of appointments and the nature of the consultation. A woman may only share the physical components of the midwifery consultation in a superficial discussion about fetal movements, backache, heartburn or constipation if the midwife expresses 'busy behaviour'. Emotional issues may not be raised. The midwife can alter this by creating a non-threatening, trusting and safe environment in which she expresses genuine empathy and respect for and confidentiality towards the woman and the information she shares.

Establishing open dialogue during any consultation with a woman and her family is a prerequisite to effective health promotion. It can help to reduce communication barriers that are often perceived when topics which need behaviour change are raised. Without such open dialogue the environment may be perceived as closed and non receptive and delicate issues that require a relationship of honesty and trust can be overlooked or not disclosed (Dunkley 2000).

Evidence suggests that economically deprived women are treated differently from articulate, economically secure women during antenatal consultations (Stapleton et al 2002). They are less likely to be made aware of choices available to them and were given less information than more advantaged women. Although pregnancy is often viewed as a period when women can be targeted with health messages, the medium used to convey information can have unintended consequences. For example, simply dispensing leaflets has been equated with giving information but leaflets have been used to block or pre-empt discussion rather than to encourage or enhance it. This has been described as a practice that serves to silence women (Stapleton et al 2002).

Midwives should be aware of the interventions used to reduce inequality in health and healthcare provision and their application to antenatal care. Smith (1997), suggests that the following have been found to be effective in reducing inequalities in health:

- Targeting effective healthcare promotion and services at the groups with the greatest health needs.
- Providing social, financial, and psychological support during pregnancy and childbirth.
- Providing smoking cessation programmes to pregnant women.
- Providing folic acid supplements before and around the time of conception.
- Providing personal support for breastfeeding.
- Providing free school milk.
- Targeting effective interventions to reduce accidents at children in deprived communities.

- Providing sex education and available, accessible, and acceptable services to reduce teenage pregnancy.
- Improving oral hygiene, reducing sugar intake, and promoting use of fluoride among people in deprived communities.

DISADVANTAGED WOMEN HAVE DISADVANTAGED BABIES

An intergenerational cycle of health inequality has been clearly demonstrated (Secretary of State for Health 2004). Health and life expectancy are linked to social circumstances and childhood poverty. People in lower socio-economic groups have a greater incidence of premature and low birthweight babies, heart disease and stroke. Risk factors for poor health associated with lower socio-economic status include lower rates of breastfeeding, smoking, physical inactivity, obesity, hypertension and poor diet (Philip et al 1997). Mothers living in deprived areas in England who have singleton births have a higher rate of low birth weight babies than mothers living in less deprived areas. Birthweight also is affected by ethnic group and mother's country of birth. In England in 2000, women born in West Africa and in the Caribbean had the highest rate of babies weighing less than 1500 g (Kmietowicz 2004). The following section explores several areas of health disadvantage where the midwife has the potential to influence individual and family behaviour to improve health and wellbeing (Department of Health 2003).

SMOKING AND DISADVANTAGE

More than any other identifiable factor smoking tobacco contributes to the gap in healthy life expectancy between those most in need, and those most advantaged. In the United Kingdom 24% of women smoke (Lader & Meltzer 2002); overall smoking rates have fallen over the decades but for the least advantaged the reduction in smoking cessation is minimal (Secretary of State for Health 1998). The close link between smoking and health inequalities was highlighted in the report of the independent inquiry into health inequalities (Acheson 1998).

Over a quarter of pregnant women who smoke continue to do so during pregnancy in the UK (Coleman 2004). These women tend to be young, single, of lower educational achievement, and in manual occupations (Coleman 2004). If they have a partner, their partner is also more likely to smoke. Smoking in pregnancy is associated with increased rates of fetal and perinatal death and reduced birth weight for gestational age (Table 15.1) (Donaldson & Donaldson 2000, Royal College of Physicians 2000). Barker (1997), maintained that low birth weight not only impacts on a child's life during the first few years but also that infants weighing less than 2.5 kg are at increased risk of developing coronary heart disease, non-insulin dependent diabetes and cardiovascular accident in later life. One of the explanations for these findings is that nutritional deficiencies at critical periods of fetal and infant growth may induce permanent changes in physiological function (Barker 1992). Women from poorer social backgrounds are one and a half times more likely to give birth to a low birthweight baby or suffer a perinatal death than those in other social classes.

The causal link between smoking and low birthweight is well documented but other potentially modifiable factors include diet and nutrition, weight, exercise, alcohol consumption, substance misuse and domestic violence. A meta-analysis of eight studies found that women who reported physical, sexual or emotional abuse

Table 15.1 The effects of smoking tobacco on the pregnancy and fetus

The effects of smoking	Reference	Physiological response
Reduced fetal growth and low birthweight	Royal College of Physicians 2000	Nicotine induces vasoconstriction, affects the function of the placenta, restricting blood flow and reducing the supply of nutrients and oxygen to the fetus
Placental complications	Williams et al 1999 Voight et al 1990 Cnattingius & Nordstrom 1996	Constriction of blood vessels and high levels of carbon monoxide induce hypoxia and cause placental abruption or cause over enlargement of the placenta and cause placenta previa. Stillbirth is linked with growth restriction and placental complications
Premature birth and premature rupture of membranes	Hadley et al 1990 Wisborg 1996	Vasoconstriction may lead to mechanical stress and disrupt the integrity of the membranes triggering labour. Smoking may cause higher levels of catecholamines that could precipitate labour
Passive smoking may cause a reduction in birth weight and premature birth and cot deaths could be caused by mothers smoking	US Department of Health and Human services 2001, Windham 2000, British Medical Association 2002	A 2.5 fold increase in the toxins in unfiltered sidestream smoke causes the effects detailed above

Children whose parents smoke are much more likely to develop lung illness than children of non-smoking parents |
| Breastfeeding mothers have lower levels of prolactin than non smoking counterparts | Fuxe 1989 | Nicotine has been found to inhibit prolactin levels. Prolaction is released from the anterior pituitary gland and stimulates the alveolar cells in the breast tissue to produce milk (Blackburn 2003) |

during pregnancy were more likely to have a low birth weight baby than women who were not abused (Murphy 2001). Passive smoking is associated with cot death and respiratory disease in childhood and lung cancer, heart disease, and stroke in adults (Edwards 2004).

Making a difference – supporting women to quit

Pregnancy is an ideal time for women and their partners who smoke to consider quitting. Most women are motivated to do everything they can to make sure their baby is healthy and are receptive to information and keen to make changes to their lifestyle (Dunkley 2000).

The government target in England is to reduce the percentage of women who smoke during pregnancy from 23% to 15% by the year 2010; with a fall to 18% by the year 2005. This will mean approximately 55 000 fewer women in England who smoke during pregnancy (Secretary of State for Health 1998). The proposed strategy for achieving this target is detailed in Smoking Kills a white paper on tobacco (Secretary of State for Health 1998), and pregnant women who smoke will be a key focus of action at local level as new NHS smoking cessation services are developed. Since April 1999, a reported £60 million in newly allocated money has been directed to help pregnant women who are disadvantaged stop smoking. Although specialist smoking cessation support is available midwives need to be confident and competent to bring up the subject of smoking and be able to provide support to women who smoke prior to referring on to such services. Evidence suggests that prenatal counselling involving ten minutes of person-to-person contact with written materials specifically designed for pregnant women can double quit rates (University of York 1998). Postnatally midwives can continue their advice and support to new mothers by providing education about the passage of nicotine through breast milk and advice on reducing the risks of cot death (see Table 15.1).

Many smokers are unaware of the immediate and long term health benefits of quitting at any age. The excess risk of death from smoking falls soon after cessation and continues to do so for at least 10–15 years thereafter. Former smokers live longer than continuing smokers, no matter what age they stop smoking, although the impact of quitting on mortality is greatest at younger ages. For smokers who stop before age 35, survival is about the same as that for non-smokers (Edwards 2004).

There are several different approaches to helping pregnant women stop smoking. For example, in some areas smoking cessation counsellors provide specialist services, but where this support is sparse or unavailable midwives take the lead and play an active role. Midwives may need further training to have the competence and confidence to take opportunities to offer the best evidenced based advice to women who smoke during pregnancy. The Royal College of Midwives (RCM) guide 'helping women stop smoking'(Royal College of Midwives 2002) provides a supportive practical guide for midwives to help women and their families reduce the harmful effects of cigarette smoke.

The following example describes a multi-agency approach to helping pregnant women who want to quit smoking (Box 15.1).

PRACTICE POINTERS

Think about the following questions:

> What strategies do you use to encourage pregnant women who smoke to quit?
> How useful are these strategies in helping women to maintain their cessation behaviour?

The web based document Delivering the Best, Midwives Contribution to the NHS Plan (Department of Health 2003) offers further examples of midwifery services that help pregnant women to quit smoking.

POOR DIET AND DISADVANTAGED SOCIAL GROUPS

Poor diet affects the health of socially disadvantaged people from the cradle to the grave. The social and economic reasons are complex, but the potential for health gain through improved diet is enormous (Philip et al 1997). A poor diet in pregnancy together with other contributing risk factors

Box 15.1   Helping pregnant women to stop smoking

The smoking cessation service of a large teaching hospital in south east London has worked collaboratively with the smoking cessation counsellors from the local Primary Care Trusts to deliver a programme of education to all midwives on smoking cessation during pregnancy. The programme includes education on how to bring up the question of smoking without creating barriers to further communication. Family members who smoke are considered to be an integral part of the process together with the provision of basic information and advice about stopping smoking. Midwives attended the training in their own time, they were paid additional money for the hours they attended. Eighty percent of the midwives were trained in smoking cessation techniques. Those women who wished to be referred for specialist support had the opportunity to do so. Referrals to the smoking cessation counsellors increased and success rates are currently being calculated. Smoking cessation counsellors support women and their partners and made contact in the home. Improvements to this service are constantly being made; one example is the new 'opt out service'. At the antenatal booking appointment women who smoke are now asked.

Do you object to being contacted by the stop smoking support services?

This new approach to offering stop smoking support is expected to increase the numbers of women who are referred to the smoking cessation counsellors during pregnancy and as a consequence influence quit rates.

et al 1995) and limits placental function and fetal growth.

It has been suggested that low birth weight perpetuates the intergenerational cycle of poor health by programming children toward the potential of adult diseases including hypertension, diabetes, obesity, and coronary heart disease (Barker 1992). People in lower socio-economic groups may have a diet high in cheap energy foods including, meat products, full cream milk, fats, sugars, preserves and potatoes with very little intake of vegetables, fruit, and wholewheat bread (Philip et al 1997). Such a diet is lower in essential nutrients such as calcium, iron, magnesium, folate, and vitamin C than that of the higher socio-economic groups. In terms of the protective role of antioxidants and other dietary factors there is scope for considerable health gain if a diet rich in vegetables, fruit, unrefined cereal, fish, and small quantities of quality vegetable oils could be more accessible to poor people (Philip et al 1997). However healthy lifestyle choices are not always accessible and/or affordable to people on low incomes or who live in areas where, for example, shops do not offer fresh fruit and vegetables. Strategies to enhance folate in affordable food products were encouraged by the Health Education Authority in 1996. During the three year folic acid health promotion initiative, certain breads and cereal were fortified with folic acid (Health Education Authority 1996). However it is important that health professionals discourage the over reliance on foodstuff to supply their recommended daily requirement of folic acid as dietary supplementation is still required to protect against neural tube defects. It is now generally accepted that increased folate intake before and during pregnancy reduces the occurrence and recurrence of neural tube defects, namely spina bifida, anencephaly and encephalocoele (Medical Research Council 1991). It is recommended that women take 400 µg of folic acid daily prior to conception and during the first trimester of pregnancy (Department of Health 1999). Simply delivering a healthy eating message and providing supporting information in the form of a leaflet does not complete the health education process. Health promotion that focuses on information about healthy eating alone is futile if economic disadvantage is ignored. Other strategies should be used for the healthy eating message to be effec-

including smoking tobacco is associated with low birthweight (Barker 1992). A diet low in folate around the time of conception not only predisposes to neural tube defects but also to lower birth weight and a shorter pregnancy (Scholl et al 1996). There is evidence to suggest that a lack of n-3 fatty acids from fish, affects brain development, shortens pregnancy, reduces fetal weight gain (Olsen

tive and bring about an adjustment to existing behaviour. This may include discussion about the current diet, factors that influence its maintenance and strategies that would encourage and sustain behaviour change such as raising awareness about how to buy healthy food on a low income budget. This could further be supported by referring women to the local Sure Start programmes where nutritionists frequently run sessions on eating and cooking healthy foods that involve cooking groups.

Encouraging and supporting increased intake of fresh fruit and vegetables should be introduced with the aim of achieving lifetime behaviour modification. There are a range of ways in which midwives could support such changes for women and their families, including working with nutritionists and women to explore ways of buying healthy foods on a low income. Supporting women to understand how to cook in ways that maintain the nutritional value of food may also be key to increasing life-long skills. Setting up services within an established Sure Start programme would focus care within the community setting to a target audience that is already defined and can maximize the impact of this approach, (see Box 15.2).

There are a range of welfare entitlements for eligible women and families. As key health workers midwives need to be knowledgeable and up-to-date about the range of welfare entitlements and other benefits available for pregnant women and their families. Such support is offered from government sources and from other agencies, such as charities. In the United Kingdom from December 2004 women and families who qualify for welfare food schemes have been offered an increase in vouchers that can be exchanged for a range of fresh foods including, fresh fruit and vegetables. These options are in addition to infant formulae entitlement (Department of Health 2004a). At the time of writing this chapter it is proposed that the vouchers will be introduced in August 2005 in Devon and Cornwall, England. At this time the Welfare Food Scheme will continue outside of Devon and Cornwall with only a few minor changes. After a six month evaluation period the new vouchers will be rolled out across the United Kingdom. It is proposed that vouchers will be exchanged at registered retailers.

Box 15.2   Supporting women and families to better diet and nutrition

Midwives should ensure that they are familiar with their local Sure Start/Children's Centre programme for nutrition and refer women where appropriate.

Sure Start programmes feature a range of interventions designed to improve the diet and nutrition of disadvantaged families. Activities include:

- Setting up initiatives such as 'Get cooking groups' looking at healthy eating on a budget.
- Nutrition and cookery taught as a part of Sure Start's parenting skills programmes.
- Securing the advice of community nutritionists or dieticians to develop good practice.
- Setting up community garden/allotment schemes where people can grow their own vegetables.
- Employing black and minority ethnic (BME) community food workers to address the diverse needs of the BME community.
- Setting up initiatives to highlight the importance of physical activity amongst the early years and how this, as well as a good diet, can have a positive influence on obesity.

http://www.surestart.gov.uk/surestartservices/health/dietandnutrition

---

BREASTFEEDING AMONG WOMEN FROM POORER SOCIO-ECONOMIC GROUPS

The benefits of breastfeeding are not in doubt. It is the safest, most economical and most convenient way to promote infant health and nutrition, encouraging a close relationship between a mother and her baby. The advantages of breast milk to the neonate are well-documented (Hanson 1998, Lawrence 1997, National Health Service Centre for Reviews and Dissemination 2000, Riordian 1997). Benefits include, protection of babies from middle ear, upper respiratory and gastrointestinal infection (Howie 1990). There is also a significant reduction in the risk of childhood asthma at age

6 years if exclusive breastfeeding is continued for at least four months after birth (Oddy et al 1999).

In addition breastfeeding has many benefits for the woman including a reduced risk of pre-menopausal and postmenopausal breast cancer (Collaborative Group on Hormonal Factors in Breast Cancer 2002), pre-menopausal ovarian cancer (Siskind et al 1997) and positive effects on bone density (Melton et al 1993). Despite such benefits and efforts to encourage breastfeeding, the breastfeeding rate, in the United Kingdom, has remained static for the past 20 years, with a strong disparity between socio-economic groups. Eighty four per cent of new mothers with partners in non-manual occupations initiated breastfeeding in 2000, compared with only 64% of those with partners in manual occupations (National Statistics 2004). Overall, 69% of infants born in 2000 were initially breastfed (Hamlyn et al 2000). By four months only 28% were still given any breast milk (Hamlyn 2002). Each year, 75 000 mothers stop breastfeeding in the first postnatal week. Only 1% suggest that breastfeeding for one week was their primary intention. The reasons most women have given for stopping, relate to problems that could be avoided or solved if they were better supported for example, the kind of help with feeding suggested in the Baby Friendly Initiative (UNICEF 2000).

IMPROVING BREASTFEEDING RATES

Several strategies have been used to promote breastfeeding in the UK, including public education through media campaigns, and peer led initiatives to support individual mothers (Kramer et al 2001, Sikorski et al 2002, Tedstone et al 1998). Voluntary organizations including the National Childbirth Trust, Breastfeeding Network, and La Leche League have long played a part in supporting women to breastfeed. In 2000 such organizations offered breastfeeding advice and support to 8% of mothers in the United Kingdom (Hamlyn 2002).

The joint World Health Organization and Unicef Baby Friendly Hospital initiative set standards for maternity services (UNICEF 1999, WHO/UNICEF 1989). The underlying principle behind the Baby Friendly initiative is that best practice standards should be adopted enabling health professionals to support mothers in their chosen feeding method. Healthcare providers that implement best practice, the 10 steps to successful breastfeeding for the maternity services (WHO/UNICEF 1989), or the seven point plan for the protection, promotion, and support of breastfeeding in community healthcare settings (UNICEF 1999) can be assessed and accredited as Baby Friendly. The standards encapsulate good practice, policy, training and information. The changes to practice include, skin to skin contact, rooming in, exclusive breastfeeding and good cooperation between the different parts of the health service and the voluntary sector. A survey of 21 baby friendly hospitals has found an increase of more than 10% in breastfeeding initiation. Two years before the maternity units received their baby friendly award, the breastfeeding rate was 60% and this rose to 70.6% a year after their accreditation. Some of the largest increases were found in hospitals serving inner city or deprived areas, which traditionally have low rates (Kmietowicz 2000).

MEANINGFUL HEALTH PROMOTION

Strategies for enhancing the uptake of breastfeeding are well documented (Dykes 2003). Several different approaches have been used including workshops, one-to-one support and peer support programmes. A study to investigate whether offering volunteer support from counsellors in breastfeeding, would result in more women breastfeeding, revealed interesting findings. Seven hundred and twenty women considering breastfeeding were recruited from 32 general practices in London and south east Essex. The results showed women valued the support of a counsellor in breastfeeding, but the intervention did not significantly increase breastfeeding rates. Offering additional support does not increase the duration of breastfeeding, perhaps because those who stopped were less likely to seek help (Graffy 2004). Small, informal group discussions on the merits of the practicalities of breastfeeding have been found to significantly impact on breastfeeding uptake. Health education approaches that encourage women to participate in small discussion groups and one-to-one advice sessions have achieved the best results, in some cases tripling the rate of breastfeeding (Kmietowicz 2000).

Dykes (2003) evaluated 79 breastfeeding practice projects to synthesize the key challenges and findings. Breastfeeding practice projects detailed in the report include:

- Breastfeeding peer support programme.
- Breastfeeding support centres.
- Antenatal workshops/education programmes.
- Healthcare assistant role.
- Projects primarily involving qualified breastfeeding counsellors/supporters.
- Education and training for health professionals.
- School education.

The key recommendations of the report state that, acute Trusts, Primary Care Trusts and Sure Start programmes should continue to collaborate with and fund projects such as: schemes that specifically reach and support women from minority ethnic communities, breastfeeding peer support programmes that are carefully co-ordinated through interagency partnerships, antenatal interactive workshops developed with sensitivity to the local socio-cultural needs, prison outreach programmes and development of the healthcare assistant role in supporting breastfeeding women across the hospital community interface (Dykes 2003).

Further information about support to enhance the uptake and success of breastfeeding can be obtained from the Good Practice and Innovations in Breastfeeding Guide (Department of Health 2004b), which provides practical evidence-based resources for health professionals, with a particular focus on reaching disadvantaged women.

The following sections present difficult, important issues that midwives may be exposed to when women and young girls book for maternity care. It is important that midwives are conversant with the subjects presented but there must be acknowledgement that specialist roles, and support services are sometimes best placed to support women in the situations described below. Appropriate referral, collaboration and multidisciplinary working is key in situations like this as detailed below.

VIOLENCE AGAINST WOMEN

Any act of gender-based violence that results in, or is likely to result in physical, sexual or psychological harm or suffering to women, is referred to as violence against women. Violence against women includes marital rape, rape, sexual abuse of children in the household, battering by partners, female genital mutilation, psychological abuse and forced prostitution (Amnesty International 2004). The consequences of violence go beyond the physical damage to the survivor. The threat of further violence and psychological damage not only reduces the woman's self esteem but can also lead to long term effects including, mental ill health, alcohol and substance misuse and suicide. It is estimated that at least one in three women have experienced violence in the course of their lifetime (Mirlees-Black1999). It is inevitable therefore that the midwife will at some point provide maternity care for women within this category. The following sections may present situations that are difficult to comprehend and may be shocking to some readers.

ASYLUM SEEKERS AND REFUGEES

Britain is a signatory to the 1951 Geneva Convention and therefore committed to offer asylum to people fleeing persecution. In the United Kingdom an asylum seeker is a person who has submitted an application for protection under the Geneva Convention (1951) and is waiting for their claim for asylum to be decided by the Home Office. A refugee is a person who has fled their country of origin or is unable to return because s/he fears persecution due to race, religion, nationality, political opinion or membership of a social group. The term 'refugee' is used to describe displaced people all over the world (Burnett & Peel 2001). In the legal context in the UK, a person is a refugee when their asylum claim has been accepted by the UK Home Office. Refugee status means that an individual's claim has been accepted under the Geneva Convention and granted indefinite leave to remain, which means permanent residence in the UK. Exceptional leave to remain is a discretionary status that falls outside of the Immigration Rules.

It may be granted on human rights grounds. For example, if a person is likely to experience inhumane treatment or would not receive a fair trial in their home country. From 1st April 2003 this type of status was changed and asylum seekers were granted either Humanitarian Protection or Discretionary Leave. Humanitarian Protection is granted where the Home Office recognizes that there is a real risk of death, torture, or other inhumane treatment, which falls outside the strict terms of the 1951 Refugee Convention (Refugee Council 2005. Applying for Asylum. Online. Available: http://www.refugeecouncil. org.uk 29th December 2005).

Refugees and asylum seekers and those with exceptional leave to remain are exempt from charges for medical treatment under the NHS. They are able to register with a GP, receive medical prescriptions and register with an NHS dentist and optician. They have free access to all other NHS services. Section 55 of the Asylum Act 2002 allows denial of benefits to asylum seekers who fail to register their application within 3 days of arrival in the UK. In the London area it has been estimated that the effect of denying benefits will mean that around 10 000 asylum seekers each year are likely to be made destitute (Singer 2004). A proportion of these will be pregnant women who may feel unable to speak out on arrival in the UK and complete the application for asylum because they are fearful of the process. As systems are subject to change it may be useful to contact the refugee council to receive up-to-date information at www.refugeecouncil.org.uk. The Department of Health provides a comprehensive list of exemptions from charges for hospital treatment, that may also be useful. This information can be accessed via the Department of Health website: www.Department of Health.gov.uk.

Many women seeking asylum are of reproductive age, pregnant and/or have dependent children. Those who are pregnant find it difficult to access maternity services because their knowledge of the NHS process is limited. Their attempts to register with a GP as the only means of accessing maternity services can be problematic (Mcleish 2002). Many find self referral to midwifery services difficult. As a consequence such women tend to book late for maternity care. A study that observed the antenatal booking patterns of 61

seeking asylum showed that 40 (61%) had antenatal care for the first time at ≥22 weeks gestation and 23 (38%) at ≥30 weeks gestation (Kennedy & Murphy-Lawless 2001).

The National Asylum Support Service (NASS) dispersal system for asylum seekers means that women in this situation may be sent anywhere in the UK and receive care in the local maternity unit. The total number of women dispersed from London ports of entry into England, Scotland and Wales by NASS between April 2001 and July 2001 was 2510 out of a total 28 000 asylum seekers dispersed at that time.

Maternal death is rare in the UK, however, women who are from socially excluded groups and/or are economically poor are disproportionately affected. Of the three hundred and ninety one maternal deaths reported to the Confidential Enquiries into Maternal Deaths and Deaths in Infancy between 2000–2002 (Department of Health 2004a) fourteen were women who were asylum seekers and recent immigrants. Four of these women had not accessed any antenatal care and five had booked after 28 weeks gestation. There is a clear need for systems to be put in place to ensure that women seeking asylum are empowered to reveal their pregnancy status without fear of reprisal so that they are supported in accessing maternity services early. The Government response to the Inequality in Health report (Secretary of State for Health 2004), recommended that accommodation centres, which house asylum seekers whilst their application for asylum status is processed, should ensure that there is a gateway to maternity services so that asylum seeking women can have equal access to maternity care provision and therefore receive early antenatal care (Secretary of State for Health 2004).

ASYLUM SEEKERS PREGNANT AS A RESULT OF RAPE

The Black Women's Rape Action Project is a project in London that provides advice, counselling, help and support services to black women, and other women of colour including immigrant and refugee women and girls who have been raped, sexually assaulted or experienced domestic violence. Other help includes, applying for asylum and immigration status and claiming compensation and other resources. This project estimates that at least half of all women asylum seekers are pregnant as a result of rape (Cowen 2001). This is likely to be a substantial underestimation as it is based on those who disclose their experience and many rape crimes are unreported (Rape, Abuse and Incest National Network 2004). In South East London a specialist clinic provides support for vulnerable women including asylum seekers who are pregnant as a result of rape (Dunkley-Bent 2004). In 2003 forty-two women who were seeking asylum were referred to the clinic. Their countries of origin included Congo, Nigeria, Angola, Ghana, Sierra Leone, Burundi, Uganda, Somalia, Eritrea and South Africa. Approximately 50% of women were first referred to the clinic because of trauma they experienced in their countries of origin. Each initial consultation was scheduled to take place for one hour but disclosure of rape and limited discussion often did not take place during the first consultation because women were fearful that the information disclosed would impact negatively on their asylum claim. Consultations that took place with the support of an interpreter took longer than the hour allotted. Counselling through an interpreter presented many challenges, for example, the natural pause moments and silences that form part of a counselling interaction, were frequently interrupted by the interpreter who would promptly repeat the questions asked. Such unnecessary interruptions did not help the disclosure process. Women who spoke English were given time to think, many cried and there were long periods of silence after which they spoke freely when they felt able and ready.

All women seen in the clinic had started to experience flashbacks and vivid dreams about the rape and torture since becoming pregnant and welcomed the opportunity to discuss their experiences. They wanted practical information on how to make the nightmares stop and the memories fade. They were fearful of what would happen to them in labour and how they would cope with a newborn baby in a strange country with no family, friends or resources.

The nature of support offered to women was flexible and reflective of individual need and included: rape trauma counselling, discussion on invasive hospital procedures, flashback, triggers,

coping mechanisms, discussion tours of the birth centres, preparation for labour, support during labour, postnatal debriefing and follow up support in the postpartum period (Dunkley-Bent 2004). Timely links were made with the health visitor, GP, refugee community group, Sure Start programmes and social services when appropriate. The Medical Foundation for the Care of Victims of Torture was also used when deemed appropriate. This organization founded in 1985, provides care and rehabilitation to survivors of torture and other forms of organized violence. (More information about the foundation can be found by accessing the website at www.torturecare.org.uk).

Amongst women who came to the clinic only 11% agreed to be referred to outside agencies for further counselling support, this included trauma counselling for post-traumatic-stress-disorder (Dunkley-Bent 2004).

Agapia's story (Box 15.3) describes one young woman's personal account of rape which she gave at her fourth consultation with the consultant midwife who runs the clinic. The consultant midwife is a rape and sexual assault counsellor with several years experience of sexual abuse counselling. It is vitally important that midwives do not enter a counselling relationship with women in this situation if they have not been trained to do so as there is the potential to do more harm. Her story may be disturbing, but presents a shocking reality of the extent of violence toward women and girls.

FEMALE GENITAL MUTILATION (FGM)

The World Health Organization defines FGM as all procedures involving partial or total removal of the external female genitalia or other injury to the female genital organs for cultural or non-therapeutic reasons (Momoh 2004). Carrying out FGM has been illegal in the UK since the prohibition of the Female Circumcision Act 1985. It was possible for people to undermine the act by having the procedure performed outside the country until the 2003 FGM Act prohibited removal of children from the UK to have the procedure performed.

Worldwide FGM affects 120 million women and an estimated 2 million girls are circumcised each year (Momoh 2003). An example of an initia-

---

Box 15.3   Rape and pre-practice issues of this nature

Agapia is a 14-year-old girl from the Congo who arrived in the UK with her aunt. Two months after arrival she booked for maternity care, she was 26 weeks pregnant. The pregnancy was a result of a gang rape in her country of origin. Her account is as follows:

I thought I was safe and they couldn't get me, I didn't want this you must believe me, I couldn't move I couldn't fight I didn't want this. My people said I should fight but I couldn't. They killed my father, he is not a spy but they killed him after they made him touch me where he shouldn't, that was not good. My mother was killed when they came to our village, we all ran when we heard the guns but they killed her. I thought I was safe when we got to the camp. I made a friend — she was 13 years old, we played, we knew that one day we would leave the country. We waited in the camp. One night the rebels came in and beat my aunt and killed some people. They took me and my friend. I was frightened, she started to fight them and bit them as they tried to do bad things to her. They shot her in

her head in front of me. I could not move I was frightened. I heard screaming all around me. They told me that the same fate would befall me if I did not do what they wanted. They tied me to a chair and for a whole week they raped me one by one. I was in pain, so much pain. I fainted most of the time. They untied me and I could not move for many days. Now I have this (pointed to the pregnant uterus). I don't want it, I want to be a child and get a good education. I have been here for many weeks and I cannot find a school. Why won't they take me? I don't want this. At night my friend comes to visit me. She tells me that it is better to come to her where we can play, she has told me how to leave this world. I must go because every night I try and sleep the rebels come in and do that to me again, I feel the pain every night. They will come and find me soon when I am not sleeping. I believe it. I like it when my friend comes to see me. I know how to take my life she told me.

N.B. pause, moments of silence and crying have not been reflected in the transcription.

---

tive which was designed to support eradication of this practice and promote the health of those women who have undergone FGM is the African Well Woman's Clinic, opened within a busy teaching hospital in south east London in 1997. The clinic is supported by a specialist FGM midwife. Women who have experienced FGM are referred to the clinic by midwives, doctors, health visitors and voluntary organizations. Women also self refer and the primary source of their information about the service is usually from other women who have attended the clinic. An official referral is not necessary and nobody is turned away.

Services provided at the African Well Woman's Clinic include, health education, counselling, surgical de-infibulation, and a plan of care for labour. The surgical de-infibulation service is available to both pregnant and non-pregnant women and it can be carried out under local anaesthetic on the same day that a woman seeks it. A total of 116 women attended the clinic in 1997, its first year of operation (Momoh et al 2001). Complete case records were available for 108 of those women. For

84 (78%) of the women an unqualified medical person had performed the FGM procedure. This had usually taken place in the child's home at an average age of seven years. Eighty nine women (82%) who attended the clinic were pregnant and had surgical de-infibulation. None requested re-infibulation after delivery, but 6 were considering taking their daughters to have the procedure performed outside of the UK. Eighteen non pregnant women attended the clinic for advice and/or de-infibulation (Momoh et al 2001). Forty women attended the clinic and had de-infibulation in 2001, this number increased to sixty in 2004 (Momoh personal communication 2005).

The health education component of the clinic service is as important as the procedure used to achieve reversal of FGM. Women are strongly discouraged from planning FGM of their daughters abroad, which is an illegal act that now carries a prison sentence (Department of Education and Skills 2003). The midwife who runs the clinic has campaigned tirelessly, working at a local, national and international level with community groups and religious leaders to help eradicate the practice of FGM. The increasing number of women who now attend the clinic, particularly those who are not pregnant, demonstrates a willingness from local communities to learn more about the health education benefits of de-infibulation and suggests a possible rejection of the practice (Momoh 2004).

DOMESTIC VIOLENCE

Domestic violence is defined as the physical, sexual or emotional abuse of an adult by an adult perpetrator in the context of an intimate relationship (Dunkley 2000). The perpetrator is usually male but domestic violence may occur in same sex relationships or by a woman to a man. In the UK one in three women experience domestic violence at some point in their lives (Mirlees-Black 1999).

The Council of Europe has stated that domestic violence is the major cause of death and disability for women aged sixteen to forty four and accounts for more death and ill health than cancer or road traffic accidents (Amnesty International 2004).

Factors that appear to place women at increased risk of domestic violence include being single, separated or divorced, the presence of children in the household, being a younger age (Mirlees-Black 1999) and pregnancy (Department of Health 2000, Mezey 1997). It is estimated that 30% of domestic violence starts in pregnancy (Department of Health 2000). The reasons for this are complex and varied and include, jealousy, over possessiveness of the perpetrator and denial of the woman having any other role but spouse. Pregnant teenagers are reported to have higher rates of domestic violence than adult women but the violence has been found to be less severe (Quinlivan & Evans 2001). It is suggested that teenagers may be more vulnerable than adults to violent and coercive relationships because they lack the experiences of dealing with interpersonal relationships (Parker 1993). Abuse experienced during pregnancy can predict abuse in the postnatal period. Stewart (1994) found that 95% of women battered during pregnancy were also battered during the first three months postpartum.

Women who experience domestic violence during pregnancy are at increased risk of physical and psychological harm. Domestic violence may result in premature labour (Shumway et al 1999) fetal distress and fetal death (Dye et al 1995). Maternal depression is not uncommon. In domestic violence situations there is a natural concern for the safety of the newborn baby. The midwife has a responsibility to protect the wellbeing of the child and as such collaboration with social services must be a priority during pregnancy if the child is to be taken back to the abusive home where there is potential for harm (Department of Health 2001). Antenatal liaison with the health visitor and other members of the women's primary care team should form part of routine practice, so that a relationship can be developed with the mother and further support offered (Department of Health 2004b).

Of the 391 maternal deaths detailed in the 2000–2002 Confidential Enquiries into Maternal And Child Health report (CEMACH) (Department of Health 2004a), 51 women (13%) had a known history of domestic violence. This proportion is thought to be an underestimation of the true prevalence of domestic violence as routine questions were not asked at the booking or subsequent antenatal visits of any of the cases reported. Evidence suggests that routine questioning for domestic violence significantly increases the rate of identification of abused women antenatally (Covington et al 1997, Wiist & McFarlane 1999), and forms part of the key recommendations proposed by the CEMACH report.

Midwives are in a unique position to support women who are experiencing domestic violence. Pregnancy provides a window of opportunity for the woman to have a relationship with someone other than the perpetrator. The woman may choose to disclose the violence and ask the midwife for help. Conversely she may seek assistance for vague complaints or symptoms including abdominal pain, or reduced fetal movements or she may be accompanied by an over-dominant partner who is reluctant to let her speak for herself. Guidance documents including the Royal College of Midwives position paper on domestic abuse (Royal College of Midwives 1999) and the Department of Health Domestic Violence Resource Manual (Department of Health 2000), are extremely useful in guiding midwives in their care of women experiencing domestic violence. The CEMACH report (Department of Health 2004a) details recommendations for maternity care providers that include, developing guidelines and local multidisciplinary support networks, and developing strategies where the woman is seen alone at least once during the antenatal period. A marker for good practice identified by the National Service Framework for Children, Young People and Maternity Services (Department of Health 2004b) includes the need for services to be developed for women who request support for coping with domestic violence.

Support services for women experiencing domestic violence include Women's Aid. This is the national domestic violence charity which co-ordinates and supports a UK wide network of over 300 local projects, providing over 500 refuges, help lines, outreach services and advice centres (Women's Aid 2005). Women's Aid aims to advocate for abused women and children and ensure their safety by working locally and nationally. Midwives should be familiar with this organization that can provide practical accommodation support within twenty four hours of making initial contact with the woman.

ACUTE STRESS REACTION AND POST-TRAUMATIC-STRESS DISORDER

Women who have experienced violence including any of the circumstances described above may show signs of post-traumatic-stress disorder (PTSD). The symptoms of PTSD, can be categorized into three: re-experiencing of the traumatic event including intrusions, dreams and re-experiencing emotions associated with the trauma; avoidance of stimuli associated with the trauma and numbing of emotional responsiveness, e.g. avoiding thoughts and feelings about the trauma, avoiding activities associated with trauma and emotional changes such as detachment from others; symptoms of hyper-arousal such as difficulty sleeping, concentrating, irritability and excessive startle responses (American Psychiatric Association 1994). PTSD usually develops within 3–6 months of the traumatic event and lasts for more than 1 month. Factors that pre-dispose to PTSD include, pre-existing personality or emotional disorder, family history, the individuals adaptive coping style, the severity of the actual

event and the nature of the outside support (Church & Scanlan 2002).

Acute stress reaction (ASR) is transient in nature and develops following a traumatic event. It is less severe than PTSD but is seen as a precursor. ASR is characterized by the appearance of being dazed, reduced consciousness levels, feeling agitated and overactive, appearing withdrawn, temporary amnesia is common, the appearance of disorientation and distress. Symptoms begin within minutes and should dissipate within hours (Church & Scanlan 2002). Midwives should be vigilant in observing and listening to women who express symptoms that may relate to previous trauma. If this is disclosed then the woman should be offered the opportunity to have trauma counselling from a trained specialist.

TEENAGE PREGNANCY AND HEALTH DISADVANTAGE

The teenage pregnancy rate in the UK is 29.2 births per 1000 women aged between fifteen and nineteen years of age (National Statistics 2004). In 2001 the teenage pregnancy rate was 3% lower than in 2000 and 9% lower than in 1998 (Department of Health 2002). Unfortunately the rate remains the highest in Europe. In the year 2000 Korea, Japan, Switzerland, the Netherlands, and Sweden had a teenage pregnancy rate of less than seven births per 1000 teenagers (Kmietowicz 2000). It is suggested that the move away from traditional family values in some countries and how these countries prepare their young people to cope with modern life, influence the teenage pregnancy rates (Kmietowicz 2000).

Three-quarters of teenage pregnancies are unplanned (Social Exclusion Unit 1999). In 1999 the Social Exclusion Unit produced a report on teenage pregnancy and parenthood. One of the action points detailed in the report is to halve the rate of conceptions of women aged under 18 years of age in England by 2010 and to reduce the risk of long-term social exclusion of teenage parents and their children. The report suggested collaborative working involving local organizations, community groups and primary care colleagues would be key in progressing the action needed to achieve these aims.

Babies of teenage mothers have a higher risk of growth restriction and low birth weight (Botting et al 1998), they also have a higher risk of pre-term birth (Hediger et al 1997). Growth restriction and pre-term delivery are associated with a greater risk of mortality and morbidity. Evidence suggests that infants born in this category are also pre-programmed to develop cardiovascular disease and diabetes in later life (Godfrey & Barker 2001), perpetuating health disadvantage over future generations. The Office for National Statistics suggests that the risk of becoming a teenage mother is almost ten times higher for a girl whose family is socio-economically disadvantaged than those who are in the higher social groups and economically advantaged (National Statistics 2004). Risk factors relating to poverty and social exclusion influence the health profiles of teenagers embarking on a pregnancy. This is further compounded by the higher rate of smoking amongst teenage girls and poor nutrition (Gregory et al 2000).

Below is an anonymized case profile of Melanie, a teenager who was unable to keep her family together due to multiple factors relating to socio-economic disadvantage and lack of support services. This is a real case that I was actively involved in (Box 15.4).

CONCLUSION

Inequality in health and healthcare provision continues despite efforts by Government agencies to inform healthcare policy and practice. The Black Report (Black et al 1982) found that there were large differentials in both morbidity and mortality that favoured the economically advantaged members of society. Women and their families in the lowest income brackets have the poorest health, the highest infant mortality rate, the shortest life expectancy and the greatest morbidity. Socio-economic deprivation is directly linked

---

Box 15.4   Vulnerable teenager and her children

Melanie was a 19-year-old; this was her fourth pregnancy and she had given birth to three babies. She lived alone in a high rise council flat. She had no social support, and had an estranged relationship with her mother. Her mother was a drug addict, who had bipolar disease and whose own five children either had been or were currently in the care of social services.

Melanie had lived in and out of foster care since the age of 7 and felt that she had had to bring herself up without any parental guidance. Her biological father left the family home once she was conceived. Her mother's boyfriends had been surrogate fathers, some better than others, one raped her when she was 6 years old.

As a teenage parent she longed to be in a stable relationship, but each of her babies' fathers had all left, either during the pregnancy or after the birth. She felt isolated and alone. Her oldest child had been kept secured in a pushchair for the majority of the time and as a consequence could not walk at 2 years of age. Her second child was 1 year old and was emotionally vacant and listless and could not crawl. Her third child was 8 months old, under-

weight and not reaching developmental milestones. Melanie was 18 weeks pregnant with her fourth child when I first met her.

She did not have a washing machine at home and therefore used a launderette monthly to wash all the clothes. To visit the launderette she had to take her 2 year old down several flights of stairs in the pushchair (the lift in her flats did not work) and left the child at the bottom of the stairs whilst she climbed back up to her flat to collect the 1 year old and 8 month old. She mostly ate out with the children because she could not carry shopping. She managed to buy milk, bread and butter to have at home.

After the birth of her fourth baby, all of her children were removed from Melanie's care by social services.

Think about the following questions:

Who should have been involved in Melanie's care?

How could Melanie be helped to enhance her lifestyle and that of her children?

with stillbirths, neonatal deaths, perinatal morbidity and delayed effects impinge on wellbeing and health in adult life. A significant proportion of maternal and perinatal adverse outcomes are avoidable and the midwifery commitment to provide focused support to women and their families can make a positive difference. Midwives play an important role in influencing the health of women and their families and have the potential to influence positively the inter-generational cycle of poor health. It is however important to acknowledge that an individualistic approach to reducing inequalities in health and healthcare provision will not change this negative picture. Adopting a multidisciplinary, multi agency approach will have greater impact. Close collaboration involving for example, primary care trust commissioners and managers, public health practitioners, primary care colleagues, social services and voluntary organizations is essential to achieve the most effective midwifery contributions to public health and improving the health of local communities. Clearly identifying the scope and purpose of the midwife's role when addressing inequalities in health and healthcare provision, will focus care toward the areas of greatest need and enhance maternity care to women and their families.

PRACTICE POINTS

- Maternity services should be proactive in designing services that engage all women particularly those from vulnerable and disadvantaged groups.
- Midwives should harness every opportunity to work in collaboration with primary care colleagues and community organizations to enhance the holistic provision of care to women and their families.
- Sure Start midwifery programmes that have been effective should be maintained and continued within Children's Centres.
- Midwives should continue to strengthen their public health role by identifying key public health issues and working with primary care trusts, public health practioners and commissioners of maternity services.
- Midwives should be conversant with local community resources including community groups and specialist services enabling appropriate and timely referrals when necessary.

References

Acheson D (Chair) 1998 Independent inquiry into inequalities in health. The Stationery Office, London

American Psychiatric Association 1994 Diagnostic and statistical manual of mental disorders. 4th edn. American Psychiatric Association, Washington, DC

Amnesty International 2004 It's in our hands, stop violence against women. Amnesty International, Oxford, UK

Barker D 1997 The long term outcome of retarded fetal growth. Clinical Obstetrics and Gynaecology 40(4): 853–863

Barker D J P (ed.) 1992 Fetal and infant origins of adult diseases. BMJ Books, London

Barker D, Gluckman P, Godfrey K 1993 Fetal nutrition and cardiovascular disease in later life. Lancet 2341: 938–941

Black D, Morris J N, Smith C, Townsend P 1982 Inequalities in health: the Black report. Penguin, Harmondsworth (first published by the Department of Health and Social Security, 1980. New introduction by P Townsend and N Davidson)

Blackburn S 2003 Maternal, fetal and neonatal physiology- A clinical perspective. WB Saunders, Philadelphia

Botting B, Rosato M, Wood R 1998 Teenage mothers and the health of their children. Population Trends 93: 67–68

Burnett A, Peel A 2001 The health needs of asylum seekers and refugees. British Medical Journal 322: 544–547

Church S, Scanlan M 2002 Post-traumatic stress disorder after childbirth so midwives have a preventative role. The Practising Midwife 5(6): 10–13

Cnattingius S, Nordstrom M L 1996 Maternal smoking and feto-infant mortality: biological pathways and public health significance. Acta Paediatrica 85: 1400–1402

Coleman T 2004 ABC of smoking cessation special groups of smokers. British Medical Journal 328: 965–966

Collaborative Group on Hormonal Factors in Breast Cancer 2002 Breast cancer and breastfeeding: collaborative reanalysis of individual data from 47 epidemiological studies in 30 countries, including 50,302 women with breast cancer and 96,973 women without the disease. Lancet 360 (9328): 187–195

Cooper Y 2004 More children to be given a sure start in life. DoH, London

Covington D L, Diel S J, Wright B D, Piner M H 1997 Assessing for violence during pregnancy using a systematic approach. Maternal and Child Health Journal 1: 129–132

Cowen T 2001 Unequal treatment: findings from a refugee health survey in Barnet. Refugee Health Access Project, London

Department for Education and Employment 2000 Sure Start: a guide. DfEE, London

Department for Education and Skills 2003 Female Genital Mutilation Act (LASSL 2004)4. Department of Health, London

Department of Health 1999 Saving lives: our healthier nation: a contract for health. The Stationery Office, London

Department of Health 2000 Domestic violence: a resource manual for healthcare professionals. NHS Executive, London

Department of Health 2000 The NHS plan a plan for investment and a plan for reform. DoH, London

Department of Health 2001 Children Act Report. DoH, London

Department of Health 2002 Government response to the 1st Annual Report of the Independent Advisory Group on Teenage Pregnancy. DoH, London

Department of Health 2003 Delivering the best midwives contribution to the NHS Plan. Online. Available: www.doh.gov.uk/deliveringthenhsplan accessed 8th March 2005

Department of Health 2004a Why mothers die. Confidential enquiry into maternal and child health improving the health of mothers, babies and children 2000–2002. RCOG, London

Department of Health 2004b National service framework for children. Department for Education and Skills, DoH, London

Donaldson L, Donaldson R 2000 Essential public health. 2nd edn. Tobeapharm, Newbury

Dunkley J 2000 Health promotion in midwifery practice. Baillière Tindall, London

Dunkley-Bent J 2004 A consultant midwife's community clinic. British Journal of Midwifery 12(3): 144–171

Dye T D, Tollivert N J, Lee R V, Kennedy C J 1995 Violence, pregnancy and birth outcome in Appalachia. Paediatric and Perinatal Epidemiology 9: 35–47

Dykes F 2003 Infant feeding initiative a report evaluating the breastfeeding practice projects 1999–2002. DoH, London

Edwards R 2004 ABC of smoking cessation. The problem of tobacco smoking. British Medical Journal 328: 575–577

Fuxe K 1989 Neuroendocrine actions of nicotine and of exposure to cigarette smoke: medical implication. Psychoneuroendocrinology 14: 19–41

Godfrey K, Barker D 2001 Fetal programming and adult health. Public Health Nutrition 4: 611–624

Graffy J, Taylor J, Williams A 2004 Randomised controlled trial of support from volunteer counsellors for mothers considering breastfeeding. British Medical Journal 328: 26–30

Gregory J, Lowe S, Bates CJ et al 2000 National diet and nutrition survey: young people aged 4–18 years. Volume 1: report of the diet and nutrition survey. TSO, London

Hadley C B, Main D M, Gabbe S G 1990 Risk factors for preterm premature rupture of the fetal membranes. American Journal of Obstetrics and Gynaecology 103: 800–805

Hamlyn B, Brooker S, Oleinikova K, Wands S 2002 Infant feeding 2000. Stationery Office, London

Hanson L A 1998 Breastfeeding provides passive and likely long lasting active immunity. Annals of Allergy, Asthma & Immunology 81(6): 523–537

Health Education Authority (HEA) 1996 folic acid campaign, local activity handbook. HEA, London

Hediger M L, O'Scholl T, Schall J, Krueger P 1997 Young maternal age and preterm labour. Annals of Epidemiology 7: 400–406

Heller R F, Heller T, Patterson S 2003 Putting the public back into public health. Part 1. A re-definition of public health. Public Health 117: 63–66

Howie P W, Forsyth J S, Ogston S A et al 1990 Protective effects of breastfeeding against infection. British Medical Journal 300: 11–16

Kennedy P, Murphy-Lawless J 2001 The maternity care needs of refugee and asylum seeking women Women's Health Unit, Eastern Region Health Authority, London

Kmietowicz Z 2000 Breastfeeding programmes should be targeted. British Medical Journal 321: 467

Kmietowicz Z 2004 Removing extreme poverty by 2015 is under threat. British Medical Journal 329: 642

Kramer M S, Chalmers B, Hodnett E D, Sevkovskaya Z, Dzikovich I, Shapiro S et al 2001 Promotion of breastfeeding intervention trial (PROBIT). Journal American Medical Association 285: 413–20

Lader D, Meltzer H 2002 Smoking related behaviour and attitudes 2002. Office for National Statistic, London. Online. Available: www.statistics.gov.uk/lib2001/index.html accessed 8th March 2005

Lawrence R A 1997 Breastfeeding is more than just good nutrition. International Journal of Childbirth Education 12(1): 16

McLiesh J 2002 Mothers in exile: maternity experiences of asylum seekers in England. Maternity Action 90: 2–3

Medical Research Council. Vitamin study research group 1991 Prevention of neural tube defects, results of the medical research council vitamin study. Lancet 338: 131–137

Melton L J 3rd, Bryant S C, Wahner H W et al 1993 Influence of breastfeeding and other reproductive factors on bone mass in later life. Osteoporosis International 3: 76–83

Mezey G C 1997 Domestic violence in pregnancy. In: Bewley S, Friend J, Mezey G (eds) Violence against women. Royal College of Obstetrics and Gynaecologists, London, pp 191–198

Mirlees-Black C 1999 Domestic violence: findings from a new British crime survey self completion questionnaire. Research Study 191. Home Office, London

Momoh C 2003 Female genital mutilation In: Squire C (ed.) The social context of birth. Radcliffe Medical, Abingdon, pp 121–135

Momoh C 2004 Female genital mutilation. Current Opinion in Obstetrics and Gynaecology 16(6): 477–480

Momoh C, Ladhani S, Lochrie P et al 2001 Female genital mutilation: analysis of the first twelve months of a southeast London specialist clinic. British Journal of Obstetrics and Gynaecology 108: 186–191

Murphy C Schei B, Myhr T 2001 Abuse a risk factor for low birth weight? A systematic review and meta-analysis. Canadian Medical Association Journal 164(11): 1667–1672

National Health Service Centre for Reviews and Dissemination 2000 Promoting the initiation of breastfeeding. Effective Healthcare Bulletin 6(2): 1–12

National Statistics 2004 Teenage conception rates: by age at conception and outcome: Social Trends 32

Oddy W, Holt P, Sly T et al 1999 Association between breastfeeding and asthma in 6-year-old children: findings of a prospective birth cohort study. British Medical Journal 319: 815–819

Olsen S F, Hansen H S, Secher N J, Jensen B, Sandstrom B 1995 Gestation length and birth weight in relation to intake of marine n-3 fatty acids. British Journal Nutrition 73: 397–404

Parker B 1993 Abuse of adolescents: What can we learn from pregnant teenagers? AWHONN's Clinical Issues in Perinatal and Women's Health Nursing 4: 363–370

Philip W, James T, Nelson M, Ralph A, Leather S 1997 Socio-economic determinants of health: The contribution of nutrition to inequalities in health. British Medical Journal 314: 1545–1547

Quinlivan J A, Evans S F 2001 A prospective cohort study of the impact of domestic violence on young teenage pregnancy outcomes. Journal of Paediatric and Adolescent Gynaecology 14: 17–23

Rape, Abuse and Incest National Network (RAINN) 2004 Online. Available: http://www.rainn.org/index.html accessed 10th March 2005

Royal College of Midwives (RCM) 2000 Vision 2000. RCM, London

Royal College of Midwives (RCM) 2001 The midwives role in public health position paper No. 24. RCM, London

Royal College of Midwives (RCM) 2002 Helping women stop smoking a guide for midwives. RCM, London

Royal College of Midwives 1999 Domestic abuse in pregnancy. Position Paper 19a. RCM, London

Royal College of Physicians 2000 Nicotine addiction in Britain. Royal College of Physicians, London

Scholl T, Hediger M L, Schall J I, Khoo G-S, Fischer R L 1996 Dietary and serum folate: their influence on the outcome of pregnancy. American Journal of Clinical Nutrition 63: 520–525

Secretary of State for Health 1998 Smoking kills a white paper on tobacco. The Stationery Office, London

Secretary of State for Health 2004 Government response to House of Commons Health Committee reports, fourth session 2002–03, provision of maternity services, eighth report session 2002–03, inequalities in access to maternity services and ninth report session 2002–03, choice in maternity services CM 6140. The Stationery Office, London

Shumway J, O'Campo P, Gielen A et al 1999 Preterm labour, placental abruption and premature rupture of membranes in relation to maternal violence or verbal abuse. Journal of Maternal-Fetal Medicine 8: 76–80

Sikorski J, Renfrew M J, Pindoria S, Wade A 2002 Support for breastfeeding mothers. Cochrane Library, Issue 3. Update Software, Oxford

Singer R 2004 Asylum seekers: an ethical response to their plight. Lancet 363: 1904

Siskind V, Green A, Bain C et al 1997 Breastfeeding, menopause and epithelial ovarian cancer. Epidemiology 8(2): 188–191

Smith R 1997 Evidence based interventions that reduce inequalities in health. British Medical Journal 314: 695

Social Exclusion Unit (SEU) 1999 Teenage pregnancy. The Stationery Office, London

Stapleton H, Kirkham M, Curtis P, Thomas G 2002 Framing information in antenatal care. British Journal of Midwifery 10(4): 197–201

Stewart D E 1994 Incidence of postpartum abuse in women with a history of abuse during pregnancy. Canadian Medical Association Journal 151: 1601–1604

Sure Start 2005 Children's centres. Online. Available: http://www.surestart.gov.uk accessed 8th March 2005

Sure Start Scotland Scottish Executive 2005. Online. Available: http://www.scotland.gov.uk/home accessed 8th March 2005

Sure Start Wales 2005 Web page. Online. Available: http://www.scotland.gov.uk/home 9th March 2005

Tedstone A, Dunce N, Aviles M, Shetty P, Daniels L 1998 Effectiveness of interventions to promote healthy feeding in infants under one year of age: a review. Health Education Authority, London

Unicef UK Baby Friendly Initiative 1999 The baby friendly initiative in the community an implementation guide. Unicef UK Baby Friendly Initiative. UNICEF, London

Unicef UK Baby Friendly Initiative 2000 Baby friendly hospitals show strong increase in breastfeeding rates. Baby Friendly News No 6. UNICEF

University of York NHS Centre for Reviews and Dissemination 1998 Effectiveness matters, Vol 3, Issue 1. University of York, York

US Department of Health and Human Services 2001 Report of the science of tobacco on health. Her Majesty's Stationery Office, London

Voight L, Hollenbach K, Krohn M, Daling J, Hickok D 1990 The relationship of abruptio placentae with maternal smoking for gestational age infants. Obstetrics and Gynaecology 75: 771–774

Walters R, Sim F, Schiller G 2002 Mapping the public health workforce 1: a tool for classifying the public health workforce. Public Health 116: 201–206

Welsh National Service Framework for Children 2004 Online. Available: http://www.wales.nhs.uk/nsf accessed 8th March 2005

WHO/UNICEF 1989 Protecting, promoting and supporting breast-feeding. The special role of maternity Services. A Joint WHO/UNICEF Statement 1989. Non serial Publication

Wiist W H, McFarlane J 1999 The effectiveness of an abuse assessment protocol in public health prenatal clinics. American Journal of Public Health 89: 1217–1221

Williams M A, Mittendorf R, Lieberman E, Monson R R et al 1999 Cigarette smoking during pregnancy in relation to placenta previa. American Journal of Obstetrics Gynaecology 165: 28–32

Windham G C, Hopkins B, Swan S 2000 Pre-natal active or passive tobacco smoke exposure and the risk of pre-term delivery. Epidemiology 11: 427–433

Wisborg K, Henrikson T B, Hedegaard M et al 1996 Smoking during pregnancy and pre-term birth. British Journal of Obstetrics and Gynaecology 103: 800–805

Women's Aid 2005 Online. Available: http://www. womensaid.org.uk accessed 11th March 2005

Chapter 16

Keeping birth normal

Tina Lavender and Carol Kingdon

WHAT DOES 'NORMAL' MEAN?

Midwives are the only professionals who specialize in the overall care of childbearing women and their babies when there are no complications, in what is usually called 'normal' pregnancy and birth. It is generally accepted that midwives are required to refer to a doctor if complications arise, yet in technology dependent societies decreasing attention has been paid to the need for midwives to confirm the normal and to be able to support, protect and encourage healthy birth without unnecessary intervention. The unprecedented rises in the number of caesarean sections performed during the 1970s and 1980s led the World Health Organization (WHO) to hold a consensus conference on appropriate technology for birth, which concluded that there was no justification for any region to have a rate higher than 10–15% (World Health Organization 1985). In England, the national caesarean section rate surpassed the WHO's recommended 15% in 1995 (Macfarlane et al 2000) and by 2001 the rate had reached 21.3% (Thomas & Paranjothy 2001). Birth through an abdominal incision was fast becoming a 'normal event' (Amu et al 1998) with vaginal, rather than caesarean birth viewed as inherently hazardous (Weaver 2000).

However, this situation may be changing as individual midwives, their professional bodies, and consumer groups have all increasingly challenged the role of midwifery in obstetric units. The International Confederation of Midwives has put its weight behind a call to 'take normal birth off the list of endangered species' (International Confederation of Midwives 2002) and in the UK, the Royal College of Midwives has put normal birth back at the pinnacle of its agenda 'championing normality' through its 'Campaign for Normal Birth' (Royal College of Midwives, 2004). Figures from midwifery-led birth settings have shown women are significantly less likely to have induced labours, instrumental deliveries, epidurals and planned caesareans (Walker 2001). In England, during 2002–2003 the national caesarean section rate levelled out at around 22% (BirthChoiceUK 2004). This was the first time in two decades that the caesarean section rate had not increased year on year. If this trend is to be continued in the UK and replicated in other countries, there has never been a greater need for midwives to protect and support normal processes. The Maternity module of the National Service Framework for Children, Young People and Maternity Services recognizes that 'women's reactions to their birth experiences can influence their emotional wellbeing, relationship with the baby and their future parenting relationships' (Department of Health 2004, p. 27).

The designation 'normal' to describe labour and childbirth has been used for centuries (Towler & Bramhall 1986). But what is 'normal'? What is meant by the words 'normal' and 'natural' is affected by the culture in which we live and practice and have ambiguous meanings both within and between countries. While the debate about rising caesarean section rates has become more prevalent, there has been little general discussion of, or agreement about, what constitutes normal birth (Downe et al 2001, p. 605). In 1997 the WHO defined normal birth as:

> ... spontaneous in onset, low risk at the start of labour and remaining so throughout labour and delivery. The infant is born spontaneously in the vertex position between 37 and 42 completed weeks of pregnancy. After birth both mother and infant are in good condition.
>
> World Health Organization 1997

Whereas Gould (2000) proposes an alternative definition based on a concept analysis of normal birth:

> Physiologically normal labour naturally follows a sequential pattern. The woman experiences painful regular uterine contractions stimulating progressive effacement and dilatation of the cervix and descent of the fetus, culminating in the spontaneous vaginal birth of a healthy baby and expulsion of placenta and membranes with no apparent complications in mother or baby. It is strenuous work. Movement has a crucial role.

In neither the WHO's (1997) nor Gould's (2000) definition of normal birth is there any reference to use of technological intervention. However, to assume we may simply define 'normal birth' as 'natural birth' without intervention is problematic, because the society and culture in which birth takes place affect what is considered to be natural. Local customs and values all affect the behaviour and expectations surrounding birth as well as the outcomes of birth. Sociologists have argued natural childbirth does not exist because human childbirth is always shaped by culture (Oakley 1983, p. 107). For example, in the UK natural birth may be routinely monitored by regular vaginal examinations or the use of the partogram. Does this mean the majority of pregnancies are abnormal or it is normal to intervene? Anderson (2002) has argued midwives should categorize their interventions according to their severity of impact upon normal processes.

Downe (2001) acknowledged the viability in definitions of normal birth based on at least five distinct perspectives. She describes these as being:

- normal birth is purely physiological;
- normal birth is physiological but with the addition of human intervention;
- normal birth is physiological with the addition of naturopathic interventions (e.g. aromatherapy, massage);
- normal birth is best phrased in a way which would be politically useful and highlights the issue of increased use of technology;
- normal birth is rooted in cultural norms, this would mean that in some countries technological intervention would be a normal feature of birth.

Downe (2001) also described three alternative new definitions, outlined below, and argued that they can be defended logically using the current evidence-base for non-intervention and intervention in low-risk labour and delivery. She said that normal birth may be:

1. 'supported physiological birth'; which is spontaneous in onset, no pharmacological pain relief is administered, accepts that labour supporters will attend women, and ends with spontaneous third stage;
2. 'moderated physiological birth': which is the same as above but with the inclusion of a managed third stage in the light of the (contested but currently mainstream) evidence (Prendville et al 1988, Rogers & Wood 1996) in this area;
3. 'salutogenic birth': a birth that generates positive short and long term wellbeing for the mother, baby, family and care-giver.

While the focus on evidence-based practice is well-developed in the field of pregnancy and childbirth (Audit Commission 1997, p. 72), there remain areas of maternity care where evidence is contested, inconclusive, or not available. Midwives must simultaneously be guardians of normal birth whilst at the same time knowing when to interfere with nature, and at what point to use intervention. To simply say that midwives believe in natural birth, and natural birth should be allowed to take its course is not the answer because nature can be cruel as well as kind. Intervention will at times be necessary to maintain safety. In the first edition of this book, Lesley Page (2000) wrote:

The definition of normal is so problematic that I have found it simpler to be guided by two simple principles:

Intervention should only be used if there are clear evidence-based clinical indicators and clear evidence that the intervention is more likely to do good than harm in the particular situation, or if a woman asks for it.

The provision of adequate support, which includes providing enough and appropriate information to women, is fundamental to avoiding unnecessary intervention in pregnancy and birth.

At present the 'rules' of the UK, and of most other countries, that govern midwifery practice usually require that midwives should be able to refer or call medical help when there is what the Nursing and Midwifery Council refers to as 'a deviation from the norm' (Nursing and Midwifery Council 2004). Page (2000) has advocated she would like to see the first rule of midwifery being the need to 'confirm the absence of any real, evidence-based indicators for intervention' and the second as the need 'to refer to a medical colleague when there is an evidence-based indicator for medical intervention'. This is not dissimilar to the two basic principles used by Enkin et al (1999, p. 389) in their Guide to Effective Care in Pregnancy and Childbirth. These were: 'firstly, that the only justification for practices that restrict a woman's autonomy, her freedom of choice, and her access to her baby, would be clear evidence that these restrictive practices do more good than harm, and secondly, that any interference with the natural process of pregnancy and childbirth should also be shown to do more good than harm'. Getting this balance right is so important because the decisions that the midwife makes at this time will affect the mother, baby and family in a number of ways for years to come. Her approach to the woman in her care, may make a difference not only between life and death, good health and severe disability, but also in the emotional wellbeing of the woman and her family.

Memories of good and poor care tend to be profound, and memories of birth are in themselves an important outcome. This is not intended to downplay the importance of midwifery care in the antenatal and postnatal period, and this is discussed in other chapters. However, the birth of a baby is like no other event in human life. As Simkin (1992, p. 64) reminds us:

The birth of a child, especially a first child, represents a landmark event in the lives of all involved. For the mother particularly, childbirth has a profound physical, mental, emotional and social effect. No other event involves pain, emotional stress, vulnerability, possible physical injury or death, and permanent role change, and includes responsibility for a dependent, helpless human being. Moreover, it generally all takes place within a single day. It is not surprising that women tend to remember their first birth experiences vividly and with deep emotion.

It is so important that midwives do not lose sight of the immensely special, unique and life-changing event each and every birth is, and this is why Downe's (2001) third definition of normal birth 'salutogenic birth' is so potentially powerful. The concept recognizes each individual woman and her way of seeing and of birthing, it also respects the hormonal dance between mother and infant, which is intrinsic and essential to the wellbeing of both in the future (Downe 2001, p. 32). The interplay between the hormones produced by the mother and baby are thought to have an impact on the labour, the neonate itself and through the first months of life.

In this chapter, we will do two things: indicate the importance of the practical aspects of midwifery by the use of examples drawn from experience, and use the best available evidence to show how midwives might 'keep birth normal'. Other chapters emphasize the critical analysis of evidence, clinical decision-making, the importance of relationships and some of the science that is the foundation of midwifery. However, the practical work that is the focus of this chapter emphasizes that hands and heart as well as head are fundamental to midwifery practice. The work of midwifery is, by its very nature, very practical. The practical aspects taken as an example in this chapter are concerned with supporting women so that they may give birth to their children without unnecessary interference. We will focus on six discrete areas:

- Creating a positive atmosphere and arranging furniture.
- Presence, comfort and encouragement.
- Assessment of labour.
- Assessment of health of the fetus.
- Mobility and positions for labour and birth.
- Helping women to cope with the pain of labour.

Reviews of evidence are available which can be used as a source of information about how care offered by midwives can be used to keep birth normal. These include the MIDIRS Informed Choice leaflets (MIDIRS 2004a–2004f) and the Cochrane Library (2005). However, the art of midwifery is more than the application of scientific rules that dictate practice and are used only if based on evidence from randomized controlled trials. Evidence must be used in conjunction with skills learnt in practice, to actively support a woman to achieve her normal birth.

CREATING A POSITIVE ATMOSPHERE AND ARRANGING FURNITURE

One of the basic ways of reducing anxiety and tension, and of helping women to cope with the pain of labour, may be by intentionally creating a calm, positive, welcoming atmosphere. Over the past decade, midwives in diverse parts of the world have expressed their views about this. What many of them, particularly those who work in large hospitals, have said is that the delivery suite or labour ward is a place that evokes anxiety in them. Furthermore, when community midwives are rotated into the delivery suite to upgrade their skills, they sometimes find it a frightening experience. In contrast, the atmosphere of a home birth is usually very different. Home is home; a sense of home is personal and can *never* be created in an institution or birth centre, although such a centre certainly can, and should be, more homely. Home is a place in which the woman is in her own surroundings, supported by chosen people and loved ones, in which it is far easier to get comfortable. Usually, only one or two professionals are in attendance.

It is far harder to create a positive calm atmosphere in a hospital. This is possibly because of the combined effect of having so many people in one area, people who are often overworked and rushed, constantly dealing with such a critical event, constantly looking after women in severe pain, so that anxiety spreads from one person to another. It is also difficult with conventional patterns of staffing to have long enough to care for one mother and baby at a time, adding to the sense of frustration and crisis. The area is often more like an intensive care unit than a place where babies are brought into the world.

It is important to think consciously about the atmosphere in which you practise because it is likely to affect you and other staff, who will in turn affect the women they are caring for. The atmosphere will also have a direct effect on the woman herself. A midwife working permanently in a delivery suite may be in a position to do something to make the atmosphere calmer, for example setting up strategies for staff support, such as getting all the staff (both midwives and doctors) together to talk and find time for reflection.

Even if the atmosphere as a whole cannot be altered, midwives can do something about the room or rooms in which they work and about protecting themselves from the atmosphere if it is unsupportive. They can be aware of their feelings and reactions, and carry out deep breathing when they go into or return to a room. Concentrating on the woman (or women) for whom they are caring at that moment will consciously keep them calm. It is also important not to have strangers wandering in and out of the room when a woman is in labour. She should feel that she is in a protected environment where she is able to focus on herself and put all her energy into coping with labour. As midwives, we tend to underestimate the intimacy of the birthing situation and how important it is for the woman to have privacy. Go out of the room to talk to doctors and colleagues about the woman's progress if that is expected; if you think you may need to make a referral or require advice, invite them in to meet the woman at an early stage, at an appropriate time and in a prearranged way.

Despite the efforts of many midwives over recent years, delivery rooms can be very ugly places. The bed is often dominant (and uncomfortable!) and right in the centre of the room. Altering the position of furniture will encourage women to move about. Put the bed against the wall and make a space that invites the woman to move and walk around, also leaving room for 'props' to support her in adopting different positions. Such props may include people, beanbags, rocking chairs, over-bed tables and the end of the bed itself. In one hospital in Iceland, padded swings are used, high enough for the woman to lean on and rock herself during contractions. Units in the United Kingdom have also made efforts to create more pleasurable environments. During a project exploring different models of maternity care, one of us (TL) visited 14 NHS maternity units in the UK and observed the environments. What was striking was the amount of effort that midwives had put into creating more 'homely' and less 'medical' environments. For example, one unit had decorated their labour rooms in themes. Other units had created small changes, which had made large differences, such as having visual stimuli (e.g. bubble lamps, an aquarium) to create ambiance, baby resuscitaire equipment that folded into the wall when not in use, and oxygen outlets concealed behind pictures. But even if a delivery suite has not had any physical transformation, turning down the lighting may help in creating a more aesthetic and calm atmosphere. Despite all this, it must be remembered that it is probably the people working in the suite who will make the most difference in the long run.

In the 1980s, there was a noticeable change in many delivery suites in response to the work of Frederic Leboyer (1975). Some of the impact of his work seems to have been lost and forgotten now, but it is worth reconsideration. A paediatrician, he wrote of how traumatic it could be for the baby to be born. He proposed that there should be silence for the birth of the baby, the cord should not be clamped and cut until pulsation had stopped, and the baby should have skin-to-skin contact on the mother's abdomen after birth. He said that the baby should be massaged and given a bath after birth in order to adjust to a totally new environment (Leboyer 1975). The silent, darkened delivery room makes sense for the baby, but also makes sense for the woman in labour, who will be given the chance to draw in on herself, and her own resources, for the challenge of labour and birth. The idea of the calm, quiet, darkened room is very different from that of the hospital hustle and bustle that is often observed.

PRESENCE, COMFORT AND ENCOURAGEMENT

One of the most important and effective things we can do for women who are in labour is to ensure that they have constant support. Such support has been shown not only to provide a woman with emotional back-up, so that she is happier and more likely to be relaxed, but also to have a strong positive effect on the physiology and outcomes of labour (MIDIRS 2004d). In recognizing the importance of this constant attendance in labour, Changing Childbirth (Department of Health 1993) recommended that:

> The aims of the maternity service should be for every woman to have a midwife with her throughout her labour, if she wishes. If possible the same midwife should stay with the woman throughout.

A range of people in addition to the woman's partner – family members, friends, trained lay people (doulas), student midwives and midwives – can provide this support (MIDIRS 2004d). A young woman may want her mother as main supporter rather than her male partner, and in some cultures it is traditional for only female family members to be present at birth.

In some maternity units the number of visitors are restricted. The individual needs of the woman should be paramount when making judgements about social support for a woman in labour. Midwives work with the woman and her supporters to achieve the companionship she needs. However, sometimes visitors have a detrimental effect on the woman and her labour. When this happens the midwife may consider asking the visitors to leave temporarily, while she discusses with the woman her specific support needs. In some cases the woman may ask the midwife to recommend that the visitors leave.

A constant presence

Staying in the room is not enough as it is easy to be 'there' without really *being* present. It is important to be able to give all one's attention to the woman. In most hospital systems, there is a major deterrent to attending properly and being 'with' the woman in labour, even when staffing is adequate. This deterrent is the paperwork and administration, which is often irrationally organized, with documentation being repeated in a number of places, which requires much duplication to complete. Yet meaningful recording of progress and decisions made and actions taken is crucial to good care. If possible records should be made 'midwife friendly'. If this cannot be done, the midwife should be aware that keeping records may take her concentration away from the woman and her supporters, and should try to combat this. Everything possible should be done to organize midwifery so as to allow this one-to-one presence in labour and birth.

Hodnett et al (2004) undertook a systematic review of 15 randomized controlled trials that included over 12000 women to assess the effects on mothers and their babies of continuous, one-to-one intrapartum support compared with usual care. They found that women who had continuous intrapartum support had more favourable outcomes. Despite the different countries and conditions covered by the studies in the review, 'there was a remarkable consistency in the description of the experimental intervention across all trials'. In all instances the support intervention included continuous or nearly continuous presence, at least during active labour. Thirteen of the 15 trials also included specific mention of comforting touch and words of praise and encouragement.

Thirty outcomes were considered; with between 1 and 15 trials contributing to the analyses of each outcome. Because of the large number of outcomes, the following summary of results is restricted to data collected and reported in at least four trials involving at least 1000 women. Women who had continuous, one-to-one support during labour were less likely to have regional anaesthesia, any analgesia/anaesthesia, an operative vaginal birth or a caesarean section. Furthermore, they were less likely to report dissatisfaction with or negative rating of the childbirth experience and more likely to have a spontaneous vaginal birth. Continuous support was not associated with decreased likelihood of artificial oxytocin during labour, low 5-minute Apgar scores, admis-

sion of the newborn to a special care nursery, or postpartum reports of severe labour pain. Nor was continuous support associated with a significant decrease in labour length.

However, there were interesting findings in the subgroup analyses which revealed that in general continuous intrapartum support was associated with greater benefits when the provider was not a member of the hospital staff, when it began early in labour, and in settings in which epidural analgesia was not routinely available. Three aspects of the birth environment – routine use of electronic fetal monitoring, availability of epidural analgesia, and policies about the presence of additional support people of the woman's own choosing – were chosen as proxies for environmental conditions that may mediate the effectiveness of labour support. Although Hodnett et al (2004) advise that the results of their subgroup analyses should be interpreted with caution, consistent patterns suggest that the effectiveness of continuous intrapartum support may be enhanced or reduced by policies in the birth setting, type of provider, and timing of onset of support. Importantly, there were no negative outcomes associated with support in labour.

All the research included in this review took place in hospitals and focused on support given by women, with or without the male partner being present. The most beneficial effect was found to be when the constant support was provided by a woman who had some experience of supporting other women in labour, either through having given birth herself and/or through education and practice as a nurse, midwife, doula, or childbirth educator. However, regardless of who the support person is 'Every effort should be made to ensure that women's birth environments are empowering, non-stressful, afford privacy, communicate respect, and are not characterized by routine interventions that add risk without clear benefit' (Hodnett et al 2004).

A constant presence is easier to ensure when there is an effective 'continuity of care' scheme in operation in which a midwife will offer care before birth and follow a woman into labour. In the One-to-One practice, over 90% of women receiving One-to-One care received constant attendance from a midwife whilst in labour compared with 50% of those in the conventional service. Despite

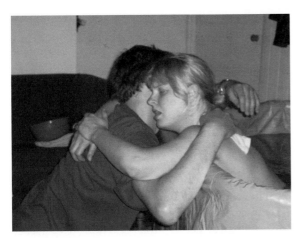

Figure 16.1 Support from partner or companion during labour is vital.

this, the One-to One service did not cost more than the provision of conventional care (McCourt & Page 1996) (Fig. 16.1).

Words of praise, comfort, encouragement and reassurance

It would be wrong to reduce the way in which we may use words of encouragement and support to that of a 'technique'. As with most communication, the importance is in listening and attending to the individual needs and preferences of a woman and her partner, and in responding to those individual needs. Robertson (1997), in her excellent book on supporting women in labour, calls it 'tuning in to women'.

Sometimes, when you have a good rapport with a woman, it helps at difficult times, for example the transition to the second stage of labour, to stand still for a moment and try to imagine how the woman is feeling. Lesley Page, in an earlier edition of this chapter (Page 2000), recalled one time that was particularly difficult because she had been torn between the care of a number of women. She was looking after a first-time mother she had never met before who really wanted to avoid analgesia. The woman had been making good progress, but then Lesley was called into another room, and when she got back the woman was in the second stage, distressed and apparently not making the progress Lesley had expected. She stood quietly for a moment trying to imagine what the woman was feeling. Lesley suspected

that the woman was finding the contractions so painful that she was frightened to follow her urge to push. She seemed to be poised at that moment when there is no turning back and the pain has to be endured, when it hurts not to push and it hurts as much if you do. Lesley simply touched her hand and said, 'I wonder if you are frightened to push because you are in so much pain; I know it is painful, but there is no turning back, you have to go on'. At that point, the woman looked at her husband, took a deep breath and started to bear down with contractions, spontaneously following her own urges. She wrote to Lesley later saying how her sensitive words had helped her to give birth to her baby. She and her husband were ecstatic; pleased too that she had managed the birth without analgesia.

How words of praise, comfort and reassurance are used and given will vary from midwife to midwife, and different women need different approaches. They may include giving information about progress in a positive rather than a negative way, telling a woman that she and her baby are doing well, and, if there are concerns, letting the woman know in a way that is not frightening. It is discouraging, for example following vaginal assessments to hear midwives saying to women 'you are *only* 3 cms dilated'. While this may be the case, presented this way can have a negative effect on the woman's ability to cope. It would be preferable to highlight the positive points of the assessment. For example, a woman may be 3 cms dilated, but her cervix may have effaced or the head may have descended, in this situation these points should be highlighted rather than the dilatation. Asking for permission before undertaking any procedure and talking through decisions in an appropriate way is crucial. It is also important to know when to be quiet.

Talking in a kind of shorthand, and being often silent can be helpful. These are the kind of phrases that might be used: 'You are doing well', 'You are breathing well', 'This contraction will soon be over', 'I can see some of the baby's head', 'Would you like to feel your baby's head?', 'Would it help you to relax more if I rubbed your shoulders?'.

The midwife's facial expressions alone can have an impact on the woman's feelings. For example, a midwife who genuinely smiles at the woman and her partner during communications says so many things: everything is fine, there is nothing to worry about, we will soon see your baby, and I am enjoying what I am doing.

All of this is far easier if you have met the woman before and have some kind of working relationship with her. Meeting before labour means having the chance to talk about some important decisions, particularly how the woman feels about using analgesia and electronic fetal monitoring. Then, during labour, discussion about these issues can be in the shorthand that is possible between two people who know and understand each other.

Comforting through touch, massage and physical support

In her chapter Authoritative Touch in Childbirth, Kitzinger (1977) reminds us that, within Western culture, great stress is placed on verbal communication, while the unspoken elements in discourse tend to be trivialized and ignored. Yet touch is an important element in the interaction of human bodies. In an account of the way in which touch has been used in childbirth through different times and across different cultures, Kitzinger classifies the different types of touch as:

blessing touch, comfort touch, physically supportive touch, diagnostic touch, manipulative touch, restraining touch and punitive touch (Fig. 16.2)

Most babies are now born in hospital settings. This context for birth takes a woman away from the potential to be surrounded by her natural circle of family and friends who may, in their own surroundings, be more likely to use physical contact and touch in a spontaneous way. In addition, the rituals of medicalized birth may restrict and alter the way in which we use touch to comfort, support and encourage women through labour, particularly where there is a reliance on technology to enhance and monitor labour. This is especially so where staff working in hospitals are rushed and overworked, and have no prior bond or relationship with the women in labour for whom they are caring.

Kitzinger (1997) pointed out that touch may be used to restrain and punish, and may cause pain. For example, touch during contractions and vaginal examinations may be very painful or invasive. Consider the experience of vaginal examination; this is often performed by staff whom the woman has never met before, to whom she has barely had an introduction, and sometimes without full consent. In everyday life, such touch would be seen as one of the worst forms of assault. Therefore, touch should be a response to the woman's needs rather than a routine or protocol to be followed; otherwise it can be distressing, irritating and painful.

When touch is used with the intention of comforting and supporting, and when it is sensitive to the woman's needs and reaction, experience teaches that it is extremely powerful. Touch used for physical support may be close contact, cradling of the woman for comfort and to help her to maintain her posture or position, or providing a neck or shoulders to lean on. Touch may be slight, for example when lightly placing a hand on the forehead, or by massage stokes that may be either gentle or firm.

Touch can cause unwanted emotional responses. In a study conducted by one of the authors (TL) a woman in the postnatal period discussed the anxiety she felt when the midwife moved away when she had tried to hold her hand (Lavender & Walkinshaw 1998). The woman felt bad, but the situation may have also been difficult for the midwife. In Western society, where touch is restricted by culture, massage may be an acceptable form of touch and considered less invasive and more acceptable than hand-holding with someone you don't know intimately. Touch elicits different responses. While massage may be an effective form of pain relief in itself, a light touch may simply be a way of saying, 'I am here with you, and you are not alone'.

ASSESSMENT OF LABOUR

DIAGNOSING LABOUR

The importance of correct diagnosis of labour cannot be emphasized sufficiently. Misdiagnosis may lead to wrongly diagnosing dysfunctional labour, consequent use of unnecessary treatment and intervention (O'Driscoll et al 1984). Although recognized as an arbitrary starting point, the most useful and frequently used marker of the onset of labour is the time when the woman is admitted to labour ward/labour care (Enkin et al 2000). For women giving birth at home, the time of the midwife's arrival may similarly be used.

However, it is well reported that many women who seek admission to hospital in labour are not considered to be in labour by the staff (Bonovich 1989, O'Driscoll et al 1973). Midwives must be careful not to dismiss women who seek support early. In Hunt and Symonds' (1995) ethnography of a hospital delivery suite, direct observation, interview and medical notes examination were used to explain the problem of women being admitted too early in labour. The 'in-house' talk classified these women as 'nigglers' who exacerbated the workload without being genuine cases. Observation of interactions with these women revealed how their perspectives on their labours was re-interpreted to fit this category and finally the medical notes recorded the diagnosis as 'false' or spurious labour. One could see that women's actual experience was not driving midwives' care but a pre-determined diagnostic category with quite specific parameters. We know from Kirkham's (1989) work that many women are dissatisfied with this aspect of their care.

Women may present themselves early because they are not aware of the signs that labour has commenced, they are not coping with the pain that they are experiencing, or they are fearful of labour events. This highlights the importance of having access to appropriate information and education in preparation for labour and birth. Where a woman seeks care when not in established labour her midwife must be sensitive to the woman's experience and feelings. Acknowledging how she is feeling and giving her information about the changes to her body which are taking place in preparation for birth can provide her with ways to contextualize what she is experiencing without disempowering or demoralizing her. This way a woman can remain confident that her own body is preparing her for active labour and birth. Carrying out assessment of whether labour has started in the woman's home can prevent unnecessary upheaval and feelings of embarrassment and deflation sometimes expressed by women when they have sought to access labour care and are then encouraged to return home from hospital.

One aspect of labour, which remains poorly understood, is the latent phase. There is a lack of evidence to guide midwives on the significance of this phase and the best policy for care of women at this time. Some consider it to be the end of pre-labour (Hendricks et al 1970), while others believe it to be a true entity (Koontz & Bishop 1982). The mean length of the latent phase is debatable with many midwives adopting the World Health Organization (1994) suggestion of an 8-hour latent phase. However, this is of little clinical significance because there is large variation between individual women. Furthermore some health professionals do not believe in the existence of a latent phase at all. O'Driscoll, Meagher and Boylan (1993), suggest that terms such as *labour not established* or *latent labour* serve only as stratagems to relieve the doctor or midwife of the onus of having to make a decision' (O'Driscoll et al 1993, p. 36). The philosophy of the National Maternity Hospital labour ward, where O'Driscoll worked, is that a woman is either in labour or she is not. Regardless of whether professionals believe a latent phase exists or not, midwives need to value women's experiences.

One of the commonest problems in labour care is differentiating between a prolonged latent phase and false labour (Crowther et al 1989). Failure of the cervix to respond to uterine contractions may be interpreted as a failure to progress, where in fact, as Porreco (1990) points out, it may be that the obstetricians and midwives have failed, by not waiting for adequate cervical effacement and dilatation of the cervix before diagnosing labour.

Several physiological changes occur prior to commencement of the active phase that may contribute to incorrect diagnoses of labour. Before effacement the cervix undergoes a process of 'ripening' that is known to be promoted by oestrogens and prostaglandins (Gee & Glynn 1997). During this period, a gel composed of glycoproteins, which normally binds the collagen fibres of the cervix, changes composition thus changing the cervical state (Osmers et al 1993). This process can be recognized clinically by using semi-objective means, such as assigning a score to assessment of cervical consistency, dilatation, length, position within the pelvis and station of the presenting part (e.g. Bishop Score).

Incorrect diagnosis of active labour can lead to unnecessary intervention and/or maternal distress. Therefore if women are admitted to labour care only once labour has been confirmed, misdiagnosisis of problems such as prolonged labour would be less likely. Midwives have supported this approach for many years, recommending that during the latent phase women are best left in their own environment (Flint 1986). McNiven et al (1998) provided some evidence through a randomized controlled trial of the impact of correct labour diagnosis on clinical outcomes. In their study of 209 low-risk nulliparous women in Canada the outcomes of women who attended a labour assessment programme were compared with those who were directly admitted to the labour ward. The study found that women who were randomized to the labour assessment unit spent less time on the labour ward, and were less likely to receive intrapartum oxytocics and analgesia than women who were admitted directly to the labour ward. Women in the labour assessment group were also more likely to report higher levels of control during labour.

Vaginal examinations

Vaginal examinations are an integral part of caring for women in labour, the regularity of which has created a routine process, which is rarely questioned. The flippant way that midwives communicate about the procedure has been demonstrated in Mavis Kirkham's work (Kirkham 1989). However, what has become routine to midwives, is far from routine to women who can find the ritual painful, embarrassing and disempowering (Bergstrom et al 1992). In some instances vaginal examinations have been associated with Traumatic Stress Disorder (Menage 1996). This is often compounded when the woman has a past history of being sexually abused (Robohm & Buttenheim 1996). Nevertheless, rightly or wrongly, some women seek reassurance from vaginal examinations, some even suggesting that more frequent examinations should be performed (Lavender et al 1998). This may occur when the woman does not feel supported, reassured and encouraged in labour.

There is no clear guidance from the literature regarding the most appropriate time to perform a vaginal examination. Friedman (1954) measured cervical dilatation at the peak of the contraction, whereas Richardson, Sutherland and Allen (1978) reported that the cervix was maximally dilated 15 seconds after the peak of each contraction. As there is insufficient evidence to guide midwives, then perhaps signs of increasing maternal discomfort should be the factor determining when examination should be timed in relation to contractions (Crowther et al 1989).

Another important issue is the frequency of performing vaginal examinations, as routinely repeating vaginal examinations is thought to be of no proven value (Devane 1996, Enkin 1992). Like many other issues surrounding labour management, a consensus has not yet been reached. Philpott and Castle (1972b) advised 4 hourly assessments, and if delay was detected, 2 hourly. O'Driscoll et al (1993) and Duignan (1985) recommend that progress is assessed one hour after admission to the labour ward then one to two hourly thereafter. Although, conventionally a minimum of 2 hours is required to diagnose arrest of cervical dilatation (Cohen & Brennan 1995), there are those who believe that one hour is sufficient (Bottoms et al 1981, Friedman & Neff 1987), particularly if the examinations have been performed by the same practitioner. Studd, Cardozo and Gibb (1982) advised three hourly assessments; and Cardozo and Studd (1985) recommended three to four hourly examinations. A survey of English labour ward policies by Garcia, Garforth and Ayers (1986) found that 70 percent of units had policies on cervical assessment, 36% of which had a fixed routine and 34% had a more flexible approach. In the units with a fixed policy, over half had a four-hourly policy, 15% had an 'at least four-hourly policy' and 5% had a 'not greater than four-hourly policy'. These variations highlight the inconsistencies in labour management.

Midwives need to treat every woman sensitively and ask the following questions prior to every vaginal examination:

- Is this examination really necessary? (i.e. are the findings of this examination going to influence the care I provide and/or benefit this woman?)

- Have I explained the procedure adequately to this woman?
- Will the examination take place at an optimum time for this woman (e.g. following analgesia, micturition)?
- Is this woman in the optimum environment (e.g. the most comfortable position, curtains drawn and door closed, engaged sign on the door, door locked, necessary attendants only in the room, partner given the option to leave)?
- Have I explained my findings in a way in which this woman understands?
- Have I accurately documented my findings in this woman's records?

Assessing progress

Labour is initiated, and progress maintained, by the contractions of the uterus (Crowther et al 1989). Confirmation of progress, however, is usually determined by the identification of increasing cervical dilatation and cervical effacement. The cervix plays an important part in the progress of labour and the generation of intrauterine pressure (Olah et al 1993). Correction of prolonged labour is therefore dependant on regular cervical assessment. However this measure, although generally accepted, is not precise or reliable. Factors such as the variation in estimation of cervical dilatation between practitioners and in estimations carried out by the same practitioner demonstrate the high level of subjectivity in this test. As pointed out by Downe (1994), midwives and obstetricians can all agree that a major degree of placenta praevia or a clear cephalopelvic disproportion should be classified as abnormal. However, there is little consensus concerning the labouring primigravidae who has made slow but steady progress for 20 hours in the absence of maternal or fetal distress.

The acceptable rate of cervical dilatation has also been debated (Beazley & Kurjak 1972, Cowan et al 1982, Friedman 1955, Gibb et al 1984; National Consensus Conference on Aspects of Caesarean section Planning Committee 1985, O'Driscoll et al 1973), with the majority of midwives currently being guided by the World Health Organization's (1994) recommendation of 1 cm/hour.

Many studies have described the duration and velocity of labour in various groups of women (Cardozo et al 1982, Friedman 1955, Hendricks et al 1970; O'Driscoll et al 1970; Tuck et al 1983). These descriptions range from Duignan et al (1975) who described the total duration of labour for a primigravidae being 5.6 hours to the World Health Organization (1994) suggesting that 18 hours is more appropriate. Albers et al (1996), in her study of 1473 low risk women at term, found that active labour lasted longer than is widely appreciated, with the mean length for nulliparous being 7.7 hours and for multiparous being 5.7 hours (statistical limits 19.4 and 13.7 hours, respectively).

In the struggle to balance early diagnosis and correction of prolonged labour with the use of unnecessary intervention, no consensus has yet been reached amongst midwives and obstetricians to provide a workable definition of normality. Perhaps it is time to acknowledge that the individuality of each woman makes it inappropriate to use objective markers, such as cervical dilatation, in isolation. In the absence of any fetal compromise, a more flexible approach to supporting labouring women is required which takes into account her physical and emotional wellbeing as well as her verbal and non verbal communications.

Role of the Partogram

It is unsurprising, given the lack of consensus on labour progress, that the introduction of the partogram (or partograph) was welcomed by midwives and obstetricians. The partogram is now used worldwide to enable practitioners to record intrapartum details in a pictorial way and to enable the early detection of pathological labour. Most partograms have three distinct sections where observations are entered on maternal condition, fetal condition and labour progress; this last section assists in the detection of prolonged labour.

The first obstetrician to provide a tool for recording individual labours was Friedman (1954) following his study of the cervical dilatation of 100 African primigravidae at term. These women were given frequent rectal examinations and their progress was recorded in centimetres of dilatation per hour, producing a slope resembling a sigmoid curve. This became know as the cervicograph. In an attempt to utilize midwives and assistants extensively in a hospital in Zimbabwe (then Rhodesia), where doctors were in short supply, Philpott (1972) developed a partogram from this original cervicograph. This provided a practical tool for recording all intrapartum details, not just cervical dilatation. An 'alert line' was added following the results of a prospective study of 624 women (Philpott & Castle 1972a). The alert line was straight not curved and was a modification of the mean rate of cervical dilatation of the slowest 10% of primigravid women who were in the active phase of labour. This line represented a progress rate of 1 cm per hour. Should a woman's cervical dilatation progress more slowly the graph would be shown to cross this alert line and arrangements were made to transfer her from a peripheral unit to a central unit where prolonged labour could be managed actively.

The next stage of partogram development was the introduction of an 'action line', four hours to the right of the alert line (Philpott& Castle 1972b). This line was developed on the premise that correction of primary inefficient uterine action would lead to a vaginal birth.

More than twenty years after its introduction, and using a partogram adapted from that formulated by Philpott and Castle (1972a, 1972b), the World Health Organization (1994) conducted a prospective study of 35 484 women in South East Asia and concluded that the partogram was a necessary tool in the management of labour and recommended its universal application.

There are many different partogram designs. However much of the available evidence of their effectiveness is methodologically weak (Neilson et al 2003). Midwives must especially bear in mind that the data derived from previous research has been population dependant and current partograms do not always allow for the individuality of each woman. By assuming that all women will progress in labour at the same rate, unthinking use of the partogram could have adverse effects such as increased rates of artificial rupture of the membranes, oxytocin augmentation and use of analgesia resulting in a more negative labour experience. In the light of such potential hazards the partogram can only ever be a guide to intrapartum wellbeing.

The process of maintaining records can act as a barrier to effective communication between midwife and woman. However, if used correctly, the partogram can assist midwives to compile efficient and comprehensive records. There is some evidence to suggest that midwives find the partogram to have practical benefits in terms of ease of use, time management, continuity of care and educational assistance (Lavender & Malcolmson 1999). These positive aspects may contribute to improving maternal and fetal outcomes. On the other hand, it has also been reported that the partogram's status within some obstetric units is such that they may restrict clinical practice, reduce midwife autonomy and limit the flexibility to treat each woman as an individual (Lavender & Malcolmson 1999), factors which could also impact on clinical and psychological outcomes. Unfortunately, the partogram can be used to dictate and constrain practice as opposed to inform and support it. The partogram is just one of the many tools available to help identify when there are deviations from the normal. Used incorrectly, it can lead to a cascade of unnecessary intervention. In our opinion, one of the fundamental problems with the partogram is the emphasis on routinely plotting cervical dilatation. This makes the vaginal examination the focal point of progress and detracts from the individual woman. Although, in many units, regular vaginal examinations are common practice, an experienced midwife will also measure progress in other ways, such as by abdominal palpation to find out how the baby's descent into the mother's pelvis is going, the way a woman is moving, the noises she is making and her facial expressions.

ASSESSMENT OF FETAL WELLBEING IN LABOUR

We listen to the fetal heart in labour to screen for hypoxia in the fetus. This can be done by electronic fetal monitoring (either periodic or continuous) or intermittent auscultation. The evidence indicates that the use of intermittent auscultation in labour is associated with a higher rate of spontaneous vaginal birth and that the outcome for the baby is not generally compromised (Royal College of Obstetricians and Gynaecologists 2001). We should be aware, when deciding how to monitor the baby's heart beat in labour, that the method chosen might affect not only the overall normal vaginal birth rate, but also the nature of the birth and a woman's particular experience. Whatever method chosen the most effective monitor is the constant presence of a competent and attentive midwife who can interpret the data relating to fetal wellbeing health.

The use of continuous electronic fetal monitoring in labour makes the experience more like that of an intensive care unit experience, limits mobility in the woman and may deflect attention from the labouring woman to the monitor. Belts, transducers and pressure gauges are extremely uncomfortable and need constant reapplication with movement of the mother or the baby.

Moreover, the accuracy of fetal monitoring in screening for fetal distress has been questioned. Interpretation of the cardiotocograph (CTG) is often inaccurate. Electronic fetal monitoring has a low specificity, this means that a large number of babies are diagnosed from their fetal heart rate trace as having fetal distress but do not have this problem. There are also babies for whom no fetal distress is identified but in whom it actually exists (false negative results). For years, there has been considerable efforts made to improve the reliability of interpretation of CTGs through professional clinical education, yet the problems remain. Given that electronic fetal monitoring is a screening tool that is more likely to be accurate in high-risk pregnancies its routine use in low-risk pregnancies increases the problems of mis-diagnosis, and a higher rate of operative delivery, including caesarean section.

The MIDIRS Informed Choice leaflet on fetal heart rate monitoring in labour (MIDIRS 2004f) includes the following information on electronic fetal monitoring (EFM), summarized from the best evidence:

When compared with intermittent auscultation:

- EFM, even when combined with fetal blood sampling (FBS), has not been shown to reduce perinatal mortality.
- EFM, even when combined with FBS, has not been shown to reduce the incidence of cerebral palsy. Indeed, what evidence we have indicates a slight increase in cerebral palsy among infants who have been monitored.

- EFM alone increases the caesarean section rate by about 160%. When used with FBS the rate of caesarean section increases by 30%.
- EFM reduces the rate of neonatal seizures. However, those babies suffering neonatal seizures did not have any long-term problems, suggesting that the type of seizures prevented were not those which presage cerebral palsy.
- EFM increases the operative vaginal delivery rate by 30%.
- There is no evidence of any benefit arising from the use of EFM in relation to the number of babies with low or very low Apgar scores or admissions to SCBU.

A review and meta-analysis of nine trials, including 18 561 women of fetal monitoring in labour indicates similar findings. There was no difference in Apgar score between groups receiving electronic fetal monitoring and intermittent auscultation, an increase in the rate of seizure in association with intermittent auscultation, and a higher incidence of operative delivery in association with electronic fetal monitoring (Thacker et al 2004).

The National Institute for Clinical Excellence's guidelines (Royal College of Obstetricians and Gynaecologists 2001) for Electronic Fetal Monitoring (EFM) made the following recommendations:

Use of EFM:

- Current evidence does not support the use of admission CTG in low-risk pregnancy.
- For a woman who is healthy and has had an otherwise uncomplicated pregnancy, intermittent auscultation should be offered and recommended in labour.
- Continuous fetal monitoring should be offered and recommended for high-risk pregnancies where there is an increased risk of perinatal death, cerebral palsy or even perinatal death.
- Continuous fetal monitoring should be used where oxytocin is being used.
- Continuous EFM should be offered and recommended in pregnancies previously monitored with intermittent auscultation:
- If there is evidence of a baseline less than 110 beats per minute (bpm) or greater than 160 bpm.

- If there is evidence on auscultation of any decelerations.
- If any intrapartum risk factors develop.

Care of women:

- Women should be given evidence-based information to make informed choices regarding monitoring.
- Women should have the same level of care and support regardless of mode of monitoring.
- Clear lines of communication and consistent terminology is required to convey urgency regarding fetal wellbeing.
- Prior to any fetal monitoring, maternal pulse should be palpated simultaneously with FHR to differentiate between maternal and fetal heart rates.
- If fetal death is suspected, viability should be confirmed by ultrasound.
- With regard to intermittent auscultation:
  - the FHR should be auscultated for one complete minute beginning immediately after the end of a contraction, repeated every 15 minutes during first stage and every 5 minutes in the second stage;
  - any intrapartum events that may affect the FHR should be noted contemporaneously in the maternal notes, signed and the time noted.

With regard to the conduct of EFM:

- the date and time of clocks on the EFM machine should be correctly set;
- traces should be labelled with the mother's name, date and hospital number;
- any intrapartum events that may affect the FHR should be noted contemporaneously on the EFM trace, signed and the date noted (e.g. vaginal examination);
- any member of staff who is asked to provide an opinion on a trace should note their findings on both the trace and maternal case notes, together with time and signature;
- following the birth, the care-giver should sign and note the date, time and mode of birth on the EFM trace;
- the EFM trace should be stored securely with the maternal notes.

SUPPORTING A WOMAN TO CHOOSE WHICH METHOD OF FETAL MONITORING TO USE IN LABOUR

We feel the following hints may help to give you information to discuss with a woman when she is deciding which method of monitoring to use for her baby's heart beat.

- If the woman has no objection to its use, a Doppler device (Sonicaid) will aid in listening to the fetal heart and can be used easily when she adopts different positions for labour and birth.
- During your first assessment of a woman in labour, palpate carefully to determine the place where the heart will be heard (over the baby's shoulder and on the same side as the back).
- Auscultate the fetal heart while the woman is recumbent (but not flat on her back) so that you know where to find it when the woman is mobile and in different positions.
- Count the heart rate during a contraction as well as afterwards, listening for any accelerations, or decelerations; note the baseline rate.
- Record all values carefully.
- Apply the learning and knowledge you have gained from the interpretation of CTGs to interpret the fetal heart rate (Fig. 16.2).

One of the advantages of intermittent auscultation is that it encourages a regular direct contact

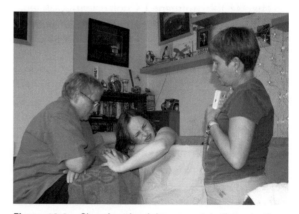

Figure 16.2 Choosing the right moment to listen to the fetal heart.

between midwife and mother through touch and words. It provides an opportunity for the midwife to give feedback to the labouring woman and to think about what she is assessing. It is also a point at which to use encouragement and support, for example 'Your baby sounds fine'.

In contrast, using a monitor for continuous electronic monitoring can allow the midwife to absent herself from the woman. In some delivery suites CTGs from individual rooms are relayed onto central monitoring systems, to allow surveillance from outside of the individual rooms. Such systems work well if used as a way of minimizing the number of clinicians who may wish to enter a room for fetal heart surveillance. However, the attending midwives need to prevent themselves from falling into the trap of monitoring women from a distance. It is also vital to ensure that the attention of all who enter and stay in the room is on the woman rather than the screen. Midwives can help to minimize this risk by discussing with a woman what the fetal heart monitor is recording and what it means, in the same way as she would if she were carrying out intermittent auscultation.

MOBILITY AND POSITIONS FOR LABOUR AND BIRTH

Most women being cared for in hospital will stay in bed during labour. In England and Wales 74% of women adopt a semi-recumbent position for birth (MIDIRS 2004e). This is to a great extent because of the frequent use of continuous electronic fetal monitoring, which fundamentally restrains mobility and alters the experience of labour. Yet the freedom to move and to adopt different positions is an important way of helping women to cope with the pain of labour and may aid progress (Fig. 16.3).

Research into the effect of maternal position in labour on outcome is limited. Many of the trials conducted during the first stage are methodologically poor, and most of the second-stage trials have focused only on the use of birth chairs (MIDIRS 2004e). The limited evidence available suggests that a woman being upright in the first stage of labour results in:

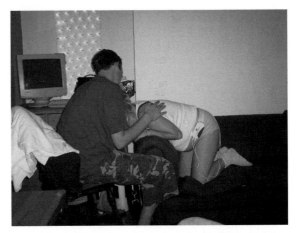

Figure 16.3   Mobility is important in labour.

- less severe pain;
- less need for epidural anaesthesia and for narcotics;
- lower rate of loss of beat-to-beat variability in the fetal heart rate;
- reduced length of the first stage of labour.

No measurable effects were detected on:

- rate of caesarean delivery;
- fetal or neonatal outcomes.

However, importantly many women in the included trials did not comply with their allocated position (Gupta et al 1989, Waldenstrom & Godvall 1991).

THE SECOND STAGE

A systematic review (Gupta & Hofmeyr 2004) of 19 trials of varying methodological quality assessed the effects of position on the second stage of labour. Use of any upright or lateral position was compared with supine or lithotomy positions. Systematic review of these trials shows that being upright in second stage results in:

- less intolerable pain;
- a shorter second stage of labour;
- fewer abnormal heart rate patterns;
- fewer assisted births;
- fewer episiotomies;
- a small increase in second degree tears;
- more women with a blood loss over 500 mL (in women using birth chairs or stools).

HELPING WOMEN TO CHOOSE APPROPRIATE POSITIONS AND MOVE FREELY

A large prospective study, which compared women who mobilized in labour with women who did not, found significantly less continuous fetal heart monitoring and use of narcotic analgesia, fewer operative deliveries and more spontaneous births in the mobile group (Albers et al 1997). However, the MIDIRS leaflet (MIDIRS 2004e) comments that while 87% of units claim that women are 'allowed' to adopt whatever position they choose, the great majority of women spend all their labour either recumbent or semi-recumbent.

This may be because of the strong cultural norm of lying down for labour and birth. Furthermore, some women may not intuitively mobilize within an unfamiliar environment and may need the midwife to give them 'permission' to do so. In this situation, the midwife needs to positively encourage and support women in adopting different positions and moving freely. Encouragement is given by suggestions, the use of props, creating enough space and active encouragement; the key is assessing what is best for the individual woman and her circumstances. However, encouraging women to move about, and to adopt the most comfortable positions, should not be taken to extremes. Some women will want and need some rest during labour, often when in advanced labour, so rest and activity should be kept in balance. The woman should never lie flat on her back because of the danger of aortocaval compression and compromised uterine blood flow.

HELPING WOMEN TO COPE WITH THE PAIN OF LABOUR

The pain associated with labour has been described as one of the most intense forms of pain that can be experienced (Melzack 1984). The purpose of pain includes that it can make a contribution to a woman's transition to motherhood, empowering her through a sense of her own achievement. Pain is also seen as being of benefit in triggering the neurohormonal cascades that keep birth normal. Given the potential complications of many of the methods of analgesia, and for the potential of a

positive birth experience without invasive methods of pain relief when adequate support is provided, exploring how midwives may both help women cope with the pain of labour and help keep birth normal is a topic of fundamental concern.

Whilst on the one hand the allure of pain relief in labour is almost irresistible in a society that sees it as a major benefit of modern living (Leap 1997), on the other, the complete removal of pain does not necessarily mean a more satisfying birth experience for women. The belief that the normal pain of childbirth is something to be erased at all costs deserves scrutiny. Leap (1997) describes what she calls the menu approach to pain relief where women are provided with a list of options. In her interviews with 10 midwives who had developed a rationale for not routinely offering pain relief to women in labour, she describes consistent themes. These include the importance of differentiating between normal and abnormal pain of childbirth, and the idea that most women can cope with the pain of labour aided by the body's endogenous opiates, which are stimulated by pain.

Women in labour vary in their need for pain relief and their choices may change during the course of their labour. Effective and satisfactory pain management needs to be individualized for each woman (Smith et al 2004, p. 2) and this means providing women with a range of options and strategies from which they may choose. In work carried out by one of the authors (TL), on women's views of factors contributing to a positive birth experience, women reported the co-existence of both positive and negative feelings towards pain in labour (Lavender et al 1998, p. 42–43). Women in this study used various methods of pain relief for their very individual needs, at different times during their labour. The following quotes are from women who had experienced different forms of pain relief to help them cope with the pain associated with labour and illustrate each woman's individuality:

> I enjoyed being in the [birthing water] pool. The warm water helped with the pain and helped me to be more mobile. The aromatherapy was enjoyable. It helped build a more relaxed atmosphere and made me feel in control.

The epidural was extremely effective. I would definitely recommend it to other women. Being pain free meant I could sleep which meant my labour seemed shorter and I wasn't too tired to push the baby out.

The purpose of this section is to highlight the variety of options available, and evidence of the advantages and disadvantages of the various possibilities for pain relief in respect of keeping birth normal. We discuss four categories of pain relief, the first of which 'comfort measures and complimentary medicines and practices' is the broadest. The use of nitrous oxide, intra-muscular opioids and epidural analgesia are also discussed. The benefits of continuity of caregivers during pregnancy and birth, and continuous one-to-one labour support, which can also help women cope with pain during labour, as discussed earlier in the chapter.

COMFORT MEASURES AND COMPLIMENTARY MEDICINES AND PRACTICES

The broad categories of comfort measures and complimentary medicines are not mutually exclusive. The MIDIRS Informed Choice Leaflet 'Non-epidural strategies for pain relief in labour' (MIDIRS 2004a) uses the term 'comfort measures' to encompass the use of maternal positioning/activity, massage/touch, application of heat or cold, use of water, cognitive therapies, hypnosis, acupuncture, acupressure and transcutaneous electrical nerve stimulation (TENS). The Cochrane Review of Complimentary and Alternative Therapies for Pain Management in Labour states the most commonly cited complementary medicines and practices associated with providing pain management in labour can be categorized into mind-body interventions (e.g. yoga, relaxation therapies), alternative medical practice (e.g. homoeopathy, traditional Chinese medicine), manual healing methods (e.g. massage, reflexology), pharmacologic and biological treatments, bioelectromagnetic applications (e.g. magnets and herbal medicines) (Smith et al 2004, p. 2). For the purposes of this chapter, we use the terms 'comfort measures' and 'complimentary practices' to mean alternatives to conventional medical analgesics. These alternatives work in a number of different ways:

- masking pain by the use of alternative sensations (e.g. applying heat and cold, for example using an ice pack or a hot water bottle) or deep massage (e.g. hard pressure to or massage of the sacral area during contractions);
- soothing pain and helping the woman adopt different positions with greater ease (e.g. by using water in a shower, bath or birthing pool);
- affecting the transmission of impulses along nerve pathways (e.g. transcutaneous nerve stimulation; TENS);
- acting as a diversion so that a woman is distracted from the experience of her pain.

Despite the increasing use of comfort measures and complimentary therapies the research evidence supporting their use is limited. There is a lack of well-designed randomized controlled trials (RCTs) to evaluate the effectiveness of these therapies for pain management in labour. The data currently available suggest that only hypnosis and acupuncture may be helpful, with the efficacy of aromatherapy and other non-conventional medical analgesics yet to be established (Smith et al 2004, p. 9). Furthermore, Tiran (2004) cautions midwives not to use complimentary therapies unless appropriately trained. Nonetheless comfort measures and cognitive strategies have a long history of use in practice, where pain has been eased in individuals with very little or no potential to do harm. The MIDIRS informed choice leaflet for non-epidural strategies for pain relief during labour (MIDIRS 2004b) lists the following shared perceived advantages of comfort measures and cognitive strategies:

- short or no time lag between deciding to use and putting the measure/strategy into effect (water pools are the exception);
- can be combined or sequenced with other pain relief options, which can increase effectiveness;
- offer unparalleled flexibility and variety. They can be used;
  - in the woman's home;
  - in combination with pain medication;
  - while awaiting the administration of epidural analgesia;
  - in circumstances where pain medication is not advisable or the birth is imminent;

- have no effect on state of consciousness;
- do not interfere with labour progress or a woman's ability to push;
- foster a sense of accomplishment and capability. Unlike pain relief, this is a key element for a satisfying experience (Hodnett 2002);
- may enable a woman to avoid pain medication during labour and therefore the possibility of encountering adverse effects of such medication, e.g. nausea and drowsiness;
- may allow labouring women to postpone or limit medication use. Pain medications are more likely to cause problems if multiple doses are taken, and when different types of drugs are used, and/or used over many hours;
- can be immediately discontinued if they fail to help or in the unlikely event that they cause a problem. This may avoid the need for other drugs and procedures to remedy unwanted effects, e.g. the need for anti-emetics;
- do not require medical staff to administer and monitor;.
- are inexpensive or cost nothing, with the exception of water pools, tub baths and showers which require considerable capital expenditure to install.

When offering women one or more of the many alternatives to conventional medical analgesics the most important factor to consider is the individual woman herself and her preferences and choices. For example, the results of one small RCT of periodic massage by partners versus usual care showed that women who receive massage by their partners report less anxiety and pain (Field et al 1997). However, many women may not want to be touched at all and simply want to be left to close their eyes, shut out external stimuli and turn themselves inwards during a contraction. Kitzinger (1997) describes the 'birth dance' that women do when they are left to their own devices and encouraged to move. Rocking, hip circling and adjustments of position may help to relieve pain and aid the progress of the baby through the birth canal.

The midwife's role is to ascertain what the woman wants and be sensitive to the possibility that she may change her mind during the course of labour. The midwife can assess these needs through verbal and non-verbal communication.

Furthermore, she can renegotiate pain management during discussions following clinical assessments. Being openly receptive to changes in women's decisions can limit potential feelings of self-reproach that original plans and expectations have changed.

Many women intuitively initiate the use of water to cope with the pains of labour by having a bath or shower at home before seeking the care of a midwife. A systematic review of eight trials (Cluett et al 2004) indicated a statistically significant reduction in the use of pain relief, overall. Reviews of existing evidence conclude that more large scale research is needed to explore the physiological effects, clinical outcomes and economic impact of water use (Woodward & Kelly 2004). In practice, women clearly find water helpful to relieve pain in the first stage (Fig. 16.4).

NITROUS OXIDE INHALATION

Nitrous oxide inhalation, also known as 'gas and air' or 'Entonox' (at 50/50 administration), can be used alone or to supplement other methods of analgesia. A systematic review of eleven randomized controlled trials concluded 'nitrous oxide is not a potent labour analgesic, it is safe for parturient women, their newborns, and healthcare workers in attendance during its administration' (Rosen 2002). It appears to provide adequately effective pain relief for many women, and a British survey by Carstoniu et al (1994) found women reported high satisfaction with its use. The advantages of nitrous oxide include that its is inexpen-

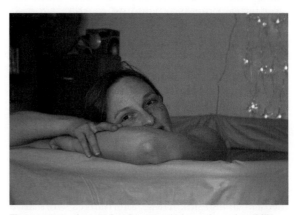

Figure 16.4   Immersion in water helps pain and mobility.

sive, easy to administer, has a rapid onset and rapid termination (Rosen 2002). However, many studies have found that timing is crucial to the successful pain relief. The MIDIRS Informed Choice Leaflet (MIDIRS 2004b) acknowledges the limitations of existing research evidence and lists a number of perceived advantages and disadvantages based on observation in clinical practice. The perceived advantages of nitrous oxide inhalation that may help keep birth normal include:

■ it increases the woman's sense of personal control as it is self-administered;
■ it does not interfere with labour progress or ability to push;
■ it may allow women to postpone or avoid opioids or epidural analgesia.

One of the perceived disadvantages of nitrous oxide inhalation with regard to keeping birth normal is that it restricts mobility because of the mechanics of using it and because it can cause drowsiness, dizziness, nausea and vomiting.

INTRA-MUSCULAR OPIOIDS

Pethidine is the most widely used intra-muscular opioid for the relief of labour pain (Elbourne Wiseman 2004). Studies of pethidine have, however, consistently cast doubt on its effectiveness for maternal pain relief and raised concerns about its potential maternal, fetal and neonatal side-effects. A review of twenty trials comparing intra-muscular opioids found that dissatisfaction with labour pain relief varied widely among trials (27–87%) (Bricker & Lavender 2002). These concerns have been translated into a search for alternative opioids, including partial agonists (meptazinol, pentazinol, nalbuphine, butorphanol), phenazocine, weak opioids (tramadol), and the potent fast acting opioids (fentanyl and remifentanil). However, a systematic review of forty-eight trials of parenteral opioids for pain relief in labour suggested the risks associated with normal physiological changes in labour might be exacerbated, e.g. respiratory alkalosis, increased gastric acid secretion, decreased gastrointestinal motility. The review found that when different opioids, different doses of the same opioid, or different modes of administration of opioids were compared, there was no impact on

the length of labour, or frequency and type of obstetric intervention (Bricker & Lavender 2002, p. S105). However, three studies of the effects of pethidine on neonatal behaviour have reported adverse effects, which included decreased alertness, and inhibition of breastfeeding initiation (Hodgkinson et al 1978, Kuhnert et al 1985, Righard & Alade 1990).

EPIDURAL ANALGESIA

Epidural analgesia involves injection of local anaesthetic into the lumbar region of the spine, close to the nerves that transmit the pain associated with uterine contractions. The research evidence relating to epidurals is far from adequate, although major adverse effects are rare (MIDIRS 2004c). Epidural analgesia was used by approximately 24% of women for their labour and/or at the time of birth in the UK in 2000–2001 (Department of Health 2002). Studies have found that women express greater satisfaction when the analgesia is administered as a combined spinal-epidural block. This method of administration of analgesia does not cause complete loss of sensation in the woman's legs and feet and therefore has the advantage that she can still be ambulant if she wishes. However, whilst women have expressed satisfaction with this method of pain relief it has been associated with the occurrence of fetal bradycardia, although to date there is no evidence of an increase in adverse fetal outcome (MIDIRS 2004c).

A patient controlled epidural is another option, which has the advantage of empowering a woman to administer her own analgesia as she feels she needs. In my experience (TL), the fact that the woman herself is able to control her own experience of pain increases her ability to cope, thus reducing the amount of analgesia she requires. Women who have used the patient controlled epidural analgesia have expressed satisfaction with this method of relieving the pain associated with labour without any apparent neonatal problems (Stienstra 2000, van der Vyver & Halpern 2001).

Current best evidence does not indicate that the use of epidural analgesia results in increased rates of caesarean section. However, an increase in the length of the first and second stage of labour, an increase in the need for oxytocin, an increase in the incidence of fetal malposition and an increase in the use of instrumental vaginal delivery if the analgesic block is maintained beyond the first stage of labour is indicated (Howell 2004). Halpern et al (1998) suggest all of the following outcomes are likely to be interrelated:

- An increase in the use of oxytocin to augment labour.
- A longer labour.
- An instrumental birth.

The latest version of the Cochrane Review of Epidural Versus Non-epidural Analgesia for Pain Relief in Labour (Howell 2004) concludes that given the current evidence of the effects of epidural analgesia on the dynamics of labour, a mother receiving epidural analgesia may not be considered to be having a 'normal labour'. However, it does not follow that women who choose epidurals and deliver vaginally do not consider their births to be 'normal', or that care-givers should deny women analgesia if they need it. There are a number of women who, even if they receive appropriate support, will still need anal-gesia in labour, and if they are denied it, may be traumatized by the experience of labour and birth.

It is best to have full discussions about pain relief and possible complications before labour starts. If possible, this should be between the woman and the care-givers who are likely to be with her in labour (Royal College of Obstetricians and Gynaecologists 1995). A woman will some-times decide in the antenatal period that she wishes to avoid analgesia or epidural anaesthesia; then, during labour, change her mind. If the midwife knows the woman ahead of time, and feels that the woman she is caring for may regret it afterwards if she changes her mind about pain relief in labour, she may want to encourage her to try to cope without it. This particularly applies if events in labour are right, for example not too prolonged. This is one of the trickiest areas of judgement for midwives in labour care. It involves a careful balance of supporting and encouraging the woman to manage without an epidural and knowing when the decision should be changed.

In the evaluation of One-to-One midwifery (Fig. 16.1), there was a significant reduction in the rate of uptake of combined spinal epidurals in the One-to-One group. However, women in the One-to-One group generally felt satisfied with their pain relief, and more found the experience of birth positive. More in the One-to-One group than in the control group said that birth was 'hard work but wonderful' (McCourt & Page 1996). The test of an appropriate avoidance of epidural anaesthesia is whether or not the woman feels supported and that she is involved in decision-making. Certainly, epidurals should not be denied when they are really needed and it is important to bear in mind current evidence suggests many of the effects of epidural analgesia can be minimized by the responses of midwifery, obstetric and anaesthetic staff. For example, consideration of the degree of the block before the second stage of labour; the appropriate use of Syntocinon in the first or second stage of labour; delayed pushing in the second stage; and the use of different drugs or methods of administration of the epidural block (Howell 2004) should be considered to help keep birth as 'normal' as possible.

Current evidence suggests women should be supported in such a way that they are less likely to need analgesia, particularly the more invasive methods such as epidural or combined spinal epi-dural, if we are to reduce the rates of operative delivery. Rather than use the title 'analgesia for labour' for this section, we intentionally used the phrase 'helping women to cope with the pain of labour' because all of the studies that have evalu-ated the provision of some form of extra support for women in labour have resulted in a lower use of analgesia and are often associated with higher satisfaction (Green et al 1998). Moreover, complete pain relief is not necessarily associated with greater satisfaction (Morgan et al 1982) but is linked to the extent to which a woman feels in control of her experience (Green et al 1988, Simkin 1992). Indeed, women who have coped with the pain of labour without interventions such as epidural analgesia may feel proud of their achievement if they feel that decisions have been within their control. Thus, it seems that rather than asking the question 'Should all women be offered analgesia for labour?', we should be focusing instead on the provision of adequate support.

CONCLUSION

In this chapter, we have not attempted to give a comprehensive overview of all aspects of care for labour and birth, nor have we examined clinical decision-making, which is in itself an important aspect of keeping birth 'normal'. Instead, we have chosen to suggest ways to help women to cope with the pain of labour, and have advised monitoring the fetal heart by intermittent auscultation, to increase a woman's likelihood of a non-operative vaginal birth. Furthermore, we have critically reviewed current practices of defining and assessing labour. We have also presented a summary of strong evidence indicating the need for continuous support for women during labour. The approach to support in labour we described requires integration of a constant presence, personal sensitivity and a calm atmosphere. It will be made much more likely if there is a good continuity-of-care scheme in place. Being able to support a woman in labour is a privilege that should never be taken for granted. If we remember this, we will always do our best for each individual woman. We hope that this chapter has given at least a limited indication of some of the practical ways in which midwives may help women to 'keep birth normal' (Fig. 16.5).

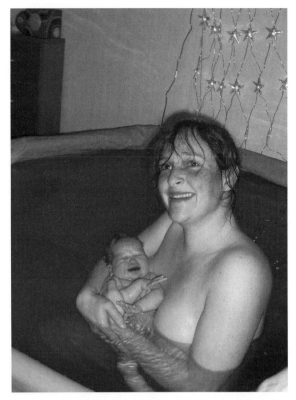

Figure 16.5 A sense of triumph.

POINTERS FOR PRACTICE

- An important function of the midwife is to confirm the normal and to support and protect physiological processes and healthy outcomes.
- The use of intermittent auscultation to monitor the fetal heart rate is associated with a lower operative delivery rate.
- Current guidelines recommend that intermittent auscultation should be used for labours at the normal end of the continuum.

- The use of epidural anaesthesia is associated with an increase in the operative delivery rate and needs a further evaluation of long-term outcomes for both mother and baby.
- Effective support is associated with a decrease in the need for analgesia.
- Midwives should stay with women in labour and use words of praise and encouragement, as well as comforting touch.

References

Albers L L, Anderson D, Cragin L 1997 The relationship of ambulation in labor to operative delivery. Journal Nurse Midwifery 42(1): 4–8

Albers L L, Schiff M, Gorwoda J G 1996 The length of active labour in normal pregnancies. Obstetrics and Gynaecology 87(3): 355–359

Amu O, Rajendran S, Bolaji I 1998 Maternal choice alone should not determine method of delivery. British Medical Journal 317: 463–465

Anderson T 2002 Peeling back the lawyers: a new look at midwifery interventions. Role of midwife in encouraging normal birth and supporting women in labour. MIDIRS Midwifery Digest 12(2): 207

Audit Commission 1997 First class delivery: improving maternity services in England and Wales. Audit Commission, London, pp 1–98

Beazley J M, Kurjak A 1972 Influence of a partogram on the active management of labour. Lancet ii:348–351

Bergstrom L, Roberts J, Skillman L, Seidel J 1992 You'll feel me touching you, sweetie: vaginal examinations during the second stage of labor. Birth 19(1):10–18; discussion 19–20

BirthChoiceUK 2004 Normal births on the increase in England. Online. Available: www.BirthChoiceUK.com/NormalBirth.htm accesses February 2005

Bonovich L 1989 Recognising the onset of labor. Journal of Obstetrics, Gynaecology and Neonatal Nursing 19: 141–145

Bottoms S F, Sokol R J, Rosen M G 1981 Short arrest of cervical dilatation: A risk for maternal/fetal/infant morbidity. American Journal of Obstetrics and Gynecology 140: 108–116

Bricker L, Lavender T 2002 Parental opioids for labor pain relief: A systematic review. American Journal of Obstetrics and Gynaecology (186)5: S94–109

Cardozo L D, Gibb D M F, Studd J W, Vasant R V, Cooper D 1982 Predictive value of cervimetric labour patterns primigravidae. British Journal of Obstetrics and Gynaecology 89: 33–38

Cardozo L D, Studd J 1985 Abnormal labour patterns. In: Studd J. (ed.) The management of labour. Blackwell Scientific, London, pp 171–187

Carstoniu J, Levytam S, Norman P, Daly D, Katz J, Sandler A N 1994 Nitrous oxide in early labor. Safety and analgesic efficacy assessed by a double blind, placebo-controlled study. Anesthesiology 80: 30–35

Cluett E R, Nikodem V C, McCandlish R E et al 2004 Immersion in water in pregnancy, labour and birth. Cochrane Database of Systematic Reviews. Issue 1. Wiley, Chichester

Cochrane Library 2005 Online. Available: www.cochrane.org

Cohan W R, Brennan J 1995 Using and archiving the labor curves. Clinics in Perinatology 22: 855–874

Cowan D B, Van Middelkoop A, Philpott R H 1982 Intrauterine pressure studies in African nulliparae: normal labour progress. British Journal of Obstetrics and Gynaecology 89: 364–369

Crowther C, Enkin M, Kierse M. Brown I. 1989 Monitoring the progress of labour. In: Chalmers I, Enkin M, Kierse M (eds.) Effective care in pregnancy and childbirth, vol. II. Oxford University Press, Oxford

Department of Health 1993 Changing childbirth. Part 1. Report of the Expert Maternity Group (Cumberlege report). HMSO, London

Department of Health 2002 NHS maternity statistics, England 1998–99 to 2000–2001. Department of Health, London

Department of Health 2004 Maternity – national service framework for children. young people and maternity services 2004 reference 40498 Department of Health, London

Devane D 1996 Sexuality and midwifery. British Journal of Midwifery 4(8): 413–416

Downe S 1994 How average is normality? British Journal of Midwifery 2(7): 303–304

Downe S 2001 Defining normal birth. MIDIRS Midwifery Digest 11(2): S31–S33

Downe S, McCormick C, Beech B 2001 Labour interventions associated with normal birth. British Journal of Midwifery 9(10): 602–604

Duignan N 1985 Active management of labour. In: Studd J (ed.) The management of labour. Blackwell Scientific Publications, Oxford, pp 146–158

Duignan N M, Studd J W W, Hughes A O 1975 Characteristics of normal labour in different racial groups. British Journal of Obstetrics and Gynaecology 82(8): 593–601

Elbourne D, Wiseman R A 2004 Types of intra-muscular opioids for maternal pain relief in labour (Cochrane Review). In: Cochrane Library, Issue 3. Wiley, Chichester

Enkin M 1992 Do I do that? Do I really do that? Like that? Commentary. Birth 19(1): 19–20

Enkin M, Keirse M, Renfrew M, Neilson J P 1999 Effective care in pregnancy and childbirth. Oxford University Press, Oxford

Enkin, M, Keirse M J N C, Neilson J, Crowther C, Duley L, Hodnett E, Hofmeyr J 2000 A guide to effective care in pregnancy and childbirth. 3rd edn. Oxford University Press, Oxford

Field T, Hernandez-Reif M, Taylor S et al 1997 Labor pain is reduced by massage therapy. Journal of Psychosomatic Obstetrics and Gynaecology 18: 286–291

Flint C 1986 Sensitive Midwifery. Butterworth Heinemann, London

Friedman E A 1954 Graphic analysis of labour. American Journal of Obstetrics and Gynecology 68: 1568–1575

Friedman E A 1955 Primigravid labour – a graphicostatistical analysis. American Journal of Obstetrics and Gynecology 6: 567–589

Friedman E A, Neff R K 1987 Labor and delivery: impact on offspring. PSG, Littleton, MA

Garcia J, Garforth S, Ayers S 1986 Midwives confined? Labour ward policies and routines. Research and the Midwife Conference. Manchester. Proceedings, pp 2–30

Gee H, Glynn M 1997 The physiology and clinical management of labour. In: Henderson C, Jones K (eds) Essential Midwifery 9: 171–202

Gibb D M F, Arulkumaran S, Lun K C, Ratnam S S 1984 Characteristics of uterine activity in nulliparous labour. British Journal of Obstetrics and Gynaecology 91: 220–227

Gould D 2000 Normal labour: a concept analysis. Journal of Advanced Nursing 31(2): 418–427

Green J, Coupland B A, Kitzinger J 1988 Great expectations: a prospective study of women's expectations and experiences of childbirth. Child Care and Development Group, Cambridge

Green J, Curtis P, Price H, Renfrew M 1998 Continuing to care: the organization of midwifery services in the UK: a structured review of the evidence. Books for Midwives Press, Cheshire

Gupta J K, Brayshaw E M, Lilford R J 1989 An experiment of squatting birth. European Journal of Obstetrics, Gynaecology and Reproductive Biology 30: 217–220

Gupta J K, Hofmeyr G J 2004 Position for women during second stage of labour(Cochrane Review). In: The Cochrane Library, Issue 3, 2004. Wiley, Chichester

Halpern S H, Leighton B L, Ohlsson A et al 1998 Effect of epidural vs. parenteral opioid analgesia on the progress of labor: a meta-analysis. Journal of American Medical Association 280: 2105–2110

Hendricks C H, Brenner W E, Kraus G 1970 Normal cervical dilatation pattern in late pregnancy and labour. American Journal of Obstetrics and Gynecology 106: 1065–1082

Hodgkinson R, Bhatt M, Wang C N 1978 Double-blind comparison of the neurobehaviour of neonates following the administration of different doses of meperidine to the mother. Canadian Anaesthesiologists Society Journal 25: 405–411

Hodnett E D 2002 Pain and women's satisfaction with the experience of childbirth: a systematic review. American Journal of Obstetrics and Gynecology 186 (suppl): S1 60–72

Hodnett E D, Gates S, Hofmeyr G J, Sakala C 2004 Continuous support for women during childbirth (Cochrane Review). In: The Cochrane Library, Issue 3, 2004. Wiley, Chichester

Howell C J 2004 Epidural versus non-epidural analgesia for pain relief in labour (Cochrane Review). In: The Cochrane Library. Issue 3. Wiley, Chichester

Hunt S, Symonds A 1995 The social meaning of midwifery. Macmillan, Basingstoke

International Confederation of Midwives 2002 Midwives at ICM Council support promotion of vaginal birth rather than caesarean section. ICM press release, April 18, 2002 Online. Available: http://www.internationalmidwives.news.htm

Kirkham M 1989 Midwives and information giving during labour. In: Robinson S, Thompson A, (eds) Midwives, research and childbirth, Vol 1. Chapman & Hall, London

Kitzinger S 1997 Authoritative touch in childbirth. In: Davis-Floyd R E, Sargent C F (eds) Childbirth and authoritative knowledge: cross cultural perspectives. University of California Press, London

Koontz W L, Bishop E H 1982 Management of the latent phase of labour. Clinical Obstetrics and Gynecology 25:111–114

Kuhnert B R, Linn P L, Kuhnert P M 1985 Obstetric medication and neonatal behavior: current controversies. Clinical Perinatology 12: 423–440

Lavender T, Malcolmson L 1999 Is the partogram a help or a hindrance? An exploratory study of midwives views. Practising Midwife 2: 23–27

Lavender T, Walkinshaw S A 1998 Can midwives reduce postpartum psychological morbidity? A randomized trial. Birth 25: 215–219

Lavender T, Walkinshaw S A, Walton I 1998 A prospective study of women's views of factors contributing to a positive birth experience. Midwifery 15: 40–46

Leap N 1997 Birthwrite: being with women in pain – do midwives need to rethink their role? British Journal of Midwifery 3(5): 263

Leboyer F 1975 Birth without violence. Alfred A Knopf, New York

Macfarlane A, Mugford M, Henderson J, Furtado, Stevens J, Dunn A 2000 Obstetric intervention rates by mothers age and parity, NHS hospital births, England and Wales, 1967, 1975, 1980, England, 1980, 1985, 1994/5. Birth Counts: Statistics of Pregnancy and Childbirth. The Stationary Office, London, pp 535–536

McCourt C, Page L 1996 Report on the evaluation of one-to-one midwifery. Thames Valley University, London

McNiven P S, Williams J L, Hodnett E, Kaufman K, Hannah M E 1998 An early labour assessment program: a randomised, controlled trial. Birth 25(1): 5–10

Melzack R 1984 The myth of painless childbirth. Pain 19: 331–337

Menage J 1996 Post traumatic stress disorder following obstetric/gynaecological procedures. British Journal of Midwifery 4(10): 532–533

MIDIRS and NHS Centre for Reviews and Dissemination 2004a Informed choice for professionals: non-epidural strategies for pain relief during labour. MIDIRS, Bristol

MIDIRS and NHS Centre for Reviews and Dissemination 2004b Informed choice for professionals: the use of water during childbirth. MIDIRS, Bristol

MIDIRS and NHS Centre for Reviews and Dissemination 2004c Informed choice for professionals: the use of epidural analgesia for women in labour. MIDIRS, Bristol

MIDIRS and NHS Centre for Reviews and Dissemination 2004d Informed choice for professionals: support in labour. MIDIRS, Bristol

MIDIRS and NHS Centre for Reviews and Dissemination 2004e Informed choice for professionals: positions in labour and delivery. MIDIRS, Bristol

MIDIRS and NHS Centre for Reviews and Dissemination 2004f Informed choice for professionals: fetal heart rate monitoring in labour. MIDIRS, Bristol

Morgan B, Bulpitt C J, Clifton P, Lewis P J 1982 Analgesia and satisfaction in childbirth (the Queen Charlotte's 1,000 mother survey). Lancet ii: 808–810

National Consensus Conference on Aspects of Caesarean Section Planning Committee 1985 Criteria used for the diagnosis of dystocia. McMaster University, Hamilton, Canada

Neilson J P, Lavender T, Wray S, Quenby S 2003 Obstructed labour: reducing maternal death and disability during pregnancy. British Medical Bulletin 67: 191–204

Nursing and Midwifery Council 2004 Midwives rules and standards. NMC, London

O'Driscoll K, Foley M, Macdonald D 1984 Active management of labour as an alternative to caesarean section of dystocia. Obstetrics and Gynaecology 63: 485

O'Driscoll K, Jackson R J A, Gallagher J T 1970 Active management of labour and cephalopelvic disproportion. British Journal of Obstetrics and Gynaecology 77: 385–389

O'Driscoll K, Meagher D, Boylan P 1993 Active Management of labour. 3rd edn. Mosby Year Book, Aylesbury

O'Driscoll K, Stronge J M, Minogue M 1973 Active management of labour. British Medical Journal 3: 135–137

Oakley A 1983 Social consequences of obstetric technology: the importance of measuring 'soft' outcomes. Birth 10(2): 99–108

Olah K S, Gee H, Brown J S 1993 Cervical contractions: The response of the cervix to oxytocic stimulation in the latent phase of labour. British Journal of Obstetrics and Gynaecology 100: 635–640

Osmers R, Rath W, Pflanz M A, Kuhn W, Stuhlsatz H, Szeverenyi M 1993 Glycosaminoglycans in cervical connective tissue during pregnancy and parturition. Obstetrics and Gynecology 81: 88

Page L 2000 Keeping birth normal. In: Page L The new midwifery. 1st edn. Elsevier, London, pp 105–121

Philpott R H 1972 Graphic records in labour. British Medical Journal 4: 163

Philpott R H, Castle W M 1972a Cervicographs in the management of labour in primigravidae. Journal of Obstetrics and Gynaecology of the British Commonwealth 79: 592–598

Philpott R H, Castle W M 1972b Cervicographs in the management of labour in primigravidae. Journal of Obstetrics and Gynaecology of the British Commonwealth 79: 599–602

Porreco R 1990 Meeting the challenge of the rising caesarean birth rate. Obstetrics and Gynaecology 75: 133–136

Prendiville W J, Harding J E, Elbourne et al 1988 The Bristol third stage trial: active versus physiological management of third stage labour. British Medical Journal 297(6659):1295–1300

Richardson J A, Sutherland I A, Allen D W 1978 A cervimeter for continuous measurement of cervical dilatation in labour. Preliminary results. British Journal of Obstetrics and Gynaecology 85: 178–184

Righard L, Alade M O 1990 Effect of delivery room routines on success of first breast-feed. Lancet 336: 1105–1107

Robertson A 1997 The midwife companion: the art of support during birth. Ace Graphics, Sydney

Robohm J S, Buttenheim M 1996 The gynecological care experience of adult survivors of childhood sexual abuse: a preliminary investigation. Women Health 24(3): 59–75

Rogers J, Wood J 1996 The Hinchingbrooke third stage randomized controlled trial. In: The art and science of midwifery gives birth to a better future. Proceedings of the International Confederation of Midwives 24th Triennial Congress, 26–31 May, Oslo. ICM, London, pp 441–444

Rosen M A 2002 Nitrous oxide for relief of labor pain: A systematic review. American Journal of Obstetrics and Gynecology 186(5): S110–130

Royal College of Midwives 2004 Campaign for Normal Birth. Online. Available: www.rcmnormalbirth.net/ accessed February 2005

Royal College of Obstetricians and Gynaecologists 2001 The use of electronic fetal monitoring. Evidence based guideline no. 8. RCOG, London

Royal College of Obstetricians and Gynaecologists, Joint Working Group of the RCOG and RCM 1995 Communication standards obstetrics. RCOG, London

Simkin P 1992 Just another day in a woman's life? Part II: Nature and consistency of women's long term memories of their first birth experiences. Birth 19(2): 64–81

Smith C A, Collins C T, Cyna A M, Crowther C A 2004 Complementary and alternative therapies for pain management in labour (Cochrane Review). In: The Cochrane Library. Issue 3. Wiley, Chichester

Stienstra R 2000 Patient-controlled epidural analgesia or continuous infusion: advantages and disadvantages of different modes of delivering epidural analgesia for labour. Current Opinion Anaesthesia 13: 253–256

Studd J W, Cardozo L D, Gibb D M F 1982 The management of spontaneous labour. In: Studd J (ed.) Progress in obstetrics and gynaecology. Churchill Livingstone, London.

Thacker S B, Stroup D F, Chang M 2004 Continuous electronic heart rate monitoring for fetal assessment during labor (Cochrane Review). In: The Cochrane Library, Issue 3. Wiley, Chichester

Thomas J, Paranjothy S 2001 Royal College of Obstetricians and Gynaecologists Clinical Effectiveness Support Unit National Sentinel Caesarean Section Audit Report. RCOG, London

Tiran D 2004 Guest editorial. Viewpoint – midwives' enthusiasm for complementary therapies: a cause for concern? Complementary Therapies in Nursing Midwifery 10(2): 77–79

Towler J, Bramhall J 1986 Midwives in history and society. Croom Helm, London

Tuck S M, Cardozo L D, Studd J W, Gibb D M F 1983 Obstetric characteristics in different racial groups. British Journal of Obstetrics and Gynaecology 90: 892–897

van der Vyver M, Halpern S 2001 Patient-controlled epidural analgesia in labor. Techniques in Regional Anesthesia and Pain Management 5: 14–7

Waldenstrom U, Godvall K 1991 A randomised trial of birthing stool or conventional semi recumbent position for second stage labour. Birth 18: 5–10

Walker J 2001 Edgeware Birth Centre: what is the significance of this model of care? MIDIRS Midwifery Digest 11(1): 8–12

Weaver J 2000 Talking about caesarean section. MIDIRS Midwifery Digest 10(4): 487–490

Woodward J, Kelly S M 2004 A pilot study for a randomised controlled trial of waterbirth versus land birth. British Journal of Obstetrics and Gynaecology 111: 537–545

World Health Organization 1985 Appropriate technology for birth. Lancet 2: 436–437

World Health Organization 1997 Care in normal birth: a practical guide. Report of a technical working party. WHO, Geneva

World Health Organization Maternal Health and Safe Motherhood Programme 1994 World Health Organization partograph in management of labour. Lancet 343: 1399–1404

Chapter **17**

Being with Jane in childbirth: putting science and sensitivity into practice

Lesley Page

INTRODUCTION

Pregnancy and birth are a time of physical change, but also a time of transition for the woman and her family, who are taking on the new roles of being responsible for the newborn, and finding a new place in the generations of the family. Midwives work closely 'with the woman', ideally acting as a companion on the journey of childbirth, supporting her, providing expertise, while allowing the woman and her partner to make their own journey, identifying their needs for support, and discovering their own internal strength. Ideally the midwife works 'with' in the sense of being alongside, of ensuring that care is focused on the needs of the woman and her family, and importantly in relation to this chapter, is able to work in the best interests of the mother and baby and family. This implies the ability to identify the forms of care and treatments and place of care that are most likely to be effective, and that will leave the woman with positive memories of her care, and sense of self and family intact.

Earlier chapters have reconceptualized midwifery to focus on the aims and principles of what I have called the New Midwifery. These are simply:

- Working in a positive relationship with women.
- Being aware of the significance of pregnancy and birth and the early weeks of life as the start of human life and the new family.
- Avoiding harm by using the best information or evidence in practice.
- Having adequate skills and knowledge to deliver effective care and support.
- Promoting health and wellbeing.

In this chapter, using an updated version of Jane's care story, which was published in the first edition of The New Midwifery (Page 2000), I will show how these principles were put into practice in this situation, illustrating the importance of relationships in midwifery care, the most fundamental being the relationship between mother, baby, father and family. In turn the most effective and sensitive midwifery is provided when there is an effective relationship of trust between the woman and her midwife/midwives. This is often described as a relationship of partnership, where each works in a reciprocal way (see Chapter 4). An important aspect of this relationship with the woman is where the midwife is working for her in the sense of being able to do her best with the use of personal, intellectual, technical and clinical skills. It is crucial to attempt to do more good than harm.

Thus evidence-based midwifery implies not only the ability to find the best information to help the woman make decisions about her care, but also the ability to 'work with' in the sense of a reciprocal relationship, and the ability to make care personal responding to the individual needs, hopes, dreams and values of the woman and her family, as well as their medical needs.

The following care story describes the values and process of the new midwifery care, with a focus on the use of evidence, and the five steps of evidenced-based midwifery to demonstrate a way of using both science and sensitivity in practice.

EVIDENCE-BASED MIDWIFERY

Evidence-based midwifery draws on the principles of Changing Childbirth (Department of Health 1993), Effective Care in Pregnancy and Childbirth (Chalmers et al 1989) and Evidence-Based Medicine (Gray 1997, Sackett et al 1997, 2000). Evidence-based midwifery is a process of involving women in making decisions about their care and of finding and weighing up information to help make those decisions. This information is drawn from knowledge of the individual needs and values of the woman and her family, information taken from the clinical examination, and evidence about treatments, place of care, and forms of support. Evidence-based midwifery is founded on an understanding that not only physical safety, but also the personal integrity of the mother, baby and family are important outcomes. Our concern is not only with the short-term outcomes, but also with an understanding that care may affect the family in a number of important ways for many years to come. Outcomes such as the form of feeding, emotional wellbeing and the love between mother, baby and family are of fundamental importance and are likely to affect the individuals involved for a lifetime. Birth is the most formative event of life, and sensitivity to the potential influence of care is crucial to evidence-based midwifery.

THE FIVE STEPS OF EVIDENCE-BASED MIDWIFERY

In this chapter, I describe the five steps that need to be taken to practise evidence-based midwifery. These are described in detail in relation to Jane's care. These steps will help bring together sensitivity to individual needs of the woman and her family and the use of scientific evidence in practice.

The five steps are as follows:

1. finding out what is important to the woman and her family;
2. using information from the clinical examination;
3. seeking and assessing evidence to inform decisions;
4. talking it through;
5. reflecting on outcomes, feelings and consequences.

These five steps will be used to tell Jane's care story, each being illustrated with examples from practice.

JANE'S CARE STORY

Jane was expecting her seventh baby. By most risk assessment scales, this grand multiparity would put her at risk of postpartum haemorrhage. In most settings, a hospital birth would be indicated. However, Jane and her husband wanted their baby to be born at home. This situation presents the midwife with a clinical dilemma. Having given birth to her last two babies at home and her older children in hospital, Jane felt that there were considerable advantages to her and her family of staying at home. In her own words (Page et al 1997):

> What appeals to me about home birth? A number of factors – each insignificant on its own, but together they make a recipe for confidence. You are already in the right place when labour starts and can arrange things around as you will want them. Life can carry on as normal with very little upset, which is an important stabilizing factor with other children around . . . Before a home birth I would never have dreamed that I could get through labour without pain control. At home I didn't need anything. The breathing I had learned was enough.

In these simple and homely words, Jane described what was important to her about the birth of her baby. Other women may want different things: some a hospital birth and technological support, others something in between. What is important is that, as midwives, we get to know what is important to each woman and use that understanding to inform our care. This chapter uses Jane's care story to illustrate an approach to practice that responds to the personal needs of women. It is an approach recognizing that the birth of a baby is one of the most important experiences of life, an experience that has profound and long-lasting consequences. This approach encourages women to become involved in making decisions about their care. It acknowledges that maternity care may do harm as well as good, however well intentioned, and thus requires that decisions are based on good information. This information includes sound evidence when it is available.

This approach, which integrates sensitivity to the individual woman and her family with scientific understanding, arises from a relationship between the woman and her midwife. This relationship is both personal and professional, often being like a friendship, but a friendship with a purpose. The midwife is an expert who uses her skill, knowledge, understanding and commitment to the women in her care in order to support them around the time of the birth of their babies. The woman is also an expert, knowing her needs and understanding the changes going on in her body, with awareness of the signals her baby is giving her, the growth, movement, and physical responses to pregnancy. The interests of the mother and baby should not be separated. Through a relationship of trust, the midwife works with the woman, integrating this personal sensitivity and personal understanding in a way that gives the mother and her family the best possible start in life.

You will remember that Jane was expecting her seventh baby and wished for a home birth. Jane's experience of home birth was similar to that of a large proportion of the women in the study of Chamberlain et al (1997). As Oakley (1997, p. 187) comments, reporting the women's follow-up survey of this large study:

> There is a contrast between accounts of hospital care that seems to remain impersonal despite the improvements of recent years and accounts of birth at home, which lead most who have experienced it to regard it as a marvellous experience.

There are a number of assumptions about a woman expecting her seventh baby. Foremost of these is the assumption that the probability of postpartum haemorrhage is greater. Turnbull and Chamberlain (1989, p. 868) stated that 'grand multiparae are prone to postpartum haemorrhage. One possible explanation is that with increasing multiparity there is an increasing amount of fibrous tissue in the myometrium hindering effective contraction of the uterus'.

In addition to postpartum haemorrhage, a number of other serious adverse outcomes have been attributed to grand multiparity. When a perception of added risk is combined with a generally held assumption that home birth is less safe than hospital birth, there is likely to be considerable pressure, on both mother and midwife, to have the woman give birth in hospital. This care history, then, is one of the most controversial examples of evidence-based midwifery I can provide.

STEP 1: FINDING OUT WHAT IS IMPORTANT TO THE WOMAN AND HER FAMILY

Providing personal care requires that we understand the values, anxieties, hopes and dreams of the woman expecting a baby. We need to start finding out what is important to the woman right at the beginning of care. It is, of course, far easier if the midwife has a continuous relationship with the woman, when this becomes a more natural process of getting to know each other.

In practice, we always seek the best outcomes. These will depend on the personal values and preferences of the family. Safety is, of course, an important underlying principle of maternity care. Mortality is, naturally, one of the most important outcome measures. However, the issue of safety may, as the Expert Maternity Group (Department of Health 1993) commented, 'become an excuse for unnecessary interventions and technological surveillance which detract from the experience of the mother'; one example of this has been the excessive reliance on electronic fetal monitoring that is common in most maternity services. Different things will be important to different women. One woman may place great value on the avoidance of analgesia in labour, while another may wish, above all else, for a pain-free labour. It is of paramount importance that the issue of safety is not used to restrict women's choices or their ability to be in control of decisions. An important concept is that of social safety. This recognizes that a mother who has formal healthcare which leaves her feeling good about her experience and herself, and which supports family integrity, is far more likely to provide the care and support her baby will require for many years to come.

Open-ended questions such as 'Tell me how you feel about being pregnant?' 'What is important to you about your care/the birth of your baby?' and 'Where would you like your baby to be born?' will usually start to clarify what the woman wants and feels. With Jane, such questions were much more a part of natural conversation than a formal interview (Page et al 1997).

I had been her midwife three times before and saw the family occasionally between pregnancies. My visits to her were in her own home, and although not long (we were both too busy), they were relaxed. We had become friends and had developed what Freeley (1995) described as 'the shorthand of a working friendship'. Although I knew Jane well, it was important to check out my assumption that she would want this baby at home. So, early on, we talked about her preferences for place of birth and why it was important to her. It was clearly a deeply felt preference. In addition, she had always made it apparent that she and her husband felt that it was important for parents to take responsibility for making decisions about their children. They were active in the work of founding a school in which parents would be involved and active in the education of their children. In this choice of place of birth, and their need to make their own decisions, they were therefore reflecting some of their core values, the need to take responsibility for the health and welfare of their children. The domination of such values gives them added weight. If, for example, Jane had felt less strongly about having her baby at home, this would carry less weight when balancing all the factors to make a decision.

STEP 2: USING INFORMATION FROM THE CLINICAL EXAMINATION

The second source of information that should be taken into account when the woman and her midwife weigh up the merits of particular courses of care is the clinical history and clinical examination. Information from these is important in interpreting the evidence and determining any increased probability of adverse outcome. With respect to general health, at a minimum the following questions should be answered by a clinical examination.

General questions

History
- Is the mother generally healthy and well nourished?
- Is she a smoker?
- Is there a habitual use of drugs or heavy alcohol consumption?
- Is there any history of illness that may be relevant?
- Is the mother well supported?
- Is she generally confident and how does she feel about pregnancy and birth?
- Are there any previous obstetric problems?
- Has she experienced or is she experiencing some form of abuse?
- Is she under social stress (for example deprivation, life style)?
- What was her experience of being parented?

Clinical
Is the mother generally healthy?

- Are the blood pressure and urine tests for protein within normal limits?
- Are the heart and lungs normal?
- Are there any signs of disease or abnormal conditions?
- Is the fetus healthy?
- Is the baby well grown, and was growth constant?
- Is there consistent fetal growth as measured by fundal height measurements and/or ultrasound scans?
- Is the baby active?
- Is the fetal heart reactive to stimulation?
- Is there a lot of amniotic fluid?
- Is it clear of meconium?

Care-specific questions

In addition to general questions to be answered by all clinical examinations, there will be specific questions for each situation, for example with regard to the probability of postpartum haemorrhage:

- Is the mother obese?
- Is the baby excessively large (over 4 kg)?
- Is there a history of postpartum haemorrhage?
- What is the haemoglobin level?

It was easier to answer the questions from the history in Jane's situation because I knew her so well. She was a healthy and self-confident woman, and had experienced no problems in her previous pregnancies or births. She had none of the clinical risk factors for postpartum haemorrhage. In addition to the answers to these questions, I took into account the fact that Jane had always had short labours, with strong contractions. At the end of her pregnancy, her haemoglobin levels were normal. The baby was active and, according to fundal height measurements, had grown consistently, being estimated to be of an average size. Neither was the fetus estimated to be large for dates by Jane's scan and abdominal palpation. All of these were reassuring factors in assessing the health of the baby before labour started.

STEP 3: SEEKING AND ASSESSING EVIDENCE TO INFORM DECISIONS

In Jane's situation, major questions fell around two key areas: *place of birth* and the increased probability of adverse outcome because of *grand multiparity*. Three general questions were important:

1. What is the evidence on the relative safety of different places of birth?
2. Is there an increased probability of any adverse outcome in Jane's case?
3. In particular, is there an increased probability of postpartum haemorrhage?

Place of birth

While home birth remains one of the most contentious issues in maternity care in much of the Western world, since the early 1990s national policy in the UK has confirmed the importance of enabling women to have a choice of place of birth including the right to give birth to their babies at home (see MIDIRS 2005). This was restated in the most recent policy document The Maternity Standard included in the National Service Framework for Children and Young People (Department of Health 2004).

In the search to evaluate the safety of home birth a complicating factor has been the quality of studies including the need to define adequately what was being evaluated. For example, many studies include both unplanned and unbooked cases in the out-of-hospital category. The outcomes of such births are generally poor, and their inclusion in studies of home birth skews the results. Nevertheless, such studies have been presented as evidence of the lack of safety of home birth.

One study illustrates the poor outcomes from unplanned, unbooked out-of-hospital births. In the UK's Northern Region Perinatal Mortality Survey (Northern Region Perinatal Mortality Survey Coordinating Group 1996), which took place between 1981 and 1994, the overall perinatal mortality rate for births occurring outside hospital was over four times higher than the average for the total population (38.7 versus 9.7 deaths per 1000 births). However, of the 134 perinatal deaths, only three had occurred in women with planned home deliveries. The others had either been planned for hospital (64 out of 134) or had not been planned at all (67 out of 134).

It has been suggested that the best way to research the relative safety of home versus hospital birth would be to conduct a randomized controlled trial (RCT). However, conducting a study of this sort would involve many practical problems, and there is considerable debate about the feasibility and advisability of using an RCT to evaluate the outcomes of home birth (Chamberlain et al 1996, Dowswell et al 1996, Macfarlane 1996, Newburn & Dodds 1996, Raisler 1996, Settattree 1996, Wiegers et al 1996a, Young 1996). One problem is that, given the low mortality rates in most developed countries, a trial would need to be very large (e.g. encompassing over 20,000 participants) in order to answer questions about safety. Given the current organizations of maternity care, a trial of this size would be almost impossible to mount. Some attempts are being made to conduct RCTs in which the outcome measures do not include mortality. Olsen (1997a) has proposed criteria for reviewing RCTs comparing home with hospital birth. A small trial has been completed and reported. However it includes only 11 women (1998) and was too small to draw any conclusions (Olsen & Jewell 1998).

We must at this point rely on non-RCT evidence to form opinions about the relative safety and merits of different places of birth. Recent high-quality studies indicate that, for low-risk women, planned home births are no less safe than planned hospital births. It is instructive to look at a number of recent studies in detail.

Olsen (1997b) compared the outcomes of planned home births (backed up by a modern hospital system) with those of planned hospital births for women with similarly low-risk pregnancies. He completed a meta-analysis of six controlled observational studies that included the perinatal outcomes of 24,092 selected and primarily low-risk pregnancies. The results were analysed to shed light on both mortality and morbidity. Confounding was controlled through restriction and matching, or in the statistical analysis. Together, these studies provide data on over 24,000 low-risk pregnancies.

The UK Northern Region Perinatal Mortality Survey was a retrospective follow-up study of 558,691 newborns registered to mothers living in a health region of North England between 1981 and 1994. The Weigers et al (1996b) study was, in contrast, a prospective cohort study of mothers in the Gelderland province of the Netherlands. Of the women studied, 1140 had chosen home birth and 696 hospital birth.

Chamberlain et al (1996) aimed to obtain a contemporary account of booked home births from midwives and from the women having babies in the UK during the year 1994. This was a prospective study of all women who were booked for home birth at 37 weeks gestation, irrespective of where the birth actually took place. Those planning home birth were matched with women of similar background, resident locality, age group, parity and obstetric history who at 37 weeks had planned to have their baby in hospital. Data were collected on 7571 women who had planned to give birth at home, as well as on 1600 who had not planned to give birth at home. In total, the study includes over 60% of all home births in 1994.

The Ackerman-Liebrich et al (1996) study similarly was a follow-up prospective cohort study with matched pairs (489 versus 385). The study was situated in Switzerland.

None of these studies found an increase in the perinatal death rate in planned home births, and there is no indication that home birth is less safe for low-risk women than hospital birth, at least when the back-up of a modern hospital system is available.

Interestingly, there appear to be a number of benefits to home birth. Intervention rates were significantly lower, and there were significantly fewer low Apgar scores in the home birth groups than in the control groups (Ackermann-Liebrich et al 1996, Olsen 1997b, Wiegers et al 1996b). There was a slightly higher intervention rate in the births planned for home but occurring in hospital than in the matched controls. However, these controls in themselves have a lower rate of intervention than average (Chamberlain et al 1996).

It is important to note that these studies must be interpreted with caution. In general, women having home births are well educated and healthy, and this may be a major factor influencing the outcomes of such studies. We must also be careful in generalizing from the results of population-based studies, particularly those carried out in other countries or communities, in which risk assessment and the management of home births may differ. On the other hand, it is important to remember that the hospital may introduce factors into care that may constitute a risk. As Campbell and MacFarlane (1996) noted, 'the iatrogenic risk associated with institutional delivery may be greater than any benefit conferred'.

As Olsen (1997b, pp 9–10) comments, it cannot be claimed 'that birth in hospital is safe for all babies – nor can it be claimed that home birth is safe for all babies'.

The evidence presented above was reviewed in the process of the care of Jane. In the revision of this chapter for the second edition I have reviewed recent evidence to see if decisions might have been different in the light of current evidence. What is apparent is a growing awareness of the complexities of evaluating the outcomes of home vs. hospital birth. Nonetheless, the best evidence available indicates that there is still no evidence that home birth is any less safe for mother or baby where the woman's pregnancy is uncomplicated and the home birth takes place in the context of integrated services where there is appropriate support for home birth, and where practitioners are skilled and knowledgeable. In a commentary on the appropriateness of a meta-analysis to synthesize the results of disparate studies of home vs. hospital birth, MacFarlane (1996) comments on the difficulties of the dichotomous divide between home and hospital birth, when the study of out of hospital births covers a range of places of birth. Moreover, some of the studies included in the Olsen meta analysis were undertaken across long periods of time, in very different healthcare settings, and where different definitions for outcome measures existed. MacFarlane suggests that a more appropriate way of reviewing studies of place of birth would be 'a critical structured review of research that describes the studies according to both their similarities and their differences' (MacFarlane 1996, p. 15). Other methodological difficulties include the impossibility of comparing rates of perinatal and maternal mortality now that the incidence of these is so low. In the paper based on studies drawn from the UK the conclusion is reached that 'the practice of not allowing a woman to book for her birth outside a consultant unit is unethical, contrary to government policy and not justifiable in the light of the available evidence' (MIDIRS 2005).

Recent studies of home birth reported since the first publication of this chapter (Page 2000), including a study of home birth in British Columbia, Canada (Janssen et al 2002) and a large study of home births in North America (Johnson & Daviss 2005). These indicate broadly similar findings to earlier studies. In the Canadian prospective comparison between 862 planned home births attended by midwives with those of hospital births attended by either midwives (N=571) or physicians (N=743) there was no increased mortality or neonatal risk associated with planned home birth under the care of a regulated midwife. Intervention rates were also lower. The authors warn that the rates of some adverse outcomes were too low to draw statistical comparisons, and that the ongoing evaluation of home birth is warranted (Janssen et al 2002).

The USA study was conducted in 2000 and is one of the largest cohort studies to evaluate planned home births in comparison with hospital births. It included 5418 women who were supported by midwives with a common certification and who planned to deliver at home when labour began and concluded that planned home birth for low risk women in North America using certified professional midwives was associated with lower

rates of medical interventions but similar intrapartum and neonatal mortality to that of low risk hospital births in the United States (Johnson & Daviss 2005).

When considering whether the findings of such studies are applicable in your practice, it is important to think about whether there are important differences about issues such as the environment in which they were conducted compared to where you work. Clearly both Canadian and USA midwives work in systems where home birth is far less integrated than it is for example in the Netherlands or in the UK. However, the consistency of outcomes which have emerged from the main body of evidence form different parts of the resource rich world is striking. The recent MIDIRS informed choice leaflet (MIDIRS 2005) gives a summary from a systematic review of place of birth, confirming the importance of giving women a choice about where their babies should be born.

While in general those women who choose to give birth at home are more satisfied with the experience, a good quality of experience is not guaranteed by home birth, unless the midwives are appropriately sensitive to the needs of the woman and her family, and confident and pleased to be attending births at home (see Chapter 5). Factors that will influence the outcomes of home births include the skills of the practitioner, and an established system of support from the healthcare system, in case of unexpected outcomes and emergencies.

Discussion with women about the choice of place of birth should include consideration of such issues as the rate of transfer. One of the findings from a number of the studies is that the outcomes of high risk births at home may be worse than those undertaken in hospital, and that appropriate screening is required (Bastion et al 1998). A major question for us in regard to Jane's care was therefore whether or not she would be considered to be 'low risk'.

Grand multiparity

In Jane's case, the decision about place of birth was complicated by the fact that she had given birth to more than five babies. Did she then have a higher chance of adverse outcome because of her 'grand multiparity'? There is a long-held belief that there is a greater chance of adverse outcome in 'grand multiparous' woman. In particular, many believe that such a woman has a higher probability of postpartum haemorrhage.

Framing clear questions

In this situation, I thought it was important for both Jane and I to find out whether or not current evidence supported the link between grand multiparity and an increased risk of postpartum haemorrhage. Sackett et al (1997, 2000) recommend that the first step in finding evidence-based information to inform decisions is to frame a clear question that will help in a literature search. The questions with regard to Jane's care were as follows:

- Is there a higher probability (chance) of adverse consequences because of her grand multiparity?
- Is there an increased probability (chance) of postpartum haemorrhage for a woman who is gravida 8 para 6 (i.e. 8 pregnancies with 6 babies born after 24 weeks' gestation)?
- Are there any other factors that would increase the probability of postpartum haemorrhage?

Searching for the evidence

I looked for studies in the following categories:

- risks of grand multiparity;
- factors associated with postpartum haemorrhage.

For this, population-based studies describing the prevalence of particular conditions in a defined group of women were needed. I asked the Midwives Information Resource Service (MIDIRS) to do a standard search for 'Grand multiparity and postpartum haemorrhage'. I searched using the MIDIRS database at two separate times, once around the time of Jane's pregnancy (Page et al 1997) and later to update the information for this book, using the abstracts provided to decide which would be useful. Studies from extremely poor, non-industrialized countries where there was a poorly developed health service (e.g. Nigeria) were omitted. Eleven relevant studies on grand multiparity and adverse outcome were discovered, as were four additional studies that

concentrated on risk factors for postpartum haemorrhage.

The studies presented were conducted in a number of different countries with different social, religious and economic conditions. The settings included Israel (Eidelman et al 1988, Goldman et al 1995, Kaplan et al 1995, Seidman et al 1988), the United Arab Emirates (Hughes & Morrison 1994), Saudi Arabia (Al-Sibai et al 1987, Fayed et al 1993), Malaysia (Tai & Urquhart 1991), Hong Kong (King et al 1991), England (Henson et al 1987) and the USA (Toohey et al 1995).

The dramatically different features of these countries and their healthcare systems must be taken into account when considering the results. Care must be taken not to make assumptions about the conditions in the different countries. Two of the studies took place in relatively affluent countries: England and the USA. Both, however, included immigrant women from deprived home countries – Bangladesh (Henson et al 1987) and a Hispanic population living in California (Toohey et al 1995).

Participants and methodology

Goldman et al (1995) aimed to evaluate the management of grand multiparous patients in contemporary obstetrics and to assess whether grand multiparas were still at risk. Their study was conducted over 3 years (1988–1990) in Jerusalem. The participants included primiparous women, multiparous women (2–3 deliveries) and grand multiparous women (five or more deliveries). It was a retrospective cohort study, comparing the grand multiparous women with the two control groups that were randomly selected. Statistical analysis was by the chi-square test. There was no adjustment for other factors that might have affected the study group.

Kaplan et al (1995) investigated the perinatal and obstetric complications of women delivering for the tenth or more time ('grand-grand multiparas', in whom parity ranged from 10 to 19), compared with the general population, between January 1990 and June 1994 in Israel. Tests of statistical significance were applied.

Toohey et al (1995) compared the incidence of intrapartum complications among grand multiparous women (para >5) with that of age-matched controls who were multiparous (2–4 births). This was a low socio-economic Hispanic group of women living in California who delivered between July 1989 and September 1991.

Hughes & Morrison (1994) aimed to document the reproductive performance of grand multiparous women receiving modern antenatal care through a cross-sectional study. Participants included grand multiparous women delivering after the 20th week of pregnancy after seven or more viable pregnancies and all para 1–6 mothers. A total of 2784 multiparous women were studied. Of these, 882 were grand multiparas. The highest parity in this series was 17, that is, the eighteenth pregnancy. Of this grand multiparous group, 22.8% were in the 40+ age range.

Fayed et al (1993) studied the obstetric performance and outcome of 228 patients of extreme multiparity (mothers of 10 pregnancies or more) against a control group of 3349 women of parity between two and five in a hospital in Saudi Arabia. Stratified sampling was used to adjust for confounding variables. Analysis combined crude calculated odds ratios and tests for significance.

Tai and Urquhart (1991) compared a parous group of women aged less than 35 years, para 5 and 6 (N = 406), and a very highly parous group of women less than 35 years of age (para 7 and above) (N=71), with all women under 35 having their babies in the same period of time (1.1.88–21.12.88). Tests of statistical significance were applied and relative risks with confidence intervals calculated. This study took place in Malaysia but consisted of a highly mixed race group of women.

King et al (1991) compared the outcomes of all grand multiparous (over para 5, average parity 6 and highest parity 11) women who gave birth in a hospital in Hong Kong over the 5-year period 1984 to 1988 inclusive with the rest of the hospital population (168 [0.57%] versus 29,048 deliveries). No tests of significance were applied.

Seidman et al (1988) studied the population of the Bikin Cholin Hospital, Jerusalem between January 1984 and June 1986. This study included 5916 deliveries, 893 (13%) of the mothers being over para 7. This was an ultra-orthodox Jewish community that the authors believed would have avoided the confounding variables of low income, mixed race and low income. The women in this population were relatively young (39.8% being above 35-years of age).

Eidelman et al (1988) studied a population of 7785 women in Jerusalem. This population comprised 889 (11.5%) grand multiparas. Of these grand multiparas, 23% were in their ninth delivery or more. Seventy-eight per cent of the population were of social class 1–3, and 35% were over 35 years. Tests of statistical significance were applied.

Al-Sibai et al (1987) surveyed 1330 grand multiparous women who were para 7 or more and compared outcomes with those of the rest of the population (N = 11,687) between January 1982 and December 1986 in the Al-Khoban University teaching hospital in Saudi Arabia. The mean age was 34.6 years, and the oldest participant was para 19 at the age of 51 years. No tests of statistical significance were applied.

Henson et al (1987) undertook a retrospective study of 216 grand multiparae and compared them with controlled patients who were matched for maternal age and ethnic origin. Tests of statistical significance were applied. There was no adjustment or analysis for confounding variables. Grand multiparity was defined as five previous pregnancies progressing beyond 28 weeks.

Results. Of the 11 studies, four reported an association between grand multiparity and adverse outcome in the intrapartum period. Of these Al-Sibai et al (1987) reported increased rates of stillbirth, perinatal mortality, postpartum haemorrhage, breech presentation, unstable lie, uterine rupture, caesarean section and maternal mortality in the grand multiparous group. Henson et al (1987) found a higher rate of perinatal mortality and postpartum haemorrhage in the grand multiparous group, while Tai & Urqhart (1991) reported a higher rate of perinatal mortality, low birth weight and preterm delivery in the over para 7 group. Goldman et al (1990) found an association between grand multiparity and postpartum haemorrhage (not defined).

Assessing the evidence

There is an inherent problem with interpreting the results of any population-based study with an individual in mind. This problem is particularly marked when studies have been situated in different locations with different healthcare systems and different populations. Because grand multi-parity is so uncommon in much of the industrialized world, much of the research has been undertaken among populations of women, and in places, that are very different from Jane and her place of care. There were a number of concerns about the validity of these studies.

Moreover, the outcomes of grand multiparity are very likely to be confounded by other factors that affect outcomes for example, age and chronic medical conditions, socio-economic status and having had a number of previous pregnancy losses. One of the factors that is likely to affect outcome is the management and quality of care. Especially in relation to postpartum haemorrhage, this can range from very aggressive treatment, including routine intravenous oxytocin, to the physiological management of third stage. Few studies give enough detail to understand the type of care provided. In addition, facilities vary from one institution to another, and few reports give any description of facilities available or of routine management. It was important, then, to make some assessment of the quality of the studies.

Sackett et al (1997, p. 86) propose three major questions for assessing evidence on prognosis before it is applied in practice:

1. Are the results of this prognosis study valid (i.e. close to the truth)?
2. Are the valid results of this prognosis study important?
3. Can you apply this valid important evidence in caring for your patient?

Criteria for validity of the studies. As with any study, there are a number of general questions to be asked with regard to the validity of prognostic studies. Is the study likely to be biased? Is it powerful enough to detect any difference. Are estimates of differences precise and not likely to be the result of chance? Has confounding been controlled for?

Adapting some of the criteria for validity proposed by Sackett et al (1997), I assessed the studies against five criteria:

- *A study group compared with a control group, which may be matched, specified or random.* A control group acts as a basis for comparison with groups who do not have the condition being studied. RCTs, in which people are randomly assigned to the study group or the control group, are the least likely to be biased, but it is not always possible to assign study participants randomly, and matched or specified groups are often used instead in an attempt to control for bias.
- *A pre-study intention of the outcomes to be measured.* The outcomes to be studied should be specified in advance because a study that looks for any differences is likely to find some simply by chance.
- *An analysis or adjustment for confounding variables.* This aims to determine whether or not the condition being studied is causally related to outcomes or whether they are associated with other variables (e.g. a number of previous perinatal losses when the perinatal mortality rate is high; see, for example, Henson et al 1987).
- *Number.* The study should be powerful enough to detect any important differences, and tests of significance should be applied to ensure that differences do not arise by chance alone. Studies of prognosis may give a relative risk or odds ratios, indicating precision in measurement.
- *What are the characteristics of the population studied?* Is this likely to affect the outcomes?
- *Were objective criteria applied in a blind fashion?* Some element of interpretation is always necessary in taking data from records. Blinding the auditor guards against his or her being influenced in this interpretation.
- *Was a defined representative group of patients assembled at a common (usually early) point in the course of the disease?* Prospective studies are less likely than retrospective studies to be biased.

Are the results of these studies on grand multiparity valid?

Was there a control group and was it restricted or matched? In pregnancy, the adverse outcomes that are likely to occur in grand multiparous women are also possible in women of lower parity so a basis for comparison is necessary to determine any increase in risk. The question is, then, how much more probable is this adverse outcome in grand multiparity than in lower-parity women? For this reason, control groups are necessary. Control groups are most useful when they are comparable for other relevant factors in the study group. Thus, matched case controls are likely to be the most useful studies. For a number of the studies, the control was the rest of the population (Al-Sibai et al 1987, Eidelman et al 1988, Fayed et al 1993, Hughes & Morrison 1994 [cross-sectional], Kaplan et al 1995, King et al 1991, Tai & Urquhart 1991 [all women having a second baby]). Seidman and colleagues (1988) compared two groups: women having given birth to seven or more infants and women having given birth to 2–6 infants.

Only the studies of Henson et al (1987; on age and ethnic origin) and Toohey et al (1995; age matched) had matched controls and that of Goldman et al (1995), controls who were randomly selected. The studies defined grand multiparity in a number of ways, from more than 5 live births after 20 weeks to more than 10 live births. Within these studies, there was a wide range in parity.

Was there a clear pre-study intention of outcomes to be measured? Were there clear definitions? Only seven of the studies gave pre-specified outcome measures or clear objectives. One study involved no tests of significance.

Was there an analysis or adjustment for confounding variables? Reports claiming one sub-group of patients has a different prognosis from others should ensure that the outcome is not being distorted by the unequal occurrence of another prognostic factor (Sackett et al 1997, p. 89). This is particularly important in grand multiparity, where other factors that are prognostic of poorer outcome (for example, socio-demographic characteristics) may confound the study. Sackett et al recommend looking for an adjustment for other prognostic factors. This adjustment is evident in stratified analyses (e.g. were older women more likely to have hypertension?; was macrosomia associated with higher rates of postpartum haemorrhage?) and multiple regression analyses (that could take into account age and economic factors). Of the studies described, only a few undertook any kind of analysis or adjustment for the control of confounding variables. Such studies included those of Eidelman et al (1988; maternal age and trisomy 21), Toohey et al (1995), to address whether or not there was enough distinction between study group and controls, Fayed et al (1993), who stratified women for example according to age in relation to hypertension and fetal weight, and Seidmanet al (1988), who submitted the four perinatal factors that were found to differ significantly

to further analysis in an attempt to determine the relationship between maternal age and parity.

Were enough women included in the studies to detect a difference in the outcomes? It is important to remember that these studies may not be powerful enough (e.g. large enough) to reach any firm conclusions about the prevalence of the less common but clinically highly important complications, such as maternal mortality or uterine rupture.

Only two studies reported the use of power calculations. Where these are not reported, it is difficult to know whether the lack of a significant finding is the result of insufficient numbers, particularly when the incidence of a particular outcome is rare.

What are the characteristics of the population being studied? This question has been addressed above. In general, the characteristics of the populations are likely to have affected the outcome.

Were objective criteria applied in a blind fashion? None of the studies reported blinding for the audit of records. The criteria for multiparity and postpartum haemorrhage varied between studies.

Was a defined sample of patients assembled at a common (usually early) point in the course of their disease? None of the studies was prospective.

Applying these criteria, I could find no evidence from the strongest of these studies to support the assumption that postpartum haemorrhage is more probable in women who are grand multiparous.

Are the valid results of this study important?

Measures include maternal and perinatal death, and trauma including uterine rupture, as well as other life-threatening conditions. One of the studies (Al Sibai et al 1987) reports an increased incidence of perinatal mortality postpartum haemorrhage and uterine rupture. Henson et al (1987) show an increased incidence of perinatal mortality and postpartum haemorrhage, and Goldman et al (1995) reports an increased incidence of postpartum haemorrhage.

Let us look at the incidence of these outcomes and what the authors have to say about them. In Al-Sibai et al's (1987) study, the perinatal mortality rate was 62 per 1000 in the series compared with

21 per 1000 in the general hospital population. There were 50 stillbirths and 32 neonatal deaths. Of the 50 stillbirths, 41 occurred in the antenatal period. The description of this group indicates a high rate of macrosomia, a large number of congenital abnormalities and medical problems. There was one maternal mortality, which occurred in a woman who was gravida 11, para 10, and who had never attended the antenatal clinic; she suffered intrauterine death and, following a number of complications, died, probably of infection. The incidence of postpartum haemorrhage was double that seen with other deliveries. This may have been associated with the high incidence of large babies, macrosomia and induction reported in the study. There were four uterine ruptures, two being associated with obstructed labour and two with induction. The rate of trauma or adverse outcome in this population appears to be generally high. This raises a number of questions about the population and management of care in this study.

Henson et al's (1987) study reports a very high rate of perinatal mortality of 31.8 per 1000 compared with 4.1 per 1000 in the controls. There were 5 stillbirths and 4 neonatal deaths in the group of grand multiparas and 1 neonatal death among the controls. Two of the neonatal deaths were caused by rhesus iso-immunization. There was a high rate of previous perinatal death in the grand multiparous group, which had a high number of Bangladeshi women who had lost babies in Bangladesh before moving to London. Henson et al (1987) also report a higher rate of postpartum haemorrhage. A blood loss of more than 500 mL occurred in five grand multiparae (out of a total of 216) but no controls. However, the incidence of blood transfusion and anaemia was similar in both groups. The similar rates of anaemia and blood transfusion might indicate that the blood loss was within the physiological range.

Tai and Urquhart's (1991) evidence suggests that the perinatal deaths in the highest parity group are most probably a function of low birth weight and preterm labour.

Thus, although these studies show an increased incidence of the most important outcomes, the higher rate may be a result of confounding by other factors.

The Goldman study (Goldman et al 1995) reports a significantly different, higher rate of postpartum haemorrhage associated with grand multiparity. Postpartum haemorrhage is not defined, and there is no control for possible confounding variables in this study. It is possible that the higher incidence of macrosomia in the grand multiparous group is associated with the higher rate of postpartum haemorrhage.

Can you apply the results to the patient in your care? The three studies reporting adverse outcomes in association with grand multiparity are likely to be confounded by other factors, such as ethnicity, locality and cultural characteristics occurring independently of the grand multiparity. Many of the studies indicate a perinatal mortality rate that is far higher than that of the UK overall, indicating some fundamental difference in either the population or the care provided. It is difficult to know how far it is appropriate to apply the findings in this particular situation. There was very little similarity between the populations described and Jane. Thus, any application of findings to Jane's situation could be made only with great caution. Although overall the findings indicated that, in healthy, higher socio-economic group women, where relevant factors had been controlled for, there was little evidence of an association between grand multiparity and adverse outcome in the intrapartum period.

More recent evidence, found to revise for the second edition of this book, presents some contradictory results (Bai et al 2002), In general recent results undertaken in industrialized countries (Humphrey 2003, Roman et al 2004) indicate that women with grandmultiparity do not have a greater risk of poor pregnancy outcomes and that the decisions that Jane made would still be sound. The most relevant recent study for Jane (from studies reported since 2000) was undertaken in the UK to compare the incidence of antenatal and intrapartum complications and neonatal outcomes among women who had previously delivered five or more times (grand multiparous) with that of age matched women who had delivered two or three times. This was a matched cohort study undertaken in an inner city university maternity hospital, that included 397 grand multiparous women and 397 matched multiparous women. It found that grand multiparity was associated with a significantly higher body mass index at booking (P<0.01) and at the last antenatal clinic an increased incidence of anaemia (22% vs.16%, OR 1.8, 95% CI 1.2–2.8) was observed, and a decreased incidence of elective caesarean section (6% vs.11%, OR 0.5, 95% CI 0.3–0.9). The conclusion to the study was that in a developed country with satisfactory healthcare conditions, grand multiparity should not be considered dangerous, and risk assessment should be based on past and present history and not simply on the basis of parity (Bugg et al 2002).

Postpartum haemorrhage

From the general studies of grand multiparity and postpartum haemorrhage, I moved to a review of the studies of risk factors for postpartum haemorrhage.

Four studies of factors associated with postpartum haemorrhage have been reviewed, all calling into question a relationship between grand multiparity and a greater probability of postpartum haemorrhage.

One study was an RCT to evaluate active versus physiological management of the third stage of labour. From the data collected from the physiologically managed group, the factors that increase the risk of postpartum haemorrhage were identified. The authors of the study concluded that postpartum haemorrhage fell with increasing parity and was highest in primiparous women (Begley 1991).

In a case control study of 9598 deliveries to find risk factors for postpartum haemorrhage, there was an association with nuliparity (an adjusted odds ratio of 1.56) but no association with grand multiparity (Combs et al 1991).

In a retrospective review of data relating to 37 497 women in London, intrinsic factors associated with significant risk factors were identified. There was no association with high parity (Stones et al 1993).

Tsu undertook a study of two groups of women, one group consisting of those with postpartum haemorrhage after a normal vaginal delivery and the other of women with a normal unassisted delivery without postpartum haemorrhage. The women shared similar socio-economic characteristics and height–weight measures. Relative risks were estimated by multivariate logistic regression. The study called into question the significance

of grand multiparity. The significantly elevated crude risks for high parity seen in these data virtually disappear once they are adjusted for maternal age (Tsu 1993).

Assessing the evidence for validity and importance. None of the studies reviewed demonstrated a direct association between grand multiparity and a higher probability of postpartum haemorrhage.

Can you apply this valid, important evidence about prognosis in caring for your patient? The largest study (Stones et al 1993) was conducted in a substantial region of London. It included 37,497 women and was the most likely of all the studies to have participants who would be similar to Jane.

Reaching conclusions

I could find no sound evidence to support the belief that grand multiparity on its own is a predictor of severe adverse outcome and the four studies of postpartum haemorrhage indicated no association between grand multiparity and postpartum haemorrhage. None of the risk factors for postpartum haemorrhage identified by these studies (weight of baby, ethnicity, previous postpartum haemorrhage and pre-eclampsia for example) applied to Jane. Given her clinical history of short labours and strong contractions, I decided that Jane did not have a higher probability of postpartum haemorrhage than other less parous women in the population.

STEP 4: TALKING IT THROUGH

Individual women will differ in the amount of detail they want to consider with regard to information taken from evidence. Some, for example, may lead the search for evidence themselves and approach healthcare professionals with searches of databases and the internet. Others may leave it up to their professional carers to stay up to date and informed on recent evidence. Women need information, and they should be given every chance of asking questions and requesting help with interpreting information. For some topics, aids such as the MIDIRS (2005) informed choice leaflets may be helpful. However, there are a number of topics for which no materials are available.

Jane knew of my search for evidence on grand multiparity. I told her of my interpretation that I had found no evidence to support the belief that grand multiparity was in itself a cause of adverse consequences and that I did not believe her to be in a high-risk group.

STEP 5: REFLECTING ON FEELINGS, OUTCOMES AND CONSEQUENCES

Much of my care of Jane was against 'usual practice'. Usual practice nowadays is dominated by routines of technological intervention and hospital care, and frequent medical treatment. As in any walk of life, there is likely to be difficulty in challenging the usual way of doing things, difficulty in doing something a little different. Such care is likely to attract attention and scrutiny. This is particularly so if there are adverse outcomes, which are always possible no matter how low the probability. It is important therefore to document discussions, decisions, actions, treatments and rationale very carefully in the woman's midwifery and medical records.

One of the difficulties for any midwife who is trying to use evidence in practice is that the perspective used in clinical research, is very different from the perspective of any midwife in practice. The midwife in practice is not making a population-based assessment but an assessment for an individual, with more direct consequences. For example, although perinatal mortality rates may be so low that any differences arising from place of birth are likely to be small (MacFarlane 1996), the possibility of death of a particular mother or baby is of enormous consequence for the individual parents, their families and friends and their carer(s). In practice, an individual is not a statistic.

Decisions to be made by a midwife who wishes to meet the individual needs of women and to avoid unnecessary intervention are finely tuned. There has to be enough confidence not to over diagnose complications, but the decisions should be made within the parameters of safety while recognizing that there is no such thing as absolute safety. These decisions are also made in a system in which intensive surveillance and hospital birth are the norm. There is little tolerance for any decision that upsets these norms, even when there is no indication of a problem. Once there is any indication of a potential problem, however slight, it becomes difficult to find any support for the decision to continue to avoid technological intervention and not to transfer to hospital.

Jane went into labour at term early in the evening. On arrival at her house, all was going well. Her baby continued to be active, and contractions were regular, ranging from mild to moderate in intensity. Jane was still feeling that to stay at home was the right decision for her. However, early in labour, her membranes ruptured spontaneously and there was meconium in the amniotic fluid, which was greenish brown with no particulate matter. There was, however, copious amniotic fluid, and on auscultation the fetal heart was reactive, with a rate of between 120 and 140. Accelerations occurred with movement. These were reassuring signs that the baby was coping with labour. I decided that, in Jane's case, the meconium was not an indicator of fetal distress. The decision to transfer to hospital was made on the side of caution.

After a 30 minute cardiotocograph when Jane was admitted to hospital, I monitored the fetal heart carefully according to the evidence-based guidelines that were then current published by the Royal College of Obstetricians and Gynaecologists (1993). The more recently published national clinical guidelines for the NHS advise that continuous electronic fetal monitoring should be used where there is meconium in the amniotic fluid (Royal College of Obstetricians and Gynaecologists 2001).

Baby Esther was born after a short labour less than 2 hours after admission, with Apgar scores of 9 at 1 minute and 10 at 5 minutes. Mother and baby were both well. Jane wished to go home immediately after birth, and her postpartum recovery was normal.

For all of us, the transfer was unpleasant. In common with many women who have planned home birth but need to be transferred (Chamberlain et al 1996), Jane was disappointed by this turn of events. In retrospect, I felt that I might more strongly have encouraged Jane to consider the slight possibility of the need for transfer in advance. In addition to the disappointment of transfer, Jane found the electronic fetal monitoring uncomfortable, feeling that attention was being diverted from her to the monitor, even though it was only used for 30 minutes.

It can be seen that there were a number of decisions to be made about Jane's pregnancy, labour and birth, most of which were quite complex. This is one of the most complex fields of evidence-based healthcare because, although a considered judgement can be made on the probability of adverse outcomes, adverse outcomes, including death and cerebral palsy, can never be entirely ruled out. We should not forget, however, that high-quality, sensitive care will make even the most unthinkable outcome – the death of the baby – more bearable. Perhaps what is most important is that parents make a genuine choice. From Chamberlain et al's study (1996, p. 108) one woman who lost her baby said:

We found the staff all cared for us with real thought and compassion in the most difficult of circumstances. Our main concern now is that we receive a full detailed account of what went wrong with the pregnancy. We hope no information will be withheld, and the truth will help us come to terms with our grief. This was to be our first home birth having experienced three pretty awful hospital experiences previously. I was wonderfully relaxed and well in control of labour with breathing exercises alone. I would recommend a home birth to anybody.

Midwives practising in countries such as the UK and North America need to be aware of the legal context in which they practise. Evidence is not weighted heavily in most legal proceedings; there is greater weight put on professional opinion and usual practice. This is entirely contrary to evidence-based clinical practice, which is a movement away from care based on professional opinion. Ultimately, the midwife is obligated to do the best for the woman in her care and must therefore be guided by the wishes of the woman and good information based on sound evidence. Decisions and the reasons for them should always be recorded in the notes alongside notes of discussion with the parents in case of any future scrutiny of care.

In conclusion, I had balanced information from the clinical examination, from the evidence available to me, in the light of Jane and the father John's values and preferences, and the context of care. The evidence alone is never enough to make decisions about the management of care. Individual women are not a population, and clinical factors, particularly in this case a history of good contractions and fast, problem-free labours, need to be borne in mind when making decisions about care.

LOOKING BACK

In reviewing this chapter I asked Jane if she wanted to change her responses to her care. After rereading the chapter she said that she felt the comments she made originally were still true, and she did not need to change them. What I have attempted to convey in this chapter is the crucial interplay of a trusting relationship, the use of evidence in practice and the use of clinical knowledge and skills. It is clear from this example that the kind of personal care given to Jane would be more difficult if there had not been continuity in our relationship. I am also aware that there are many challenges to the kind of care described. In many situations midwives are caring for women who may not share the same mother tongue, or who are living in extremely adverse circumstances. This may make the principles of care I have tried to illustrate in this chapter more difficult; yet still, observance of the principles of care that meets the individual needs of the woman and her family, that support their autonomy, that aim to provide care that is more likely to be beneficial than harmful, and that recognize the significance of the event, are important for everyone.

This chapter is published with the consent of Jane Phillips. (Fig. 17.1)

POINTERS FOR PRACTICE

■ In order to provide care that meets the parents' most deeply felt needs, and in order to use science, we can in practice never take anything for granted. Putting science and sensitivity into practice relies on the ability of the midwife to think, to ask and to answer questions.

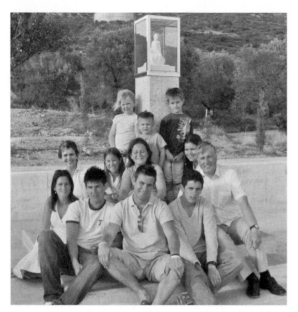

Figure 17.1 A recent picture of Jane, John and family.

- In this chapter, I have described five steps for ensuring that:
  - the preferences and values of the woman are known and that she is involved in making decisions about her care;
  - harm is, as far as possible, avoided;
  - evidence is sought and assessed;
  - the four sources of information, individual values, the clinical history and examination and strong evidence and policy are taken into account;
  - there is a process of reflection on care.
- The review of evidence outlined in this chapter is provided to give an example of the process. By the time this book goes to print, there may be new evidence available.

References

Ackerman-Liebrich U, Voegeli T, Gunter-Witt K et al 1996 Home versus hospital deliveries: follow-up study of matched pairs for procedures and outcome. British Medical Journal 313: 1313–1318

Al-Sibai M H, Rahman M S, Rahman J 1987 Obstetric problems in the grand multipara: a clinical study of 1330 cases. Journal of Obstetrics and Gynaecology 8: 135–138

Bai J, Wong F W S, Bauman A, Mohsin M 2002 Parity and pregnancy outcomes. American Journal of Obstetrics and Gynecology 186: 274–278

Bastion H, Keirse M J N C, Lancaster P A L 1998 Perinatal death associated with planned home birth in Australia: population based study. British Medical Journal 317: 384–388

Begley C M 1991 Postpartum haemorrhage – who is at risk? Midwives Chronicle and Nursing Notes (Apr) 102–106

Bugg G J, Atwal G S, Maresh M 2002 Grandmultiparae in a modern setting. British Journal of Obstetrics and Gynaecology 2002: 249–253

Campbell R, MacFarlane A 1996 Where to be born: the debate and the evidence. National Perinatal Epidemiology Unit, Oxford

Chalmers I, Enkin M, Kierse M J N C 1989 Effective care in pregnancy and childbirth. Oxford University Press, Oxford

Chamberlain G, Wraight A, Crowley P 1996 Home births. The report of the 1994 Confidential Enquiry of the National Birthday Trust Fund. Parthenon, London

Combs C A, Murphy E L, Laros R K 1991 Factors associated with postpartum haemorrhage with vaginal birth. Obstetrics and Gynecology 77: 69–76

Department of Health 1993 Changing childbirth. Part 1. Report of the Expert Maternity Group (Cumberlege report). HMSO, London

Department of Health 2004 National service framework for children and young people and maternity service: the maternity standard. Department for Education and Skills, Department of Health, London

Dowswell T, Thornton J G, Hewison J, Lilford R J L 1996 Should there be a trial of home versus hospital delivery in the United Kingdom? British Medical Journal 312: 753–757

Eidelman A L, Kamar R, Schimmel M S, Bar-on E 1988 The grandmultipara: is she still at risk? American Journal of Obstetrics and Gynecology 158: 389–392

Fayed H M, Abid S F, Stevens B 1993 Risk factors in extreme grand multiparity. International Journal of Gynecology and Obstetrics 41: 17–22

Freely M 1995 Team midwifery – a personal experience. In: Page L A (ed.) Effective group practice in midwifery: working with women. Blackwell Science, Oxford

Goldman G A, Kaplan B, Neri A, Hecht-Resnick R, Harel L, Ovadia J 1995 The grand multipara. European Journal of Obstetrics and Gynecology 61: 105–109

Gray M J A 1997 Evidence-based healthcare: how to make health policy and management decisions. Churchill Livingstone, Edinburgh

Henson G L, Knott P D, Colley N V 1987 The dangerous multipara: fact or fiction? Journal of Obstetrics and Gynaecology 8: 130–134

Hughes P F, Morrison J 1994 Grandmultiparity – not to be feared? Analysis of grandmultiparous women receiving modern antenatal care. International Journal of Gynecology and Obstetrics 44: 211–217

Humphrey M D 2003 Is grand multiparity an independent predictor of pregnancy risk? A retrospective observational study. Medical Journal of Australia 179: 294–296

Janssen P A, Lee S Koran E M, Etches D J, Fraquharson D F, Peacock D, Klein M C 2002 Outcomes of planned hospital births versus planned hospital births after regulation of midwifery in British Columbia. Canadian Medical Association Journal 166: 315–323

Johnson K C, Daviss A 2005 Outcomes of planned home births with certified professional midwives: large prospective study in North America. British Medical Journal 330: 1416

Kaplan B, Harel L, Neri A, Rabinerson D, Goldman G A, Chayen B 1995 Great grand multiparity – beyond the 10th delivery. International Journal of Gynecology and Obstetrics 50: 17–19

King P A, Duthie S J, Ma H K 1991 Grand multiparity: a reappraisal of the risk. International Journal of Gynecology and Obstetrics 36: 13–16

MacFarlane A 1996 Trial would not answer key question, but data monitoring should be improved. British Medical Journal 312: 754

MIDIRS 2005 Place of birth. Midwives information and research service and NHS centre for reviews and dissemination: informed choice leaflets. MIDIRS, Bristol. Online. Available: www.midirs.org accessed July 2005

Newburn M, Dodds R 1996 Such trial should not limit the choices of women who already have a preference. British Medical Journal 312: 756

Northern Region Perinatal Mortality Survey Coordinating Group 1996 Collaborative survey of perinatal loss in planned and unplanned home births. British Medical Journal 313: 1306–1309

Oakley A 1997 The follow-up study In: Chamberlain G, Wraight A, Crowley P (eds) Home births. The report of the 1994 confidential enquiry by the National Birthday Trust Fund. Parthenon, London

Olsen O 1997a Home vs. hospital birth [protocol]. Cochrane Library, Issue 1. Update Software, Oxford

Olsen O 1997b Meta-analysis of the safety of home birth. Birth 24: 4–13

Olsen O, Jewell M D 1998 Home versus hospital birth. The Cochrane Database of Systematic Reviews 1998, Issue 3. Art.No.:CD000352.DOI:10.1002/14651858.CD000352. Wiley, Chichester

Page L A 2000 The new midwifery. Science and sensitivity in practice. Churchill Livingstone, Edinburgh

Page L A, Phillips J, Drife J O 1997 Changing childbirth: changing clinical decisions. British Journal of Midwifery 5(4): 203–206

Raisler J 1996 Evidence from US suggests that trials will not alter obstetric behaviour. British Medical Journal 312: 754

Roman H, Robillard P-Y, Verspyck E, Hulsey T C, Marpeau L, Barau G 2004 Obstetric and neonatal outcomes in grand multiparity. Obstetrics and Gynecology 103:1294–1298

Royal College of Obstetricians and Gynaecologists 1993 Recommendations arising from the 26th RCOG Study Group. In: Spencer J A D, Ward R H T (eds) Intrapartum fetal surveillance. RCOG, London

Royal College of Obstetricians and Gynaecologists 2001 The use of electronic fetal monitoring. RCOG, London, p. 31

Sackett D L, Rosenberg W M C, Gray J A M, Haynes R B, Richardson S S 1997 Evidenced-based medicine: what it is and what it isn't. Churchill Livingstone, Edinburgh

Sackett D L, Strauss S E, Richardson W S, Rosenberg W, Haynes R B 2000 Evidenced-based medicine: what it is and what it isn't. Churchill Livingstone, Edinburgh

Seidman D S, Armond Y, Roll D, Stevenson D K, Gale R 1988 Grandmultiparity: an obstetric or neonatal risk factor? American Journal of Obstetrics and Gynecology 158: 1034–1039

Settatree R S 1996 Mortality is still important, and hospital is safer. British Medical Journal 312: 756–757

Stones R W, Paterson, C M, St G Sanders N 1993 Risk factors for major obstetric haemorrhage. European Journal of Obstetrics, Gynecology, and Reproductive Biology 48: 15–18

Tai C, Urquhart R 1991 Grandmultiparity in Malaysian women. Asia-Oceania Journal of Obstetrics and Gynaecology 17(4): 327–334

Toohey J S, Keegan K A, Morgan M A, Francis J, Task S, deVeciana M 1995 The 'dangerous multipara'. Fact or fiction? American Journal of Obstetrics and Gynecology 172: 683–686

Tsu V D 1993 Postpartum haemorrhage in Zimbabwe: a risk factor analysis. Journal of Obstetrics and Gynaecology 100: 327–333

Turnbull A, Chamberlain G 1989 Obstetrics. Churchill Livingstone, Edinburgh

Wiegers T A, Keirse M J N C, Berghs G A H, van der Zee J 1996a An approach to measuring quality of midwifery care. Journal of Clinical Epidemiology 49: 319–325

Wiegers T A, Keirse M J N C, van der Zee J, Berghs G A H 1996b Outcome of planned home and planned hospital births in low risk pregnancies: prospective study in midwifery practices in the Netherlands. British Medical Journal 313: 1309–1311

Young G 1996 Uncertainty is likely to persist, but some knowledge would be better than none. British Medical Journal 312: 755

Index